Essentials of Paramedic Care

Canadian

WORKBOOK

Robert S. Porter, *M.A., NREMT-P*
Kevin Branch, *BHSc.PHC, ACP*
Coordinator, Paramedic Programs, Cambrian College

Bryan E. Bledsoe, D.O., F.A.C.E.P., EMT-P
Emergency Department Staff Physician
Baylor Medical Center—Ellis County
Waxahachie, Texas
and
Clinical Associate Professor of Emergency Medicine
University of North Texas Health Sciences Center
Fort Worth, Texas

Robert S. Porter, M.A., NREMT-P
Senior Advanced Life Support Educator
Madison County Emergency Medical Services
Canastota, New York
and
Flight Paramedic
AirOne, Onondaga County Sheriff's Department
Syracuse, New York

Richard A. Cherry, M.S., NREMT-P
Clinical Assistant Professor of Emergency Medicine
Assistant Residency Director
SUNY Upstate Medical University
Syracuse, New York

Dwayne E. Clayden, M.E.M., Paramedic
Assistant to the Medical Director
The City of Calgary Emergency Medical Services
Calgary, Alberta

PEARSON
Prentice
Hall
Toronto

Original edition, entitled *Workbook Essentials of Paramedic Care*, published by Pearson Education, Inc., Upper Saddle River, New Jersey, USA. Copyright © 2003 by Pearson Education, Inc. This edition is authorized for sale only in Canada.

ISBN 0-13-120308-8

Executive Editor: Samantha Scully
Developmental Editor: Pamela Voves
Production Editor: Marisa D'Andrea
Production Coordinator: Patricia Ciardullo

28 16

Printed and bound in Canada.

NOTICE ON CARE PROCEDURES

It is the intent of the authors and publishers that this workbook be used as part of a formal paramedic education program taught by a qualified instructor. The care procedures presented here represent accepted competencies and practices in Canada. They are not offered as a standard of care.

Paramedic-level pre-hospital care in Canada is to be performed under the specific paramedic competencies available in each province. These competencies are specific for Primary Care Paramedics (PCP), Advanced Care Paramedics (ACP), and Critical Care Paramedics (CCP). Medically delegated acts can only be performed by a paramedic certified by a licensed medical physician or base hospital physician. It is the reader's responsibility to know and follow local protocols and follow their scope of practice associated to the system to which they belong. Also, it is the reader's responsibility to remain current of emergency care procedures and changes to their scope of practice. The material in this workbook contains the most current information available at the time of publication. However, federal, provincial, and local guidelines concerning clinical practices, including, without limitation, those governing infection control and universal precautions, change rapidly. The reader should note, therefore, that the new regulations may require changes in some procedures.

It is the responsibility of the reader to familiarize himself or herself with the policies and procedures set by national, provincial, and local agencies as well as the institution or agency where the reader is employed. The authors and the publisher of this workbook disclaim any liability, loss, or risk resulting directly or indirectly from the suggested procedures and theory, from any undetected errors, or from the reader's misunderstanding of the text. It is the reader's responsibility to stay informed of any new changes or recommendations made by any national, provincial, or local agency as well as by his or her employing institution or agency.

Contents

Introduction

To the Self-Instructional Workbook
Essentials of Paramedic Care

Welcome to the self-instructional workbook for *Essentials of Paramedic Care*. This workbook is designed to help guide you through an educational program for initial or refresher training that follows the specific paramedic competencies available in each province. The workbook is designed to be used either in conjunction with your instructor or as a self-study guide you use on your own.

This workbook features many different ways to help you learn the material necessary to become a paramedic, including those listed below.

FEATURES

Review of Chapter Objectives

Each chapter of *Essentials of Paramedic Care, Volume 1 and 2,* begins with objectives that identify the important information and principles addressed in the chapter reading. To help you identify and learn this material, each workbook chapter reviews the important content elements addressed by these objectives as presented in the text.

Content Self-Evaluation

Each chapter of *Essentials of Paramedic Care* presents an extensive narrative explanation of the principles of paramedic practice. The workbook chapter (or chapter part) contains between 10 and 90 multiple-choice, true/false, and matching questions to test your reading comprehension of the textbook material and to give you experience taking typical emergency medical service examinations.

Chapter Parts

Several chapters in *Essentials of Paramedic Care* are long and contain a great deal of subject matter. To help you grasp this material more efficiently, the workbook breaks these chapters into parts with their own objectives and content review.

How to Use
The Self-Instructional Workbook

The self-instructional workbook accompanying *Essentials of Paramedic Care, Canadian Edition, Volume 2* may be used as directed by your instructor or independently by you during your course of instruction. The recommendations listed below are intended to guide you in using the workbook independently.

• Examine your course schedule and identify the appropriate text chapter or other assigned reading.

• Read the assigned chapter in the text carefully. Do this in a relaxed environment, free of distractions, and give yourself adequate time to read and digest the material. The information presented in *Essentials of Paramedic Care* is often technically complex and demanding, but it is very important that you comprehend it. Be sure that you read the chapter carefully enough to understand and remember what you have read.

• Carefully read the Review of Chapter Objectives at the beginning of each workbook chapter (or part). This material includes both the objectives listed in *Essentials of Paramedic Care* and narrative descriptions of their content. If you do not understand or remember what is discussed from your reading, refer to the referenced pages and reread them carefully. If you still do not feel comfortable with your understanding of any objective, consider asking your instructor about it.

• Take the Content Self-Evaluation at the end of each workbook chapter (or part), answering each question carefully. Do this in a quiet environment, free from distractions, and allow yourself adequate time to complete the exercise. Correct your self-evaluation by consulting the answers at the back of the workbook, and determine the percentage you have answered correctly (the number you got right divided by the total number of questions). If you have answered most of the questions correctly (85 to 90 percent), review those that you missed by rereading the material on the pages listed in the answer key and be sure you understand which answer is correct and why. If you have more than a few questions wrong, (less than 85 percent correct), look for incorrect answers that are grouped together. This suggests that you did not understand a particular topic in the reading. Reread the text dealing with that topic carefully, and then retest yourself on the questions you got wrong. If incorrect answers are spread throughout the chapter content, reread the chapter and re-take the Content Self-Evaluation to assure that you understand the material. If you don't understand why your answer to a question is incorrect after reviewing the text, consult with your instructor.

• When you have completed *Essentials of Paramedic Care, Canadian Edition Volume 2* and its accompanying workbook, prepare for a course test by reviewing both the text in its entirety and your class notes.

If, during your completion of the workbook exercises, you have any questions that either the textbook or workbook doesn't answer, write them down and ask your instructor about them. Prehospital emergency medicine is a complex and complicated subject, and answers are not always black-and-white. It is also common for different EMS systems to use differing methods of care. The questions you bring up in class, and your instructor's answers to them, will help you expand and complete your knowledge of prehospital emergency medical care.

Guidelines to Better Test-Taking

The knowledge you will gain from reading the textbook, completing the exercises in the workbook, listening in your paramedic class, and participating in your clinical and field experience will prepare you to care for patients who are seriously ill or injured. However, before you can practice these skills, you will have to pass several classroom written exams and your state's certification exam successfully. Your performance on these exams will depend not only on your knowledge but also on your ability to answer test questions correctly. The following guidelines are designed to help your performance on tests and to better demonstrate your knowledge of prehospital emergency care.

1. Relax and be calm during the test.

A test is designed to measure what you have learned and to tell you and your instructor how well you are doing. An exam is not designed to intimidate or punish you. Consider it a challenge, and just try to do your best. Get plenty of sleep prior to the examination. Avoid coffee or other stimulants for a few hours before the exam, and be prepared.

Reread the text chapters, review the objectives in the workbook, and review your class notes. It might be helpful to work with one or two other students and ask each other questions. This type of practice helps everyone better understand the knowledge presented in your course of study.

2. Read the questions carefully.

Read each word of the question and all the answers slowly. Words such as "except" or "not" may change the entire meaning of the question. If you miss such words, you may answer the question incorrectly even though you know the right answer.

EXAMPLE:
The art and science of Emergency Medical Services involves all of the following EXCEPT:
- **A.** sincerity and compassion.
- **B.** respect for human dignity.
- **C.** placing patient care before personal safety.
- **D.** delivery of sophisticated emergency medical care.
- **E.** none of the above

The correct answer is C, unless you miss the "EXCEPT."

3. Read each answer carefully.

Read each and every answer carefully. While the first answer may be absolutely correct, so may the rest, and thus the best answer might be "all of the above."

EXAMPLE:
Indirect medical control is considered to be:
- **A.** treatment protocols.
- **B.** training and education.
- **C.** quality assurance.
- **D.** chart review.
- **E.** all of the above

While answers A, B, C, and D are correct, the best and only acceptable answer is "all of the above," E.

4. Delay answering questions you don't understand and look for clues.

When a question seems confusing or you don't know the answer, note it on your answer sheet and come back to it later. This will ensure that you have time to complete the test. You will also find that other questions in the test may give you hints to answer the one you've skipped over. It will also prevent you from being frustrated with an early question and letting it affect your performance.

5. Answer all questions.

Even if you do not know the right answer, do not leave a question blank. A blank question is always wrong, while a guess might be correct. If you can eliminate some of the answers as wrong, do so. It will increase the chances of a correct guess.

EXAMPLE:
When a paramedic is called by the patient (through the dispatcher) to the scene of a medical emergency, the medical control physician has established a physician/patient relationship.
>
> **A.** True
> **B.** False

A true/false question gives you a 50 percent chance of a correct guess.

The hospital health professional responsible for sorting patients as they arrive at the emergency department is usually the:
>
> **A.** emergency physician.
> **B.** ward clerk.
> **C.** emergency nurse.
> **D.** trauma surgeon.
> **E.** both A and C (correct)

A multiple-choice question with five answers gives a 20 percent chance of a correct guess. If you can eliminate one or more incorrect answers, you increase your odds of a correct guess to 25 percent, 33 percent, and so on. An unanswered question has a 0 percent chance of being correct. Just before turning in your answer sheet, check to be sure that you have not left any items blank.

Essentials of Paramedic Care

Division 3

Trauma Emergencies

Chapter 16

Trauma and Trauma Systems

Review of Chapter Objectives

With each chapter of the Workbook, we identify the objectives and the important elements of the text content. You should review these items and refer to the pages listed if any points are not clear.

After reading this chapter, you should be able to:

1. Describe the prevalence and significance of trauma.   pp. 3-4

Trauma is the fourth most common cause of mortality and the number one killer for persons under the age of 45 in Canada. It may be the most expensive medical problem of society today. Traumas can be divided into those caused by blunt and penetrating injury mechanisms, with only 10 percent of all trauma patients experiencing life-threatening injuries and the need for the services of the trauma center/system.

2. List the components of a comprehensive trauma system.   pp. 3-6

The trauma system consists of a province-level agency that coordinates regional trauma systems. The regional systems consist of regional, area, and community trauma centers and, in some cases, other facilities designated and dedicated to the care of trauma patients. The trauma system also consists of injury prevention, provider education, data registry, and quality assurance programs.

3. Identify the characteristics of community, area, and regional trauma centers.   pp. 5-6

Community or Tertiary Trauma Center. This is a general hospital with a commitment to provide resources and staff training specific to the care of trauma patients. Such centers are generally located in rural areas and will stabilize the more serious trauma patients, and then transport them to higher level trauma centers.

District or Secondary Trauma Center. This is a facility with an increased commitment to trauma patient care including 24-hour surgery. A Level II center can handle all but the most critical and specialty trauma patients.

Primary Trauma Center. This is a facility, usually a university teaching hospital, which is staffed and equipped to handle all types of serious trauma 24 hours a day and 7 days a week, as well as to support and oversee the regional trauma system.

4. Identify the trauma triage criteria and apply them to several narrative descriptions of trauma patients. pp. 6-10

Trauma triage criteria include a listing of mechanisms of injury and physical findings suggestive of serious injury. The criteria identify patients likely to benefit from the care offered by the primary or secondary trauma center. They include:

Mechanism of Injury

Falls greater than 6 metres (3x victim's height)	Pedestrian/bicyclist vs. auto collisions
Motorcycle accidents (over 34 kmph)	Ejections from vehicles
Severe vehicle impacts	Rollovers with serious impact
Death of another vehicle occupant	Prolonged extrications

Physical Findings

Revised Trauma Score less than 11	Pediatric Trauma Score less than 9
Glasgow Coma Scale less than 14	Systolic blood pressure less than 90
Pulse greater than 120 or less than 50	Penetrating trauma (non-extremity)
Multiple proximal long bone fractures	Flail chest
Pelvic fractures	Limb paralysis
Respiratory rate greater than 29 or less than 10	Airway or facial burns
Burns greater than 15% body surface area (BSA)	

5. Describe how trauma differs from medical emergencies in the scene size-up, assessment, pre-hospital emergency care, and transport. pp. 6-10

Scene size-up of the trauma incident differs from that with the medical emergency in that it is usually associated with more numerous scene hazards and involves an analysis of the mechanism of injury, using the evidence of impact to suggest possible injuries (the index of suspicion).

Assessment employs an initial assessment examining the risk of spinal injury, a quick mental status check, and an evaluation of airway, breathing, and circulation (ABCs), followed by a rapid trauma assessment looking to the head and torso and any sites of potential serious injury suggested by the index of suspicion or patient complaint.

Prehospital care and transport of the trauma patient is designed to provide expedient and supportive care and rapid transport of the patient to the trauma center or other appropriate facility.

6. Explain the "Golden Hour" concept and describe how it applies to pre-hospital emergency medical service. pp. 8-9

Research has demonstrated that the seriously injured trauma patient has an increasing chance for survival as the time from the injury to surgical intervention is reduced. Practically, this time should be as short as possible, ideally less than one hour. This "Golden Hour" concept directs pre-hospital care providers to reduce on-scene and transport times by expeditious assessment and care at the scene and by the use of air medical transport when appropriate and available.

7. Explain the value of air medical service in trauma patient care and transport. pp. 8-9

Air medical transport can move the trauma patient more quickly and along a direct line from the crash scene to the trauma center, thereby reducing transport time and increasing the likelihood that the patient will reach definitive care expeditiously. Air medical transport units are usually helicopters are usually staffed by Critical Care Paramedic (CCP) or Advanced Care Paramedics (ACP).

CONTENT SELF-EVALUATION

Multiple Choice

_____ 1. Firearm injuries account for how many deaths each year in Canada?
  A. 1 300   **D.** 1 100
  B. 1 500   **E.** 110
  C. 13 000

_____ 2. The legislation that led to the development of today's Emergency Medical Services system was the:
  A. Trauma Care Systems Planning and Development Act of 1990.
  B. Consolidated Emergency Services Act of 1971.
  C. Highway Safety Act of 1966.
  D. Trauma Systems Act of 1963.
  E. National Readiness Act of 1960.

_____ 3. The trauma system is predicated on the principle that serious trauma is:
  A. a frequent occurrence.
  B. usually a medical emergency.
  C. inevitable.
  D. a surgical disease.
  E. fatal if the patient is not seen by a qualified physician in less than 30 minutes.

_____ 4. A primary trauma center is usually a(n):
  A. community hospital.
  B. teaching hospital with resources available full-time for emergency cases.
  C. emergency department with 24-hour service.
  D. non-emergency health care facility.
  E. stabilizing and transport facility.

_____ 5. The small community hospital or healthcare facility in a remote area, designated as a receiving facility for trauma, a:
  A. district   **D.** tertiary
  B. primary   **E.** elite
  C. secondary.

_____ 6. Trauma centers may also be designated for provision of which of the following special services?
  A. pediatric trauma center   **D.** hyperbaric center
  B. burn center   **E.** all of the above
  C. neurocenter

_____ 7. The period of time between the occurrence of serious injury and surgery suggested as a goal for pre- hospital care providers is the:
  A. platinum 10 minutes.   **D.** bleed-out equation.
  B. golden hour.   **E.** critical differential.
  C. trauma time differential.

_____ 8. The reduction in the incidence and seriousness of trauma in recent years can be credited to:
  A. better highway design.
  B. better auto design.
  C. use of auto restraint systems.
  D. development of injury prevention programs.
  E. all of the above

9. The standardized data retrieval system used to evaluate and improve the trauma system is the:
   A. pre-hospital care report system.
   B. trauma triage system.
   C. trauma registry.
   D. trauma quality improvement program.
   E. CISD.

True/False

10. Quality Improvement is a significant method of assessing system quality and providing for its improvement.
    A. True
    B. False

11. Although trauma poses a serious threat to life, its presentation often masks the patient's true condition.
    A. True
    B. False

12 Some 90 percent of all trauma patients do not have serious, life-endangering injuries.
    A. True
    B. False

13. Trauma triage criteria are mechanisms of injury or physical signs exhibited by the patient that suggest serious injury.
    A. True
    B. False

14. In applying trauma triage criteria, it is best to err on the side of precaution.
    A. True
    B. False

15. Trauma triage criteria are designed to over-triage trauma patients to ensure those with more subtle injuries are not missed.
    A. True
    B. False

Matching

Write the letter of the term in the space provided next to the appropriate description.

A. trauma   **D.** less than 10 minutes
B. golden hour   **E.** index of suspicion
C. mechanism of injury

_____ 16. the maximum acceptable time between injury and surgery

_____ 17. physical injury or wound caused by external force

_____ 18. ideal time of assessment, stabilization, packaging, and initiation of transport of a trauma patient

_____ 19. the anticipation of an injury based on analysis of mechanism of injury

_____ 20. the processes and forces that cause trauma

Chapter 17

Blunt Trauma

Review of Chapter Objectives

After reading this chapter, you should be able to:

1. **Identify, and explain by example, the laws of inertia and conservation of energy. pp. 13-14**

Inertia is the tendency for objects at rest or in motion to remain so unless acted upon by an outside force. In some cases, that force is the energy exchange that causes trauma. For example, a bullet will continue its travel until it exchanges all its energy with the tissue it strikes.
Conservation of energy is the physical law explaining that energy is not lost but changes form in the auto or other impact. An example is the deformity in the auto when it impacts a tree.

2. **Define kinetic energy and force as they relate to trauma. pp. 14-15**

Kinetic energy is the energy any moving object possesses. This energy is the potential to do harm if it is distributed to a victim.
Force is the exchange of energy from one object to another. It is determined by an object's mass (weight) and the velocity of rate change (acceleration or deceleration). This force induces injury.

3. **Compare and contrast the types of vehicle impacts and their expected injuries.
   pp. 16-19, 21-34**

There are basically five types of vehicle impacts—frontal, lateral, rotational, rear-end, or rollover impacts. There are four events within each impact. First, the vehicle impacts the object and quickly comes to rest. Then, the vehicle occupant impacts the vehicle interior and comes to rest. Meanwhile, various organs and structures within the occupant's body collide with one another causing compression and stretching and injury. In the fourth event, objects within the vehicle may continue their forward motion until they impact the slowed or stopped occupant. In some instances, secondary vehicle impacts occur; these are impacts that may subject the injured occupant to additional acceleration, deceleration, and injury.

Frontal impact is the most common type of auto collision, although it also offers the most structural protection for the occupant. The front crumple zones of the auto absorb energy and the restraints—seat belts and airbags—provide additional protection. The anterior surface of the victim impacts the steering wheel, dash, windshield and/or firewall resulting in chest, abdominal, head, and neck injuries as well as knee, femur, and hip fractures.
Lateral impacts occur without the benefit of the front crumple zones, thereby permitting transmission of more energy directly to the occupant. The occupant is turned 90 degrees to the impact, resulting in fractures of the hip, femur, shoulder girdle, clavicle, and lateral ribs. Internal injury may result to the aorta and spleen on the driver's side or liver on the passenger's side. An unbelted occupant may impact the other occupant, causing further injury.
Rotational impacts result from oblique contact between vehicles, spinning as well as slowing the autos. This mediates the deceleration and reduces the expected injury. Injury patterns resemble a mix of those associated with frontal and lateral patterns though the severity is generally reduced.

Rear-end impacts push the auto, auto seat, and finally the occupant forward. The body is well protected, though the head may remain stationary while the shoulders move rapidly forward. The result may be hyperextension of the head and neck and cervical spine injury. Once the vehicle begins deceleration, other injuries may occur as the body contacts the dash, steering wheel, or windshield if the occupant is unbelted.

Rollovers occur as the roadway elevation changes or a vehicle with a high center of gravity becomes unstable around a turn. The vehicle impacts the ground as it turns, exposing the occupants to multiple impacts in places where the vehicle interior may be not designed to absorb such impacts. The result may be serious injuries to anywhere on the body or ejection of the occupants. Restraints greatly reduce the incidence of injury and ejection, while ejection greatly increases the chance of occupant death.

4. Discuss the benefits of auto restraint and motorcycle helmet use.   pp. 19-21, 31-32

Lap belts and shoulder straps control the deceleration of the vehicle occupant during a crash, slowing them with the auto. The result is a great reduction in injuries and deaths. However, when improperly worn, serious injuries may result. Shoulder straps alone may account for serious neck injury while the lap belt worn too high may injure the spine and abdomen.

Airbags inflate explosively during an impact and provide a cushion of gas as the occupant impacts the steering wheel, dash, or vehicle side. This slows the impact, reduces the deceleration rate, and reduces injuries. The airbag may entrap the driver's fingers and result in fractures or may impact a small driver or passenger who is seated close to the device and result in facial injury.

Child safety seats provide much needed protection for infants and small children for whom normal restraints do not work adequately by themselves because of the children's rapidly changing anatomical dimensions. The seat faces rearward for infants and very small children and then should be replaced with a model facing forward as the child grows. This positioning permits the seat belt to provide restraint, similar to that provided for the adult. Child safety seats should not be positioned in front of airbag restraint systems because inflation of those devices may push the rear-facing child forcibly into the seat.

Motorcycle helmet use can significantly reduce the incidence and severity of head injury, the greatest cause of motorcycle crash death. Helmets do not, however, reduce the incidence of spinal injury.

5. Describe the mechanisms of injury associated with falls, crush injuries, and sports injuries. pp. 40-43

Falls are a release of stored gravitational energy resulting in an impact between the body and the ground or other surface. Injuries occur at the point of impact and along the pathway of transmitted energy, resulting in soft tissue, skeletal, and internal trauma.

Crush injuries are injuries caused by heavy objects or machinery entrapping and damaging an extremity. The resulting wound restricts blood flow and allows the accumulation of toxins. When the pressure is removed, blood flow may move the toxins into the central circulation and hemorrhage from many disrupted blood vessels at the wound site may be hard to control.

Sports injuries are commonly the result of direct trauma, fatigue, or exertion. They often result in injury to muscles, ligaments, and tendons and to the long bones. Special consideration must be given to protecting such an injury from further aggravation until it can be seen by a physician.

6. Identify the common blast injuries and any special considerations regarding their assessment and proper care. pp. 34-40

The blast injury process results in five distinct mechanisms of injury—pressure injury, penetrating objects, personnel displacement, structural collapse, and burns.

Pressure injury occurs as the pressure wave moves outward, rapidly compressing, then decompressing anything in its path. A victim is impacted by the wave and air-filled body spaces such as the lungs, auditory canals, and bowels may be damaged. Hearing loss is the most frequent result of pressure injury, though lung injury is most serious and life threatening. The pressure change may damage or rupture alveoli resulting in dyspnea, pulmonary edema, pneumothorax, or air embolism.

Care includes provision of high-flow oxygen, gentle positive-pressure ventilation, and rapid transport. The hearing loss patient needs careful reassurance and simple instruction.

Penetrating objects may be the bomb casing or debris put in motion by the pressure of the explosion. They may impale or enter the body, resulting in hemorrhage and internal injury. Care specific to the resulting injury should be provided, and any hemorrhage controlled by direct pressure. Any impaled object should be immobilized and the patient rapidly transported to a trauma center.

Personnel displacement occurs as the pressure wave and blast wind propel the victim through the air and he or she then impacts the ground or other surface. Blunt and penetrating trauma may result, and such injuries are cared for following standard procedures.

Collapse of a structure after a blast may entrap victims under debris and result in crush and pressure injuries. The collapse may make victims hard to locate and then extricate. Further, the nature of the crush-type wounds may make control of hemorrhage difficult, while the release of a long-entrapped extremity may be dangerous as the toxins that accumulated when circulation is disrupted are distributed to the central circulation.

Burns may result directly from the explosion or as a result of secondary combustion of debris or clothing. Generally the initial explosion will cause only superficial damage because of the short duration of the heat release and the fluid nature of the body. However, incendiary agents and burning debris or clothing may result in severe full-thickness burns.

7. **Identify and explain any special assessment and care considerations for patients with blunt trauma. pp. 16-43**

Blunt injury patients must be carefully assessed because the signs of serious internal injury may be hidden or absent. Careful analysis of the mechanism of injury and the development of an index of suspicion for serious injury may be the only way to anticipate the true seriousness of the injuries.

8. **Given several preprogrammed and moulaged blunt trauma patients, provide the appropriate scene size-up, initial assessment, rapid trauma or focused physical exam and history, detailed exam, and ongoing assessment, and provide appropriate patient care and transportation. pp. 16-43**

During your training as a Paramedic, you will participate in many classroom practice sessions involving simulated patients. You will also spend some time in the emergency departments of local hospitals as well as in advanced-level ambulances gaining clinical experience. During these times, use your knowledge of the mechanisms of blunt trauma to help you assess and care for the simulated or real patients you attend.

CONTENT SELF-EVALUATION

Multiple Choice

1. The study of trauma is related to a branch of physics called:
   A. kinetics.
   B. velocity.
   C. ballistics.
   D. inertia.
   E. heuristics.

2. The anticipation of injuries based upon the analysis of the collision mechanism is referred to as the:
   A. mechanism of injury.
   B. index of suspicion.
   C. trauma triage criteria.
   D. mortality potential.
   E. RTS.

3. The tendency of an object to remain at rest or remain in motion unless acted upon by an external force is:
   A. kinetics.
   B. velocity.
   C. ballistics.
   D. inertia.
   E. deceleration.

4. Two autos accelerate from a stop sign to a speed of 50 kmph, the first one by normal acceleration and the second when it was struck from behind by another vehicle. Assuming that both vehicles have the same weight, which vehicle gained the most kinetic energy?
- **A.** the vehicle in normal acceleration
- **B.** the vehicle struck from behind
- **C.** both vehicles gained the same kinetic energy
- **D.** cannot be determined since the kinetic energy is not known
- **E.** cannot be determined since the force is not known

5. Which of the following is an example of energy dissipation from an auto accident?
- **A.** sound of the impact
- **B.** bending of the structural steel
- **C.** heating of the compressed steel
- **D.** internal injury to the occupant
- **E.** all of the above

6. Which of the following increases the kinetic energy of a collision most quickly?
- **A.** the temperature of the object
- **B.** increasing object speed
- **C.** decreasing object speed
- **D.** increasing object mass
- **E.** decreasing object mass

7. Blunt trauma may cause:
- **A.** rupture of the bowel.
- **B.** bursting of the alveoli.
- **C.** crushing of blood vessels.
- **D.** contusion of the liver or kidneys.
- **E.** all of the above.

8. Which of the following is a common cause of blunt trauma?
- **A.** auto collisions
- **B.** falls
- **C.** sports injuries
- **D.** pedestrian impacts
- **E.** all of the above

9. In which order do the events of an auto collision usually occur?
- **A.** body collision, vehicle collision, organ collision, secondary collisions
- **B.** organ collision, vehicle collision, body collision, secondary collisions
- **C.** vehicle collision, secondary collisions, body collision, organ collision
- **D.** vehicle collision, body collision, organ collision, secondary collisions
- **E.** body collision, vehicle collision, secondary collisions, organ collision

10. A supplemental restraint system (SRS) refers to which of the following?
- **A.** shoulder belts
- **B.** airbags
- **C.** lap belts
- **D.** child seats
- **E.** all of the above

11. Which of the following restraint systems is likely to induce hand fractures?
- **A.** shoulder belts
- **B.** passenger airbags
- **C.** driver-side airbags
- **D.** child seats
- **E.** lap belts

12. The type of auto impact that occurs most frequently in rural areas is:
- **A.** lateral.
- **B.** rotational.
- **C.** frontal.
- **D.** rear-end.
- **E.** rollover.

13. Which type of auto impact occurs most frequently in the urban setting?
- **A.** lateral
- **B.** rotational
- **C.** frontal
- **D.** rear-end
- **E.** rollover

14. The down-and-under pathway is most commonly associated with which type of auto collision?

A.	lateral	**D.**	rear-end
B.	rotational	**E.**	rollover
C.	frontal		

15. Which of the following injuries are associated with significant lateral impact?

A.	aortic aneurysms	**D.**	vertebral fractures
B.	clavicular fractures	**E.**	all of the above
C.	pelvic fractures		

16. The most common injury associated with the rear-end impact is to the:

A.	abdomen.	**D.**	femur.
B.	pelvis.	**E.**	head and neck.
C.	aorta.		

17. Which of the following is a hazard commonly associated with auto collisions?

A.	hot liquids	**D.**	sharp glass or metal edges
B.	caustic substances	**E.**	all of the above
C.	downed power lines		

18. In fatal collisions, about what percentage of the drivers are legally intoxicated?

A.	40 percent	**D.**	50 percent
B.	20 percent	**E.**	83 percent
C.	35 percent		

19. The most common body area associated with vehicular mortality is the:

A.	head.	**D.**	extremities.
B.	chest.	**E.**	spine.
C.	abdomen.		

20. In motorcycle accidents, the highest index of suspicion for injury should be directed at the:

A.	neck.	**D.**	pelvis.
B.	head.	**E.**	femurs.
C.	extremities.		

21. Use of a helmet in a motorcycle crash reduces the incidence of neck injury by about:

A.	25 percent.	**D.**	75 percent.
B.	35 percent.	**E.**	85 percent.
C.	58 percent.		

22. Which of the mechanisms below can cause patient injury in a blast?

A. the pressure wave
B. flying debris
C. the patient being thrown into objects
D. heat
E. all of the above

23. Underwater detonation of an explosive generally increases its lethal range by:

A.	10 percent.	**D.**	300 percent.
B.	25 percent.	**E.**	500 percent.
C.	100 percent.		

24. The arrow-shaped projectiles in military-type explosives that are designed to extend the injury power of a bomb are called:

A.	ordinance.	**D.**	oatmeal.
B.	casing material.	**E.**	granulation.
C.	flechettes.		

25. Which of the following are secondary blast injuries?

A. heat injuries D. injuries caused by structural collapse
B. pressure injuries E. both A and B
C. projectile injuries

26. The most serious and common traumas associated with explosions affect the:

A. heart. D. lungs.
B. bowel. E. brain.
C. auditory canal.

27. Severe injury is generally associated with a fall from:

A. three times the patient's own height D. more than 2 metres
B. twice the patient's own height. E. none of the above
C. greater than 4 metres.

28. Sports injuries are frequently associated with:

A. fatigue. D. rotation.
B. extreme exertion. E. all of the above
C. compression.

29. Air bags can be located in:

A. steering column. D. seat sides.
B. front dash E. all of the above
C. headliners above doors

30. Physical contact made with athletes wearing cleats usually result in injuries to the:

A. neck. D. humerus.
B. pelvis E. scapula
C. knee

31. In contact sports injuries, a patient should be evaluated at the emergency department if the collision leads to:

A. any period of unconsciousness D. all of the above.
B. neurologic deficit E. none of the above
C. lowered level of orientation.

32. Accounting for most injury deaths and disabilities, blunt trauma includes all but which of the following:

A. crush injuries. D. falls.
B. gun shot wounds E. blast injuries
C. sports injuries

33. Which is the most common injury sustained from rapid deceleration?

A. internal jugular may be twisted D. tympanic membrane rupture.
B. femoral artery occlusion E. lacerated liver
C. lacerated diaphragm

34. Seat belts that are improperly worn or when lap belts alone are worn can lead to a spinal fracture at:

A. T2-T8. D. L5 to S2.
B. T12 to L2 E. T10-T12
C. L1 to L5

35. Likely injuries in motorcycle accidents include:

A. skull fractures. D. abdominal injuries
B. internal thoracic injuries E. all of the above
C. spinal fractures

36. During a frontal impact car accident, ejection is responsible for _____ percent of all vehicular fatalities.

A.	22%	**D.**	27%
B.	20%	**E.**	35%
C.	15%		

37. The major types of vehicles most often involved in recreational vehicle collisions are:

A.	snowmobiles.	**D.**	jet-skis or other water craft
B.	boats	**E.**	all of the above
C.	all-terrain vehicles		

38. Frontal collisions are common with ATVs and snowmobiles. The highest suspicion of injury should be directed at:

- **A.** head, spine, upper and lower extremities
- **B.** head, chest, lower extremities
- **C.** lower extremities only
- **D.** head, upper and lower extremities
- **E.** pelvis, spine and upper extremities

True/False

39. Penetrating trauma is the most common type of trauma associated with patient mortality.
- **A.** True
- **B.** False

40. The major effect of the seat belt during the auto collision is to slow the passenger with the auto.
- **A.** True
- **B.** False

41. While less convenient than a child carrier, holding a child in the arms is relatively safe except in the most severe of crashes.
- **A.** True
- **B.** False

42. When analyzing the lateral impact injury mechanism, you must assign a higher index of suspicion for serious life-threatening injury than with other types of impact.
- **A.** True
- **B.** False

43. With rotational impacts, the seriousness of injury is often less than vehicle damage would suggest.
- **A.** True
- **B.** False

44. With modern vehicle construction that incorporates crumple zones, you can dependably use the amount of vehicular damage to approximate the patient injuries inside.
- **A.** True
- **B.** False

45. In an auto vs. child pedestrian accident, you would expect the victim to turn toward the impact.
- **A.** True
- **B.** False

46. In addition to the danger of trauma, the boating collision patient is also likely to suffer possible hypothermia and near-drowning.
- **A.** True
- **B.** False

_____ **47.** A victim's orientation to the blast does not effect the nature and severity of the injuries he or she sustains from an explosion.
    A.   True
    B.   False

_____ **48.** When victims are within a structure that contains an explosion, like a building, the effects of the blast are concentrated and the severity of the expected injuries increases.
    A.   True
    B.   False

_____ **49.** Jet skis are especially dangerous in the hands of inexperienced riders.
    A.   True
    B.   False

_____ **50.** In crush injuries, prolonged pressure can disrupt blood flow and cause aerobic metabolism and some tissue death.
    A.   True
    B.   False

Matching

Write the letter of the term in the space provided next to the appropriate description.

A.	pressure wave	**F.**	inertia
B.	hemoptysis	**G.**	ATV
C.	flechettes	**H.**	velocity
D.	exsanguination	**I.**	paper bag syndrome
E.	kinetics	**J.**	Newton's Second Law

_____ **51.** tendency of an object to remain at rest or remain in motion unless acted on by an external force

_____ **52.** the branch of physics that deals with motion, taking into consideration mass and force

_____ **53.** all terrain vehicle

_____ **54.** the result of the compression of the chest against the steering column

_____ **55.** expectoration of blood from the respiratory tract

_____ **56.** the rate of motion in a particular direction in relation to time

_____ **57.** the draining of blood to the point at which life cannot be sustained

_____ **58.** area of over pressure that radiates outward from an explosion

_____ **59.** Force=Mass x Acceleration or Deceleration

_____ **60.** arrow shaped projectiles found in some military ordinance

Chapter 18

Penetrating Trauma

Review of Chapter Objectives

After reading this chapter, you should be able to:

1. **Explain the energy exchange process between a penetrating object or projectile and the object it strikes. pp. 45-49**

The kinetic energy of a bullet is dependent upon its mass and even more so on its velocity according to the kinetic energy formula ($KE = \dfrac{M \times V^2}{2}$).

This energy is distributed to the body tissues in the form of damage as the bullet slows. Due to the semifluid nature of body tissue, the passage of a bullet causes injury as the bullet directly strikes tissue and contuses and tears it and as it sets the tissue in motion outward and away from the bullet's path (cavitation). The faster the bullet and the larger its presenting surface (profile), the more rapid the exchange of energy and the resulting injury.

2. **Determine the effects profile, yaw, tumble, expansion, and fragmentation have on projectile energy transfer. pp. 46-49**

The rate of projectile energy exchange and the seriousness of resulting injury are dependent upon the rate of energy exchange. That rate is directly related to the bullet's presenting surface or profile. The larger the bullet's caliber (diameter), the greater its profile, the more rapid its exchange of energy with body tissue, and the greater the damage it causes. Yaw (swinging around the axis of the projectile's travel), tumble, expansion, and fragmentation all lead to a greater area of the bullet striking tissue than simply its profile, and hence these factors increase the damaging power of a bullet.

3. **Describe elements of the ballistic injury process including direct injury, cavitation, temporary cavity, permanent cavity, and zone of injury. pp. 46-49, 52-54**

As a penetrating object enters the body it disrupts the tissue it contacts by tearing it, displacing it from its path, and causing *direct injury*. As the object's velocity increases, the rate of energy exchange increases and the rate of displacement increases. A bullet's speed is so great that the bullet's passage sets the semifluid body tissue in motion away from the bullet's path. This creates a cavity behind and to the side of the projectile pathway. This *cavitation* further stretches and tears tissue as it creates a *temporary cavity*. The natural elasticity of injured tissue and the adjoining tissue closes the cavity, but an area of disrupted tissue remains (the *permanent cavity*). The *zone of injury* is the region along and surrounding the bullet track where tissue has been disrupted due to direct injury or to the stretching and tearing of cavitation.

4. Identify the relative effects a penetrating object or projectile has when striking various body regions and tissues.   pp. 55-59

The passage of a bullet (and its cavitational wave) has varying effects depending on the elasticity (resiliency) and density of the tissue the bullet strikes. Connective tissue is very resilient, stretches easily, and will somewhat resist cavitational injury. Solid organs are generally very dense and much less resilient than connective tissue. They do not withstand the force generated by the cavitational wave as well as connective tissue, and the resulting injury can be expected to be much greater. Hollow organs are resilient when not distended with fluid; if an organ is full, however, the cavitational wave may cause the organ to rupture. Direct injury can also perforate an organ and permit spillage of its contents into surrounding tissue. Lung tissue is both very resilient and air filled. The tiny air pockets (the alveoli) absorb the energy of the bullet's passage and limit lung injury. On the other hand, bone is extremely dense and inelastic. Direct contact with a bullet or, in some cases, just the cavitational wave may shatter the bone and drive fragments into surrounding tissue. Slow-moving penetrating objects do not produce a cavitational wave, and injury from them is limited to the pathway of the object.

The passage of a bullet and its associated injury are related to the bullet's path of travel and, specifically, to the body region it passes through. Extremity wounds are by far the most common, yet due to the limited major body structures in the extremities, they rarely result in life-threatening injury. If the projectile strikes the bone, however, the dramatic exchange of energy may cause great tissue disruption and vascular injury, which can result in severe hemorrhage. Abdominal penetration most commonly affects the bowel, which is reasonably tolerant of the cavitational wave. However, the upper abdomen contains the liver, pancreas, and spleen, solid organs that are subject to severe injury from direct injury and cavitation. Penetrating chest trauma may affect the lungs, heart and great vessels, esophagus, trachea, and diaphragm. The lung is rather resilient to penetrating injury, while the heart and great vessels may perforate or rupture with rapid exsanguination ensuing. Tracheal tears may result in airway compromise, while esophageal tears may release gastric contents into the mediastinum with potentially deadly results. Large penetrations of the thoracic wall may permit air to move in and out (sucking or open pneumothorax) or may open the airway internally to permit air to enter the pleural space (closed pneumothorax). Neck injuries may permit severe hemorrhage, disrupt the trachea, or allow air to enter the jugular veins and embolize the lungs. Head injuries may disrupt the airway or may penetrate the cranium and cause extensive, rarely survivable, injury to the brain.

5. Anticipate the injury types and extent of damage associated with high-velocity/high-energy projectiles, such as rifle bullets; with medium velocity/medium-energy projectiles, such as handgun and shotgun bullets, slugs, or pellets; and with low-energy/low-velocity penetrating objects, such as knives and arrows.   pp. 49-52

High-velocity/high-energy projectiles (rifle bullets) are likely to cause the most extensive injury because they have the potential to impart the most kinetic energy to the patient. Their rapid energy exchange causes the greatest cavitational wave and is most likely to produce bullet deformity and fragmentation. These characteristics cause more severe tissue damage to a greater area. The effects of these projectiles can be further enhanced if the bullet hits bone and causes it to shatter, creating additional projectiles that are driven into adjoining tissue.

Medium-velocity/medium-energy projectiles (from handguns) are likely to cause only moderate injury beyond the direct pathway of the bullet as their reduced energy does not usually cause the bullet deformity, fragmentation, and extensive cavitation waves seen with rifle projectiles. The shotgun is a particularly lethal weapon at close range because its medium-energy projectiles are numerous and their numbers cause many direct injury pathways.

Low-velocity/low-energy penetrating objects are commonly knives, arrows, ice picks, and other objects traveling at low speeds. They generally cause only direct injury along the path of their travel. They may, however, be moved about, once inserted and either left in place or withdrawn.

6. **Identify important elements of the scene size-up associated with shootings or stabbings. pp. 59-61**

Penetrating trauma, especially when associated with shootings or stabbings, presents the danger of violence directed toward others (other rescuers, bystanders, your patient, and you). It is essential that you approach the scene with great caution and ensure that the police have secured it before you approach or enter. Penetrating trauma also calls for gloves as minimum BSI precaution, with goggles and gown required for spurting hemorrhage, airway management, or massive blood contamination. During the scene size-up, you should evaluate the mechanism of injury including the type of weapon, caliber, distance, and angle between the shooter and the victim, and the number of shots fired and patient impacts.

7. **Identify and explain any special assessment and care considerations for patients with penetrating trauma. pp. 61-63**

In assessing the patient with penetrating trauma you must anticipate the projectile or penetrating object's pathway and the structures it is likely to have injured. The exit wound from a projectile may help you better approximate the wounding potential, and remember that the bullet may have been deflected along its course and damaged or completely missed critical structures. Always suspect and treat for the worst-case scenario. Be especially wary of injuries to the head, chest, and abdomen as wounds to these regions often have lethal outcomes. Cover all open wounds that enter the thorax or neck with occlusive dressings and be watchful for the development of dyspnea due to pneumothorax, tension pneumothorax, or pulmonary emboli. Be prepared to provide aggressive fluid resuscitation, but understand that doing so may dislodge forming clots and increase the rate of internal hemorrhage. Stabilize any impaled objects and only remove them when it is required to ensure a patent airway, to perform CPR, or to transport the patient.

8. **Given several preprogrammed and moulaged penetrating trauma patients, provide the appropriate scene size-up, initial assessment, rapid trauma or focused physical exam and history, detailed exam, and ongoing assessment, and provide appropriate patient care and transportation. pp. 45-63**

During your training as a Paramedic you will participate in many classroom practice sessions involving simulated patients. You will also spend some time in the emergency departments of local hospitals as well as in advanced-level ambulances gaining clinical experience. During these times, use your knowledge of the mechanisms of penetrating trauma to help you assess and care for the simulated or real patients you attend.

CONTENT SELF-EVALUATION

Multiple Choice

1. Approximately what numbers of deaths are attributable to shootings each year?
   A. 1,750
   B. 3,800
   C. 1,300
   D. 500
   E. 1,500

2. An object traveling at twice the speed of another object of the same weight has:
   A. twice the kinetic energy.
   B. three times the kinetic energy.
   C. four times the kinetic energy.
   D. eight times the kinetic energy.
   E. ten times the kinetic energy.

3. The curved tract a bullet follows during flight is called its:
   A. ballistics.
   B. cavitation.
   C. trajectory.
   D. yaw.
   E. parabola.

4. The surface of a projectile that exchanges energy with the object struck is its:
   A. caliber.
   B. profile.
   C. drag.
   D. yaw.
   E. expansion factor.

5. When a rifle bullet hits tissue, normally it will:
   A. continue without tumbling.
   B. tumble once then travel nose first.
   C. tumble quickly, the slowly rotate.
   D. wobble but not tumble.
   E. tumble 180 degrees then continue.

6. Which of the following statements accurately describes a rifle bullet in contrast to a handgun bullet?
   A. It is a heavier projectile.
   B. It travels at a greater velocity.
   C. It is more likely to deform.
   D. It is more likely to fragment.
   E. all of the above

7. Which element of the projectile injury process is related to the actual damage caused as the bullet contacts tissue?
   A. direct injury
   B. pressure wave
   C. temporary cavity
   D. permanent cavity
   E. zone of injury

8. The movement of tissue away from the bullet's path as it passes through the body results in:
   A. direct injury.
   B. the pressure wave.
   C. a temporary cavity.
   D. fragmentation.
   E. referred injury.

9. The passage of a projectile through the body results in a region where tissues are disrupted and not functioning normally that is known as the:
   A. direct injury.
   B. pressure wave.
   C. temporary cavity.
   D. permanent cavity.
   E. zone of injury.

10. The temporary cavity formed as a high-velocity/high-energy bullet passes may be how large?
    A. 12 times the projectile's profile
    B. 14 times the projectile's profile
    C. 16 times the projectile's profile
    D. 100 times the projectile's profile
    E. rarely more than the projectile's profile

11. The tissue structure that is very resilient, yet dense, and usually sustains limited damage with the passage of a projectile is:
    A. a solid organ.
    B. a hollow organ.
    C. connective tissue.
    D. bone.
    E. a lung.

12. The tissue structure that is likely to rupture and spill its contents when struck by a projectile is:
    A. a solid organ.
    B. a hollow organ.
    C. connective tissue.
    D. bone.
    E. a lung.

13. The abdominal organ most tolerant to the passage of a projectile is the:
    A. bowel.
    B. liver.
    C. spleen.
    D. kidney.
    E. pancreas.

14. The body region in which a penetrating wound has the greatest likelihood of drawing air into the venous system is the:

A. abdomen.
B. thorax.
C. head.
D. neck.
E. none of the above

15. Which of the following is NOT associated with an entrance wound?

A. tattooing
B. a small ridge of discoloration around the wound
C. a blown outward appearance
D. subcutaneous emphysema
E. propellant residue on the surrounding tissue

16. Which of the following information should you gain through the scene size-up, if possible?

A. the gun caliber
B. the angle of the gun to the victim
C. the type of gun used
D. assurance that no other weapons are involved
E. all of the above

17. As you care for a patient at a potential crime scene, actions you take to help preserve evidence should include:

A. cutting through, not around bullet or knife holes in clothing.
B. moving what you can away from the patient.
C. removing obviously dead patients from the scene as quickly as possible.
D. disturbing only the items necessary to provide patient care.
E. all of the above

18. Frothy blood at a bullet exit or entrance wound suggests a(n):

A. simple pneumothorax.
B. open pneumothorax.
C. tension pneumothorax.
D. pericardial tamponade.
E. mediastinum injury.

19. A projectile entering the small or large bowel may result in which of the following:

A. hemothorax
B. peritoneal irritation
C. hepatomegaly
D. thoracic spine fracture
E. splenic rupture

20. The damage pathway that a high-velocity projectile inflicts results in which of the three specific factors?

A. pressure shock wave, cavitation and direct energy
B. zone of injury, permanent cavity and temporary cavity
C. pressure shock wave, penetrating zone, and zone of incidence
D. resiliency, pressure shock wave and cavitation
E. pressure shock wave, infection, and direct energy

21. Approximately how many times greater pressure than the normal atmospheric pressure can high-velocity rifle bullets produce?

A. 60 times greater
B. 100 times greater
C. 40 times greater
D. 80 times greater
E. 200 times greater

22. In recent military experiences, extremity injuries account for what percentage of injuries?

A. between 50 and 70 per cent
B. between 40 and 80 per cent
C. less than 10 per cent
D. 50 per cent
E. between 60 and 80 per cent

_____ 23. Of the high percentage of extremity trauma in recent military experience, what
percentage accounts for fatalities?
- **A.** 5 per cent
- **B.** 10 per cent
- **C.** 15 per cent
- **D.** 20 per cent
- **E.** 50 per cent

_____ 24. All open penetrating chest wounds should be covered with a(n):
- **A.** sterile pressure dressing.
- **B.** sealed dressing.
- **C.** non-occlusive dressing.
- **D.** occlusive dressing.
- **E.** triangular bandage.

_____ 25. The body region(s) deserving special attention with penetrating trauma include:
- **A.** neck
- **B.** abdomen
- **C.** thorax
- **D.** head
- **E.** all of the above

True/False

_____ 26. Wounds from rifle bullets are considered two to four times more lethal than handgun
bullets.
- **A.** True
- **B.** False

_____ 27. While handgun bullets are made of relatively soft lead, their kinetic energy is generally
not sufficient to cause significant deformity.
- **A.** True
- **B.** False

_____ 28. Civilian hunting ammunition is designed to deform and will frequently fragment when
striking soft tissue.
- **A.** True
- **B.** False

_____ 29. The shotgun is limited in range and accuracy; however, injuries it inflicts at close range
can be very severe or lethal.
- **A.** True
- **B.** False

_____ 30. Penetrating wounds to the extremities account for about 70 percent of all penetrating
wounds yet account for less than 10 percent of fatalities related to this injury mechanism.
- **A.** True
- **B.** False

_____ 31. Because of the pressure-driven dynamics of respiration, any large wound to the chest may
compromise breathing.
- **A.** True
- **B.** False

_____ 32. The entrance wound is more likely to reflect the actual damaging potential of the
projectile than the exit wound.
- **A.** True
- **B.** False

_____ 33. With shotgun shells, the larger the shot number, the smaller the number of projectiles.
- **A.** True
- **B.** False

34. Trying to reconstruct the event at the scene of a shooting may help you determine the angle at which a bullet entered the victim.
   A. True
   B. False

35. Penetrating injuries, especially those associated with gunshot wounds, are responsible for a high incident of death.
   A. True
   B. False

Matching

Write the letter of the term in the space provided next to the appropriate description.

A.	drag	F.	calibre
B.	resiliency	G.	cricothyrotomy
C.	prognosis	H.	yaw
D.	trajectory	I.	profile
E.	ballistics	J.	cavitation

36. the outward motion of tissue due to a projectile's passage, resulting in a temporary cavity and a vacuum

37. a surgical incision into the cricothyroid membrane, usually to provide an emergency airway

38. the path a projectile follows

39. the forces acting on a projectile in motion to slow it down

40. the study of projectile motion and its interactions with a gun

41. swing or wobble around the axis of a projectile's travel

42. the diameter of a bullet expressed in hundredths of an inch

43. The size and shape of a projectile as it contacts a target

44. the anticipated outcome of a disease or injury

45. the connective tissue strength and elasticity of an object or fabric

Chapter 19

Hemorrhage and Shock

Review of Chapter Objectives

After reading this chapter, you should be able to:

1. **Describe the epidemiology, including the morbidity/mortality and prevention strategies, for shock and hemorrhage. pp. 72-74, 82-84**

Shock is the transitional stage between normal physiologic function of the body and death. It is the underlying killer of all trauma patients and is prevented using the strategies described for each of the types of trauma addressed by the following seven chapters. Hemorrhage is loss of the body's precious medium, blood, and is a common cause of shock and death in the trauma patient. Strategies to prevent hemorrhage are those designed to prevent trauma as discussed in the next seven chapters.

2. **Discuss the anatomy, physiology, and pathophysiology of the cardiovascular system as they apply to hemorrhage and shock. (see Chapters 12 and 13)**

The cardiovascular system is a closed system of interconnected tubes (blood vessels) that direct blood to the essential organs and tissues of the body. Arteries distribute blood to the various organs and tissues of the body. Arterioles determine the amount of blood perfusing the tissue of an organ and together constrict and increase peripheral vascular resistance or dilate and reduce peripheral vascular resistance. Progressive vasoconstriction can help maintain blood pressure and circulation to the most critical organs as the body loses blood during hemorrhage or fluid during other forms of shock. The venous system collects blood and returns it to the heart. It contains about 60 percent of the total blood volume and, when constricted, can return a relatively great volume (up to 1 liter) to the active circulation.

The cardiovascular system is powered by the central pump, the heart. It circulates the blood and, against the peripheral vascular resistance, drives the blood pressure. Its output is a factor of preload (the blood delivered to it by the venous system), stroke volume (the amount of blood ejected into the aorta with each contraction), rate, and afterload (the peripheral vascular resistance). The heart can help compensate for blood loss by attempting to maintain cardiac output by increasing its stroke volume (which is hard to do in hypovolemic states) or by increasing its rate.

Finally, the cardiovascular system contains the precious fluid, blood. Blood provides oxygen and nutrients to the body cells and removes carbon dioxide and waste products of metabolism. Blood also contains clotting factors that will occlude blood vessels if they are torn or disrupted.

The central nervous system provides control of the cardiovascular system using baroreceptors in the carotid arteries and aortic arch to sense fluctuations in blood pressure. It will maintain blood pressure by increasing heart rate, cardiac preload, and peripheral vascular resistance. Hormones from the kidneys and elsewhere help control blood volume and electrolytes as well as the production of erythrocytes.

3. **Define shock based on aerobic and anaerobic metabolism. (see Chapter 13)**

Cells are the elemental building blocks of the body and ultimately carry out all body functions. They derive their energy from a two-step process. The first step, called glycolysis, requires no oxygen (anaerobic) and generates a small amount of energy. The second step, called the citric acid or Krebs cycle, requires oxygen (aerobic) and generates about 95 percent of the cell's energy. In shock, which is inadequate tissue perfusion that does not adequately supply the cells with oxygen, the cells produce energy in an inefficient way and toxins accumulate.

4. Describe the body's physiologic response to changes in blood volume, blood pressure, and perfusion. pp. 83-86

Increased peripheral resistance is caused by the constriction of the arterioles and provides two mechanisms that combat shock. The arterioles constrict and maintain the blood pressure, and they divert blood to only the critical organs. This reduction in perfusion to the less critical organs results in the increased capillary refill time and the cool, clammy, and ashen skin often associated with shock states. It also results in reduced pulse pressure and weak pulses.

Venous constriction compensates for some blood loss and helps maintain cardiac preload. Since the veins account for about 60 percent of the blood volume, this is reasonably effective in minor to moderate blood loss.

As the cardiac preload drops, the heart rate increases in an attempt to maintain cardiac output and blood pressure. In the presence of significantly reduced preload, this may not be effective. Peripheral vascular shunting directs the blood away from the skin, conserves body heat, and reduces fluid loss through evaporation. It also redirects blood to more critical areas.

Fluid shifts are the result of drawing fluid from the interstitial and cellular spaces. Fluid moves into the vascular space. While this is a slow mechanism, it can provide the vascular system with several liters of fluid.

5. Describe the effects of decreased perfusion at the capillary level. pp. 83-84

Decreased capillary perfusion limits the amount of oxygen and nutrients delivered to the body cells. It usually causes the release of histamine that, in turn, causes precapillary sphincter dilation and an increase in perfusion. However, in shock states this is not effective, and the cells must revert to anaerobic metabolism while the byproducts of metabolism accumulate and the available oxygen is exhausted. Carbon dioxide, metabolic acids, and other waste products accumulate while body cells begin to die.

6. Discuss the cellular ischemic, capillary stagnation, and capillary washout phases related to hemorrhagic shock. pp. 83-84

Ischemia. As shock ensues, decreased perfusion, first to the non-critical organs, then to all organs, diminishes blood flow through the microcirculation. At the cellular level this diminishes the supply of oxygen and nutrients to the cells and restricts the removal of carbon dioxide and the waste products of metabolism. The cells quickly exhaust their supply of oxygen and begin to use anaerobic metabolism as their sole source of energy to remain alive. This produces an accumulation of pyruvic acid, which in turn, converts to lactic acid and the cells become more acidotic. As cells begin to die, their decomposition releases even more toxins that then begin to affect other cells.

Capillary stagnation. With diminished capillary flow, coupled with the increasingly hypoxic and acidic environment caused by the ischemic cells, the red blood cells become sticky and clump together. They form columns of coagulated erythrocytes called rouleaux that either block the capillary to further flow of blood or will wash out and cause microemboli.

Capillary washout. The toxic environment of the ischemic tissue associated with severe shock finally causes the post-capillary sphincters to dilate and release the hypoxic and acidotic blood as well as the rouleaux into the venous circulation. As this washout becomes extensive, it further reduces the effectiveness of the cardiovascular system and the body moves quickly toward irreversible shock.

7. Discuss the various types and degrees of shock and hemorrhage. pp. 72-74, 84-86

Hemorrhage can be divided into four stages as a patient moves through compensated, decompensated, and irreversible shock.

Stage 1 blood loss is a loss of up to 15 percent of the patient's blood volume. It generally presents with some nervousness, cool skin, and slight pallor. It is difficult to detect as the body compensates well for blood loss in this range.

Stage 2 blood loss is a loss of up to 25 percent of the patient's blood volume. Signs and symptoms become more apparent as the body finds it more difficult to compensate for the loss. The patient may display thirst, anxiety, restlessness, and cool and clammy skin.

Stage 3 blood loss is a loss of up to 35 percent of the patient's blood volume. It presents with the signs of stage 2 blood loss and air hunger, dyspnea, and severe thirst. Survival is unlikely without immediate intervention.

Stage 4 blood loss is a blood loss in excess of 35 percent of the patient's blood volume. The patient begins to display a deathlike appearance with pulses disappearing and respirations becoming very shallow and ineffective. The patient becomes very lethargic and then unconscious and survival becomes unlikely.

8. Predict shock and hemorrhage based on mechanism of injury. pp. 74-75, 86-87

Shock due to internal blood loss can be a very silent killer if not recognized and the patient brought to definitive care (surgery) quickly. Severe blunt and deep penetrating trauma can induce internal hemorrhage that is both difficult to identify and treat. If you wait until the frank signs of shock appear, too much time may have passed for care to be effective. Hence it is very important to both analyze the mechanism of injury to anticipate shock and to recognize the very early signs of shock.

A large hematoma may account for up to 500 ml of blood loss, while fractures of the humerus or tibia/fibula may account for 500 to 750 ml. Femoral fractures may account for up to 1,500 ml of blood, while pelvic fractures often involve hemorrhage of up to 2,000 ml. Internal hemorrhage into the chest or abdomen may contribute even greater losses. In penetrating or severe blunt trauma to the chest or abdomen, suspect the development of shock. Also suspect the rapid development of shock in the patient who begins to display the early signs of shock (an increasing pulse rate, decreasing pulse pressure, and anxiety and restlessness) very quickly after the trauma event.

9. Identify the need for intervention and transport of the patient with hemorrhage or shock. pp. 74-79, 86-89

Hemorrhage and shock are progressive pathologies that eventually become irreversible. To be effective in care, we must carefully assess our patients for the earliest of signs and intervene with rapid transport to a facility that can rapidly provide surgical intervention (to halt the internal bleeding). We also must immediately halt any external hemorrhage and provide supplemental high-flow oxygen. Intravenous fluids may be run to replace volume, but extreme care must be used to prevent increased internal hemorrhage and hemodilution.

10. Discuss the assessment findings and management of internal and external hemorrhage and shock. pp. 74-79, 86-89

Tachycardia is a compensatory cardiac action to maintain cardiac output when a reduced preload is present. A weak pulse reflects a narrowing pulse pressure and increasing peripheral vascular resistance to maintain systolic blood pressure. Cool, clammy skin is due to the redirection of blood to more critical organs than the skin. Ashen, pale skin may present due to hypoxia and peripheral vasoconstriction. Agitation, restlessness, and reduced level of consciousness occurs as the brain receives a reduced flow of oxygenated blood. The hypoxia causes the defense mechanisms of agitation and restlessness, followed by a noticeable reduction in the level of consciousness. Dull, lackluster eyes occur secondary to low perfusion and hypoxic states. Rapid, shallow respiration may occur as shock progresses, the respiratory muscles tire in the hypoxic state, and respiratory effort becomes less efficient. Dropping oxygen saturation may also provide evidence to support developing shock. As the peripheral circulation slows, the readings may drop or become erratic. Falling blood pressure heralds the progression from compensated to decompensated shock. As a late sign, it should not be used to determine the presence of shock.

External hemorrhage must be controlled by direct pressure. If direct pressure alone does not work, use elevation, pressure points or, as a last resort, the tourniquet, to stop the hemorrhage. If all sites of hemorrhage are controlled and you can rule out internal hemorrhage, provide fluid resuscitation to return the blood pressure and vital signs to normal.

Should the mechanism of injury or any early development of shock signs or symptoms suggest internal hemorrhage, or external hemorrhage cannot be controlled, transport should be expedited and care initiated immediately. Provide high-flow oxygen and ventalitory support as needed and infuse fluids to maintain the blood pressure just below 100 mmHg, ensuring it does not drop below 50 mmHg.

11. Differentiate between the administration rate and volume of IV fluid in patients with controlled versus uncontrolled hemorrhage. pp. 89-92

If hemorrhage has been controlled (as with external hemorrhage) then fluid resuscitation can be aimed at returning the blood pressure and other vital signs toward normal. However, if the hemorrhage is internal, and especially if it involves the chest, abdomen, or pelvis, great care must be exercised not to enhance the hemorrhage or excessively dilute the remaining blood. Resuscitation is generally aimed at stabilizing the blood pressure somewhere just below 100 mmHg and preventing it from dropping below 50 mmHg. To maintain these parameters, lactated Ringer's solution (preferred) or normal saline should be run rapidly through trauma or blood tubing and large-bore short catheters. Pressure infusers may be necessary as the blood pressure begins to fall below 50 mmHg. Usually pre-hospital care is limited to between 1 and 3 liters of crystalloid.

12. Relate pulse pressure and orthostatic vital sign changes to perfusion status. pp. 77-78, 88

Pulse pressure is the difference between the systolic and diastolic blood pressures and is responsible for the pulse. It is a relative measure of the effectiveness of cardiac output against peripheral vascular resistance. One of the early signs of shock is a decreasing pulse pressure, occurring as cardiac output begins to fall and the body increases peripheral vascular resistance in an attempt to maintain blood pressure.

Normally the body can maintain blood pressure and perfusion despite rapid changes from one position to another. However, in hypovolemia the body is already in a state of compensation so it becomes more difficult to maintain the pulse rate and blood pressure as someone moves from a supine to a seated or a standing position. If hypovolemic compensation exists, this movement will cause an increase in pulse rate and a drop in systolic blood pressure (usually by 20 points or more).

13. Define and differentiate between compensated and decompensated hemorrhagic shock. pp. 84-86

Compensated shock is a state in which the body is effectively compensating for fluid loss, or other shock-inducing pathology, and is able to maintain blood pressure and critical organ perfusion. If the original problem is not corrected or reversed, compensated shock may progress to decompensated shock.

Decompensated shock is a state in which the cardiovascular system cannot maintain critical circulation and begins to fail. Hypoxia affects the blood vessels and heart so they cannot maintain blood pressure and circulation.

Irreversible shock is a state of shock in which the human system is so damaged that it cannot be resuscitated. Once this stage of shock sets in, the patient will die, even if resuscitation efforts restore a pulse and blood pressure.

14. Discuss the pathophysiological changes, assessment findings, and management associated with compensated and decompensated shock. pp. 84-92

As the body experiences a stressor that induces shock, the cardiovascular system is quick to compensate. The venous system constricts to maintain a full vascular system and preload. The heart rate increases to maintain cardiac output, and the arterioles constrict, increasing peripheral vascular resistance to maintain blood pressure (the pressure of perfusion). As these actions become significant, the patient becomes anxious and slightly tachycardic, and the skin becomes cool and pale (circulation is shunted from the skin to more vital organs). With increasing blood loss, the compensation becomes more significant, and thirst, a rapid, weak pulse, and restlessness become apparent. These signs become more apparent as greater compensation is required to maintain the blood pressure. When the body reaches the limits of its compensation and it can no longer maintain the blood pressure, BP drops precipitously, circulation all but stops, and the patient moves very quickly into irreversible shock.

Care for the shock patient includes high-flow oxygen, hemorrhage control, and fluid resuscitation to maintain vital signs when hemorrhage is controlled, with a stable blood pressure just below 100 mmHg (88 mmHg may be optimal with continuing hemorrhage), or use aggressive fluid resuscitation if the blood pressure drops below 50 mmHg.

15. Identify the need for intervention and transport of patients with compensated and decompensated shock. pp. 86-92

The body's ability to compensate for shock is limited. While it can maintain blood pressure, the compensation is not without cost. As the arterioles constrict, they deny blood flow to some organs and themselves use energy and tire. The venous vessels tire as they constrict to reduce the volume of the vascular system. If compensation is significant or prolonged, the body may move into decompensation, especially if the hemorrhage is not controlled. Most serious internal hemorrhage can only be halted with surgical intervention, most commonly at a trauma center. In the time between our recognition of shock and arrival at the trauma center, we can help the body with its compensation by providing oxygen and fluid resuscitation.

16. Differentiate among normotensive, hypotensive, or profoundly hypotensive patients. pp. 86-92

A normotensive patient is one who has a systolic blood pressure of at least 100 mmHg. Hypotension is the patient with a blood pressure of less than 100 mmHg, while a blood pressure of less than 50 mmHg is considered profound hypotension. However, these figures apply to the young healthy adult and must be adjusted to the norms for the patient you are treating. (For example, a small young female may normally have a blood pressure below 100 mmHg and may not need fluid resuscitation.)

17. Describe the differences in administration of intravenous fluid in normotensive, hypotensive, or profoundly hypotensive patients. pp. 89-91

Administration of intravenous fluids in the normotensive patient without hypovolemia permits the rapid administration of medications and may be indicated when hypovolemia is anticipated (the burn patient). In the patient who is in compensated shock and maintains a relatively normal systolic blood pressure, fluid resuscitation is indicated if hemorrhage is controlled. If the hemorrhage is internal and cannot be controlled in the field, aggressive fluid resuscitation may lead to increased internal hemorrhage and hemodilution making perfusion and clotting less effective. Generally, the administration of intravenous fluids in the normotensive patient is limited.

In the patient who is hypotensive (BP <100 mmHg), intravenous fluids are administered to maintain, not increase, the blood pressure. Here again aggressive fluid resuscitation would dilute the blood and decrease the effectiveness of perfusion and clotting. An increase in blood pressure would also likely break apart clots that are reducing the internal hemorrhage.

In the patient who is profoundly hypotensive (absent pulses and you are unable to determine a blood pressure, or it is < 50 mmHg), aggressive fluid resuscitation is indicated. Here the consequences of severe hypoperfusion outweigh the risks of further hemorrhage.

18. Discuss the physiologic changes associated with application and inflation of the pneumatic anti-shock garment (PASG). pp. 91-92

The pneumatic anti-shock garment (PASG) is an air bladder that circumferentially applies pressure to the lower extremities and abdomen. In theory, it compresses the venous blood vessels, returning some blood to the critical circulation, and compresses the arteries, increasing peripheral vascular resistance. These actions increase circulating blood volume and blood pressure, which should help the patient in shock. However, in some cases of shock, this may increase the rate of internal hemorrhage and may disrupt the clotting mechanisms that are restricting blood loss associated with internal injury.

19. Discuss the indications and contraindications for the application and inflation of the PASG.
pp. 91-92

With current pharmacological interventions the PASG has become virtually redundant since better treatments are now available. The PASG was indicated for any patient who displays internal or external hemorrhage in the lower abdomen, pelvis, or lower extremities. It was recommended for the stabilization of any pelvic fracture and may be helpful with bilateral femoral fractures with the signs and symptoms of shock.

The PASG should not be used in the patient who is experiencing pulmonary edema or has a head or penetrating chest injury. It should be used with caution on any patient who is experiencing dyspnea as it may increase intra-abdominal pressure and restrict the movement of the diaphragm. The abdominal section should not be employed if the patient is in the third trimester of pregnancy, has an abdominal evisceration, or an impaled object in the abdomen.

Prior to application of the PASG, the patient's blood pressure, pulse rate and strength, and level of consciousness should be assessed and recorded. The abdomen, lower back, and lower extremities should be visualized to ensure that no sharp debris that could harm either the patient or the garment is present.

20.   Given several preprogrammed and moulaged hemorrhage and shock patients, provide the appropriate scene size-up, initial assessment, rapid trauma or focused physical exam and history, detailed exam, and ongoing assessment, and provide appropriate patient care and transportation.   pp. 65-92

During your training as a Paramedic you will participate in many classroom practice sessions involving simulated patients. You will also spend some time in the emergency departments of local hospitals as well as in advanced-level ambulances gaining clinical experience. During these times, use your knowledge of hemorrhage and shock to help you assess and care for the simulated or real patients you attend.

CONTENT SELF-EVALUATION

Multiple Choice

1. Which of the following types of hemorrhage is characterized by bright red blood?
   A.   capillary bleeding   D.   both A and C
   B.   venous bleeding   E.   both A and B
   C.   arterial bleeding

2. Which of the following types of hemorrhage is characterized by dark red blood?
   A.   capillary bleeding   D.   both A and C
   B.   venous bleeding   E.   none of the above
   C.   arterial bleeding

3. Which of the following is NOT a stage in the clotting process?
   A.   intrinsic phase
   B.   vascular phase
   C.   platelet phase
   D.   coagulation phase
   E.   All of the above are phases in the clotting process.

4. Which of the following represents the phase of clotting where blood cells are trapped in fibrin strands?

A. intrinsic phase
B. vascular phase
C. platelet phase
D. coagulation phase
E. marrow phase

5. The clotting process normally takes about what length of time?

A. 1 to 2 minutes
B. 3 to 4 minutes
C. 4 to 6 minutes
D. 7 to 10 minutes
E. 10 to 12 minutes

6. Which of the following is likely to adversely affect the clotting process?

A. aggressive fluid resuscitation
B. hypothermia
C. movement at the site of injury
D. drugs such as aspirin
E. all of the above

7. Fractures of the femur can account for a blood loss:

A. from 500 to 750 mL.
B. up to 1 500 mL.
C. in excess of 2 000 mL.
D. less than 500 mL.
E. in excess of 2 500 mL.

8. In which stage of hemorrhage does the patient first display ineffective respiration?

A. the first stage
B. the second stage
C. the third stage
D. the fourth stage
E. the terminal stage

9. The intravascular fluid accounts for what percentage of the total body water?

A. 7 percent
B. 15 percent
C. 35 percent
D. 45 percent
E. 75 percent

10. In which stage of hemorrhage does the patient first display thirst?

A. the first stage
B. the second stage
C. the third stage
D. the fourth stage
E. none of the above

11. In which stage of hemorrhage does the patient first display air-hunger?

A. the first stage
B. the second stage
C. the third stage
D. the fourth stage
E. none of the above

12. Which of the following react differently to blood loss than the normal, healthy adult?

A. pregnant women
B. athletes
C. the elderly
D. children
E. all of the above

13. The late pregnancy female is likely to have a blood volume:

A. much less than normal.
B. slightly less than normal.
C. slightly greater than normal.
D. much greater than normal.
E. that is normal and does not change with pregnancy.

14. Obese patients are likely to have a blood volume:

A. much less than normal.
B. slightly less than normal.
C. slightly greater than normal.
D. much greater than normal.
E. none of the above

15. Fractures of the pelvis can account for a blood loss:
- **A.** from 500 to 750 mL.
- **B.** up to 1 500 mL.
- **C.** in excess of 2 000 mL.
- **D.** up to 500 mL.
- **E.** of none because the pelvis does not bleed.

16. A black, tarry stool is called:
- **A.** hemoptysis.
- **B.** melena.
- **C.** hematuria.
- **D.** hematochezia.
- **E.** ebony stool.

17. A positive tilt test demonstrating orthostatic hypotension is positive when:
- **A.** the blood pressure rises by at least 20 mmHg.
- **B.** the blood pressure falls by at least 20 mmHg.
- **C.** the pulse rate rises by at least 20 beats per minute.
- **D.** the pulse rate falls by at least 20 beats per minute.
- **E.** both B and C

18. For the patient in compensated shock, you should perform an ongoing assessment:
- **A.** every five minutes.
- **B.** every fifteen minutes.
- **C.** after every major intervention.
- **D.** after noting any change in signs or symptoms.
- **E.** all except B

19. Which of the following is a technique used to help control hemorrhage?
- **A.** direct pressure
- **B.** elevation
- **C.** pressure points
- **D.** limb splinting
- **E.** all of the above

20. When applying a tourniquet, you should inflate the cuff:
- **A.** until the bleeding slows.
- **B.** to the diastolic blood pressure.
- **C.** to the systolic blood pressure.
- **D.** to 30 mmHg above the systolic blood pressure.
- **E.** none of the above

21. Which of the following is NOT a pulse pressure point?
- **A.** the brachial artery
- **B.** the carotid artery
- **C.** the femoral artery
- **D.** the popliteal artery
- **E.** the radial artery

22. The column of coagulated erythrocytes caused by capillary stagnation is called:
- **A.** ischemia.
- **B.** rouleaux.
- **C.** capillary washout.
- **D.** hydrostatic reflux.
- **E.** compensated reflux.

23. Which list places the stages of shock in the order of their occurrence.
- **A.** irreversible, decompensated, compensated
- **B.** compensated, decompensated, irreversible
- **C.** compensated, irreversible, decompensated
- **D.** decompensated, irreversible, compensated
- **E.** decompensated, compensated, irreversible

24. Which stage of shock ends with a precipitous drop in blood pressure?
- **A.** compensatory
- **B.** decompensatory
- **C.** irreversible
- **D.** hypovolemic
- **E.** none of the above

25. Which of the following does NOT occur during the compensated stage of shock?
  A.   increasing pulse rate
  B.   decreasing pulse strength
  C.   decreasing systolic blood pressure
  D.   skin becomes cool and clammy
  E.   the patient experiences thirst and weakness

26. Which of the following suggests shock?
  A.   a pulse rate above 100 in the adult
  B.   a pulse rate above 140 in the school-age child
  C.   a pulse rate above 160 in the preschooler
  D.   a pulse rate above 180 in the infant
  E.   all of the above

27. When using a pulse oximeter, you should use oxygen and ventilation to keep the reading above which oxygen saturation value?
  A.   45 percent   D.   95 percent
  B.   80 percent   E.   99 percent
  C.   85 percent

28. During assessment you note that the patient's lower extremities and lower abdomen are warm and pink while the upper extremities, thorax, and upper abdomen are cool and clammy. This presentation is consistent with which type of shock?
  A.   hypovolemic   D.   cardiogenic
  B.   neurogenic   E.   respiratory
  C.   obstructive

29. Which of the following may be an indication to employ overdrive respiration?
  A.   severe rib fractures   D.   head injury
  B.   flail chest   E.   all of the above
  C.   diaphragmatic respirations

30. Which of these fluid replacement choices would be most desirable for the patient who is losing blood through internal bleeding?
  A.   packed red blood cells   D.   colloids
  B.   fresh frozen plasma   E.   crystalloids
  C.   whole blood

31. Most of the solutions used in prehospital care for infusion are:
  A.   hypotonic colloids.   D.   hypotonic crystalloids.
  B.   isotonic colloids.   E.   isotonic crystalloids.
  C.   hypertonic colloids.

32. Which of the following characteristics of a catheter will ensure that fluids run rapidly through it?
  A.   short length, small lumen
  B.   short length, large lumen
  C.   long length, small lumen
  D.   long length, large lumen
  E.   large lumen and either long or short length

33. In the patient that has internal bleeding and hypovolemia, the objective blood pressure to maintain by PASG and fluid infusions is:
  A.   120 mmHg.   D.   below 50 mmHg.
  B.   100 mmHg.   E.   at a steady level.
  C.   50 mmHg.

34. The PASG may return what volume of blood to the central circulation?

A.	250 mL		**D.**	1 000 mL
B.	500 mL		**E.**	none at all
C.	750 mL			

35. Which of the following factors may hinder the clotting process?

A.	aggressive fluid therapy		**D.**	low body temperatures
B.	warfarin, ASA, or heparin		**E.**	all of the above
C.	movement of the wound site			

True/False

36. Cleanly and transversely cut blood vessels tend to bleed very heavily.
- **A.** True
- **B.** False

37. Bleeding from capillary or venous wounds is easy to halt because the pressure driving the hemorrhage is limited.
- **A.** True
- **B.** False

38. The risk of transmitting disease to your trauma patient is probably much greater than the risk of obtaining a disease from him.
- **A.** True
- **B.** False

39. The sooner the signs and symptoms of shock appear in your patient, the greater the hemorrhage rate and the likelihood that the patient will move into the later stages of shock.
- **A.** True
- **B.** False

40. Once the patient becomes profoundly unconscious and loses his vital signs, he moves into irreversible shock.
- **A.** True
- **B.** False

41. The color, temperature, and general appearance of the skin can indicate shock before there are changes in the blood pressure.
- **A.** True
- **B.** False

42. Fibrin are protein fibres that trap white blood cells as part of the clotting process.
- **A.** True
- **B.** False

43. Uric acid is a compound produced from pyruvic acid during anaerobic glycolysis
- **A.** True
- **B.** False

44. Pulse pressure is the drop in blood pressure when a patient takes a deep breath.
- **A.** True
- **B.** False

45. Orthostatic hypotension is an increase in blood pressure when a person moves from a supine to an upright position
- **A.** True
- **B.** False

Matching

Write the letter of the term in the space provided next to the appropriate description.

A.	shock	**F.**	hematoma
B.	rouleaux	**G.**	ischemia
C.	anaerobic	**H.**	melena
D.	hematochezia	**I.**	homeostasis
E.	catacholamine	**J.**	washout

_____ **46.** the natural tendency of the body to maintain a steady and normal internal environment

_____ **47.** a passage of stools containing red blood

_____ **48.** a hormone that strongly effects the nervous and cardiovascular systems, metabolic rate, temperature and smooth muscle

_____ **49.** able to live without oxygen

_____ **50.** a group of red blood cells that are stuck together

_____ **51.** a blockage in the delivery of oxygenated blood to the cells

_____ **52.** a state of inadequate perfusion

_____ **53.** black, tar-like feces due to a gastrointestinal bleed

_____ **54.** the release of accumulated lactic acid, carbon dioxide, potassium and rouleaux into the venous circulation

_____ **55.** a collection of blood beneath the skin or trapped within a body compartment

Chapter 20

Soft-Tissue Trauma

Review of Chapter Objectives

After reading this chapter, you should be able to:

1. Describe the incidence, morbidity, and mortality of soft-tissue injures. p. 95

Soft tissue injuries are by far the most prevalent type of injuries to occur, accounting for over 10 million visits to the emergency department yearly. Any mechanism of injury affecting the human system must first penetrate the skin and then the soft tissues to injure any organ. However, soft-tissue injuries rarely by themselves threaten life. Open injuries to the skin may permit pathogens to enter and infection to develop, and significant wounds may cause cosmetic and, to some degree, functional disruption of the skin. Injuries to the skin may also permit significant hemorrhage.

2. Describe the anatomy and physiology of the integumentary system. (see Chapter 12)

The integumentary system is the largest body organ, accounting for about 16 percent of weight. It provides the outer barrier for the body and protects it against environmental extremes, fluid loss, and pathogen invasion. The three-layer structure consists of:

a. Epidermis
The epidermis is the most superficial layer of the skin and consists of numerous layers of dead or dying cells. The epidermis provides a flexible covering for the skin and a barrier to fluid loss, absorption, and the entrance of pathogens.

b. Dermis
The dermis is the true skin. It is made up of connective tissue and houses the sensory nerve endings, many of the specialized skin cells that produce sweat, oil, etc., and the upper-level capillary beds that allow for the conduction of heat to the body's surface.

c. Subcutaneous tissue
The subcutaneous layer, although not a true part of the skin, works in concert with the skin to insulate the body from heat loss and the effects of trauma. It consists of connective and adipose (fatty) tissues.

3. Identify the skin tension lines of the body. pp. 98-99

The skin is a flexible cover for the body and as such is firmly connected to some parts of the anatomy while at other locations it is somewhat mobile. Its elasticity permits a wide range of motion by the musculoskeletal system while maintaining its own integrity. This elasticity creates tension along lines (called skin tension lines) that will cause a wound to gape or remain somewhat closed based upon its orientation to the skin tension lines. Please see the illustration (Figure 20-6) on page 99 of the textbook.

4. Predict soft-tissue injuries based on mechanism of injury. pp. 113-117

Blunt trauma is most likely to produce closed soft-tissue injury such as a contusion or hematoma, especially when the tissue is trapped between the force and skeletal structures like the ribs or skull. Crush injury occurs as the soft tissue is trapped in machinery or under a very heavy object. Penetrating trauma occurs as an object passes through the soft tissues, introducing pathogens to the body's interior and creating the risk of infection. Penetrating injury is likely to produce lacerations, incisions, and punctures as well as internal hemorrhage. Shear and tearing injuries may result in avulsions or amputation.

5. Discuss blunt and penetrating trauma. pp. 95-101

Blunt trauma is a kinetic force spread out over a relatively large surface area and directed at the body. It is most likely to induce injuries that do not break the skin, including contusions, and internal hemorrhage between the fascia, or hematomas. The stretching forces caused by blunt trauma, if significant enough, may cause a tear in the skin (laceration) and an open wound. Compression-type injuries can cause crushing wounds where the tissues and blood vessels and nerves are crushed, stretched, and torn.

Penetrating trauma, depending upon its exact mechanism, may cause a laceration (a jagged cut), an incision (a very precise or surgical cut), or a puncture (a deep wound with an opening that closes). Tearing or shear forces may cause an avulsion (a tearing away of skin), or an amputation (a complete severance or tearing away of a digit or limb). Scraping forces may abrade away the upper layers of skin and produce an abrasion.

6. Discuss the pathophysiology of soft-tissue injuries. pp. 95-111

Soft-tissue injuries either damage blood vessels and the structure of the soft tissue (blunt trauma) or open the envelope of the skin (penetrating trauma) and may permit pathogens to enter and blood to escape. Blunt trauma includes contusions, hematomas, and crush injuries. Penetrating trauma includes abrasions, lacerations, incisions, punctures, impaled objects, avulsions and amputations. Soft-tissue wounds may also present with hemorrhage, either capillary (oozing), venous (flowing), or arterial (spurting). The hemorrhage may be external or internal. Once injured, the soft tissue has the ability to heal itself through hemostasis, inflammation, epithelialization, neovascularization, and collagen synthesis. It also is able, through the recruitment of blood cells (phagocytes), to combat invading pathogens and prevent or combat infection. Infection risk is increased with pre-existing diseases like COPD or with diseases that compromise the immune system like HIV infection and AIDS. Use of medications like the NSAIDs also affects infection risk. The contamination introduced into the wound, the wound site (distal extremities), and the nature of the wound (puncture, crush, and avulsion) also have an impact on the risk of infection.

7. Differentiate among the following types of soft-tissue injuries:

a. Closed   pp. 96-97
i. Contusion
A contusion is a closed wound caused by blunt trauma that damages small blood vessels. The blood vessels leak, and the affected area becomes edematous. The contusion is characterized by swelling, pain, and, later on, discoloration. Since the wound is closed, the danger of infection is remote.

ii. Hematoma
The hematoma is a blunt soft-tissue injury in which blood vessels (larger than capillaries) are damaged and leak into the fascia, causing a pocket of blood. Large hematomas may accumulate up to 500 mL of blood.

iii. Crush injuries
Crush injuries occur as the soft tissues are trapped between a compressing force and an unyeilding object and extensive injury occurs. The injury disrupts blood vessels, nerves, muscle, connective tissue, bone, and possibly internal organs. Such an injury often provides a challenge to management because there is often serious bleeding from numerous sources and

the nature of the wound makes the bleeding hard to control. Open crush injuries are frequently associated with severe infection.

b. Open   pp. 97-101

i. Abrasions

An abrasion is a scraping away of the upper layers of the skin. It will normally present with capillary bleeding, and since the wound is open and may involve an extended surface, it can be associated with infection.

ii. Lacerations

Laceration is the most common open wound. It is a tear into the layers of the skin and, sometimes, deeper. A laceration can involve blood vessels, muscles, connective tissue, and other underlying structures. Since it is an open wound, it carries with it the danger of infection and external hemorrhage.

iii. Incisions

The incision is a very smooth laceration made by a surgical or other sharp instrument. It is otherwise a laceration.

iv. Avulsions

An avulsion is a partial tearing away of the skin and soft tissues. It is commonly associated with blunt skull trauma, animal bites, or machinery accidents. The degloving injury is a form of avulsion.

v. Impaled objects

An impaled object is any object that enters and then is lodged within the soft or other tissue. While its entry poses an infection risk, removing the object risks increased hemorrhage because the impaled object may be tamponading blood loss. Removal may also cause further harm if the object is irregular in shape.

vi. Amputations

An amputation is the partial or complete severance of a body part. The injury usually results in the complete loss of the limb distal to the site of severance; however, the severed limb can sometimes be successfully reattached or its tissue may be used for grafting to extend the length and usefulness of the remaining limb.

vii. Punctures

Punctures are penetrating wounds into the skin where the nature of the wound (deep and narrow) encourages closure. Pathogens driven into the wound by the mechanism find a hypoxic environment and may thrive in the injured tissue, resulting in serious infection.

8. Discuss the assessment and management of open and closed soft-tissue injuries. pp. 113-133

In the pre-hospital setting, the assessment of soft-tissue injuries is straightforward. In fact, soft-tissue injuries may be the only physical indications of serious internal injuries underneath. The assessment of these internal injuries is only complicated because the discoloration normally associated with them takes a few hours to develop. Examine the skin for any deformity, discoloration, or variation in temperature. Visualize any noted wound and determine its nature and extent. Be able to describe it (as it will be covered by a dressing and bandaging) to the attending physician upon your arrival at the emergency department.

The management of a soft-tissue wound is simply accomplished by meeting three objectives: immobilizing the wound site, keeping the wound clean (as sterile as possible), and controlling any hemorrhage. Immobilization will assist the clotting and healing processes. Keeping the wound sterile will reduce the bacterial load and reduce the risk and severity of infection. Controlling the hemorrhage with the use of direct pressure will limit blood loss and speed the repair cycle. In most circumstances, direct pressure effectively controls hemorrhage. Occasionally both direct pressure and elevation of the limb may be necessary. In severe cases of hemorrhage, the use of pressure points will be needed in addition to direct pressure and elevation. In extreme cases, such as severe crush injury, a tourniquet may be needed.

9. Discuss the incidence, morbidity, and mortality of crush injuries. pp. 97, 128-130

Crush injury is an infrequent mechanism that often results in severe soft tissue damage. The extensive nature of the injury predisposes it to infection, which can be severe. Entrapment of a limb or body region may lead to crush syndrome in which a prolonged lack of circulation leads to the breakdown of muscle tissues and to rhabdomyolysis. Reperfusion of the affected region then transports myoglobin to the kidneys, threatening renal failure, and potassium to the heart, causing dysrhythmias or sudden death.

10. Define the following injuries:

a. Crush injury   pp. 97, 109-110, 128-130
Crush injury occurs when a part of the body is trapped between a force and an object resisting it. Such injuries may occur as a limb is trapped in machinery, under a car as a jack releases, or in a building collapse. The injury disrupts the soft, connective, vascular, and nervous tissue and may injure internal organs.

b. Crush syndrome   pp. 97, 110, 128-130   (4 hours)
Crush syndrome occurs as a body part is trapped for more than four hours. The reduced or absent circulation within the trapped part does not permit the supply of oxygen and nutrients nor does it allow removal of carbon dioxide and waste products. The tissues become hypoxic and acidotic, and waste products accumulate. Upon release of the entrapping pressure, these toxins are returned to the central circulation with very severe effects. Fluid from the blood also flows into the injured tissue, resulting in a significant contribution to hypovolemia.

c. Compartment syndrome   pp. 130-131
Compartment syndrome occurs as edema increases the pressure within a fascial compartment of the body. The pressure restricts venous flow from the extremity, capillary flow through the affected portion of the limb, and arterial return to the central circulation. The result of untreated compartment syndrome is often loss of some of the muscle mass and possibly the shortening of the muscle mass.

11. Discuss the mechanisms of injury, assessment findings, and management of crush injuries. pp. 97, 109-110, 128-130

Crush injuries occur as soft tissues are trapped between two forces. The result is damage to the soft tissues, blood vessels, nerves, muscles, and bones. The limb or region that is crushed may appear normal or may be quite disfigured. Distal sensation and circulation may be disrupted, and the wound may not bleed at all or hemorrhage severely with no distinct site of hemorrhage. The limb may also feel hard and "boardlike" as hypoxia and acidosis cause the muscles to contract. Management of the crush injury follows routine soft-tissue injury care with special emphasis on hemorrhage control (use of a tourniquet may be necessary), keeping the wound clean (as the crush injury is at increased risk for infection), and elevating the limb (to enhance venous return and distal circulation).

12. Discuss the effects of reperfusion and rhabdomyolysis on the body. pp. 110, 130

As a limb or other body region is compressed for more than 4 hours, the lack of circulation causes a destruction of muscle tissue (rhabdomyolysis). This destruction releases a protein, myoglobin, and phosphate, potassium, and lactic and uric acids. When compression is released, reperfusion returns these toxins to the central circulation. Myoglobin clogs the tubules of the kidneys, especially when the patient is in hypovolemic shock. This may result in renal failure and, ultimately, death. More immediate, however, is the effect of the release of electrolytes on the heart. That release may result in dysrhythmias or sudden death. Other effects of reperfusion include calcification of the vasculature or of nervous tissue and increased cellular and systemic acidosis as restored circulation permits the production of uric acid.

13. **Discuss the pathophysiology, assessment, and care of hemorrhage associated with soft-tissue injuries, including:**

a. Capillary bleeding   pp. 102, 120

Capillary bleeding oozes from the wound and usually continues for a few minutes as the capillaries do not have the musculature to constrict as do the arteries and veins. The hemorrhage is usually minimal and can easily be controlled with the application of a dressing and minimal pressure.

b. Venous bleeding   pp. 102, 120

Venous hemorrhage may be extensive as the volume flowing through the vessels is equivalent to the amount flowing through arteries though the pressure of flow is much less. Venous hemorrhage is limited as the injured vessel constricts and clotting mechanisms are usually effective. Simple direct pressure will easily stop most venous hemorrhage.

c. Arterial bleeding   pp. 102, 120-122

Arterial hemorrhage is powered by the blood pressure and, if the wound is open, may spurt bright red blood. The musculature of the arterial vessels will constrict to limit hemorrhage, but bleeding will likely still be heavy. Direct pressure must be applied to the bleeding site to effectively control it; in some cases, use of elevation and pressure points will be necessary.

Basically, hemorrhage can be controlled by employing direct pressure, elevation, proximal arterial pressure, and, if all else fails, a tourniquet.

Direct pressure is a very effective first-line technique for the control of hemorrhage. Since hemorrhage is powered by blood pressure, digital pressure at the site of blood loss should easily stop most blood loss.

Elevation can be used to complement direct pressure. Elevating an extremity decreases the blood pressure to the limb, and the hemorrhage may be easier to control. Use elevation only for wounds on otherwise uninjured limbs, and only after direct pressure alone has proved ineffective.

Use of a pressure point is an adjunct to both direct pressure and elevation. A proximal artery is located and compressed, reducing the pressure of the hemorrhage. Use of pressure points can be very helpful in the crush wound where the exact location of blood loss is difficult to locate.

The tourniquet is the last technique to be used in attempts to control hemorrhage. A limb is circumferentially compressed above the systolic pressure under a wide band, such as a blood pressure cuff. If a lower pressure is used, the wound will bleed more severely. The tourniquet carries with it the additional hazard of permitting toxins to accumulate in the unoxygenated limb. These toxins endanger the future use of the limb and, when released into the central circulation, the patient's life.

14. **Describe and identify the indications for and application of the following dressings and bandages: pp. 111-113**

a. Sterile/nonsterile dressing

Sterile dressings are used for wound care as it is important to reduce the amount of contamination at a wound site to reduce the risk of infection.

b. Occlusive/nonocclusive dressing

Most dressings are nonocclusive, which means they permit both blood and air to travel through them in at least a limited way. Occlusive dressings do not permit the flow of either fluid or air and are useful in sealing a chest or neck wound to prevent the aspiration of air or covering a moist dressing on an abdominal evisceration to prevent its drying.

c. Adherent/nonadherent dressing

Adherent dressings support the clotting mechanisms; however, as they are removed they will dislodge the forming clots. Most dressings are specially treated to be nonadherent to prevent reinjury when they are removed from a wound.

d. Absorbent/nonabsorbent dressing

Most dressings used to treat wounds are absorbent, and they will soak up blood and other fluids. Nonabsorbent dressings absorb little or no fluid and are used to seal wound sites when a barrier to leaking is desired, for example, with the clear membranes that are used to cover venipuncture sites.

e. Wet/dry dressing
Wet dressings may provide a medium for the movement of infectious agents and are not frequently used in prehospital care. They may be used for abdominal eviscerations and burns.

f. Self-adherent roller bandage
The self-adherent roller bandage is soft, gauze-like material that molds to the contours of the body and is effective in holding dressings in place. As its stretch is limited, it does not pose the danger of increasing the bandaging pressure with each wrap as do some other bandaging materials.

g. Gauze bandage
Gauze bandaging is a self-adherent material that does not stretch and may increase the pressure beneath the bandage with consecutive wraps or with edema and swelling from the wound.

h. Adhesive bandage
An adhesive bandage is a strong gauze, paper, or plastic material backed with an adhesive. It can effectively secure small dressings to the skin where circumferential wrapping is impractical. It is inelastic and will not accommodate edema or swelling.

i. Elastic bandage
An elastic bandage is made of fabric that stretches easily. It conforms well to body contours but will increase the pressure applied with each wrap of the bandage. These bandages are often used to help strengthen a joint or apply pressure to reduce edema but should be used with great care, if at all, in the prehospital setting.

j. Triangular bandage
A cotton triangular shaped bandage that is strong, nonelastic and commonly used to make slings and swathes and in some case to affix splints

15. Predict the possible complications of an improperly applied dressing or bandage. pp.111-113, 125

Improper application of a dressing may include use of the wrong dressing for the injury or the application of the right dressing in an incorrect manner. Use of a nonocclusive dressing with an open chest may permit air to enter the thorax, increasing the severity of a pneumothorax, or use of such a dressing for a neck wound may permit air to enter the jugular vein, creating pulmonary emboli. Use of dry dressings with an abdominal evisceration may permit tissues to dry, adding additional injury, while use of wet dressings in other circumstances provides a route for infection of wounds. Adherent dressings may facilitate natural clotting but may dislodge clots and re-institute hemorrhage as they are removed. If a dressing is too large for the wound, it may not permit application of adequate direct pressure to arrest hemorrhage. If a dressing is too small, it may become lost in the wound and again not provide a focused direct pressure to stop hemorrhage.

Improperly applied bandaging may either be insufficient to immobilize the dressing or to protect it from catching on items during care and transport. It may be too tight, restricting edema and swelling and compressing the soft tissues beneath, which can cause reduced or absent blood flow to the distal extremity. In such a case, the bandaging acts as a venous tourniquet and may actually increase the rate of hemorrhage as it increases the venous pressure. On the other hand, a bandage that is too loose may not maintain adequate direct pressure to stop bleeding or may not hold the dressing securely to the injury site.

16. Discuss the process of wound healing, including:

a. Hemostasis   pp. 102-104
Hemostasis is the process by which the body tries to restrict or halt blood loss. It begins with the constriction of the injured blood vessel wall to reduce the rate of hemorrhage. The injured tissue of the vessel wall and the platelets become sticky. The platelets then aggregate to further

occlude the lumen. Finally, the clotting cascade produces fibrin strands that trap erythrocytes and form a more durable clot to halt all but the most severe hemorrhage.

b. Inflammation p. 104
Cells damaged by trauma or invading pathogens signal the body to recruit white blood cells (phagocytes) to the injury site. These cells engulf or attack the membranes of the foreign agents. The byproducts of this action cause the mast cells to release histamine, which dilates precapillary vessels and increases capillary permeability. Fluid and oxygen flows into the region resulting in an increase in temperature and edema.

c. Epithelialization p. 104
The stratum germinativum cells of the epidermis create an expanding layer of cells over the wound edges. This layer eventually joins almost unnoticeably, or, if the wound is too large, a region of collagen may show through (scar tissue).

d. Neovascularization pp. 104-105
Neovascularization occurs as the capillaries surrounding the wound extend into the new tissue and begin to provide the new tissue with circulation. These new vessels are very delicate and prone to injury and tend to bleed easily.

e. Collagen synthesis p. 105
Collagen synthesis is the building of new connective tissue (collagen) in the wound through the actions of the fibroblasts. Collagen binds the wound margins together and strengthens the healing wound. The early repair is not as good as new but by the fourth month the wound tissue is about 60 percent of the original tissue's strength.

17. Discuss the assessment and management of wound healing. pp. 102-111

Wound healing is most commonly complicated by movement of the injury site or by infection. Injuries affecting joints, other locations associated with movement, or regions with poor circulation are most prone to improper wound healing. Immobilization can help the process. Infection is a common complication of open soft-tissue injuries and results in delayed or incomplete wound healing. Wound healing is best managed by keeping the site immobilized (within reason) and keeping the site as sterile as possible, with frequent dressing changes. In some cases, wound drainage may help remove the products of pathogen breakdown and enhance the recovery and healing process.

18. Discuss the pathophysiology, assessment, and management of wound infection. pp. 105-107

Next to hemorrhage, infection is the most common complication of open soft-tissue wounds. It occurs as pathogens are introduced into the wound site and grow, usually in the damaged, warm, and hypoxic tissues. The most common infectious agents are of the Staphylococcus and Streptococcus bacterial families. It takes a few days for the bacteria to grow to the numbers necessary for the development of significant signs and symptoms. Consequently, infection is not usually seen during emergency care. The site of infection is generally swollen, reddened, and warm to the touch. A foul-smelling collection of white blood cells, dead bacteria, and cellular debris (pus) may drain from the wound, and visible red streaks (lymphangitis) may extend from the wound margins toward the trunk. The patient may complain of fever and malaise. The management of an infected wound includes keeping the wound clean, permitting it to drain, and administering antibiotics.

19. Formulate treatment priorities for patients with soft-tissue injuries in conjunction with:

a. Airway/face/neck trauma pp. 131-132
Soft-tissue injury to the face and neck generally heals well due to the more than adequate circulation in the area. However, these wounds, due to their prominence, deserve special attention because of their cosmetic implications. They also deserve special concern because of the potential danger to the airway. First, ensure that the airway is patent and not in danger of being obstructed from either hemorrhage or swelling. If an ACP, intubate early, possibly with rapid sequence intubation (CCP only), to ensure the airway remains patent. In the some severe cases, cricothyrotomy (needle or surgical) may be necessary. If there are any open wounds to the neck,

ensure they are covered with occlusive dressings to prevent the passage of air into the jugular veins.

b. Thoracic trauma (open/closed)   pp. 131-132
Anticipate internal chest injury associated with superficial soft-tissue injuries to the thorax and cover any significant open wounds with occlusive dressings sealed on three sides. Auscultate the chest frequently to monitor respiratory exchange and anticipate progressive chest pathologies, increasing edema, or pneumothorax. Also anticipate associated internal hemorrhage and abdominal injuries and move quickly to transport the patient to a trauma center.

c. Abdominal trauma   p. 132
In cases of abdominal trauma, consider the possibility of internal injury and dress all open wounds. Anticipate internal hemorrhage and move quickly to transport the patient to a trauma center. Cover any abdominal eviscerations with moistened sterile dressings, and then cover with occlusive dressings.

20. Given several preprogrammed and moulaged soft-tissue trauma patients, provide the appropriate scene size-up, initial assessment, rapid trauma or focused physical exam and history, detailed exam, and ongoing assessment, and provide appropriate patient care and transportation. pp. 113-133

During your training as a Paramedic you will participate in many classroom practice sessions involving simulated patients. You will also spend some time in the emergency departments of local hospitals as well as with Advanced Care Paramedics in ambulances, gaining clinical experience. During these times, use your knowledge of soft-tissue injuries to help you assess and care for the simulated or real patients you attend.

CONTENT SELF-EVALUATION

Multiple Choice

1. About what percentage of soft-tissue wounds become infected, with a significant resultant morbidity?
   - **A.**   2 percent
   - **B.**   7 percent
   - **C.**   15 percent
   - **D.**   50 percent
   - **E.**   75 percent

2. Which of the following types of wounds are unlikely to heal well?
   - **A.**   wounds that gape
   - **B.**   wound associated with static tension lines
   - **C.**   wounds associated with dynamic tension lines
   - **D.**   wounds perpendicular to tension lines
   - **E.**   all except B

3. The type of wound characterized by erythema usually seen during the pre-hospital setting is the:
   - **A.**   abrasion.
   - **B.**   contusion.
   - **C.**   laceration.
   - **D.**   incision.
   - **E.**   avulsion.

4. Which of the following wounds is not considered open?
   - **A.**   laceration
   - **B.**   abrasion
   - **C.**   contusion
   - **D.**   puncture
   - **E.**   avulsion

5. Which of the following wound types is characterized as a very clean, open wound?
   A. abrasion
   B. contusion
   C. laceration
   D. incision
   E. avulsion

6. Crush injuries usually involve injury to:
   A. blood vessels.
   B. nerves.
   C. bones.
   D. internal structures.
   E. all of the above

7. Which of the following is NOT usually considered an open wound?
   A. abrasion
   B. crush injury
   C. incision
   D. degloving injury
   E. avulsion

8. The wound that poses the greatest risk for serious infection is the:
   A. puncture.
   B. laceration.
   C. contusion.
   D. incision.
   E. hematoma.

9. The injury in which the skin is pulled off a finger, hand, or extremity by farm or industrial machinery is called a(n):
   A. amputation.
   B. incision.
   C. complete laceration.
   D. degloving injury.
   E. transection.

10. The natural tendency of the body to maintain its normal environment and function is called:
    A. anemia.
    B. homeostasis.
    C. hemostasis.
    D. coagulation.
    E. metabolism.

11. The agents that recruit cells responsible for the inflammatory response are called:
    A. macrophages.
    B. lymphocytes.
    C. chemotactic factors.
    D. granulocytes.
    E. fibroblasts.

12. The cells that attack invading pathogens directly or through an antibody response are:
    A. macrophages.
    B. lymphocytes.
    C. white blood cells.
    D. granulocytes.
    E. fibroblasts.

13. The stage of the healing process in which the phagocytes and lymphocytes are most active is:
    A. inflammation.
    B. epithelialization.
    C. neovascularization.
    D. collagen synthesis.
    E. none of the above

14. Regenerated skin, after about four months, is about how strong as compared to the original skin?
    A. 20 percent
    B. 30 percent
    C. 40 percent
    D. 50 percent
    E. 60 percent

15. Infection usually appears how long after the initial wound?
    A. 12 to 24 hours
    B. 1 to 2 days
    C. 2 to 3 days
    D. 4 to 6 days
    E. 7 to 10 days

16. Which of the following is an infection risk factor with soft-tissue wounds?
- **A.** advancing age
- **B.** crush injury
- **C.** NSAIDs use
- **D.** cat bites
- **E.** all of the above

17. It is common practice to provide tetanus boosters if the patient's last booster was over:
- **A.** 1 year ago.
- **B.** 2 years ago.
- **C.** 3 years ago.
- **D.** 4 years ago.
- **E.** 5 years ago.

18. Which of the following can interfere with normal clotting?
- **A.** aspirin
- **B.** warfarin
- **C.** streptokinase
- **D.** penicillin
- **E.** all of the above

19. The location at greatest risk for compartment syndrome is the:
- **A.** calf.
- **B.** thigh.
- **C.** forearm.
- **D.** arm.
- **E.** ankle.

20. The excessive growth of scar tissue within the boundaries of the wound is called:
- **A.** hypertrophic scar formation.
- **B.** keloid scar formation.
- **C.** anatropic scar formation.
- **D.** residual scar formation.
- **E.** regressive scar formation.

21. A crush injury that produces crush syndrome usually requires what minimum time of entrapment?
- **A.** 1 hour
- **B.** 2 hours
- **C.** 4 hours
- **D.** 6 hours
- **E.** 10 hours

22. Which of the following is likely with the release of entrapment in the patient suffering crush syndrome?
- **A.** kidney failure
- **B.** cardiac dysrhythmias
- **C.** hypovolemia
- **D.** abnormal vascular calcifications
- **E.** all of the above

23. The type of dressing that prevents the movement of fluid or air through the dressing is:
- **A.** sterile.
- **B.** nonadherent.
- **C.** absorbent.
- **D.** occlusive.
- **E.** nonocclusive.

24. The bandages that increase pressure beneath the bandage with each consecutive wrap are:
- **A.** elastic bandages.
- **B.** self-adherent roller bandages.
- **C.** gauze bandages.
- **D.** adhesive bandages.
- **E.** triangular bandages.

25. Which of the following are important factors to consider in the assessment and management of external hemorrhage?
- **A.** type of bleeding
- **B.** rate of hemorrhage
- **C.** volume of blood lost
- **D.** stopping further hemorrhage
- **E.** all of the above

26. Which of the following is one of the primary objectives of bandaging?
- **A.** neat appearance
- **B.** hemorrhage control
- **C.** allowing easy movement of the wound
- **D.** debridement
- **E.** aeration

27. The restoration of circulation once a tourniquet is released may cause which of the following?
   A. shock
   B. hypovolemia
   C. lethal dysrhythmias
   D. renal failure
   E. all of the above

28. After bandaging a patient's severely hemorrhaging forearm wound, you notice that the limb is cool, capillary refill is slowed, and the radial pulse cannot be found. You should:
   A. apply more dressing material and increase the pressure.
   B. leave the bandage as it is.
   C. loosen the bandage.
   D. elevate the extremity and assess circulation again.
   E. remove the bandage.

29. To alleviate pain associated with soft-tissue injury, you should administer morphine sulfate:
   A. 10 mg IV.
   B. 2 mg every 5 minutes titrated to pain relief.
   C. 5 mg every 5 minutes titrated to pain relief.
   D. 10 mg every 10 minutes times 2.
   E. 20 mg every 5 minutes titrated to pain relief.

30. With a large and gaping wound to the neck, use a(n):
   A. large absorbent dressing.
   B. large nonadherent dressing.
   C. occlusive dressing.
   D. nonabsorbent dressing.
   E. triangular bandage.

31. The type of dressing recommended for blood and fluid leaking from the auditory canal is a(n):
   A. nonocclusive dressing.
   B. nonadherent dressing.
   C. occlusive dressing.
   D. gauze dressing.
   E. wet dressing.

32. Which of the following is NOT a distal sign that a circumferential bandage is too tight?
   A. diaphoresis
   B. pallor
   C. loss of pulses
   D. tingling
   E. swelling

33. You find a patient who has suffered a finger amputation. You should keep the amputated part:
   A. warm and dry.
   B. warm and moist.
   C. cool and dry.
   D. cool and moist.
   E. packed in ice.

34. In which of the following situations is removal of an impaled object allowed or required?
   A. The object obstructs the airway.
   B. The object prevents performance of CPR.
   C. The object is impaled in the cheek.
   D. The object is impaled in the chest of a trauma patient who needs resuscitation.
   E. all of the above

35. Care for the patient with crush syndrome includes:
   A. rapid transport.
   B. fluid resuscitation.
   C. diuresis.
   D. possibly systemic alkalinization.
   E. all of the above

36. The most ideal fluid for the resuscitation of the crush syndrome patient, prior to extrication, is:
A.   hetastarch.   D.   5 percent dextrose in 1/2 normal saline.
B.   normal saline.   E.   Dextran.
C.   lactated Ringer's solution.

37. It is recommended that you infuse what volume of fluid to the crush syndrome patient per hour of entrapment?
A.   200 mL   D.   600 mL
B.   400 mL   E.   1 000 mL
C.   500 mL

38. Sudden cardiac arrest care after extrication of the entrapped patient with crush syndrome should include the routine cardiac drugs and:
A.   potassium for hypokalemia.   D.   dopamine for low blood pressure.
B.   calcium chloride for hypokalemia.   E.   none of the above
C.   sodium bicarbonate for hypokalemia.

39. The most prominent symptom of compartment syndrome is:
A.   pain out of proportion to physical findings with the injury.
B.   reduced or absent distal pulses.
C.   increased skin tension in the affected limb.
D.   paresthesia.
E.   paresis.

40. Compartment syndrome is most likely to occur:
A.   immediately after injury.   D.   within 4 hours of injury.
B.   within 2 hours of injury.   E.   6 to 8 hours after injury.
C.   within 3 hours of injury.

41. The most effective treatment in the prehospital setting for compartment syndrome is:
A.   a fasciectomy.   D.   massaging the extremity.
B.   the application of cold packs.   E.   none of the above
C.   elevation of the extremity.

42. A wound involving which of the following requires transport?
A.   nerves   D.   ligaments
B.   blood vessels   E.   all of the above
C.   tendons

43. Which types of patients are prone to a delay in wound repair or healing?
A.   diabetics   D.   the chronically ill
B.   the elderly   E.   all of the above
C.   the malnourished

44. During the injury process, the material released from the injured cells, and the debris released as the phagocytes destroy invading cells cause the mast cells to release _____ .
A.   histamine.   D.   pathogens
B.   leukocytes   E.   none of the above
C.   erythrocytes

45. Which of the following is NOT a reaction to the release of histamine in the body?
A.   blood vessel dilation   D.   increased capillary permeability
B.   decreased blood flow   E.   edema
C.   increase body temperature

True/False

_____ 46. Amputations that occur cleanly are likely to be associated with severe hemorrhage.
  A.   True
  B.   False

_____ 47. When torn or cut, the muscles in the capillaries constrict, thereby limiting hemorrhage.
  A.   True
  B.   False

_____ 48. Closing wounds with staples or sutures increases the risk of infection.
  A.   True
  B.   False

_____ 49. The patient is not likely to experience injury, even when immobilized for a long period on a long spine board, PASG, or rigid splint.
  A.   True
  B.   False

_____ 50. The nature of crush injury produces an injury area that is an excellent growth medium for infection.
  A.   True
  B.   False

_____ 51. Not only is the skin the first body organ to experience trauma, it is often the only one to display the signs of injury.
  A.   True
  B.   False

_____ 52. Insufficient tourniquet pressure may increase the rate and volume of hemorrhage.
  A.   True
  B.   False

_____ 53. If the amputated part cannot be immediately located, wait only a few minutes at the scene as its transport with the patient is extremely important.
  A.   True
  B.   False

_____ 54. Tourniquets should only be used as a last resort, when bleeding cannot be controlled by any other means.
  A.   True
  B.   False

_____ 55. Treatment of edema caused by soft-tissue injuries should include the use of cold packs.
  A.   True
  B.   False

Matching

Write the letter of the term in the space provided next to the appropriate description.

A.	erythema	F.	neovascularization
B.	gangrene	G.	contusion
C.	hematoma	H.	keloid
D.	tension lines	I.	hemostasis
E.	ecchymosis	J.	phagocytosis

_____ 56. a collection of blood beneath the skin or trapped within a body compartment

_____ 57. process in which a cell surrounds and absorbs a bacterium or other particle

_____ **58.** general reddening of the skin due to dilation of the superficial capillaries

_____ **59.** the body's natural ability to stop bleeding

_____ **60.** a formation resulting from overproduction of scar tissue

_____ **61.** blue-black discoloration of the skin due to leakage of blood into the tissues

_____ **62.** deep space infection usually caused by the anaerobic bacterium Clostridium perfringens

_____ **63.** natural patterns in the surface of the skin revealing tensions within

_____ **64.** new growth of capillaries in response to healing

_____ **65.** closed wound in which damage has occurred to the tissue immediately beneath

Chapter 21

Burns

Review of Chapter Objectives

After reading this chapter, you should be able to:

1. **Describe the anatomy and physiology of the skin and remaining human anatomy as they pertain to thermal burn injuries. (see Chapter 12)**

The skin or integumentary system is the largest organ of the body and consists of three layers, the epidermis, the dermis, and the subcutaneous layer. It functions as the outer barrier of the body and protects it against environmental extremes and pathogens. The outer-most layer is the epidermis, a layer of dead or dying cells that provides a barrier to fluid loss, absorption, and the entrance of pathogens. The dermis is the true skin. It houses the sensory nerve endings, many of the specialized skin cells that produce sweat, oil, etc., and the upper-level capillary beds that allow for the conduction of heat to the body's surface. The subcutaneous layer, although not a true part of the skin, works in concert with the skin to insulate the body from heat loss and the effects of trauma.

2. **Describe the epidemiology, including incidence, mortality/morbidity, and risk factors for thermal burn injuries as well as strategies to prevent such injuries. p. 136**

The incidence of burn injury has been declining over the past few decades but still accounts for over 200 000 burn injuries in Canada each year. Those at greatest risk are the very young, the elderly, the infirm. Burns are the second leading cause of death for children under 12 and the second leading cause of trauma death, after motor vehicle collisions.

Much of the decline in burn injury and death is attributable to better building codes, improved construction techniques, and the use of smoke detectors. Educational programs that teach children not to play with matches or lighters and that instruct the family to turn the water heater down to below 130ºF have also helped reduce burn morbidity and mortality.

3. **Describe the local and systemic complications of a thermal burn injury.**
   pp. 136-138, 148-151

Thermal burn injury results as the rate of molecular movement in a cell increases, causing the cell membranes and proteins to denature. This causes a progressive injury as the heat penetrates deeper and deeper through the skin and into the body's interior. At the local level, the injury disrupts the envelope of the body, permitting fluid to leak from the capillaries into the tissue and evaporate, resulting in dehydration and cooling. Serious circumferential burns may form an eschar and constrict, restricting ventilation or circulation to a distal extremity.

The systemic effects of serious burns include severe dehydration and infection. Fluid is drawn to the injured tissue as it becomes edematous and then may evaporate in great quantities as the skin loses its ability to contain fluids. Infection can be massive and can quickly and easily overwhelm the body's immune system. The products of cell destruction from the burn process may enter the bloodstream and damage the tubules of the kidneys, resulting in failure. Organ failure due to burn byproducts may also affect the liver and the heart's electrical system. Lastly, the burn injury and the associated evaporation of fluid may cool the body more rapidly than it can create heat. The result is a lowering of body temperature, hypothermia.

4. Identify and describe the depth classifications of burn injuries, including superficial burns, partial-thickness burns, and full-thickness burns. pp. 146-147

Superficial (first-degree) burns involve only the upper layers of the epidermis and dermis. The effects are limited to an irritation of the upper sensory tissues with some pain, minor edema, and erythema. = Redness

Partial-thickness (second-degree) burns penetrate slightly deeper than first-degree burns and cause blistering, erythema, swelling, and pain. Since the cells that reproduce the skin's upper layers are still alive, complete regeneration is expected.

Full-thickness (third-degree) burns penetrate the entire dermis, causing extensive destruction. The burned area may display a variety of appearances and colors, the site is anesthetic, and healing is prolonged. Third-degree burns may involve not only the skin, but also underlying tissues and organs. (Organ and other tissue involvement is sometimes called fourth-degree burn)

5. Describe and apply the "rule of nines," and the "rule of palms" methods for determining body surface area percentage of a burn injury. pp. 147-148

The "rule of nines" approximates the body surface area burned by assigning each body region nine percent of the total. These regions include: each upper extremity, the anterior of each lower extremity, the posterior of each lower extremity, the anterior of the abdomen, the anterior thorax, the upper back, the lower back, and the entire head and neck. The remaining one percent is assigned to the genitalia. For children, the head is given 18 percent, and the lower extremities are assigned 13 1/2 percent.

The "rule of palms" method of approximating burn surface area assumes the victim's palm surface is equivalent to one percent of the total body surface area. The paramedic then estimates the burn surface area by determining the number of palmar surfaces it would take to cover the wound.

6. Identify and describe the severity of a burn including a minor burn, a moderate burn, and a critical burn. pp. 153-156

BSA = Body Surface Area

Minor burns are those that are superficial and cover less than 50 percent of the body surface area (BSA), partial-thickness burns covering less than 15 percent of the BSA, or full-thickness burns involving less than two percent of the body surface area.

Moderate burns are classified as superficial burns over more than 50 percent of the BSA, partial-thickness burns covering less then 30 percent of the BSA; or full-thickness burns covering less than 10 percent of the BSA.

Critical burns are those partial-thickness burns covering more than 30 percent of the BSA, full-thickness burns over 10 percent of the BSA, and any significant inhalation injury. Critical burns also include any burns that involve any partial or full-thickness burn to the hands, feet, genitalia, joints, or face.

7. Describe the effects age and pre-existing conditions have on burn severity and a patient's prognosis. pp. 150, 155

Burn patients who are very young, very old, or have a significant pre-existing disease are at increased risk for the systemic problems associated with burn injury. They cannot tolerate massive fluid losses often associated with burns because they have smaller fluid reserves and they cannot effectively fight the ensuing massive infection commonly associated with large burns. They should be considered one step closer to critical than consideration of their burn type and BSA would normally place them.

8. Discuss complications of burn injuries caused by trauma, blast injuries, airway compromise, respiratory compromise, and child abuse. pp. 144-146, 151-153, 159

Traumatic injury, in the presence of burn injury, is a complicating factor that interferes with the burn healing process and may exacerbate hypovolemia. Any time these injuries coexist, the patient should be considered a higher priority than both injury would suggest, and the paramedic must care for both conditions.

Blast mechanisms produce injury through thermal burns, the pressure wave, projectile impact, and structural collapse (crush) mechanisms. When burns coexist with these other injuries, the patient priority for care and transport must be elevated at least one priority level and all injuries must be cared for. Again, the patient will have to heal from multiple injuries, making the recovery process more difficult.

Airway and respiratory compromise associated with burn injury is an extremely serious complication. The airway must be secured early, possibly with intubation as an ACP, and adequate ventilation with supplemental oxygen ensured. Swelling of the upper or lower airway may rapidly occlude it, preventing both ventilation and intubation. In extreme circumstances, cricothyrotomy may be required (ACP/CCP). Also be watchful for carbon monoxide poisoning as it can reduce the effectiveness of oxygen transport without overt signs.

Burns associated with child abuse often result from scalding water immersion, open flame burns, or cigarette-type injuries. The child presents with a history of a burn that does not make sense, such as stove burns when he or she cannot yet reach the stove, multiple circular burns (cigarettes), or burns isolated to the buttocks, which occur as the child lifts his or her legs during attempts at immersion in hot water.

9. Describe thermal burn management including considerations for airway and ventilation, circulation, pharmacological and nonpharmacological measures, transport decisions, and psychological support/communication strategies.   pp. 151-159

The management of the burn patient is a rather complicated, multifaceted process. The first consideration is to extinguish the fire to ensure the burn does not continue. If necessary, use water from a low-pressure hose and remove all jewelry, leather, nylon, or other material that may continue to smolder or hold heat and continue to burn the patient. Also consider removing any restrictive jewelry or clothing, as such an item may act as tourniquet, restricting distal blood flow as the burn region swells.

Then assess and ensure that the airway remains adequate. With any history suggestive of an inhalation burn or injury, carefully assess and monitor the airway for any signs of restriction. If they are found, move to protect the airway with intubation early (ACP/CCP), before the progressive airway swelling prevents intubation or significantly restricts the size of the endotracheal tube you can introduce. Small and painful burns may be covered with wet dressings to occlude airflow and reduce the pain; however, any extensive burn should be covered with a sterile dry dressing to prevent body cooling and the introduction of pathogens through the dressing.

Resuscitation for extensive burns must include large volumes of prehospital as burns often account for massive fluid loss into and through the burn. The patient must also be kept warm because by their nature burns account for rapid heat loss.

Any burns on opposing tissue, such as between the fingers and toes, should be separated by nonadherent dressings, as the burned surfaces are likely to adhere firmly together and cause further damage as they are pulled apart. In painful burns consider morphine, in 2 mg increments, for pain relief as long as there is no evidence of hypotension or respiratory depression.

Watch for any constriction from eschar formation that may reduce or halt distal circulation or restrict respiration. Medical direction may request a surgical incision to relieve the pressure (an escharotomy).

Any burn patient with serious injury should be transported to the burn center where he or she can receive the specialized treatment needed. Also ensure that the burn patient receives therapeutic communication while you are at the scene and during transport. The burn injury is very painful and the appearance can be very frightening. Constantly talk with the patient. Try to distract him or her from the injury, and monitor level of consciousness and anxiety level throughout your care and transport.

10. Describe special considerations for a pediatric patient with a burn injury and describe the criteria for determining pediatric burn severity.   pp. 147-148, 150, 155

To determine the severity of a burn for a pediatric patient, you must first examine the depth of burn (superficial, partial, or full thickness) and then determine the BSA affected. With children the head is given a greater percentage of BSA (18%) and the legs are given less (13.5%). (Please note that there are several more specific methods to determine BSA for children that better take into account their changing anatomy, but they are more complicated and age- and size-specific and harder to use.) Once the BSA and depth of burn are determined, the pediatric patient is assigned a level of severity one place higher than that for the adult. Any serious burn to the airway, face, joint, hand, foot, or any circumferential burn is considered serious or critical as is the pediatric burn patient with another pre-existing disease or traumatic injury.

11. Describe the specific epidemiologies, mechanisms of injury, pathophysiologies, and severity assessments for inhalation, chemical, and electrical burn injuries and for radiation exposure. pp. 159-166

Inhalation injuries are commonly associated with burn injuries and endanger the airway. According to University of Toronto, smoke inhalation is the most common cause of death (30%) among those who suffer major burns. They are caused by the inhalation of hot air or flame, which cause limited damage, by superheated steam, which results in much more significant thermal damage, or by the inhalation of toxic products of combustion, which results in chemical burns. Inhalation injury can also involve carbon monoxide poisoning and the absorption of chemicals through the alveoli and systemic poisoning. Any sign of respiratory involvement during the burn assessment process is reason to consider early and aggressive airway care and rapid transport.

Chemical burn injury is most frequently found in the industrial setting and is frequently associated with the effects of strong acids or alkalis. Both mechanisms destroy cell membranes as they penetrate deeper and deeper. The nature of the wounding process is somewhat self-limiting, though alkali burns tend to penetrate more deeply. Any chemical burn that disrupts the skin should be considered serious.

Electrical burn injuries are infrequent but can be very serious. As electricity passes through body tissue, resistance creates heat energy and damage to the cell membranes. The blood vessels and nerve pathways are especially sensitive to electrical injury. The heat produced can be extremely high and cause severe and deeply internal burn injury, depending upon the voltage and current levels involved.

Any electrical burn that causes external injury or any passage of significant electrical current through the body is reason to consider the patient a high priority for transport, even if no overt signs of injury exist. Electrical injury can also affect the muscles of respiration and induce hypoxia or anoxia if the current remains. Electrical disturbances can also affect the heart, producing dysrhythmias. A special electrical injury is the lightning strike. Extremely high voltage can cause extensive internal injury, though often the current passes over the exterior of the body, resulting in limited damage. Resuscitation of the patient struck by lightning should be prolonged as this mechanism of injury may permit survival after lengthy resuscitation.

Radiation exposure is a relatively rare injury process caused by the passage of radiation energy through body cells. The radiation changes the structure of molecules and may cause cells to die, dysfunction, or reproduce dysfunctional cells. Radiation hazards cannot be seen, heard, or felt, yet they can cause both immediate and long-term health problems and death. The objective of rescue and care is to limit the exposure for both the patient and rescuer. Radiation exposure is cumulative. The less time in an area of hazard, the less effect radiation will have on the human body. The greater the distance from a radiation source, the less strength and potential it has to cause damage. Radiation levels are diminished as the particles travel through dense objects. By placing more mass between the source and patient and rescuers, the exposure is reduced. Since it is very difficult to determine the extent of exposure, gather what information you can and transport the patient for further evaluation.

12. Discuss special considerations that impact the assessment, management, and prognosis of patients with inhalation, chemical, and electrical burn injuries and with exposure to radiation. pp. 159-166

When assessing an inhalation injury, you should examine the mechanism of injury to identify any unconsciousness or confinement during fire or any history of explosive stream expansion and inhalation. Study the patient carefully for signs of facial burns, carbonaceous sputum, or any hoarseness. Should there be any reason to suspect inhalation injury, monitor the airway very carefully and consider oxygen therapy and transport to the hospital without delay. As an ACP/CCP, early intubation early, as needed. The airway tissues can swell quickly and result in serious airway restriction or complete obstruction.

Chemical burn injury is indicated by the signs or history of such exposure and should begin with an identification of the agent and type of exposure. Remove contaminated clothing and dispose of it properly. The site of exposure should be irrigated with copious amounts of cool water and, once the chemical is completely removed, covered with a dry sterile dressing. Special consideration should be given to contact with phenol (soluble in alcohol), dry lime (brush off before irrigation), sodium metal (cover with oil to prevent combustion), and riot control agents (emotional support). The prognosis for a serious chemical burn is related to the agent, length of exposure to it, and depth of damage. These injuries are often severe and will leave damaged or scar tissue behind.

With an electrical burn injury, direct your assessment to seeking out and examining entrance and exit wounds and to trying to determine the voltage and current of the source. The wounds should be covered with dry sterile dressings and the patient monitored for dysrhythmias. Even if the entrance and exit wounds seem minor, consider this patient for rapid transport as the internal injury may be extensive.

Radiation is invisible and otherwise undetectable by human senses. When radiation exposure is suspected, ensure that you and the patient remain as remote from the source (distance) with as much matter as possible between you and the source (shielding) and that you spend as little time close to the source as possible. Attention to these factors will reduce the amount of radiologic exposure for both you and the patient. Assessment of the patient exposed to a radiation source is very difficult because the signs of injury are delayed except in cases of extreme exposure. Any suggestion of exposure to radiation merits examination at the emergency department and assessment of the risk by specially trained experts in the field. Limited radiation exposure does not often result in medical problems, but more severe doses may cause sterility or, later in life, cancer. Extensive exposure may cause severe illness or death.

13. Differentiate between supraglottic and infraglottic inhalation burn injuries. pp. 144-146

A supraglottic inhalation burn is a thermal injury to the mucosa above the glottic opening. It is a significant burn because the tissue is very vascular and will swell very quickly and extensively. Because of the moist environment and the vascular nature of the tissue, it takes great heat energy to cause burn injury. When such injury occurs, however, the associated swelling can quickly threaten the airway.

Infraglottic (or subglottic) inhalation burns occur much less frequently because the moist supraglottic tissue absorbs the heat energy and the glottis will likely close to prevent the injury from penetrating more deeply. However, superheated steam, as is produced when a stream of water hits a particularly hot portion of a fire, has the heat energy to carry the burning process to the subglottic region. There, airway burns are extremely critical, as even slight tissue swelling will restrict the airway.

Special consideration should also be given to the toxic nature of the hot gasses inhaled during the inhalation burn. Modern construction materials and the widespread use of synthetics are products that release toxic agents when they burn (cyanide, arsenic, hydrogen sulfide, and others). Often these agents will combine with the moisture of the airway and form caustic compounds that induce chemical burns of the airway, or they may be absorbed into the bloodstream, causing systemic poisoning. The risk for inhalation injury increases with a history of unconsciousness or with being within a confined space during a fire.

14. Describe the special considerations for a chemical burn injury to the eye. p. 163

Chemicals introduced onto the surface of the eye threaten to damage the delicate corneal surface. It is imperative that you consider these injuries when chemicals are splashed and that the eye is irrigated for up to 20 minutes. Irrigation may be accomplished by running normal saline through an administration set into the corner of the eye and directed away from the other eye if it is not affected. If both eyes are involved, a nasal cannula may be helpful in directing fluid flow to both eyes simultaneously. Be alert for contact lenses, as they may trap chemicals under their surface and prevent effective irrigation.

15. **Given several preprogrammed, simulated thermal, inhalation, electrical, and chemical burn injury and radiation exposure patients, provide the appropriate scene size-up, initial assessment, rapid trauma or focused physical exam and history, detailed exam, and ongoing assessment, and provide appropriate patient care and transportation. pp. 151-166**

During your training as a Paramedic you will participate in many classroom practice sessions involving simulated patients. You will also spend some time in the emergency departments of local hospitals as well as in advanced-level ambulances gaining clinical experience. During these times, use your knowledge of burn trauma to help you assess and care for the simulated or real patients you attend.

CONTENT SELF-EVALUATION

Multiple Choice

1. A preventative action that will reduce the incidence of scalding injuries is:
   A. use of child-proof faucets.
   B. education of children on the dangers of hot water.
   C. placing caution stickers on water faucets.
   D. lowering the water heater temperature to 130°F.
   E. none of the above

2. The area of a burn that suffers the most damage is generally the:
   A. the zone of hyperemia.   D. the zone of coagulation.
   B. the zone of denaturing.   E. the zone of most resistance.
   C. the zone of stasis.

3. The theory of burns that explains the burning process is:
   A. the thermal hypothesis.
   B. Jackson's theory of thermal wounds.
   C. the Phaseal discussion of burns.
   D. the Hypermetabolism dynamic.
   E. none of the above

4. The order in which the phases of the body's response to a burn would normally be expected to occur is:
   A. emergent, fluid shift, hypermetabolic
   B. fluid shift, hypermetabolic, emergent
   C. fluid shift, emergent, hypermetabolic
   D. hypermetabolic, fluid shift, emergent
   E. emergent, hypermetabolic, fluid shift

5. Which of the following skin types has the greatest resistance to the passage of electrical current?
   A. mucous membranes   D. the skin on the inside of the arm
   B. wet skin   E. the skin on the inside of the thigh
   C. calluses

6. Electrical injury is likely to cause which of the following?
   A. serious injury where the electricity enters the body
   B. serious injury where the electricity exits the body
   C. damage to nerves
   D. damage to blood vessels
   E. all of the above

7. Which of the following radiation types is least powerful?
   A. neutron
   B. alpha
   C. gamma
   D. beta
   E. delta

8. Which of the following radiation types is the most powerful type of ionizing radiation?
   A. lambda
   B. alpha
   C. gamma
   D. beta
   E. delta

9. Which of the following is a type of radiation present only inside nuclear reactors and bombs?
   A. neutron
   B. alpha
   C. gamma
   D. beta
   E. delta

10. To protect themselves from radiation exposure, EMS personnel should:
    A. limit the duration of exposure.
    B. increase the shielding from exposure.
    C. increase the distance from the source.
    D. ensure that the patient is decontaminated.
    E. all of the above

11. The radiation dose that is lethal to about 50 percent of those exposed is:
    A. 0.2 Gray.
    B. 100 rads.
    C. 1 Gray.
    D. 4.5 Grays.
    E. 200 rads.

12. Which one of the following statements is true regarding radiation exposure?

    A. as radiation exposure increases, the signs of exposure become less evident and only reappear later in the course of the disease.
    B. hiding under a chair or desk will prevent further injury
    C. as radiation exposure increases, the signs and symptoms of exposure become more evident
    D. the strength of the radiation increases the further away you move form the source

13. Which of the following is commonly associated with inhalation injury?
    A. carbon monoxide poisoning
    B. toxic inhalation
    C. supraglottic injury
    D. subglottic injury
    E. all of the above

14. Which type of circumstance is most likely to cause subglottic thermal burn injury?
    A. inhalation of hot air
    B. inhalation of flame
    C. inhalation of superheated steam
    D. standing in a burn environment
    E. inhalation of toxic substances

15. What percentage of burn patients who die have associated airway burn injury?
    A. 20 percent
    B. 35 percent
    C. 50 percent
    D. 60 percent
    E. 80 percent

16. The burn characterized by erythema, pain, and blistering is the:
    A. superficial burn.
    B. partial-thickness burn.
    C. full-thickness burn.
    D. electrical burn.
    E. chemical burn.

17. The burn characterized by discoloration and lack of pain is the:
   A. superficial burn.
   B. partial-thickness burn.
   C. full-thickness burn.
   D. electrical burn.
   E. chemical burn.

18. An adult has received burns to the entire anterior chest and to the entire left upper extremity, circumferentially. Using the rule of nines, the percentage of body surface (BSA) area involved is:
   A. 9 percent.
   B. 18 percent.
   C. 27 percent.
   D. 36 percent.
   E. 48 percent.

19. A child has received burns to the entire left lower extremity and the genitals. Using the rule of nines, the percentage of the body surface area involved is:
   A. 9 percent.
   B. 10 percent.
   C. 141/2 percent.
   D. 19 percent.
   E. 211/2 percent.

20. An adult has received burns to the entire left lower extremity and the genitals. Using the rule of nines, the percentage of the body surface area involved is:
   A. 9 percent.
   B. 10 percent.
   C. 18 percent.
   D. 19 percent.
   E. 21 percent.

21. A child receives burns to his entire head and neck and upper back. What percentage of body surface area is involved?
   A. 9 percent
   B. 10 percent
   C. 18 percent
   D. 19 percent
   E. 27 percent

22. Which of the following systemic complications should you suspect with all serious burns?
   A. hypothermia
   B. hypovolemia
   C. infection
   D. eschar formation
   E. all of the above

23. Which of the following conditions would increase the impact a burn has on a patient?
   A. being very young
   B. being very old
   C. having the flu
   D. emphysema
   E. all of the above

24. Which of the following should NOT be removed from any burned area of a patient?
   A. nylon clothing such as a windbreaker
   B. small pieces of burned fabric lodged in the wound
   C. shoes and socks
   D. rings, watches, and other articles of jewelry
   E. leather belts

25. Your assessment reveals an area of burn that is reddened, painful, and just beginning to display blisters. What burn classification would you give this burn?

   A. superficial burn
   B. partial-thickness burn
   C. full-thickness burn
   D. first degree burn
   E. A or D

26. The patient you are attending has her entire left upper extremity seriously burned. The forearm and hand are very painful and reddened, while the upper arm is relatively painless and a dark red color. What percentage of the BSA and burn depth would you assign this patient?

A. 9 percent full-thickness burn
B. 9 percent partial-thickness burn
C. 41/2 percent full-thickness burn
D. 41/2 percent partial-thickness burn
E. 41/2 percent partial-thickness and 41/2 percent full-thickness burn

27. Your assessment reveals a burn patient with superficial burns to 27 percent of the body. To which classification of burn severity would you assign her?

A. minor
B. moderate
C. serious
D. critical
E. none of the above

28. Your assessment reveals a burn patient with full-thickness burns to the entire left thigh and calf. What classification of burn severity would you assign him?

A. minor
B. moderate
C. serious
D. critical
E. none of the above

29. Your assessment reveals a burn patient with partial-thickness burns to all of both lower extremities. What classification of burn severity would you assign her?

A. minor
B. moderate
C. serious
D. critical
E. none of the above

30. Your assessment reveals a burn patient with partial-thickness burns to her entire lower extremities and a suspected femur fracture. What classification of burn severity would you assign her?

A. minor
B. moderate
C. serious
D. critical
E. none of the above

31. Cool water immersion may reduce the depth and significance of small burns if applied within:

A. 1 to 2 minutes.
B. 2 to 4 minutes.
C. 4 to 5 minutes.
D. 10 minutes.
E. 20 minutes.

32. In general, moderate to severe burns should be covered with:

A. moist occlusive dressings.
B. dry sterile dressings.
C. cool water immersion.
D. plastic wrap covered by a soft dressing.
E. warm water immersion

33. The Parkland formula for fluid administration calls for administration of 4 mL of fluid to a patient multiplied by the patient's BSA involved. What other factor(s) determines the total fluid administered in the first 24 hours?

A. patient's age
B. patient's weight
C. depth of burns
D. age of the patient
E. all of the above

34. Which of the following is the preferred fluid for resuscitation of the severely burned patient?

A. normal saline
B. 1/2 normal saline
C. dextrose 5 percent in water
D. lactated Ringer's solution
E. dextrose 5 percent in normal saline

35. Which of the following drugs may be given to the patient with severe burns in the pre-hospital setting?

A. ipratropium   D. furosemide
B. morphine   E. haloperidol
C. epinephrine

36. Which of the following may be appropriate when a forming eschar is restricting distal blood flow to an extremity?

A. elevating the extremity
B. incising the eschar to relieve the pressure
C. wrapping the extremity in dry sterile dressings
D. administering morphine
E. immersing the limb in cold water

37. A patient was found unconscious in a burning mobile home. Your assessment discovers severe dyspnea, no airway restriction, chest pain, altered mental status, and some seizure activity. What condition would you suspect?

A. carbon monoxide poisoning
B. cyanide poisoning
C. chemical burns to the lungs
D. hypoxia due to inhalation of oxygen- deprived air
E. superheated steam inhalation

38. If an IV line is not yet established in a patient with suspected cyanide poisoning you should administer which of the following?

A. amyl nitrate   D. haloperidol
B. sodium nitrate   E. ipratropium
C. sodium thiosulfide

39. In addition to the entrance and exit wounds normally expected with the passage of electrical current through the human body, the paramedic should expect:

A. ventricular fibrillation.   D. smoldering clothing.
B. cardiac irritability.   E. all of the above
C. internal damage.

40. In Canada, lightning strikes hit about how many people per year?

A. 2   D. 26
B. 10   E. 90
C. 16

41. In general, caustic chemical contamination should be cared for by:

A. dry sterile dressings.   D. cool water irrigation.
B. chemical antidotes.   E. rapid transport.
C. rigorous scrubbing.

42. The chemical phenol is soluble in:

A. water.   D. ammonia.
B. dry lime.   E. none of the above
C. normal saline.

43. Which chemical agent reacts vigorously with water?

A. phenol   D. riot control agents
B. bleach   E. ammonia
C. sodium

44. How long should you irrigate a patient's eye contaminated with chemicals of an unknown nature?

A. less than 2 minutes   D. up to 20 minutes
B. up to 5 minutes   E. none of the above
C. up to 15 minutes

_____ 45. If the source of radiation cannot be contained or moved away from the patient:
    A.   the patient should be brought to you.
    B.   care should be offered by you in protective gear.
    C.   care should be offered by specialists in protective gear.
    D.   care should be offered by the highest ranking officer.
    E.   A or C

True/False

_____ 46. The incidence of burn injury has been on the decline over the past decade.
    A.   True
    B.   False

_____ 47. Burns result from the disruption of the proteins found in cell membranes.
    A.   True
    B.   False

_____ 48. Prolonged contact with alternating current may result in respiratory paralysis.
    A.   True
    B.   False

_____ 49. Chemical burns involving strong alkalis are likely to be deep due to coagulation necrosis.
    A.   True
    B.   False

_____ 50. Burns due to strong acids are likely to be less deep than burns due to strong alkalis because they produce liquefaction necrosis.
    A.   True
    B.   False

_____ 51. When considering intubation of the patient with suspected airway injury due to inhalation of the byproducts of combustion, you should have a supply of several smaller than normal endotracheal tubes ready.
    A.   True
    B.   False

_____ 52. In severe inhalation injury due to airway burns it may be necessary to perform a cricothyrotomy to secure an adequate airway.
    A.   True
    B.   False

_____ 53. High-flow oxygen therapy is very helpful in cases of carbon monoxide poisoning because it will then be carried in sufficient quantities in the plasma to maintain life.
    A.   True
    B.   False

_____ 54. The patient with any full-thickness burn should be considered for administration of tetanus toxoid as the wound is an open one.
    A.   True
    B.   False

_____ 55. Adjacent full-thickness burns, such as those affecting the fingers and toes, should be held together without dressings to ensure rapid healing.
    A.   True
    B.   False

Matching

Write the letter of the term in the space provided next to the appropriate description.

A. zone of stasis
B. current
C. coagulation necrosis
D. BSA
E. Gamma

F. eschar
G. subglottic
H. blepharospasm
I. supraglottic
J. emergent phase

_____ **56.** hard, leathery hard product of a deep full thickness burn

_____ **57.** first stage of the burn process, characterized by a pain-mediated reaction

_____ **58.** twitching of the eyelids

_____ **59.** referring to the upper airway

_____ **60.** the process in which an acid, while destroying tissue, forms an insoluble layer limiting further damage

_____ **61.** the rate of flow of an electric charge

_____ **62.** referring to the lower airway

_____ **63.** area of a burn characterized by decreased blood flow

_____ **64.** Body Surface Area

_____ **65.** the most powerful ionizing radiation

Chapter 22

Musculoskeletal Trauma

Review of Chapter Objectives

After reading this chapter, you should be able to:

1. Describe the incidence, morbidity, and mortality of musculoskeletal injuries. pp. 168-169

In trauma, musculoskeletal injuries are second in frequency only to soft-tissue injuries. They account for thousands of injuries ranging from strains to fractures and dislocations and are rarely, by themselves, life threatening. However, significant musculoskeletal injuries are found in 80 percent of patients who suffer multi-system trauma and may account for significant disability.

2. Discuss the anatomy and physiology of the muscular and skeletal systems. (see Chapter 12)

The skeletal system is a living body system that protects vital organs, acts as a storehouse for body salts and other materials needed for metabolism, produces erythrocytes, permits us to have an upright stature, and permits us to move with relative ease through the environment. The skeletal system consists of the axial and appendicular skeletons.

The common long bone consists of a diaphysis, metaphysis, and epiphysis. The diaphysis is the hollow skeletal shaft of the long bone and contains the yellow bone marrow. It is covered by the periosteum, which contains sensory nerve fibers and initiates the bone repair cycle. The metaphysis is the transitional region between the diaphysis and the epiphysis. In this region, the thin layer of compact bone of the diaphysis shaft becomes the honeycomb of the weight-bearing epiphyseal region. The epiphysis is the articular end of the bone. Through the widening of the metaphysis and the cancellous bone underneath, the weight-bearing, articular surface distributes support over a large surface area.

Bones join at an area called a joint, where they move together to permit articulation. The actual surface of movement is the articular surface and is covered with cartilage, a smooth, shock-absorbing surface that allows free movement between the two ends of the adjoining bones. It is the actual joint surface. The joint is held together with ligaments, which are bands of connective tissue attaching bones to each other. These bands encapsulate the joint and allow some stretch, while holding the articulating bones firmly together.

Muscles make up most of the body's mass, are the driving power behind body motion, and also provide most of the body's heat energy. They only have the ability to contract with force, hence are usually paired with one opposing the motion of the other. Muscles are usually attached by strong connective tissue called tendons. The point of attachment that remains stationary with muscle contraction is the origin, while the point of attachment that moves is the insertion.

3. Predict injuries based on the mechanism of injury, including: pp. 169-175

• **Direct.** Direct injury can be caused by blunt or penetrating mechanisms that deliver kinetic energy to the location of injury and may account for fractures, dislocations, muscle contusions, strains, sprains, subluxations, or combinations of the above.

• **Indirect.** Indirect injuries are injuries that occur as energy is transmitted along the musculoskeletal system to a point of weakness. For example: A person falls forward and braces the fall on an outstretched arm. The energy is transmitted up the extremity to the clavicle, where a fracture occurs. Another example is the football player whose cleated shoe remains stationary while contact with an opposing player turns his body, resulting in an injury to the ligament of the knee.

• **Pathologic.** Pathologic injury results from tumors of the periosteum, bone, articular cartilage, ligaments, tendons, or muscles. Diseases that affect the musculoskeletal structures may also cause injuries as may radiation treatment. Bones or joint structures injured in this way are not likely to heal well.

4. Discuss the types of musculoskeletal injuries, including:

• Fractures (open and closed)   **pp. 172-174**

A fracture is a break in the continuity of the bone. It may present with pain, false motion, angulation, and, possibly, an open wound.

• Dislocations/fractures   pp. 171-172

A dislocation is a displacement of one of the bones of a joint from the joint capsule. The area is noticeably deformed, the limb is usually fixed in position, and the injury is very painful. Due to the proximity of blood vessels and nerves, there is a concern for involvement of these structures and loss of distal circulation and sensation. A fracture is a disruption in the continuity of a bone. In a closed fracture, bone ends do not penetrate the skin. In an open fracture, they do. Other types of fractures include hairline, impacted, transverse, oblique, comminuted, spiral, fatigue, greenstick, and epiphyseal. Fractures may also occur in the proximity of joints and present in a similar fashion with similar dangers.

• Sprains   p. 171

A sprain is the tearing of the ligaments of a joint. The injury produces pain, swelling, and discoloration with time. Since the injury has damaged the joint's integrity, further exertion may cause joint failure. A subluxation is a transitional injury between the sprain and dislocation. The ligaments have been stretched and do not provide a stable joint. The range of motion may be limited and the site is very painful.

• Strains   p. 171

A strain is an overstretching of a muscle body that produces pain. The muscle fibers have been damaged; however, there is usually no internal hemorrhage or associated discoloration.

5. Describe the six "Ps" of musculoskeletal injury assessment.   p. 180

Pain. The patient with musculoskeletal injury may report pain, pain on touch (tenderness), or pain on movement of the injured limb.
Pallor. The skin at the injury site and distal to it may be pale or flushed and capillary refill may be delayed.
Paralysis. The patient may be unable to move the limb and/or may have diminished strength distal to the injury.
Paresthesia. The patient may complain of numbness or tingling or may have limited or no sensation distal to the injury.
Pressure. The patient may complain of a sensation of pressure at the site of injury or palpation may detect greater skin tone and tissue rigidity at the injury site.
Pulses. The distal pulses may be diminished or absent distal to the injury site.

6. List the primary signs and symptoms of extremity trauma.   pp. 177-182

The primary signs of extremity trauma include pain, mechanism of injury, deformity (angulation or swelling), soft-tissue injuries (suggesting injury beneath), unusual limb placement, inequality in limb length, and the inability of the patient to bear weight or use the extremity.

7. List other signs and symptoms that can indicate less obvious extremity injury. pp. 180-182

In addition to the six "Ps" of musculoskeletal injury, the injury may demonstrate instability of the joint or limb, inequality of sensation or limb strength, crepitus (a grating sensation), unusual motion, abnormal muscle tone, and unusual regions of warmth or coolness.

8. Discuss the need for assessment of pulses, motor function, and sensation before and after splinting.   p. 185

It is essential to monitor distal pulses, sensation, and motor function during the splinting process. You need to first determine a baseline to ensure that the distal function of the limb is intact before you begin the process. If not, minor movement of the limb may restore it. Once the process is complete, and frequently thereafter, you need to ensure that the splint does not constrict the limb too forcibly, restricting distal blood flow. The check will also ensure venous return is adequate and that the nerves remain uncompressed and functional.

9. Identify the circumstances requiring rapid intervention and transport when dealing with musculoskeletal injuries.   pp. 178-179

Because musculoskeletal injuries are not often associated with life-threatening injuries, they by themselves do not frequently require rapid intervention and transport. However, when the distal circulation or innervation is interrupted by the injury, immediate intervention and rapid transport may is indicated. If a distal pulse or nervous function deficit is noted, you may try to gently manipulate the injury site to restore pulse or function (this includes dislocation reduction in some circumstances). It is also imperative to bring the patient to the emergency department quickly if your attempts to correct the circulation or nervous problem are unsuccessful.

10. Discuss the general guidelines for splinting.   pp. 184-189

Once any patient life threats and serious injuries have been cared for, splinting may take place. The injury is assessed as are the distal pulse, sensation, and motor function. Any open wound is covered with a sterile dressing and the limb is positioned for splinting, as long as the injury is no closer than 7 cm from a joint. Provide any movement for limb positioning with gentle in-line traction unless the movement significantly increases pain or resistance is felt. Choose a device (malleable, Speed splint, traction splint, etc.) that accommodates the limb and secure it to immobilize the joint above and the joint below the injury. Secure the splint from the distal to the proximal end to ensure the best venous return and check distal circulation, sensation, and motor function in the limb at the end of the splinting process. Joint injuries are generally immobilized as found unless there is distal pulse, sensation, or motor function deficit. Then an attempt to align the injury may be indicated.

11. Explain the benefits of the application of cold and heat for musculoskeletal injuries. p. 190

The application of cold to a musculoskeletal injury in the few hours after the injury constricts the vasculature and limits edema. This ensures better circulation through the limb after the injury, especially if splinting is employed. Heat applied after 48 hours will increase the circulation to the injury site and speed the healing process.

12. Describe age-associated changes in the bones.   p. 175

As bones develop in the fetus they are almost exclusively cartilaginous in nature. This makes them extremely flexible but not very rigid. With the newborn and infants, the cartilage begins to fill with salt deposits and becomes stronger and more rigid. It is, however, still very flexible and one reason infants have a hard time standing and holding their heads up. Bones lengthen from the epiphyseal plate near the bone ends, an area where fracture may disrupt the growth process. With increasing age, children's bones become more rigid, but they are prone to fractures like the greenstick, breaking and splintering on one side but not breaking completely. By the late teen years, the bone tissue reaches its maximum strength. As an adult reaches 40 years of age, bone degeneration begins. The bones become less flexible and more prone to fracture. They also heal more slowly. With advancing age and continuing bone degeneration, fractures may occur with normal stresses and lead to falls.

13. Discuss the pathophysiology, assessment findings, and management of open and closed fractures.   pp. 173-174, 191-194

Fractures are generally traumatic events that disrupt the structure of the bone. They may be a result of blunt trauma such as a fall or an auto collision or of penetrating trauma as when a bullet slams into a rib. Assessment will reveal a patient who complains of pain and the inability to use the extremity. Physical assessment will reveal angulation, swelling, deformity, and false motion (where joint-like motion is unexpected). Distally, the limb may display pallor, coolness, diminished or absent pulses, reduced sensation or motor function, and may be shortened when compared to the opposing limb. By definition, there will be an open wound associated with an open fracture, though it may be caused by the offending force causing the fracture or by one or more of the fractured bone ends penetrating the skin. Management includes covering any open wound with a sterile dressing and then gently aligning the bone with traction and immobilizing it and the joints above and below the injury with a splinting device.

14. Discuss the relationship between the volume of hemorrhage and open or closed fractures. pp. 179, 191, 192

Fractures alone, whether open or closed, do not often account for severe and continued blood loss with the exception of pelvic and femoral fractures. Pelvic fractures may account for more than 2,000 ml of blood loss and femoral fractures, up to 1,500ml. Tibial/fibular and humeral fractures may account for 500ml of loss, and other fractures and dislocations for less. These losses do contribute to hypovolemia and shock in the multi-system trauma patient. Closed fractures have limited blood loss because of fascial containment of the hemorrhage, with the exception of the pelvis, where lack of any fascial compartment helps account for the severe hemorrhage associated with that injury. Open wounds may permit blood to be lost externally in excess of the numbers above, but hemorrhage control techniques should easily control that loss.

15. Describe the special considerations involved in femur fracture management.   pp. 191-192

The femur is the largest long bone of the body and its fracture requires great energy, resulting in a serious and very traumatic injury. The injury is generally very painful, causing the large muscles of the thigh to contract and naturally splint the site. This action pushes the broken femur ends into the muscles of the thigh, increasing the pain and causing further muscle spasm. The result is a serious and progressing injury. Gentle traction will utilizing a traction splint such as the Sager can prevent further damage and pain from the femur movement and then relax the muscle masses. This allows the femur ends to move back to a more anatomic position. This enhances blood flow through the limb and reduces soft tissue injury caused by the overriding bones. Gentle traction is applied manually and then is maintained by a traction splint device.

16. Discuss the pathophysiology, assessment findings, and management of dislocations. pp. 171-172, 195-199

Dislocations are forceful events that displace the bone ends from their proper location within a joint by stretching or tearing ligaments. The patient will complain of pain and the inability to use the joint, while you will notice deformity of the joint and unusual limb placement. Dislocations are usually immobilized as they are found unless the distal pulse, sensation, or motor function distal to the injury is disrupted or the time from injury to care at the emergency department will be long. Then attempts made at dislocation reduction may be made.

17. Discuss the pre-hospital management of dislocation/fractures, including splinting and realignment.   pp. 191-199

The objective of dislocation and fracture care is splinting to prevent further injury during transport to the emergency department. A splint should be chosen for ease in application, ability to immobilize the fracture or dislocation site (and the joint above and below), and patient comfort. The limb should be aligned to ensure adequate immobilization with the splint by bringing the distal limb in line (using gentle traction) with the proximal limb. The movement continues until the limb is aligned, you meet resistance, or the patient experiences a significant increase in pain. The devices below should be utilized only if they can accomplish the goals of splinting effectively.

Pelvis—long spine board with additional support or scoop stretcher
Hip—long spine board, scoop stretcher
Femur—Sager splint
Knee—Speed splint, padded board splints
Tibia and fibula—Speed splint, padded board splints, air splint
Ankle—Speed splint, pillow splint, padded board splint, air splint
Foot—Speed splint, pillow splint, padded board splint, air splint, malleable splint
Shoulder—sling and swathe
Humerus—Peed splint, cuff and collar sling and swathe
Elbow—Speed splint, malleable splint, padded board splint
Radius and ulna—Speed splint, malleable splint, padded board splint, air splint
Wrist— Speed splint, malleable splint, padded board splint, air splint
Hand— Speed splint, malleable splint, padded board splint, air splint
Finger—conforming splint, padded board splint

18. Explain the importance of manipulating a knee dislocation/fracture with an absent distal pulse.   pp. 195-196

The absence of distal pulses secondary to a fracture or dislocation may be due to associated pressure on the artery due to bone displacement. Gentle, controlled manipulation may move the bones enough to re-establish the distal circulation and ensure the distal tissues receive adequate perfusion during the remaining care and transport.

19. Describe the procedure for reduction of a shoulder, finger, or ankle dislocation/fracture. pp. 196-199

The general process for dislocation reduction is to use increasing traction to move the bone ends apart (distraction) and then toward a normal anatomic position. The pull is slowly increased over about 3 minutes or until you feel the bone ends "pop" into position and see the limb assume a more normal anatomic appearance. The distal circulation, sensation, and motor function are examined before and after the procedure to ensure that distal function remains normal. Generally, reduction is not attempted unless there is serious neurovascular compromise. If the procedure does not produce relocation in a few minutes, splint the limb as is and transport.

Shoulder dislocations are most commonly anterior (hollow or squared-off shoulder) or posterior (elbow and forearm held off the chest). Place a strap across the chest and under the arm and have a rescuer pull traction against the traction you pull along the arm while you draw the arm somewhat away from the chest (abduction). Some rotation along the axis of the humerus (by rotating the elbow) may facilitate reduction. For the less common inferior dislocation, have one rescuer stabilize the chest while you flex the elbow and apply a firm traction along the axis of the humerus. Gently rotate the humerus externally.

Finger dislocations are relatively common and most often displace posteriorly. Grasp the finger and apply firm distal traction, distracting the two bone ends and moving the finger toward the normal anatomic position.

Ankle dislocations present with the ankle turned outward (lateral), the foot pointing upward (anterior), and the foot pointing downward (posterior). With the anterior dislocation, grasp the toe and heel and rotate the foot toward a normal orientation. With the anterior dislocation, move the foot posteriorly, while with posterior dislocations, move the foot anteriorly.

20. Discuss the pathophysiology, assessment findings, and management of sprains, strains, and tendon injuries. pp. 171, 199

Sprains generally result from the movement of a joint beyond its normal range of motion while the ligaments holding it together are stretched or torn. The patient will complain of a mechanism of injury and pain at the joint that usually increases with any attempt to move it or put weight on it.

Management is centered around immobilizing the site and transporting the patient to rule out fracture (by x-ray).

Strains are overexertion injuries to the muscles where muscle fibers are torn. The particular muscle is sore, and pain will increase with attempts to use it. Care is centered around rest and reduced use of the muscle until the body can heal it.

Tendon injuries include tears or ruptures of the tendons, or the tendons may pull loose from their skeletal attachments. Injury is usually due to overexertion or to severe blunt or penetrating trauma. Care is usually directed at immobilizing the patient's affected limb in the position of function (neutral positioning) and transporting for assessment and possible surgical repair at the emergency department.

21. Differentiate between musculoskeletal injuries based on the assessment findings and history. pp. 177-183

It is very difficult to differentiate between muscle, joint, and long bone injuries in the pre-hospital setting. Hence, treat any suspected musculoskeletal injury found within 7 cm of a joint as a dislocation, splinting it as it is found unless there is a distal neurovascular deficit. In that case, reduction may be considered. Injuries affecting the limbs and more than 7 cm from the joint are considered fractures and are brought into alignment using gentle distal traction unless there is a great increase in pain or you meet resistance.

23. Given several preprogrammed and moulaged musculoskeletal trauma patients, provide the appropriate scene size-up, initial assessment, rapid trauma or focused physical exam and history, detailed exam, and ongoing assessment, and provide appropriate patient care and transportation. pp. 177-203

During your training as a Paramedic you will participate in many classroom practice sessions involving simulated patients. You will also spend some time in the emergency departments of local hospitals as well as in advanced-level ambulances gaining clinical experience. During these times, use your knowledge of musculoskeletal trauma to help you assess and care for the simulated or real patients you attend.

CONTENT SELF-EVALUATION

Multiple Choice

1. Musculoskeletal injuries can include injury to:
   A. bones.
   B. tendons.
   C. ligaments.
   D. muscles.
   E. all of the above

2. A specific sign associated with compartment syndrome is:
   A. deep pain.
   B. absent distal pulses.
   C. pain on passive extension.
   D. absent distal sensation.
   E. diaphoresis.

3. The condition in which exercise draws down the supply of oxygen and energy reserves and metabolic waste products accumulate, limiting the ability of a muscle group to perform is called:
   A. cramp.
   B. fatigue.
   C. strain.
   D. sprain.
   E. spasm.

4. The tissue that is normally damaged in a sprain is the:
   A. tendon. `
   B. ligament.
   C. muscle.
   D. articular cartilage.
   E. epiphyseal plate.

5. The overstretching of a muscle that presents with pain is a:
   A. strain.   D. spasm.
   B. sprain.   E. subluxation.
   C. cramp.

6. Which of the following fractures is relatively stable?
   A. hairline   D. comminuted
   B. impacted   E. both A and B
   C. transverse

7. Which of the following fractures is most likely to be open?
   A. fibula   D. humerus
   B. tibia   E. ulna
   C. femur

8. Which of the following types of fractures is likely to occur only in the pediatric patient?
   A. greenstick   D. comminuted
   B. oblique   E. spiral
   C. transverse

9. The bones of the elderly are likely to be:
   A. less flexible.   D. more slow to heal.
   B. more brittle.   E. all of the above
   C. more easily fractured.

10. The growth of bone that comes after a fracture and encapsulates the fracture site is called the:
    A. epiphyseal outgrowth.   D. natural splinting.
    B. periosteum.   E. comminution.
    C. callus.

11. Which of the following is caused by a build-up of uric acid crystals in the joints?
    A. gout   D. bursitis
    B. rheumatoid arthritis   E. tendinitis
    C. osteoarthritis

12. An inflammation of the small synovial sacs that reduce friction and cushion tendons from trauma is:
    A. gout.   D. bursitis.
    B. rheumatoid arthritis.   E. tendinitis.
    C. osteoarthritis.

13. Which of the following is an indication for the use of PASG in the patient with skeletal injury?
    A. pelvic fracture   D. hip dislocation
    B. serious tibial fracture   E. both A and D
    C. femur fracture

14. With which of the fractures below should you consider immediate transport of the patient because of possible internal blood loss?
    A. humerus   D. pelvis
    B. femur   E. both B and D
    C. tibia

15. When assessing a limb for possible fracture, you should examine distally for:
    A. sensation.   D. crepitus.
    B. motor strength.   E. all of the above
    C. circulation.

16. A patient complains of a "pins and needles" sensation between the webs of his toes and a serious crushing-type injury has caused his calf to feel "almost board hard." What injury would you suspect?
    A. tibial fracture
    B. muscular contusion
    C. compartment syndrome
    D. tendinitis
    E. subluxation

17. An elderly patient who has suffered a fracture due to bone degeneration is expected to experience what level of pain when compared to a traumatic fracture?
    A. about the same
    B. more pain
    C. less pain
    D. no pain at all
    E. extreme pain

18. In general, long bone shaft fractures should be splinted:
    A. aligned, except if resistance is experienced.
    B. as found.
    C. extended, except if resistance is experienced.
    D. flexed, except if resistance is experienced.
    E. none of the above

19. Which of the following positions is ideal for the immobilization of most extremity injuries?
    A. extended
    B. flexed
    C. hyperextended
    D. hyperflexed
    E. neutral

20. Ascending to altitude in a helicopter will cause the pressure in the air splint to:
    A. increase.
    B. decrease.
    C. remain the same.
    D. become less uniform.
    E. become more uniform.

21. The traction splint is designed to splint which musculoskeletal injury?
    A. knee dislocation
    B. hip dislocation
    C. pelvic fracture
    D. femur fracture
    E. all of the above

22. Which of the following is a disadvantage of the vacuum splint when applying it to splint fractures?
    A. It is difficult to apply.
    B. It is bulky and heavy.
    C. It shrinks during application.
    D. It takes more than two rescuers to apply.
    E. all of the above

23. Align a seriously angulated long bone fracture unless:
    A. there is an absent distal pulse.
    B. there is absent sensation.
    C. both sensation and pulses are intact.
    D. you meet with resistance.
    E. you feel crepitus.

24. If after moving a limb to alignment you notice the distal pulse is absent, you should:
    A. splint the limb, as is.
    B. gently move the limb to restore the pulse.
    C. return the limb to the original positioning.
    D. elevate the limb and then splint it.
    E. splint and apply an ice pack.

25. Early reduction of a dislocation usually results in which of the following?
    A. less stress on the ligaments
    B. less stress on the joint structure
    C. better distal circulation
    D. better distal sensation
    E. all of the above

26. Signs that a reduction of a dislocation has been effective include:
- **A.** feeling a "pop."
- **B.** patient reports of less pain.
- **C.** greater mobility in the joint.
- **D.** less deformity of the joint.
- **E.** all of the above

27. Heat may be applied to a muscular injury:
- **A.** immediately.
- **B.** after 1 hour.
- **C.** after 24 hours.
- **D.** after 48 hours.
- **E.** not at all.

28. The splinting device recommended for a painful and isolated fracture of the femur is:
- **A.** the vacuum splint.
- **B.** the PASG.
- **C.** the spine board and padding.
- **D.** long padded board splints.
- **E.** none of the above

29. The splinting device recommended for a painful and isolated fracture of the tibia is the:
- **A.** traction splint.
- **B.** PASG.
- **C.** long spine board and padding.
- **D.** padded board splint.
- **E.** sling and swathe.

30. The splinting device recommended for an isolated fracture of the humerus is the:
- **A.** traction splint.
- **B.** sling and swathe.
- **C.** air splint.
- **D.** padded board splint.
- **E.** both B and D

31. The fracture of the forearm close to the wrist that presents with the "silver fork" deformity is called:
- **A.** Richardson's fracture.
- **B.** Colles's fracture.
- **C.** Volkman's contracture.
- **D.** Blundot's inversion.
- **E.** none of the above

32. An anterior hip dislocation normally presents with the:
- **A.** foot turned outward.
- **B.** foot turned inward.
- **C.** knee flexed.
- **D.** knee turned outward.
- **E.** knee turned inward.

33. Which of the following is NOT a sign of patellar dislocation?
- **A.** knee in the flexed position
- **B.** significant joint deformity
- **C.** the extremity drops at the knee
- **D.** lateral displacement of the patella
- **E.** none of the above

34. If a patient presents with an ankle deformed with the foot turned to the side, you would suspect which type of ankle dislocation?
- **A.** anterior
- **B.** posterior
- **C.** lateral
- **D.** medial
- **E.** inferior

35. If a patient presents with an ankle deformed with the foot pointing upward, you should suspect which type of ankle dislocation?
- **A.** anterior
- **B.** posterior
- **C.** lateral
- **D.** medial
- **E.** inferior

36. When a patient's shoulder appears "squared-off," the patient complains of severe pain, and she cannot move her arm, you should suspect what type of shoulder dislocation?
- **A.** anterior
- **B.** inferior
- **C.** superior
- **D.** posterior
- **E.** lateral

37. Which of the following injuries can be adequately splinted by using the short padded board splint, placing the hand in the position of function, and slinging and swathing the extremity?

A.	radial fractures	**D.**	finger fractures
B.	ulnar fractures	**E.**	all of the above
C.	wrist fractures		

38. Nitrous oxide in the pre-hospital setting:
- **A.** is non-explosive.
- **B.** reduces the perception of pain.
- **C.** can be self-administered.
- **D.** diffuses easily into air-filled spaces.
- **E.** all of the above

39. Which of the following is NOT an analgesic that is used to control the pain of musculoskeletal injuries?

A.	meperidine	**D.**	diazepam
B.	morphine	**E.**	none of the above
C.	nalbuphine		

40. The "I" within acronym RICE used by athletic trainers stands for:

A.	immobilization.	**D.**	intensity of pain.
B.	ice for the first 48 hours.	**E.**	both A and B
C.	instability.		

True/False

41. Contusion can account for significant fluid loss into the more massive muscles of the body.
- **A.** True
- **B.** False

42. In serious long bone fractures, especially those that are manipulated after injury, there is the possibility of fat embolizing and becoming lodged in the lungs.

- **A.** True
- **B.** False

43. The dislocation, or fracture in the area of a joint, is generally less significant than the long bone shaft fracture because it does not have as high an incidence of vascular and nervous injury.
- **A.** True
- **B.** False

44. The energy and degree of manipulation needed to cause further injury after a bone has broken is much less than was initially needed to cause the fracture.
- **A.** True
- **B.** False

45. As the effects of the fight-or-flight response wear off, the symptoms of fracture will become less evident.
- **A.** True
- **B.** False

46. It is essential to tell the patient that limb alignment will cause some increased pain, as this will help maintain his or her confidence in you.
  A. True
  B. False

47. Do not attempt realignment of any fracture within 3 inches of a joint.
  A. True
  B. False

48. With joint injury you should not move the limb around, even to restore circulation or sensation.
  A. True
  B. False

49. In general, anterior dislocations of the knee can be reduced in the prehospital setting.
  A. True
  B. False

50. The elbow dislocation is a simple injury but one that it is essential to reduce in the field.
  A. True
  B. False

Matching

Write the letter of the term in the space provided next to the appropriate description.

A.	sprain	**F.**	open fracture
B.	osteoporosis	**G.**	gout
C.	dislocation	**H.**	fatigue fracture
D.	callus	**I.**	greenstick fracture
E.	subluxation	**J.**	strain

51. a broken bone in which the bone end penetrates the surrounding skin

52. inflammation of the joints due to a buildup of uric acid crystals

53. injury resulting from overstretching of muscle fibres

54. thickened area that forms at the site of a fracture as part of the healing process

55. complete displacement of a bone end from its position in a joint capsule

56. partial fracture of a child's bone

57. tearing of a joint capsule's connective tissue

58. weakening of the bone tissue due to loss of essential minerals, especially calcium

59. break in a bone associated with prolonged or repeated stress

60. partial displacement of a bone end from its position in a joint capsule

Chapter 23

Head, Facial, and Neck Trauma

Review of Chapter Objectives

After reading this chapter, you should be able to:

1. Describe the incidence, morbidity, and mortality of head, facial, and neck injures.   p. 206

Approximately 34 000 people are admitted to hospital with brain injuries each year. Head trauma is the most common cause of trauma death, being especially lethal in auto collisions. Gunshot wounds to the head are less frequent but have a mortality of 75 to 80 percent. The population most at risk for head injury is the male between 15 and 24 years of age, infants and young children, and the elderly.

2. Explain the head and facial anatomy and physiology as they relate to head and facial injuries.   (see Chapter 12)

Several layers of soft, connective, and skeletal tissues protect the brain. These include the scalp, the cranium, and the meninges. The scalp is a thick and vascular layer of tissue that is strong and flexible and able to absorb tremendous kinetic energy. Beneath it are several layers of connective and muscular fascia that further protect the skull and its contents and that are only connected to the skull on a limited basis. This permits the scalp to move with glancing blows and further protect the cranium.

The skull consists of numerous bones, fused together at fixed joints called sutures. These bones form a container for the brain called the cranium. The cranium is made up of three layers of bone, two thin layers of compact bone separated by a layer of cancellous bone. This construction makes the cranium both light and very strong. This vault for the brain is fixed in volume and does not accommodate any expansion of its contents. However, in the newborn and infant, the skull is more cartilaginous and more flexible, with two open areas, the anterior and posterior fontanelles. These spaces close by 18 months.

The meninges are three layers of tissue—the dura mater, the arachnoid, and the pia mater—that provide further protection for the brain. The dura mater is a tough, fibrous layer that lines the interior of the skull and spinal foramen and is continuous with the inner periosteum of the cranium. The pia mater is a delicate membrane covering the convolutions of the brain and spinal cord. The arachnoid is a web-like structure between the dura mater and pia mater. The cerebrospinal fluid fills the subarachnoid space and "floats" the brain and spinal cord to help absorb the energy of trauma.

The brain occupies about 80 percent of the volume of the cranium and is made up of the cerebrum, cerebellum, and brainstem. The cerebrum occupies most of the cranial vault and is the center of consciousness, personality, speech, motor control, and perception. It is separated into right and left hemispheres by the falx cerebri, extending inward from the anterior, superior, and posterior central skull. The cerebellum sits beneath the posterior half of the cerebrum and is responsible for fine tuning muscular control and for balance and muscle tone. It is separated from the cerebrum by the tentorium cerebelli, a fibrous sheath that runs transverse to the falx cerebri along the base of the cerebrum. The brainstem runs anterior to the cerebellum and central and inferior to the cerebrum. It consists of the hypothalamus, thalamus, pons, and medulla oblongata. The brainstem controls the endocrine system and most primary body functions including respiration, cardiac activity, temperature, and blood pressure.

The face, consisting of several bones covered with soft tissue, protects the special sense organs of sight, smell, hearing, balance, and taste and forms and protects the upper airway and the beginning of the alimentary canal. The brow ridge (a portion of the frontal bone), the nasal bones, and the zygoma form the eye sockets and protect the eyes. The upper jaw (the maxilla) and the moveable lower jaw (mandible) provide the skeletal structures that form the opening of the mouth. Cavities within this region (sinuses) help to provide shape to the face without increasing the weight of the head. The nasal cavity provides an extended surface to warm, humidify, and cleanse incoming air. The oral cavity houses the tongue and teeth and accommodates the early physical and chemical breakdown of food.

3. **Differentiate between the following types of facial injuries, highlighting the defining characteristics of each: (see also Chapter 12)**

a. Eye p. 222
The eye is a globe filled with a crystal-clear fluid (vitreous humor) that focuses light through a lens onto light sensitive tissue, the retina. The amount of light entering the eye is determined by the size of the opening, the pupil (as controlled by the iris). The delicate surface of the eye is covered by the cornea (over the pupil and iris) and the conjunctiva (over the white portion of the eyeball, called the sclera). The eye is well protected from most blunt trauma by the skeletal structures of the brow ridge, zygomatic arch, and nasal bones. Blunt trauma may induce hyphema (blood filling the anterior chamber), subconjunctival hemorrhage (a blood-red discoloration of the sclera), and retinal detachment. Penetrating trauma or severe blunt trauma may directly injure the eye or entrap the small muscles that control it.

b. Ear p. 221
The external portion of the ear is the pinna, a cartilaginous structure covered by skin and only minimally supplied with circulation. A natural opening into the skull, the external auditory canal channels sound to the tympanum, where it and then the ossicles (the three bones of hearing) are set in motion. The ossicles vibrate the window of the cochlea, stimulating this organ of hearing to send impulses to the brain. The inner ear also houses the semicircular canals, which serve as an organ sensing head movement and balance. The pinna is easily injured, bleeds minimally, and heals poorly. Injury to the internal structures of the ear occurs very infrequently but may be caused by pressure differentials as with the blast over-pressures of an explosion, with the unequalized pressure associated with diving, or with direct insertion of an object into the ear canal.

c. Nose p. 221
The nasal cavity is a pair of hollows formed by the junctures of the ethmoid, nasal, and maxillary bones. The external openings of the nose are the nares, formed by the nasal cartilage and anterior soft tissues. Frontal impact may fracture the nasal cartilage or bones, and severe Le Fort–type fractures may disrupt the nasal region. Since the area has a significant blood supply to warm incoming air, hemorrhage (epistaxis) can be heavy.

d. Throat   p. 224
The throat or pharynx may be injured with lower facial or upper neck injury through either blunt or penetrating mechanisms. This region is made up of predominantly soft tissue and gains some support from the structure of the jaw and hyoid bones. Injury may fracture these bones, reducing the structural integrity of the region, or may damage soft tissues, resulting in massive swelling that threatens the airway. Any serious injury to this region is likely to endanger the airway.

e. Mouth   p. 224

The mouth, or oral cavity, is made up of the upper and lower jaws, the hard and soft palates (superiorly), and the musculature and connective tissue in the base of the tongue. Fracture of the mandible and, to a lesser degree, the maxilla may reduce the structural integrity of the cavity and endanger its patency as a part of the airway. Injury may also result in severe soft-tissue swelling, hemorrhage, and in some cases, the loss of teeth.

4. Predict head, facial, and other related injuries based on mechanism of injury. pp. 206-207

Injuries to the head, face, and neck occur secondary to blunt or penetrating mechanisms. The most common cause of serious and blunt head trauma is the auto collision; other common mechanisms include falls, acts of violence, and, occasionally, sport-related activities. The neck is well protected both anteriorly and laterally, but it still may be impacted as the neck strikes the steering wheel or when the shoulder strap alone restrains movement of a vehicle's occupant. Penetrating injury is not as common as blunt injury but can still endanger life. Penetrating injuries to the cranium can be devastating to the brain tissue and are frequently not survivable, especially those injuries caused by high-energy gunshot wounds. Gunshot wounds to the face can also be life threatening as they may compromise the airway and distort facial and airway features.

5. Differentiate between facial injuries based on the assessment and history.   pp. 219-223

The greatest dangers from skeletal or soft-tissue injury to the face are related to endangering of the airway, injury to the sensory organs housed and protected there, and damage to the cosmetic appearances of the region. The region is also very vascular and prone to serious blood loss. Facial fractures are classified according to the Le Fort criteria, with Le Fort I fractures relating to simple maxillary fractures, Le Fort II to fractures extending into the nasal bones, and Le Fort III to fractures involving the facial region all the way up to the brow ridge. These fractures are usually due to serious blunt trauma.

6. Explain the pathophysiology, assessment, and management for patients with eye, ear, nose, throat, and mouth injuries. pp. 219-246

Eye injury may be due to blunt trauma and includes hyphema (blood in the eye's anterior chamber), conjunctival hemorrhage, or retinal detachment (the patient complaining of a curtain across part of the field of view). Severe blunt injury may cause orbital fracture, making it appear as though the eye was avulsed, or may entrap the ocular muscles and limit eye movement. Management includes covering both eyes with a cup over any protruding tissue or impaled object and bandaging. The patient must also be calmed and reassured because these injuries are very anxiety provoking. Penetrating eye trauma not only injures the delicate ocular tissue but also risks the loss of either aqueous or vitreous humors.

Ear injury most commonly affects the pinna and is due to glancing blows. Infrequently the internal organs of hearing and balance are damaged due to objects inserted into the ear or from dramatic pressure changes caused by explosions or diving injuries. External injury is cared for with dressing and bandaging, while with any internal injury the ear is covered with gauze to permit the drainage of any fluids from the external auditory canal.

Nasal injury can involve the nasal cartilage and bones and cause fractures or dislocations. Hemorrhage in this area (epistaxis) can be very heavy. If possible, the patient's head should be brought forward to ensure that blood from the nasal cavity drains outward and not down the throat, which could irritate the stomach and increase the likelihood of vomiting.

Injuries to the oral cavity are related to fractures of the mandible and associated soft-tissue destruction. Penetrating trauma, especially that produced by high-speed projectiles, can cause severe injury to the structures and tissues of the facial region and result in serious hemorrhage and danger to the patency of the airway. The airway should be maintained with suctioning, oral or nasal airway insertion, or with rapid sequence intubation, if necessary.

Pharyngeal injury is associated with serious risk of soft-tissue swelling and airway compromise. Use suction to remove fluids and consider early intubation because progressive swelling will restrict the airway and make later attempts at intubation more difficult.

7. Explain anatomy and relate physiology of the CNS to head injuries. pp. 211-219

The brain occupies 80 percent of the volume of the cranial vault. The brain consists of three major components: the cerebrum, the cerebellum, and the brainstem. The cerebrum is the center for conscious thought, perception, and motor control and is the largest structure within the cranium. The cerebellum fine tunes muscle movement and is responsible for muscle tone. The brainstem is made up of the thalamus, the hypothalamus, the pons, and the medulla oblongata. It is responsible for control of the vital signs and for consciousness. The central nervous system tissue is very delicate, very dependent upon adequate perfusion and a constant supply of oxygen, glucose, and thiamine, and easily injured by the forces of trauma. The contents of the cranium are protected by the scalp, the cranium, and the meninges. They are bathed in cerebrospinal fluid that floats them in a near-weightless environment.

8. Distinguish between facial, head, and brain injury. pp. 208-224

Facial injury involves the soft or skeletal structures of the face, including the facial bones and mandible, the nasal cavity, the oral cavity, and the soft tissues covering the region. Their injury threatens the airway and the patient's cosmetic appearance. Serious facial injury is also suggestive of head and brain injury.

Head injury suggests that serious blunt or penetrating forces were expressed to the head with the potential for intracranial injury. Head injury involves damage to the scalp or cranium. It may also include brain (or intracranial) injury.

Brain injury is injury to the cerebrum, cerebellum, or brainstem. It may be caused by blunt trauma, either injuring tissue and blood vessels at the point of impact (coup injury) or injuring tissue and blood vessels away from the point of impact (contrecoup injury). Injury may also occur with an expanding lesion, as with epidural or subdural hematoma, with extensive cerebral edema that causes an increase in intracranial pressure, with a decrease in intracranial perfusion, and possibly with physical brain damage from pressure and displacement secondary to hemorrhage or edema.

9. Explain the pathophysiology of head/brain injuries. pp. 206-219

Brain injury either is direct, related to the initial insult, or indirect, related to progressive pathologies secondary to the insult such as developing tissue irritation, inflammation, edema, hemorrhage, and physical displacement or by hypoxia. Direct injuries can be either coup or contrecoup in origin and include both the focal and diffuse injuries.

Focal injuries include cerebral contusion, which produces confusion and some local swelling, and intracranial hemorrhage, which produces hemorrhage as an arterial vessel above the dura mater ruptures and leads to a quickly evolving accumulation of blood and pressure (epidural hematoma) or as a venous vessel beneath the arachnoid membrane ruptures and produces a more gradual hemorrhage and build-up of pressure (subdural hematoma). Hemorrhage may also occur within the tissue of the brain (intracerebral hemorrhage) leading to a small accumulation of blood and some associated irritation, edema, and increase in intracranial pressure.

Diffuse injuries include the concussion (a mild or moderate diffuse axonal injury) and moderate and severe axonal injuries. These injuries are common and, with increasing severity, increasingly impair neurologic function and decrease the potential for return to a neurologically intact state. Diffuse injuries contuse, tear, shear, or stretch the brain tissue and cause injury that is often distributed throughout the brain.

Indirect injuries result as pressure displaces, compresses, or restricts the blood flow to regions of the brain. This secondary-type injury may induce hypoxia or ischemia that damages brain cells, causing inflammation and resulting in edema and further increases in ICP.

10. Explain the concept of increasing intracranial pressure (ICP). pp. 210-216

The cranium is a rigid container with a fixed volume. It is full and each of its contents (cerebrum, cerebellum, brainstem, cerebrospinal fluid, and blood) occupies a component of the volume. Within this container, there is a limited constant pressure, the intracranial pressure. This pressure rarely exceeds 10 mmHg and at such a low level does not restrict cerebral blood flow. However, if one of the cranial residents increases its volume (vascular, as with hematoma, or the cerebrum itself, as with edema), another resident will have to decrease its volume or a pressure increase will result. During increasing ICP, some of the venous blood will leave the cranium, and then some cerebrospinal fluid will move to the spinal cord. These compensatory mechanisms work rather well, but the volume they can compensate for is limited. If expansion continues, the pressure (ICP) begins to rise. As it does, the difference between the intracranial pressure (ICP) and the mean arterial pressure (MAP) falls. This is the pressure driving cerebral perfusion (cerebral perfusion pressure, CPP). If CPP drops below 50 mmHg, cerebral perfusion pressure is not adequate to perfuse the brain. The body will increase the blood pressure in an attempt to maintain cerebral perfusion (autoregulation), but this only increases the edema or hemorrhage in a progressively worsening cycle.

11. Explain the effect of increased and decreased carbon dioxide on ICP. pp. 215-216

Increased carbon dioxide concentrations in the blood cause the cerebral arteries to dilate and thereby provide better circulation to the contents of the cranium. This, however, can increase the intracranial pressure and increase any damage occurring due to a pre-existing elevated intracranial pressure.

Decreased carbon dioxide causes vasoconstriction in the cerebral arteries and limits blood flow to the brain. If the blood CO_2 levels are reduced excessively, this will seriously limit cerebral blood flow and cause further injury to the patient who is already suffering from reduced cerebral blood flow (as with increased intracranial pressure).

12. Define and explain the process involved with each of the levels of increasing ICP. pp. 215-216

The damage caused by increasing intracranial pressure (ICP) is progressive and limits cerebral perfusion. Normal intracranial pressure is very minimal and does not interfere with perfusion. However, as an injury (edema or an accumulation of blood) expands, it compresses the contents of the cranium. This compresses the veins and forces some venous blood from the cranium. If the pressure continues to rise, the pressure begins to move cerebrospinal fluid from the cranium (and into the spinal cord). If the pressure rise continues, arteries are compressed and cerebral blood flow suffers. This reduced circulation through the cerebrum causes a rise in the systemic blood pressure (autoregulation). This increases the cerebral blood flow but also increases the rate of intracranial hemorrhage and further increases the ICP. The result is a rapid rise in ICP, a reduction in cerebral blood flow, and cerebral hypoxia.

13. Relate assessment findings associated with head/brain injuries to the pathophysiologic process. pp. 206-219

The most noticeable findings of brain injury are associated with the vital signs and include increasing blood pressure, erratic respirations (Cheyne-Stokes, Kussmaul's, central neurologic hyperventilation, or ataxic respirations), and a slowing pulse. These things are known collectively as Cushing's reflex. These signs indicate severe injury to the medulla oblongata, possibly due to its herniation into the foramen magnum. Eye signs, such as one pupil dilating and becoming unresponsive, are due to pressure on the oculomotor nerve as it is compressed against the tentorium. Such a sign is usually related to injury on the same (ipsilateral) side. The patient frequently demonstrates a reduced level of orientation or responsiveness and a Glasgow Coma Scale score of less than 15. The patient may also display retrograde or anterograde amnesia. These are generalized signs related to either diffuse axonal injury or increased intracranial pressure.

14. Classify head injuries (mild, moderate, severe) according to assessment findings. pp. 213-214

Head injuries are classified according to the Glasgow Coma Scale. Those patients who score from 13 to 15 are considered to have received a mild injury, those from 9 to 12, a moderate injury, and those with a score of 8 or below are considered to have a severe head injury. Any change in the level of consciousness or orientation or any personality changes are signs of at least a mild head injury. Any finding that suggests the pulse rate is slowing, the respirations are becoming more erratic, and the blood pressure is rising due to head injury should be considered to indicate that the patient has a severe injury. The patient with the signs of a mild or moderate head injury must be watched very carefully because these pathologies frequently progress to more severe injuries.

15. Identify the need for rapid intervention and transport of the patient with a head/brain injury. pp. 225, 232

The pathologic processes at work in the patient with serious head injury are completely internal and cannot be repaired or stabilized in the field. High-flow oxygen administration and adequate ventilation (not hyperventilation) will ensure the best cerebral oxygenation without blowing off too much CO_2. Ensuring good cardiovascular function and maintaining blood pressure are essential. In some systems, medications are also used to reduce cerebral edema in the field. However, often the only definitive way to correct the problems affecting the patient with serious head trauma is surgical intervention. For this reason, care for head injury patients focuses on bringing them quickly to a center capable of neurosurgical intervention.

16. Describe and explain the general management of the head/brain injury patient, including pharmacological and nonpharmacological treatment.   pp. 232, 244

The general management of the patient with recognized or suspected head injury begins with immobilization of the cervical spine to ensure no aggravation of any spinal injury. This manual immobilization is maintained and augmented by the application of a cervical collar, until the immobilization is continued by mechanical immobilization with a KED and/ or long spine board, or Scoop stretcher. The airway and adequate ventilation must be ensured. High-flow oxygen is the first-line drug for the patient with suspected head injury and complements ventilation to ensure the patient has good respirations, full breaths at 12 to 20 times per minute, without hyperventilation. As a CCP , intubation may be attempted early using rapid sequence intubation with vecuronium as the paralytic of choice because succinylcholine may cause an increase in intracranial pressure. Mannitol may be beneficial as it draws fluid from the tissue with its osmotic properties and may reduce cerebral edema. Sedatives are indicated to premedicate the patient for the RSI procedure. Atropine will reduce airway secretions and may also reduce vagal stimulation and any increase in intracranial pressure that would otherwise occur during intubation attempts.

17. Analyze the relationship between carbon dioxide concentration in the blood and management of the airway in the head/brain injured patient.   pp. 210-216

In general, the higher the level of carbon dioxide in the blood, the greater the need to ventilate the patient. However, very low levels of carbon dioxide cause cerebral vasodilation, which may lead to a more rapidly increasing intracranial pressure. The objective of airway and respiratory care for the head injury patient is to ensure a patent airway and good respiratory exchange without blowing off too much CO_2. This generally means that a patient should be ventilated with full breaths up to 20 times per minute.

18. Explain the pathophysiology, assessment, and management of a patient with:

a. Scalp injury   pp. 208-229, 227-228, 232-244
Scalp injuries tend to bleed heavily because their blood vessels do not constrict as well as those elsewhere on the body. This type of hemorrhage is easy to control because of the firm skull beneath, except when skull fracture is suspected. In that case, use distal pressure points and controlled direct pressure to stop any serious bleeding. Glancing injuries may expose the skull and flap the scalp over on itself. Remove any gross contaminants and cover the exposed surfaces with a sterile dressing. These injuries will heal very well due to the more than adequate blood supply they receive.

b. Skull fracture   pp. 209-211, 227, 232-244
Skull fractures are skeletal injuries that usually heal uneventfully. The greatest concern is for the possible damage within the cranium. Skull fracture is anticipated by the mechanism of injury and should be suspected if fluids are draining out of the nose or ears. The retroauricular or bilateral periorbital ecchymosis associated with basilar skull fracture are not frequently seen in the pre-

hospital setting because they take hours to develop. Immobilize the potentially fractured skull carefully and cover the ears and nose with gauze to ensure free outward movement of any cerebrospinal fluid.

c. Cerebral contusion   pp. 211, 232-244
The cerebral contusion is usually due to direct head trauma and may be the result of coup or contrecoup injury mechanisms. The patient may experience regional related neurologic deficits that resolve with time. This patient should be suspected of severe but more slowly progressive injury and watched very carefully. Administer oxygen and transport quickly.

d. Intracranial hemorrhage (including epidural, subdural, subarachnoid, and intracerebral hemorrhage)   pp. 212-213, 232-244
Intracranial hemorrhage (be it epidural, subdural, subarachnoid [a subset of subdural], or intracerebral) is a progressive injury mechanism that occurs as blood accumulates, displaces brain tissue, and raises intracranial pressure or as bleeding irritates brain tissue, initiates an inflammatory response, and causes cerebral edema and an increase in intracranial pressure. Patients with intracranial hemorrhage will display progressively deteriorating levels of orientation and consciousness and a history of serious head trauma. The elderly and chronic alcoholics may have an increased incidence of brain injury due to a reduced cerebral mass and more room for the brain to move during head trauma. Intracranial hemorrhage management includes oxygen, airway management, ensuring adequate ventilation, ensuring adequate blood pressure, and rapid transport. As an CCP, Rapid sequence intubation may be necessary, and mannitol may relieve some of the edema associated with the injury and ease the increased intracranial pressure.

e. Axonal injury (including concussion and moderate and severe diffuse axonal injury). pp. 213-214, 232-244
Diffuse axonal injury may be anticipated by the mechanism of injury and by observation of any signs of progressively deteriorating levels of orientation and consciousness. Care is directed at oxygen administration, airway management, ensuring adequate ventilation, ensuring adequate blood pressure, and rapid transport.

f. Facial injury pp. 219-223, 228-229
Facial injury may be anticipated by the mechanism of injury or recognized by soft-tissue injuries to or structural deformities of the region. Care is directed at maintaining the airway, protecting the eyes, and controlling any significant blood loss.

g. Neck injury   pp. 223-224, 229-230, 232-244
Neck injury is anticipated by the mechanism of injury and by a quick evaluation of the region. The spine is immobilized manually, a cervical collar is applied, and eventually manual immobilization is replaced with the mechanical immobilization of the KED and/or the long spine board or Scoop stretcher. Open soft-tissue injuries are covered with sterile dressings (or occlusive dressings if the injury is significant) and the airway is assessed to ensure that it is not at risk.

19. Develop a management plan for the removal of a helmet for a head-injured patient. p. 226

A helmet is carefully removed using techniques that limit the movement of the cervical spine and head. Full-face helmets provide the greatest challenge to removal, and to deal with them you should employ the techniques described in Chapter 24, "Spinal Trauma,".

20. Differentiate between the types of head/brain injuries based on the assessment and history. pp. 206-232

The pathologies of head injury will either make your patient get progressively worse or better. Contusion and mild diffuse axonal injuries are likely to improve with time. However, as diffuse axonal injury gets more severe, the chances for recovery lessen and associated edema will likely increase the ICP and cause progressive neurologic deficit. Patients with intracranial hemorrhage (epidural and subdural) and intracerebral hemorrhage are likely to deteriorate with time. Epidural hemorrhage patients will show decreasing levels of consciousness and then the signs of increasing intracranial hemorrhage (eye signs, increasing systolic blood pressure, slowing and strengthening pulse, and erratic respirations). Patients with subdural and intracerebral hemorrhage will take longer to display these signs and may not do so in the prehospital setting. Be advised however, that one injury may be superimposed upon another. The concussion may render a patient unconscious and permit him to awaken, experience a lucid interval, and then deteriorate due to a developing epidural hematoma.

21. **Given several preprogrammed and moulaged head and facial injury patients, provide the appropriate scene size-up, initial assessment, rapid trauma or focused physical exam and history, detailed exam, and ongoing assessment, and provide appropriate patient care and transportation. pp. 225-246**

During your training as a Paramedic you will participate in many classroom practice sessions involving simulated patients. You will also spend some time in the emergency departments of local hospitals as well as in advanced level ambulances gaining clinical experience. During these times, use your knowledge of head, facial, and neck trauma to help you assess and care for the simulated or real patients you attend.

CONTENT SELF-EVALUATION

Multiple Choice

1. The most common cause of trauma-related death is due to injury to the:
   - A. head.
   - B. thorax.
   - C. abdomen.
   - D. pelvis.
   - E. extremities.

2. What percentage of penetrating wounds to the cranium result in mortality?
   - A. 30 to 40 percent
   - B. 40 to 50 percent
   - C. 65 to 70 percent
   - D. 75 to 80 percent
   - E. 90 to 95 percent

3. Which of the following statements is NOT true of scalp wounds?
   - A. They pose a risk of meningeal infection.
   - B. Wounds there tend to heal very well.
   - C. Wounds there tend to bleed heavily.
   - D. Contusions there swell outward noticeably.
   - E. Avulsion of the scalp is not a likely injury.

4. The most common type of skull fracture is:
   - A. depressed.
   - B. basilar.
   - C. linear.
   - D. comminuted.
   - E. spiral.

5. The type of skull fracture most often associated with high-velocity bullet entry is:
   - A. depressed.
   - B. basilar.
   - C. linear.
   - D. comminuted.
   - E. spiral.

6. The discoloration found around both eyes due to basilar skull fracture is:
   - A. retroauricular ecchymosis.
   - B. bilateral periorbital ecchymosis.
   - C. Cullen's sign.
   - D. the halo sign.
   - E. Gray's sign.

7. Blood and CSF draining from the ear may display a:
   - A. speckled appearance.
   - B. concentric lighter yellow circle.
   - C. congealed mass.
   - D. greenish discoloration.
   - E. none of the above

8. The type of injury that causes damage to the brain on the side opposite the impact is called:
   A. coup.
   B. subdural hematoma.
   C. subluxation.
   D. contrecoup.
   E. concussion.

9. Which of the following is considered a focal injury?
   A. cerebral contusion
   B. epidural hematoma
   C. subdural hematoma
   D. intracerebral hemorrhage
   E. all of the above

10. Which of the following injuries is most likely to cause the patient to deteriorate rapidly?
    A. cerebral contusion
    B. epidural hematoma
    C. subdural hematoma
    D. intracerebral hemorrhage
    E. concussion

11. Which of the following is an injury with venous bleeding into the arachnoid space?
    A. cerebral contusion
    B. epidural hematoma
    C. subdural hematoma
    D. intracerebral hemorrhage
    E. concussion

12. The injury that classically presents with unconsciousness immediately after the accident followed by a lucid interval and then a decreasing level of consciousness is most likely a(n):
    A. concussion.
    B. epidural hematoma.
    C. subdural hematoma.
    D. cerebral hemorrhage.
    E. both A and B

13. Which of the following head injuries would you NOT expect to get worse with time?
    A. intracerebral hemorrhage
    B. subdural hematoma
    C. concussion
    D. epidural hematoma
    E. intracranial hemorrhage

14. As intracranial hemorrhage begins, it first displaces which occupant of the cranium?
    A. cerebrospinal fluid
    B. venous blood
    C. arterial blood
    D. oxygen
    E. the pia matter

15. Perfusion through the cerebrum is a factor of intracranial pressure and:
    A. systolic blood pressure.
    B. diastolic blood pressure.
    C. mean arterial pressure.
    D. cerebral perfusion pressure.
    E. none of the above

16. High levels of carbon dioxide in the blood will cause which of the following?
    A. hyperventilation
    B. cerebral artery constriction
    C. cerebral artery dilation
    D. hypertension
    E. none of the above

17. Vomiting, changes in the level of consciousness, and pupillary dilation result from herniation of the upper brainstem through the:
    A. tentorium incisura.
    B. foramen magnum.
    C. falx cerebri.
    D. transverse sinus.
    E. tentorium cerebelli.

18. Cushing's reflex includes which of the following?
    A. erratic respirations
    B. increasing blood pressure
    C. slowing heart rate
    D. A and B
    E. A, B, and C

19. Which of the following respiratory patterns is NOT indicative of brain injury?
- **A.** eupnea
- **B.** ataxic respirations
- **C.** central neurogenic hyperventilation
- **D.** Cheyne-Stokes respirations
- **E.** agonal respirations

20. In the presence of intracranial pressure, the fontanelles of the infant will:
- **A.** withdraw.
- **B.** become stiff.
- **C.** bulge.
- **D.** pulsate.
- **E.** atrophy.

21. According to the Le Fort criteria, a fracture involving just the maxilla and limited instability is classified as:
- **A.** Le Fort I.
- **B.** Le Fort II.
- **C.** Le Fort III.
- **D.** Le Fort IV.
- **E.** Le Fort V.

22. Which type of Le Fort fracture is likely to result in cerebrospinal fluid leakage?
- **A.** Le Fort I
- **B.** Le Fort III
- **C.** Le Fort IV
- **D.** Le Fort V
- **E.** none of the above

23. Which of the following statements is TRUE regarding injuries to the pinna of the ear?
- **A.** They hemorrhage severely.
- **B.** Hemorrhage is difficult to control.
- **C.** Hemorrhage is limited.
- **D.** Wounds there do not heal very well.
- **E.** both C and D

24. Which of the following mechanisms is likely to injure the tympanum?
- **A.** basilar skull fracture
- **B.** an explosion
- **C.** diving injury
- **D.** an object forced into the ear
- **E.** all of the above

25. The collection of blood in front of a patient's pupil and iris due to blunt trauma is called a(n):
- **A.** hyphema.
- **B.** retinal detachment.
- **C.** aniscoria.
- **D.** anterior chamber hematoma.
- **E.** sub-conjunctival hemorrhage.

26. A sudden and painless loss of sight is most likely a(n):
- **A.** hyphema.
- **B.** retinal detachment.
- **C.** acute retinal artery occlusion.
- **D.** anterior chamber hematoma.
- **E.** sub-conjunctival hemorrhage.

27. Blood vessel injury in the neck region carries with it the hazards of all of the following EXCEPT:
- **A.** severe venous hemorrhage.
- **B.** severe arterial hemorrhage.
- **C.** development of subcutaneous emphysema.
- **D.** air aspiration.
- **E.** pulmonary emboli.

28. The patient with a suspected brain injury should be ventilated with full breaths:
- **A.** 8 to 10 times per minute.
- **B.** 12 to 20 times per minute.
- **C.** 20 to 24 times per minute.
- **D.** 24 to 30 times per minute.
- **E.** 30 to 36 times per minute.

29. Which of the following is a probable sign of increasing intracranial pressure?
- **A.** decreasing pulse strength
- **B.** weakening pulse strength
- **C.** slowing pulse rate
- **D.** increasing pulse strength
- **E.** both C and D

30. The major reason for allowing fluid to drain from the nose or ear is that:

A. it may slow the rise of intracranial pressure
B. its flow will prevent pathogens from entering the meninges
C. it is impossible to stop the flow anyway
D. regeneration of CSF is beneficial to the healing process
E. none of the above

31. When light intensity changes in one eye and both respond, this response is called:

A. diplopia.   D. synergism.
B. aniscoria.   E. photophobia.
C. consensual reactivity.

32. Any significant open wound to the anterior or lateral neck should be covered with a(n):

A. wet dressing.   D. adherent dressing.
B. occlusive dressing.   E. pressure dressing.
C. nonadherent dressing.

33. When a patient reports of sensitivity to light, this is an example of:

A. diplopia.   D. synergism.
B. aniscoria.   E. photophobia.
C. consensual reactivity.

34. During your assessment you determine that the patient exhibits confused speech, follows simple commands, and opens his eyes on his own. What Glasgow Coma Scale value would you assign?

A. 15   D. 10
B. 14   E. 7
C. 12

35. A patient who responds only to pain and then only flexes, mutters incomprehensible words when shouted at loudly, and opens his eyes only to pain is given what Glasgow Coma Scale score?

A. 14   D. 8
B. 12   E. 6
C. 10

36. Which of the following could be considered a component of Cushing's reflex?

A. Cheyne-Stokes respirations   D. ataxic respirations
B. decreasing pulse rate   E. all of the above
C. increasing blood pressure

37. If the head injury patient is found without any other suspected injuries, what positioning would be best for her?

A. the Trendelenburg position
B. with the head of the spine board elevated 30 degrees
C. left lateral recumbent position
D. immobilized completely and rolled to her side
E. none of the above

38. Which of the following airway techniques is NOT acceptable for the patient with suspected basilar skull fracture?

A. nasopharyngeal airway insertion   D. orotracheal intubation
B. directed intubation   E. rapid sequence intubation
C. digital intubation

39. The process of inserting an endotracheal tube increases the intracranial pressure and should only be done by the care provider most experienced in the procedure.

A. True
B. False

40. Which of the following is an acceptable method for confirming endotracheal tube placement in the head injury patient?
- **A.** use of an end-tidal CO_2 monitor
- **B.** use of a pulse oximeter
- **C.** observing bilaterally equal chest rise
- **D.** good and bilaterally equal breath sounds
- **E.** all of the above

41. Ventilation of the head injury patient should be guided by oximetry to maintain a saturation of at least:
- **A.** 80 percent.
- **B.** 85 percent.
- **C.** 90 percent.
- **D.** 95 percent.
- **E.** 98 percent.

42. In the head injury patient you must keep the blood pressure above:
- **A.** 50 mmHg.
- **B.** 60 mmHg.
- **C.** 90 mmHg.
- **D.** 120 mmHg.
- **E.** none of the above

43. Which of the following drugs is the first-line diuretic in the treatment of head injury?
- **A.** oxygen
- **B.** mannitol
- **C.** furosemide
- **D.** succinylcholine
- **E.** morphine

44. Which of the following paralytics increases ICP and should be used with caution, if at all, in head injury patients?
- **A.** diazepam
- **B.** mannitol
- **C.** vecuronium
- **D.** succinylcholine
- **E.** midazolam

45. Which of the following drugs will reverse the effects of diazepam and midazolam?
- **A.** narcan
- **B.** flumazenil
- **C.** atropine
- **D.** thiamine
- **E.** none of the above

46. Which of the following actions of atropine make it a desirable adjunct to rapid sequence intubation?
- **A.** It reduces vagal stimulation.
- **B.** It reduces airway secretions.
- **C.** It reduces fasciculations.
- **D.** It helps maintain heart rate during intubation.
- **E.** all of the above

47. Dextrose is administered to the head injury patient:
- **A.** routinely.
- **B.** for hyperglycemia only.
- **C.** for hypoglycemia only.
- **D.** for suspected diabetes or alcoholism.
- **E.** with hetastarch.

48. Dislodged teeth from a patient should be:
- **A.** wrapped in gauze soaked in water.
- **B.** wrapped in gauze soaked in sterile saline.
- **C.** wrapped in dry gauze.
- **D.** kept dry but cool.
- **E.** replaced immediately.

49. Which of the following is indicative of a brain injury?
- **A.** amnesia .
- **B.** diaphragmatic pain
- **C.** vomiting
- **D.** both A and C
- **E.** all of the above

50. Neurogenic shock from spinal trauma may cause:

    A.   hypotension   **D.**   hypertension

    B.   hyperglycemia   **E.**   all of the above

    C.   hypoglycemia

True/False

51. Scalp wounds may present in a manner that confounds assessment.

    A.   True

    B.   False

52. Serious scalp injury is unlikely to produce hypovolemia and shock as the arteries there frequently constrict and effectively limit blood loss.

    A.   True

    B.   False

53. It is common for the paramedic to observe either Battle's sign or bilateral periorbital ecchymosis in the patient who has just sustained a basilar skull fracture.

    A.   True

    B.   False

54. A cranial fracture, by itself, is a skeletal injury that will heal with time; it is the injury underneath that is of most concern.

    A.   True

    B.   False

55. Indirect brain injury occurs as a result of, but after, initial injury.

    A.   True

    B.   False

56. Increasing intracranial pressure is likely to cause pupillary dilation on the ipsilateral side.

    A.   True

    B.   False

57. With facial trauma, airway obstruction is more likely due to blood than other fluids or physical obstruction.

    A.   True

    B.   False

58. The head injury patient may vomit without warning and the vomiting may be projectile in nature.

    A.   True

    B.   False

59. For adequate ventilation through a needle cricothyrotomy, you must use a demand valve ventilator.

    A.   True

    B.   False

60. When locating the cricoid cartilage, either for Sellick's maneuver or the cricothyrotomy, it is the first hard rigid ring you feel as you move your fingers up the trachea from the suprasternal notch.

    A.   True

    B.   False

Matching

Write the letter of the term in the space provided next to the appropriate description.

A.	concussion	**F.**	ICP
B.	fasciculations	**G.**	retrograde amnesia
C.	diplopia	**H.**	subdural hematoma
D.	coup injury	**I.**	anterograde amnesia
E.	hyphema	**J.**	LeFort criteria

_____ **61.** double vision

_____ **62.** collection of blood directly beneath the dura mater

_____ **63.** inability to remember events that occurred after the trauma that caused the condition

_____ **64.** classification system for fractures involving the maxilla

_____ **65.** involuntary contractions or twitching of muscle fibres

_____ **66.** a transient period of unconsciousness, usually followed by a complete return of function

_____ **67.** an injury to the brain occurring on the same side as the site of impact

_____ **68.** blood in the anterior chamber of the eye

_____ **69.** CPP=MAP-____

_____ **70.** inability to remember events that occurred before the trauma that caused the condition

Chapter 24

Spinal Trauma

Review of Chapter Objectives

After reading this chapter, you should be able to:

1. **Describe the incidence, morbidity, and mortality of spinal injuries in the trauma patient. pp. 248-249**

Spinal cord injuries account for over 1 347 hospital admission injuries, occurring most frequently in males aged from 15 to 34. Auto collisions account for almost half of the injuries, while falls, penetrating injuries, and sports-related injuries also contribute significantly to the toll. Spinal cord injuries are especially devastating because they affect the very specialized tissue of the central nervous system, which has relatively little ability to repair itself, and because the cord is the major communication conduit of the body. Injury often results in permanent loss of function below the lesion.

2. **Describe the anatomy and physiology of structures related to spinal injuries, including: (see Chapter 12)**

   a. Cervical spine C 1 - C 7
   The cervical spine is the vertebral column between the cranium and the thorax. It consists of seven irregular bones held firmly together by ligaments that both support the weight of the head and permit its motion while protecting the delicate spinal cord that runs through the central portion of these bones.

   b. Thoracic spine T 1 - T 12
   The thoracic vertebral column consists of 12 thoracic vertebrae, one corresponding to each rib pair. Like the cervical spine, it consists of irregular bones held firmly together by ligaments that support the weight of the head and neck and permit its motion while protecting the delicate spinal cord that runs through the central portion of these bones.

   c. Lumbar spine L 1 - L 5
   The lumbar spine consists of five lumbar vertebrae with massive vertebral bodies to support the weight of the head, neck, and thorax. Here the spinal cord ends at the juncture between L-1 and L-2 and nerve roots fill the spinal foramen from L-2 into the sacral spine.

   d. Sacrum
   The sacrum consists of five sacral vertebrae that are fused into a single plate that forms the posterior portion of the pelvis. The upper body balances on the sacrum, which articulates with the pelvis at a fixed joint, the sacroiliac joint.

   e. Coccyx
   The coccygeal region of the spine consists of three to five fused vertebrae that form the remnant of a tail.

f.   Spinal cord

The spinal cord is a component of the central nervous system consisting of very specialized nervous system cells that do not repair themselves very well. The cord is the body's major communications conduit, sending motor commands to the body and returning sensory information to the brain.

g.   Nerve tracts

The nerve tracts are pathways within the spinal cord for impulses from distinct areas and with distinct sensory or motor functions. The two major types of nerve tracts are ascending tracts, those that carry sensory information to the brain, and descending tracts, those that carry motor commands to the body.

h.   Dermatomes

The dermatomes are distinct regions of the body's surface that are sensed by specific peripheral nerve roots. For example, the collar region is sensed by C3, the nipple line is sensed by T4, the umbilicus is sensed by T10, and the lateral (little) toe is sensed by S1. These landmarks are useful in denoting where the loss of sensation occurs, secondary to spinal injury.

3. Predict spinal injuries based on mechanism of injury.   pp. 249-252

Most spinal trauma is related to extremes of motion. These include extension/flexion, lateral bending, rotation, and axial loading/distraction. These types of movement place stresses on the vertebral column that stretch and injure the ligaments, fracture the vertebral elements, rupture the intervertebral disks, and dislocate the vertebra. While these are all connective or skeletal tissue injuries, they threaten the protective function served by the vertebral column and endanger the spinal cord. The injury mechanism itself or further movement of the vertebral column may cause the skeletal elements to compress, contuse, lacerate, sever, or stretch the cord, resulting in neurologic injury and a deficit below the level of injury.

A frontal impact injury mechanism is likely to cause axial loading and a crushing-type injury to the spine as well as flexion injury (as may occur in the auto or diving incidents). Lateral impact auto collisions are likely to cause lateral bending injury, while rear-end impacts are likely to cause extension, then flexion injury. Hangings may cause distraction injury. Rotational injuries may occur during sporting events.

Penetrating injury is a direct type of injury that disrupts the connective and skeletal structure of the vertebral column and may directly involve the spinal cord. Deep and powerful knife injuries and bullet wounds are the most common mechanisms of this injury.

4. Describe the pathophysiology of spinal injuries.   pp. 249-255

The spinal cord, like all central nervous system tissue, is extremely specialized and delicate and does not repair itself well, if at all. The spinal cord may be injured in much the same way as the brain by mechanisms including concussion, contusion, compression, laceration, hemorrhage, and transection. The concussion is a jarring that momentarily disrupts the cord function. Contusion results in some damage and bleeding into the cord but will likely repair itself. Compression may occur due to vertebral body displacement or as a result of cord edema; it deprives portions of the cord of blood, and ischemic damage may result. The degree of injury and its permanence is related to the amount of compression and the length of time the compression remains. Laceration occurs as bony fragments are driven into the cord and damage it. If the injury is severe, the injury is probably permanent. Hemorrhage into the cord results in compression and irritation of the cord tissue as blood crosses the blood-brain barrier. The injury may also restrict blood flow to a portion of the cord, extending the injury. Transection is a partial or complete severance of the cord with its function below the lesion, for the most part, lost.

5. **Identify the need for rapid intervention and transport of the patient with spinal injuries.**
   pp. 256-261

The need for rapid intervention and transport of the spinal injury patient must take into account the key element of pre-hospital care, which is immobilizing the vertebral column to restrict motion and any further injury. Once injured, the vertebral column can no longer protect the spinal cord from injury and, in fact, becomes the source of probable injury with manipulation. It is imperative that the head be brought to the neutral position and maintained there until the injury heals, it is corrected surgically, or X-rays and CT scans rule out injury. This means that once spinal injury is suspected, the patient remains immobilized until delivered to the emergency department.

6. **Describe the pathophysiology of traumatic spinal injury related to:**

- **Spinal shock   p. 254**
Spinal shock is a transient form of neurogenic shock due to a temporary injury to the spinal cord. It results as the brain loses control over body functions including vasoconstriction, motor control, and sensory perception below the level of injury.

- **Spinal neurogenic shock p. 255**
Neurogenic shock is a more permanent result of cord injury resulting in loss of control over body functions including vasoconstriction, motor control, and sensory perception below the level of injury. The injury results in an inability to control peripheral vascular resistance and blood pressure.

- **Quadriplegia/paraplegia p. 253-254**
The loss of neurologic control over the lower extremities (paraplegia) and the loss of control over all four limbs (quadriplegia) is related to the location of the spinal cord lesion. The higher the injury along the vertebral column, the more of the body is affected. These injuries are related to the distribution of the dermatomes for sensation and myotomes for motor control. Injuries at or below the thoracic spine (T3) involve the lower extremities (paraplegia) while injuries above this level affect all four extremities (quadriplegia).

- **Incomplete and complete cord injury and cord syndromes pp. 253-254**
Injury to the spinal cord can result from the mechanisms discussed earlier. A complete cord injury completely severs the spinal cord, and the potential to send and receive nerve impulses below the site of the injury is lost. Results may include, depending on the site of injury, incontinence, paraplegia, quadriplegia, and partial or complete respiratory paralysis.

     With incomplete cord injury, the spinal cord is only partially severed. There is potential for recovery of function. There are three common types of incomplete cord syndrome:

—**Central cord syndrome   p. 254**
Central cord syndrome is related to hyperextension-type injuries and is often associated with a pre-existing disease like arthritis that narrows the spinal foramen. It usually results in motor weakness of the upper extremities and in some cases loss of bladder control. The prognosis for at least some recovery for the central cord syndrome is the best of all the cord syndromes.

—**Anterior cord syndrome   p. 254**
Anterior cord syndrome is due to damage caused by bone fragments or pressure on the arteries that perfuse the anterior portion of the cord. The affected limbs are likely only to retain motion, vibration, and positional sensation with motor and other perceptions lost.

—**Brown-Séquard's syndrome   p. 254**
Brown-Séquard's syndrome is most often caused by a penetrating injury that affects one side of the cord (hemitransection). Sensory and motor loss is noted on the ipsilateral side, while pain and temperature sensation is lost on the contralateral side. The injury is rare but often associated with some recovery.

7. Describe the assessment findings associated with and management for traumatic spinal injuries.   pp. 256-274

The primary assessment finding used to determine the need for spinal precautions is the mechanism of injury. Vertebral column injury may present with only minimal signs and symptoms of injury, often overshadowed by more painful injuries. Failure to immobilize the spine early during assessment and care may lead to vertebral column movement and damage to the spinal cord.

The signs and symptoms of spinal injury include pain or tenderness along the spinal column, any neurologic deficit, especially if it corresponds to the dermatomes and is bilateral, including any deficits in sensation to touch, temperature, motion, vibration, etc. Any loss in the ability to move (paralysis) or muscular strength (paresis) is suggestive of spinal cord injury. Special signs associated with spinal injury include an involuntary erection of the penis (priapism), loss of bowel and bladder control, and diaphragmatic breathing.

8. Describe the various types of helmets and their purposes.   pp. 266-267

Helmets are made for use in contact sports, bicycling, skateboarding, in-line skating, and motorcycling. Some helmets are partial and can be easily removed at the accident scene. Other helmets (football, for example) completely enclose the head and may be difficult to remove at the accident scene and may pose immobilization problems for pre-hospital care givers. It must be remembered that, while helmets offer some protection for the head, they have not been proven to reduce spinal injuries.

9. Relate the priorities of care to factors determining the need for helmet removal in various field situations including sports-related incidents.   pp. 266-267

Remember that while a helmet provides some protection for head injury, it does not necessarily protect the spine. Take immobilization precautions if the mechanism of injury suggests the potential for spinal injury. If the patient can be fully immobilized with the helmet on, it can be left in place. However you must remove a helmet if the helmet does not immobilize the patient's head, if the helmet cannot be securely immobilized to the long spine board, if it prevents airway care, or if it prevents assessment of anticipated injuries. The helmet should also be removed if you anticipate development of airway or breathing problems. Always be sure that helmet removal will not cause further injuries.

Procedures for helmet removal will vary with the type of helmet. The prime consideration is to continue to maintain manual immobilization of the patient throughout whatever procedure is used and then to ensure that the patient receives proper mechanical immobilization once the helmet is removed.

10. Given several preprogrammed and moulaged spinal trauma patients, provide the appropriate scene size-up, initial assessment, rapid trauma or focused physical exam and history, detailed exam, and ongoing assessment, and provide appropriate patient care and transportation.   pp. 256-274

During your training as a Paramedic you will participate in many classroom practice sessions involving simulated patients. You will also spend some time in the emergency departments of local hospitals as well as in advanced-level ambulances gaining clinical experience. During these times, use your knowledge of spinal trauma to help you assess and care for the simulated or real patients you attend.

CONTENT SELF-EVALUATION

Multiple Choice

_____ 1. Which of the following motions is likely to result from hanging?
  A. extension   D. axial loading
  B. flexion   E. distraction
  C. lateral bending

_____ 2. The region that accounts for more than half of spinal cord injuries is the:
  A. cervical spine.   D. sacral spine.
  B. thoracic spine.   E. coccygeal spine.
  C. lumbar spine.

_____ 3. The region of the vertebral column in which the spinal cord ends is the:
  A. cervical.   D. sacral.
  B. thoracic.   E. coccygeal.
  C. lumbar.

_____ 4. Which of the following is a sign associated with neurogenic shock?
  A. priapism
  B. decreased heart rate
  C. decreased peripheral vascular resistance
  D. warm skin below the injury
  E. all of the above

_____ 5. Which of the following is associated with the resolution of shock due to cord injury and results in hypertension?
  A. autonomic hyperreflexia syndrome
  B. neurogenic shock
  C. spinal shock
  D. central cord syndrome
  E. both B and D

_____ 6. Which of the following is NOT a mechanism of injury likely to cause spinal injury?
  A. fall from over three times the patient's height.
  B. high-speed motor vehicle crash
  C. serious blunt trauma above the shoulders
  D. penetrating trauma directed to the lateral thorax
  E. penetrating trauma directed to the spine

_____ 7. During the initial assessment, you should be aware that exaggerated abdominal movement and limited chest excursions often suggest:
  A. airway obstruction.
  B. the need to reposition the head and neck.
  C. diaphragmatic breathing.
  D. neurogenic shock.
  E. cardiac contusion.

_____ 8. The pulse rate in the patient with spinal injury is likely to be:
  A. fast.   D. very slow.
  B. very fast.   E. normal.
  C. slow.

9. The "hold-up" positioning of the arms is due to injury at or around:
   A.   C-3.   D.   T-10.
   B.   T-1.   E.   S-1.
   C.   T-4.

10. Which of the following is indicative of spinal injury?
    A.   increased heart rate   D.   a normal body temperature
    B.   increasing blood pressure   E.   none of the above
    C.   excessive chest expansion

11. The most ideal position for the adult head during spinal immobilization is:
    A.   2.5-5.0 cm above the spine board
    B.   level with the spine board
    C.   with padding under the shoulders and the head on the spine board
    D.   with the head slightly extended and level with the board
    E.   none of the above

12. Which of the following is a contraindication to continuing to move the head and spine
    toward the neutral, in-line position?
    A.   You meet with significant resistance.
    B.   Your patient complains of a significant increase in pain.
    C.   You notice gross deformity along the spine.
    D.   You notice an increase in the signs of neurologic injury.
    E.   all of the above

13. The ideal position for the small adult's or large child's head during spinal immobilization
    is:
    A.   2.5-5.0 cm above the spine board
    B.   level with the spine board (ground level)
    C.   with padding under the shoulders and the head on the spine board
    D.   with the head slightly extended and level with the board
    E.   none of the above

14. The standing takedown for the patient with spinal injuries requires a minimum of how
    many care providers?
    A.   two   D.   five
    B.   three   E.   no less than six
    C.   four

15. Under which of the following circumstances should a helmet be removed from a patient?
    A.   The head is not immobilized within the helmet.
    B.   The helmet prevents airway maintenance.
    C.   You cannot secure the helmet firmly to the long spine board.
    D.   You anticipate breathing problems.
    E.   all of the above

16. Which of the following circumstances would not automatically merit employment of
    rapid extrication techniques?
    A.   toxic fumes   D.   rising water
    B.   an auto collision   E.   none of the above
    C.   an immediate threat of fire

17. Which of the following is used in the pre-hospital setting for the treatment of spine
    injuries?
    A.   mannitol   D.   furosemide
    B.   methylprednisolone   E.   both B and C
    C.   dexamethasone

18. If a suspected spinally injured patient does not respond to fluid resuscitation, which drug would you consider?
- **A.** methylprednisolone
- **B.** atropine
- **C.** furosemide
- **D.** dopamine
- **E.** diazepam

19. To address bradycardia in the suspected spinally injured patient, which drug would you consider?
- **A.** methylprednisolone
- **B.** atropine
- **C.** furosemide
- **D.** dopamine
- **E.** diazepam

20. A condition usually caused from damage to one side of the spinal cord resulting in sensory and motor loss to that side of the body is called:
- **A.** central cord syndrome
- **B.** Brown-Sequard's syndrome
- **C.** anterior cord syndrome
- **D.** laceration
- **E.** spinal shock

21. At what level of the lesion does sympathetic control lead to relaxation of the blood vessels during neurogenic shock?
- **A.** 2.5-5.0 cm above the suspected fracture or lesion
- **B.** level with the fracture or lesion
- **C.** C7-T4
- **D.** 2.5 cm below the lesion site
- **E.** none of the above

22. A cervical collar should be applied:
- **A.** after splinting all other fractures
- **B.** after the primary assessment (rapid trauma assessment)
- **C.** after the secondary assessment
- **D.** during the primary assessment
- **E.** none of the above

23. The 180 degree log roll begins with:
- **A.** the placement of the long spine board on the opposite side of the patient
- **B.** the placement of the long spine board behind the paramedics back
- **C.** the placement of the KED resting on the patient's back
- **D.** the placement of the long spine board between the paramedics and the patient
- **E.** the placement of the orthopedic stretcher under the patient's lower limbs

24. The initial treatment for hypovolemia from a suspected neurogenic shock is:
- **A.** Norepinephrine
- **B.** Dopamine
- **C.** a fluid bolus
- **D.** epinephrine
- **E.** Valium

25. Signs and symptoms of a spinal injury may include all but which of the following:
- **A.** priapism
- **B.** loss of bowel of bladder control.
- **C.** bradycardia.
- **D.** paralysis of the extremities.
- **E.** tachycardia

True/False

26. Spinal cord injury can occur without injury to the vertebral column or its associated ligaments.
- **A.** True
- **B.** False

27. Spinal shock is a temporary form of neurogenic shock.
    A.   True
    B.   False

28. A spinal cord concussion is likely to produce residual deficit.
    A.   True
    B.   False

29. Helmets reduce the incidence of both head and spine injury.
    A.   True
    B.   False

30. Oral intubation is generally more difficult in the patient who requires spinal precautions because the landmarks are more difficult to visualize.
    A.   True
    B.   False

31. Proper immobilization of the patient with spinal injury should include placing a blanket roll under the knees.
    A.   True
    B.   False

32. Some gentle axial traction on the head will make cervical immobilization more effective.
    A.   True
    B.   False

33. A four-count cadence is preferable for moves as it better signals care providers when the move starts.
    A.   True
    B.   False

34. Orthopedic stretchers are not rigid enough to be used for spinal immobilization by themselves.
    A.   True
    B.   False

35. The vest-type immobilization device is meant to permit rescuers to move the patient from a seated to a supine position in an auto crash by rotating the buttocks on the seat, then tilting the patient to the supine position.
    A.   True
    B.   False

Matching

Write the letter of the term in the space provided next to the appropriate description.

A.	transection	**F.**	anterior cord syndrome
B.	priapism	**G.**	central cord syndrome
C.	parathesia	**H.**	hangman's fracture
D.	scoop	**I.**	autonomic hyperreflexia syndrome
E.	paralysis	**J.**	Brown-Sequard's syndrome

36. C1/C2 fracture

37. condition related to hyperflexion of the cervical spine that results in motor weakness usually in the upper extremities

38. condition caused by cutting of one side of the spinal cord resulting in motor and sensory loss to that side of the body

39. body's adjustment to the effects of neurogenic shock

_____ **40.** a prolonged painful erection of the penis

_____ **41.** condition that is caused by bony fragments compressing arteries of the anterior spine resulting in loss of motor function, and sensation below the injury site

_____ **42.** inability to move

_____ **43.** a cross-sectional cut

_____ **44.** tingling of the extremities

_____ **45.** orthopedic stretcher

Chapter 25

Thoracic Trauma

Review of Chapter Objectives

After reading this chapter, you should be able to:

1. **Describe the incidence, morbidity, and mortality of thoracic injuries in the trauma patient. p. 277**

Chest trauma accounts for about 25 percent of vehicular mortality and is second only to head trauma as a reason for death in the auto accident. Heart and great vessel injuries are the most common cause of death from blunt trauma. Penetrating trauma to the chest also results in significant mortality with heart and great vessel injuries, again, accounting for the greatest mortality. Modern auto and highway design, the speed at which the chest trauma patient arrives at the trauma center, and newer surgical techniques have significantly reduced chest trauma mortality in the last decade.

2. **Discuss the anatomy and physiology of the organs and structures related to thoracic injuries. (see Chapter 12)**

The ribs, thoracic spine, sternum, and diaphragm define the structure of the thoracic cage. The skeletal components allow the cage to expand as the ribs are lifted upward and outward by contraction of the intercostal muscles, and the intrathoracic volume further expands as the diaphragm contracts and moves downward. The net action of this muscle movement is to increase the volume of the thoracic cage and to reduce its internal pressure. Air from the environment moves through the airway into the alveoli to equalize this pressure, and inspiration occurs. The intercostal muscles relax and the thorax settles, while the diaphragm rises back into the thorax and the volume of the cavity decreases. This increases the intrathoracic pressure, and air rushes out to equalize with the environment. This is expiration. The pleura, two serous membranes, seal the lungs to the interior of the thoracic cage during this action and ensure that the lungs expand and contract with the changing volume of the thoracic cavity. The lungs have exceptional circulation, with capillary beds surrounding the alveoli to ensure a free exchange of oxygen and carbon dioxide between the alveolar air and the bloodstream.

The lungs fill all but the central portion of the chest cavity and are found on either side of the central structure, called the mediastinum. The mediastinum contains the heart, trachea, esophagus, major blood vessels, and several nerve pathways. The heart is located in the left central chest and is the major pumping element of the cardiovascular system. The inferior and superior vena cavae collect blood from the lower extremities and abdomen and the upper extremities, head, and neck, respectively, and return it to the heart. The pulmonary arteries and veins carry blood to and from the lungs respectively, and the aorta distributes the cardiac output to the systemic circulation. The trachea enters the mediastinum just beneath the manubrium and bifurcates at the carina into the left and right mainstem bronchi. The esophagus enters the mediastinum just behind the trachea and exits through the diaphragm.

3. Predict thoracic injuries based on mechanism of injury.   pp. 278-280

As in other regions of the body, thoracic trauma results from either blunt or penetrating mechanisms of injury. Blunt trauma may result from deceleration (as in an auto crash), crushing mechanism (as in a building collapse), or pressure injury (as with an explosion). Deceleration frequently causes the "paper bag" syndrome, lung and cardiac contusions, rib fractures, and vascular injuries. Crushing mechanisms may cause traumatic asphyxia and vascular damage and restrict respiratory excursion. Blast mechanisms may cause lung injuries or vascular tears.

Penetrating trauma may involve any structure within the thorax, although injury to the heart and great vessels is most likely to be lethal. Lung tissue is rather resilient and suffers limited injury with a bullet's passage, while the heart and great vessels are damaged explosively, especially if engorged with blood at the time of the bullet's impact. Slower velocity penetrating objects result in damage that is limited to the actual pathway of the object.

4. Discuss the pathophysiology of, assessment findings with, and the management and need for rapid intervention and transport of the patient with chest wall injuries, including:

a.   Rib fracture   pp. 281-282, 302-303
Blunt or penetrating trauma induces a fracture and possible associated injury underneath. The fracture itself is of only limited concern; however, the pain from an such injury may limit chest excursion and suggests more serious injury beneath. Care is directed to administering oxygen, considering the possibility of underlying injury, and supplying pain medication to ensure respirations are not limited by pain. These injuries do not by themselves require immediate intervention or transport.

b.   Flail segment   pp. 283-284, 303
A flail segment is the result of several ribs (three or more) broken in numerous (two or more) places. This creates a rib segment that is free to move independently from the rest of the thorax. This paradoxical motion greatly decreases the efficiency of respiration as air that would be exhaled moves to the region under the flail segment and then returns to the unaffected lung with inspiration. Care includes seeing that the section is stabilized, the patient is given oxygen, possibly using overdrive ventilation. Consider the flail chest patient a candidate for rapid transport. Because of the severity of forces required to compromise the chest wall with this injury and the likelihood of serious underlying injury, this patient is given a high priority for care and transport.

c.   Sternal fracture pp. 282-283
As with the flail chest patient, suspect the patient with sternal fracture of having serious internal injury. The kinetic forces necessary to fracture the sternum are likely to injure and contuse the heart and other structures of the mediastinum. The patient will have a history of blunt chest trauma and may complain of chest pain similar to that of a myocardial infarction. Administer oxygen, monitor the heart with an ECG, and watch the patient very carefully for any signs of myocardial or great vessel injury. This patient is a candidate for rapid transport.

5. Discuss the pathophysiology of, assessment findings with, and management and need for rapid intervention and transport of the patient with injury to the lung, including:

a.   Simple pneumothorax   pp. 285-286
A simple or closed pneumothorax is an injury caused by either blunt or penetrating trauma that opens the airway to the pleural space. Air accumulates within the space and displaces the lung, resulting in less effective respirations and reduced oxygenation of the blood. This patient has a history of trauma and progressive dyspnea. Oxygen is administered and the patient is observed for progression to tension pneumothorax.

b.   Open pneumothorax   pp. 286-287, 303
Open pneumothorax is like simple pneumothorax, though in this case the injury penetrates the thoracic wall. The injury must be significantly large in order for air to move preferentially through the wound. The patient will have an open chest wound and dyspnea. Care includes sealing the

wound on three sides to prevent further progress of the pneumothorax, provision of oxygen, and monitoring the patient for the development of tension pneumothorax.

c.   Tension pneumothorax   pp. 287-288, 304-305
Tension pneumothorax is a pneumothorax created under the mechanisms associated with simple or open pneumothorax that progresses because of a valve-like injury site. The valve permits air to enter the pleural space but not exit. This results in a progressive lung collapse, followed by increasing pressure that displaces the mediastinum and restricts venous return to the heart. The patient has a trauma history and progressive dyspnea that becomes very severe. The patient may also display subcutaneous emphysema and distended jugular veins. Care is directed at decompressing the thorax with the insertion of a catheter into the 2nd intercostal space, providing oxygen, and monitoring the patient for a recurring tension pneumothorax.

d.   Hemothorax   pp. 288-289, 305
A hemothorax is a collection of blood in the pleural space. It may occur with or without pneumothorax. Hemothorax will generally become a hypovolemic problem before it seriously endangers respiration because the amount of fluid loss necessary to restrict respiration is great. The patient may experience dyspnea and the signs and symptoms of hypovolemic compensation (shock). Provide the patient with shock care, oxygen, fluid replacement, and rapid transport.

e.   Hemopneumothorax   p. 288
A hemopneumothorax is simply the existence of blood loss into the pleura and an accumulation of air there. Its presentation includes the signs and symptoms associated with both these pathologies. Care is directed at oxygen administration and rapid transport.

f.   Pulmonary contusion   pp. 289-290
Pulmonary contusion is a blunt trauma injury to the tissue of the lung resulting in edema and stiffening of the lung tissue. This reduces the efficiency of air exchange and causes an increased workload associated with respiration. If the region involved is limited, the patient may only experience very mild dyspnea. If the area is extensive, the patient may experience severe dyspnea. Care is centered around ensuring good oxygenation, including overdrive ventilation when indicated, and rapid transport.

6. **Discuss the pathophysiology of, findings of assessment with, and management and need for rapid intervention and transport of the patient with myocardial injuries, including:**

a.   Myocardial contusion   pp. 290-291, 306
Myocardial contusion is simply a contusion to the myocardium, usually related to blunt anterior chest trauma. The patient will present with myocardial-infarction-like pain and possible dysrhythmias. Care is directed at oxygen therapy, cardiac medications as indicated, and rapid transport.

b.   Pericardial tamponade   pp. 291-293, 306
Pericardial tamponade is usually related to penetrating trauma in which a wound permits blood from within the heart to enter the pericardium. It progressively fills the pericardium and restricts ventricular filling. The cardiac output drops and circulation is severely restricted. The patient will present with a penetrating trauma mechanism and will move quickly into shock, and possibly, sudden death. Care is insertion of a needle into the pericardial sac and the withdrawal of fluid. Any patient suspected of this injury requires immediate transport to the closest hospital.

c.   Myocardial rupture   pp. 293-294, 306
Myocardial rupture is often associated with high-velocity penetrating trauma. The bullet's passage through the engorged heart causes the blood to move outward from the bullet's path (cavitation) explosively. The heart wall tears, and the patient hemorrhages extensively as cardiac output ceases. The patient will display the signs of sudden death and no resuscitation efforts will be successful.

7. **Discuss the pathophysiology of, findings of assessment with, and management and need for rapid intervention and transport of the patient with vascular injuries, including injuries to:**

a.   Aorta   pp. 294, 306

Aortic aneurysm is a ballooning of the aorta as blunt trauma shears open the tunica intima and tunica media. Blood under systolic pressure enters the injury site and begins to dissect the vessel, causing it to balloon like a tire's inner tube. The patient will have a history of blunt trauma and complain of a tearing central chest pain that may radiate into the back. Care is centered around gentle but rapid transport to the trauma center. Oxygen is administered and fluid infusion should be very minimal.

A rupture or penetrating injury to the aorta results in almost immediate death as the vessel is very large and contains great pressure. The patient will have a history of penetrating or severe blunt chest trauma and display the signs of shock and move quickly to decompensation and death. Care is directed to oxygen administration, shock management, and rapid transport to the trauma center.

b.   Vena cava   p. 294

Injury to the vena cava is only slightly less severe than aortic injury since the vessels carry the same volume of fluid, but under different pressures (less for the vena cava). The progression of injury is just slightly slower with injury to the vena cava, though the result of injury is probably the same. In the field, it may be difficult to determine the exact blood vessel involved in a penetrating injury to the chest.

c.   Pulmonary arteries/veins   p. 294

As with aortic and vena caval injuries, the patient will have a history of penetrating or severe blunt trauma and the signs and symptoms of hypovolemia and shock. Care is directed at helping the body compensate for shock, some fluid resuscitation, and rapid transport.

8. **Discuss the pathophysiology of, findings of assessment with, and management and the need for rapid intervention and transport of patients with diaphragmatic, esophageal, and tracheobronchial injuries.   pp. 295-296, 306**

Diaphragmatic injury is usually due to severe compression of the diaphragm during blunt abdominal trauma or due to penetrating trauma along the border of the rib cage. Remember that the diaphragm is a dynamic muscle that moves up and down with respiration. Injury may result in less effective respiration and/or the movement of abdominal organs into the chest cavity, most commonly the bowel. The injury may present similarly to tension pneumothorax as the abdominal contents displace the lung tissue. Bowel sounds may also be heard in the chest, though it usually takes too much time to decipher these sounds. Care is directed at treating shock and dyspnea with rapid transport indicated.

Esophageal injury does not usually present with acute symptoms other than a history of penetrating trauma to the central chest. Perforation may permit food, drink, or gastric contents to enter the mediastinum, where it either forms an excellent medium for infection (with gastric contents) or damages some of the structures within. The result is serious damage to some of the most important structures within the chest and a significant mortality rate. The patient with such injury will present with penetrating injury to the region and care is directed toward other, more immediately important pathologies. Nevertheless, suspect esophageal injury and communicate that suspicion to the attending physician.

Tracheobronchial injuries are usually related to penetrating trauma to the upper mediastinum, and they open the major airways to the mediastinum. The injuries permit air to enter the mediastinum and possibly the neck. The patient will have dyspnea (possibly severe) and may have subcutaneous emphysema. Positive-pressure ventilation may make matters worse as air is then actively "pushed" into the mediastinal space. The patient may also experience pneumothorax and tension pneumothorax.

9. **Discuss the pathophysiology of, findings of assessment with, and management and need for rapid intervention and transport of the patient with traumatic asphyxia. pp. 296, 306-307**

Traumatic asphyxia is a crushing-type injury in which the crushing mechanism remains in place and restricts both respiration and venous return to the central circulation. The patient may display bulging eyes, petechial hemorrhage, and red or blue skin above the level of compression. The injury may damage many internal blood vessels but tamponades hemorrhage because of the continuing compression. Once the compression is released, profound hypovolemia may occur and the patient may demonstrate the signs and symptoms of serious internal injury. Care is directed at oxygen administration, ventilation, fluid resuscitation, and rapid transport to the trauma center.

10. **Differentiate between thoracic injuries based on the assessment and history. pp. 296-302**

Anterior blunt trauma is most likely to cause rib fracture, pulmonary contusion, closed pneumothorax ("paper bag" syndrome) (possibly progressing to tension pneumothorax), and myocardial contusion. Sharp pain suggests rib fracture, while dull pain suggests pulmonary or myocardial contusion. Dyspnea may be present in all circumstances but will likely be progressive and become severe with pulmonary contusion or pneumothorax. Lateral impact may cause traumatic aortic aneurysm with tearing chest pain, possibly radiating to the back. Crushing injury may cause traumatic asphyxia and display with a discolored upper body and severe shock at the pressure release.

Penetrating trauma may induce an open pneumothorax but is more likely to cause closed pneumothorax unless there is a very large entrance wound. Injury to the great vessels and heart may cause immediate exsanguination, while heart injury may lead to pericardial tamponade. Penetrating trauma to the central chest may perforate any mediastinal structure, including the trachea or esophagus. Rapid hypovolemia and shock suggest great vessel or heart injury, while progressively increasing dyspnea suggests tension pneumothorax. Severe dyspnea, absent breath sounds on the ipsilateral side, and distended jugular veins confirm a probable diagnosis of tension pneumothorax. Any penetration of the thorax with possible entry into the mediastinum should suggest esophageal or tracheal injury.

11. **Given several preprogrammed and moulaged thoracic trauma patients, provide the appropriate scene size-up, initial assessment, rapid trauma or focused physical exam and history, detailed exam, and ongoing assessment, and provide appropriate patient care and transportation. pp. 296-307**

During your training as a Paramedic you will participate in many classroom practice sessions involving simulated patients. You will also spend some time in the emergency departments of local hospitals as well as in advanced-level ambulances gaining clinical experience. During these times, use your knowledge of thoracic trauma to help you assess and care for the simulated or real patients you attend.

CONTENT SELF-EVALUATION

Multiple Choice

_____ 1. Which of the following is NOT likely to be associated with blunt trauma?
A. pericardial tamponade
B. pneumothorax (paper bag syndrome)
C. traumatic asphyxia
D. aortic aneurysm
E. myocardial contusion

_____ 2. Which of the following is NOT likely to be associated with penetrating trauma?
A. open pneumothorax
B. esophageal disruption
C. traumatic asphyxia
D. cavitational lung injury
E. comminuted fracture of the ribs

_____ 3. Rib fracture is found in about what percent of significant chest trauma?
A. 10 percent
B. 25 percent
C. 35 percent
D. 50 percent
E. 65 percent

_____ 4. Which ribs are fractured the most frequently?
A. ribs 1 and 3
B. ribs 4 through 8
C. ribs 7 through 9
D. ribs 8 through 11
E. ribs 9 through 12

_____ 5. Which rib group results in mortality up to 30 percent when they are fractured?
A. ribs 1 and 3
B. ribs 4 through 8
C. ribs 7 through 9
D. ribs 8 through 11
E. ribs 9 through 12

_____ 6. Which of the following groups is more likely to experience internal injury without rib fracture?
A. the pediatric patient
B. the adult male patient
C. the adult female patient
D. the elderly female patient
E. the elderly male patient

_____ 7. Which of the following is a sign or symptom of rib fracture?
A. local pain
B. crepitus
C. limited chest excursion
D. hemothorax
E. all of the above

_____ 8. Which of the following is most frequently associated with sternal fracture?
A. hemothorax
B. myocardial contusion
C. esophageal injury
D. simple pneumothorax
E. open pneumothorax

_____ 9. Air from under the flail segment in flail chest does which of the following?
A. moves out from under the segment during expiration
B. moves toward the segment during expiration
C. does not move with the segment
D. moves out from under the segment during inspiration
E. none of the above

_____ 10. Simple pneumothorax is associated with what percent of serious thoracic trauma?
A. 5
B. 10 to 30
C. 25 to 50
D. 60
E. more than 75

11. The condition in which a part of the chest wall moves in opposition to the rest of the chest due to numerous rib fractures is called:

    A.   pneumothorax.   **D.**   atelectasis.
    B.   tension pneumothorax.   **E.**   none of the above
    C.   hemothorax.

12. The chest injury that causes the patient to experience increasing dyspnea because of an open or closed pneumothorax that has a valve-like function and allows intrathoracic pressure to increase is referred to as:

    A.   subcutaneous emphysema.
    B.   traumatic asphyxia.
    C.   hyperbaric mediastinal displacement.
    D.   tension pneumothorax.
    E.   flail chest.

13. For air to move through an open wound to create an open pneumothorax, the wound opening must be:

    A.   just large enough to permit air passage.
    B.   two-thirds the size of the tracheal opening.
    C.   the size of the trachea.
    D.   about the size of a hunting rifle bullet.
    E.   larger than the trachea.

14. Which of the following is a very late sign of tension pneumothorax?

    A.   head and neck petechiae
    B.   intercostal bulging
    C.   a narrowing pulse pressure
    D.   tracheal deviation away from the injury
    E.   distended jugular veins

15. Each hemithorax can hold up to what volume of blood from a hemothorax?

    A.   500 mL   **D.**   3,000 mL
    B.   750 mL   **E.**   4,500 mL
    C.   1,500 mL

16. Which of the following statements is NOT true regarding hemothorax?

    A.   Hemorrhage into the thorax is more severe due to decreased pressure there.
    B.   Serious hemothorax may displace an entire lung and has a 75 percent mortality rate.
    C.   Hemothorax often occurs with pneumothorax.
    D.   Hemothorax rarely occurs with simple rib fractures.
    E.   none of the above

17. Distant or absent breath sounds heard during auscultation of the chest and the signs of shock are suggestive of which pathology?

    A.   pneumothorax   **D.**   pulmonary contusion
    B.   tension pneumothorax   **E.**   hemothorax
    C.   aortic aneurysm

18. Which of the following problems would most likely result in a chest area that was dull to percussion?

    A.   pneumothorax   **D.**   subcutaneous pneumothorax
    B.   tension pneumothorax   **E.**   pericardial tamponade
    C.   hemothorax

19. Your patient has received chest trauma yet did not initially present with crackles. However, as the assessment continues, they are heard in both the lower lung fields. This condition is most likely a result of which of the following?

A. pulmonary contusion   D. aortic aneurysm
B. hemothorax   E. pericardial tamponade
C. pneumothorax

20. The most common cause of myocardial contusion is:

A. blunt anterior chest trauma.   D. blunt posterior chest trauma.
B. blunt lateral chest trauma.   E. the pressure wave of an explosion.
C. penetrating anterior chest trauma.

21. A patient presents with the signs of shock, jugular vein distention, distant heart sounds, and a narrowing pulse pressure. The lung fields are clear. Which condition is most likely the cause?

A. tension pneumothorax   D. pericardial tamponade
B. hemothorax   E. atelectasis
C. traumatic asphyxia

22. Pericardial tamponade occurs with what frequency in serious chest trauma patients?

A. less than 2 percent of the time   D. 25 percent of the time
B. 10 percent of the time   E. 30 to 45 percent of the time
C. 20 percent of the time

23. Which of the following is a sign of pericardial tamponade?

A. pulsus paradoxus   D. hypotension
B. a narrowing pulse pressure   E. all of the above
C. distended jugular veins

24. The patient with pericardial tamponade may be in hypovolemic shock due to the volume of blood lost into:

A. conus medularis   D. lung
B. pericardial sac   E. aortic arch
C. right atrium

25. A decrease in jugular vein distention during inspiration is known as:

A. Beck's triad.   D. Kussmaul's sign.
B. pulsus paradoxus.   E. electrical alternans.
C. Cushing's reflex.

26. Your patient was involved in a lateral impact auto accident. The car is greatly deformed, though the patient does not have many signs of injury. During your assessment, he complains of a tearing sensation in his central chest and numbness in his left upper extremity. Your highest index of suspicion of injury is for:

A. traumatic asphyxia.   D. myocardial contusion.
B. pulmonary contusion.   E. pericardial tamponade.
C. aortic aneurysm.

27. What percentage of patients with traumatic aortic aneurysm survive the initial impact and injury?

A. as high as 10 percent   D. 70 percent
B. as high as 20 percent   E. 73 percent
C. 50 percent

28. In a patient with a history of blunt lateral trauma and a suspected traumatic aortic aneurysm, which signs or symptoms would you expect to find?
- **A.** severe tearing chest pain
- **B.** pulse deficit between extremities
- **C.** reduced pulse strength in the lower extremities
- **D.** hypertension
- **E.** all of the above

29. A harsh systolic murmur is heard over the central chest. This is suggestive of which pathology?
- **A.** pneumothorax
- **B.** tension pneumothorax
- **C.** traumatic aortic aneurysm
- **D.** pulmonary contusion
- **E.** hemothorax

30. The traumatic diaphragmatic rupture is likely to present like which of the following thoracic injuries?
- **A.** tension pneumothorax
- **B.** pulmonary contusion
- **C.** aortic aneurysm
- **D.** pericardial tamponade
- **E.** esophageal injury

31. The two major problems associated with traumatic asphyxia are restriction of chest excursion and:
- **A.** distortion of the airway.   .
- **B.** restriction of venous return.
- **C.** atelectasis.
- **D.** hemorrhage during the compression
- **E.** massive strokes.

32. The classic signs of traumatic asphyxia include which of the following?
- **A.** bulging eyes
- **B.** conjunctival hemorrhage
- **C.** petechiae of the head and neck
- **D.** dark red or purple appearance of the head and neck
- **E.** all of the above

33. Serious penetrating trauma will likely require which of the following body substance isolation procedures?
- **A.** gloves
- **B.** face shield
- **C.** gown
- **D.** mask
- **E.** all of the above

34. During your assessment of a supine patient with blunt chest trauma, you notice slight jugular vein distention. With no other signs of injury, this suggests which of the following?
- **A.** a normal patient
- **B.** pericardial tamponade
- **C.** tension pneumothorax
- **D.** traumatic asphyxia
- **E.** B, C, and D

35. Crackles heard during auscultation of the chest are suggestive of which pathology?

- **A.** pneumothorax
- **B.** tension pneumothorax
- **C.** aortic aneurysm
- **D.** pulmonary contusion
- **E.** hemothorax

36. Hyperresonance heard during percussion of the chest is suggestive of which pathology?
- **A.** pneumothorax
- **B.** tension pneumothorax
- **C.** hemothorax
- **D.** pulmonary contusion
- **E.** both A and B

37. Which of the following thoracic structures takes the least energy to fracture and often results in a more common, yet less serious, thoracic injury?
- **A.** ribs 1 through 3
- **B.** ribs 4 through 9
- **C.** ribs 10 through 12
- **D.** the sternum
- **E.** the manubrium

38. A patient who displays subcutaneous emphysema is most likely to have which of the conditions listed below?
- **A.** traumatic asphyxia
- **B.** tension pneumothorax
- **C.** the paper bag syndrome
- **D.** pulmonary contusion
- **E.** cardiac contusion

39. Which of the following is an indication for the use of PASG?
- **A.** diaphragmatic rupture
- **B.** penetrating chest injury
- **C.** blunt chest trauma with a blood pressure below 100
- **D.** blunt chest trauma with a blood pressure below 60
- **E.** suspected pericardial tamponade

40. The patient who is suspected of a flail chest or other thoracic cage injury, without suspected spine injury, should be positioned:
- **A.** on the uninjured side.
- **B.** on the injured side.
- **C.** supine with legs elevated.
- **D.** on the left lateral side.
- **E.** on the right lateral side.

41. The open pneumothorax should be cared for using which of the following techniques?
- **A.** Pack the wound with a sterile dressing.
- **B.** Cover the wound an occlusive dressing and tape securely.
- **C.** Cover the wound with an occlusive dressing, taped on three sides.
- **D.** Attempt to close the wound with a hemostat and then cover with a sterile dressing.
- **E.** Cover the wound loosely with a sterile dressing.

42. Which location is recommended for prehospital pleural decompression?
- **A.** 2nd intercostal space, midclavicular line
- **B.** 5th intercostal space, midclavicular line
- **C.** 5th intercostal space, midaxillary line
- **D.** A and B
- **E.** A and C

43. A few minutes after you have inserted a needle and decompressed a tension pneumothorax, you notice that a patient's dyspnea is getting worse and breath sounds on the injured side are becoming diminished. Which action would you take?
- **A.** Insert a second needle.
- **B.** Remove the dressing.
- **C.** Provide overdrive ventilation.
- **D.** Consider nitrous oxide administration.
- **E.** all of the above

44. A patient is trapped in a wrecked auto for about half an hour and is suspected of having traumatic asphyxia. Care should include which of the following?
- **A.** two large-bore IVs
- **B.** normal saline or lactated Ringer's solution
- **C.** fluids run rapidly
- **D.** consideration of sodium bicarbonate
- **E.** all of the above

45. What percentage of traumatic deaths are secondary to injuries in the thoracic region?
    A.   10
    B.   15
    C.   20
    D.   25
    E.   30

True/False

46. As the pain of the flail chest increases with time, the amount of paradoxical movement will decrease due to muscular splinting.
    A.   True
    B.   False

47. Extensive pulmonary contusions may account for blood losses up to 1,500 mL.
    A.   True
    B.   False

48. If the chamber of the heart is significantly damaged yet does not rupture immediately, it is likely to rupture in around two weeks.
    A.   True
    B.   False

49. The right side is the site of most diaphragmatic ruptures as most assailants are right-handed.
    A.   True
    B.   False

50. Overdrive ventilation (bag-valve masking) of the patient with flail chest will cause the flail segment to move with, rather than in opposition to, the chest wall.
    A.   True
    B.   False

51. Meperidine, diazepam, or morphine sulfate may be given to the minor rib fracture patient to reduce pain and increase respiratory excursion.
    A.   True
    B.   False

52. A flail chest is described as three of more adjacent ribs fractured in three or more places.
    A.   True
    B.   False

53. In the absence of hypovolemia, JVD is a classic sign of a tension pneumothorax.
    A.   True
    B.   False

54. Chest wall contusion is the most common result of blunt trauma to the thorax.
    A.   True
    B.   False

55. A simple pneumothorax may present with little or no symptoms.
    A.   True
    B.   False

Matching

Write the letter of the term in the space provided next to the appropriate description.

A.	co-morbidity	**F.**	flail chest
B.	pneumothorax	**G.**	hemoptysis
C.	precordium	**H.**	tracheobronchial tree
D.	hemothorax	**I.**	pulsus paradoxus
E.	aneurysm	**J.**	hemopneumothorax

_____ 56. coughing of blood that has origin in the respiratory tract

_____ 57. the structures of the trachea and the bronchi

_____ 58. area of the chest wall overlying the heart

_____ 59. a weakening or ballooning in the wall of a blood vessel

_____ 60. associated with disease process

_____ 61. blood within the pleural space

_____ 62. air in the pleural space

_____ 63. drop of greater than 10 mmHg in the systolic BP during the inspiratory phase of respiration

_____ 64. condition where air and blood are in the pleural space

_____ 65. defect in the chest wall that allows for free movement of a segment

Chapter 26

Abdominal Trauma

Review of Chapter Objectives

After reading this chapter, you should be able to:

1. **Describe the epidemiology, including the morbidity/mortality, for patients with abdominal trauma as well as prevention strategies to avoid the injuries.**   **p. 310**

While serious abdominal trauma accounts for some mortality, it ranks behind head and chest trauma as a region associated with trauma deaths. Rapid transport to the trauma center and modern surgical techniques have accounted for a great decrease in abdominal trauma mortality and morbidity, but it still remains a serious consideration during trauma assessment and care. Highway and vehicle design and the proper use of restraints have reduced abdominal injuries greatly, however, and more correct use of seat belts by greater numbers of the population can lead to continuing decreases in both the incidence and severity of abdominal injury.

2. **Apply epidemiologic principles to develop prevention strategies for abdominal injuries.** **p. 310**

The current major causes of abdominal injury are improper seat belt use and violence. Education programs designed to promote the use and proper application of seat belts and programs to reduce unintentional or deliberate injuries resulting from handguns can help further reduce abdominal injury.

3. **Describe the anatomy and physiology of organs and structures related to abdominal injuries.** **(see Chapter 12)**

The abdomen is one of the body's largest cavities, bounded superiorly by the diaphragm, laterally by the flank muscles, inferiorly by the pelvis, posteriorly by the spine and back muscles, and anteriorly by the abdominal muscles. Since most of its border is soft tissue, it is rather unprotected from injury. The abdomen contains the continuous, muscular tube of digestion, the alimentary canal. It enters the abdomen through the hiatus of the diaphragm as the esophagus. It joins the stomach, an organ that physically mixes the food with gastric juices and then sends it out and into the small bowel. The first portion of the bowel, the duodenum, mixes the digesting food with bile (a byproduct of the liver) and pancreatic juices and then begins the process of absorption. The remainder of the small bowel draws the nutrients from the food.

As the digesting food enters the large bowel it is mixed with bacteria, releasing water and any remaining nutrients. They are absorbed, and the material is pushed by peristalsis to the rectum, awaiting defecation. The bowel is a thin and vascular tube that drains its blood supply through the liver for detoxification, where some nutrients are stored and others added to the circulation.
The liver is a large, solid organ found in the right upper quadrant, just below the diaphragm. The pancreas is a delicate organ found in the lower aspect of the upper left quadrant with a portion of it extending into the right upper quadrant. In addition to digestive juices, it manufactures insulin and glucagon. The kidneys are found deep within the flanks and filter blood to remove excess water and electrolytes. They are very vascular organs that excrete urine into the ureters through which the urine then travels to the bladder. The bladder (in the central pelvic space) rids the body of urine through the

urethra. The spleen is an organ of the immune system and is very delicate and vascular, residing in the left upper quadrant.

The abdominal cavity is lined with a serous membrane, the peritoneum. It covers the anterior abdominal organs and a double-layer sheath of it forms the omentum, which covers the anterior surface of the abdomen. The bowel is slung from the posterior wall of the abdomen by connective tissue called the mesentery that also provides perfusion to the bowel. The abdominal aorta and inferior vena cava run along the spinal column and branch frequently to serve the abdominal organs.

4. Predict abdominal injuries based on blunt and penetrating mechanisms of injury. pp. 310-318

Blunt trauma compresses, shears, or decelerates the various organs and structures within the abdomen resulting in rupture of the hollow organs, fracture or tearing of the solid organs, or tearing or severance of the abdominal vasculature. The spleen is the most frequently injured organ with the liver the second most commonly injured structure. The bowel, kidneys, and diaphragm are also common recipients of blunt injury.

Penetrating injury to the abdomen may involve low- and high-velocity objects. Bullets disrupt a larger cylinder of tissue with their passage and are especially damaging to hollow organs filled with fluid and to the extremely dense and delicate solid organs of the abdomen. Mortality is about ten times greater with high-energy bullets than with stab-type wounds. The liver is affected more frequently than the bowel, with the spleen, kidneys, and pancreas injured in descending order of frequency. A special category of penetrating injury is the shotgun blast. At short range (under 3 yards), the projectiles have tremendous energy and create numerous tracts of serious injury.

5. Describe open and closed abdominal injuries. pp. 310-313

Open wounds to the abdomen may be very small, such as those caused by a bullet or knife, or large enough to permit abdominal contents to protrude (an evisceration). Bullet wounds may cause injury beyond their direct path through cavitation and are especially harmful to the solid organs (liver, spleen, kidneys, pancreas) or to the stomach and intestinal tract when full of fluid. Shotgun blasts, especially if delivered from less than 7 feet, are extremely damaging because the many small projectiles still have significant kinetic energy and have not yet spread out to disperse their energy.

Blunt (closed) injuries may compress the internal organs of the abdomen between the offending object and the spine or posterior abdominal wall or between other organs. The force may shear solid organs and their vascular attachments or may directly cause organ fracture and hemorrhage or the spillage of organ contents or both. Hollow organs may rupture and spill their contents into the abdominal cavity. Severe abdominal compression may rupture the diaphragm and push abdominal organs into the thorax.

6. Identify the need for rapid intervention and transport of the patient with abdominal injuries based on assessment findings. pp. 318-324

The abdomen, for the most part, is bound by connective and muscle tissue rather than the skeletal structures found protecting the skull and thorax. This permits an easier transmission of traumatic forces to the internal organs and frequent injury. The abdomen also does not show the dramatic signs and symptoms of injury seen elsewhere, again because of the lack of rigid skeletal protection. Hence, it is important to carefully assess the abdominal cavity, looking for any sign of trauma (such as erythema), and to question the patient about pain or other abdominal symptoms. Blood, bacteria, and, to a lesser degree, gastric, duodenal, and pancreatic contents irritate the abdominal lining (the peritoneum) only after the passage of time, which again limits the signs and symptoms of serious abdominal injury visible during prehospital care.

7. Explain the pathophysiology of solid and hollow organ injuries, abdominal vascular injuries, pelvic fractures, and other abdominal injuries. pp. 313-318

Solid Organ Injuries

The spleen is well protected, although it is very delicate and not contained within a strong capsule. It frequently ruptures and bleeds heavily. The liver is a very dense and vascular organ in the right upper quadrant just behind the lower border of the rib cage. It is contained within a strong capsule, although it can be lacerated during severe deceleration by its restraining ligament (the ligamentum teres). The kidneys are well protected both by their location deep within the flank and by strong capsules. The pancreas is located in the lower portion of the left upper quadrant, extending just into the right quadrant. It is more delicate than either the liver or kidneys even though it lies deep within the central abdomen. When injured, it may hemorrhage and release pancreatic juices into the abdomen.

Hollow Organ Injuries

Hollow organs include the stomach, small and large bowel, rectum, gall bladder, urinary bladder, and pregnant uterus. Compression may contuse them or cause them to rupture while penetrating injury may perforate them. The gall bladder, stomach, and first part of the small bowel may release digestive juices that will chemically irritate and damage the abdominal structures. Injury can cause the rest of the bowel to release material high in bacterial load that can induce infection. The rupture of the urinary bladder will release blood and urine into the abdomen. Injury to the abdomen may cause blood in emesis (hematemesis), blood in the stool (hematochezia), or blood in the urine (hematuria).

Abdominal Vascular Injuries

The major vascular structures of the abdomen include the abdominal aorta, the inferior vena cava, and many arteries branching to the abdominal organs. These vessels may be injured by blunt trauma, though penetrating trauma is a far more frequent cause of injury. The abdomen does not develop an internal pressure against hemorrhage as do the muscles and other solid regions of the body, and bleeding may continue unabated while the accumulation of blood is difficult to recognize.

Pelvic Fractures

Pelvic fractures are addressed in Chapter 22, "Musculoskeletal Trauma," Division 3. However, remember that pelvic fracture can cause injury to the bladder, genitalia, and rectum, and to some very large blood vessels with serious associated hemorrhage.

Other Abdominal Organ Injuries

Other injuries include injuries to the mesentery and peritoneum. The mesentery supports the bowel and may be injured, most commonly at points of fixation like the ileocecal or duodenal/jejunal junctures. Hemorrhage here is often contained by the peritoneum. Peritoneal injury is generally related to irritation either by chemical action (most rapid) or by bacterial contamination (12 to 24 hours).

8. Describe the assessment findings associated with and management of solid and hollow organ injuries, abdominal vascular injuries, pelvic fractures, and other abdominal injuries. pp. 318-324

Injury to the abdominal contents is difficult to ascertain because the signs and symptoms of injury are often diffuse and around 30 percent of patients with serious abdominal injury have no clear signs or symptoms of injury. During assessment, you should seek to discover what evidence of injury exists and what it suggests about the injury's precise nature and location. Pay attention to pain, tenderness, and rebound tenderness in each quadrant and note any thirst or other signs of hypovolemia and shock.

The management of the patient with suspected abdominal trauma is basically supportive with airway maintenance, oxygen, ventilation as needed, and fluid resuscitation. Establish large-bore IVs but do not run fluids aggressively unless the blood pressure drops below 100 mmHg. Use of the PASG may be helpful, especially if the blood pressure drops below 50 mmHg. Cover any evisceration with a sterile dressing soaked in normal saline and cover that with an occlusive dressing to prevent evaporation. As with all hypovolemia patients, keep the patient warm and provide rapid transport.

9. Differentiate between abdominal injuries based on the assessment and history. pp. 318-323

As mentioned earlier, 30 percent of patients with serious abdominal injury present without signs and symptoms. Many others present with diffuse signs and symptoms, making it very hard to differentiate among the different abdominal pathologies. Try to relate the mechanism of injury or any patient complaints to the anatomic region involved and the specific organs found there. For example, left flank trauma and pain may suggest splenic injury, while right upper quadrant injury and pain may suggest liver pathology.

Penetrating abdominal trauma will present with an entrance wound and, possibly, an exit wound. It may also manifest with the signs and symptoms of blunt abdominal trauma due to the same mechanisms. Evisceration will be evident by the protrusion of bowel from an open wound involving the abdominal wall.

Blunt abdominal trauma may be recognized by abdominal tenderness, rebound tenderness, pain, or a pulsing mass. It may involve any of the abdominal or retroperitoneal organs. Signs will be superficial such as contusions or, more likely, erythema. Symptoms may result from the injury or from blood, body fluids, or bacteria (causing delayed pain) in the peritoneal cavity.

10. Given several preprogrammed and moulaged abdominal trauma patients, provide the appropriate scene size-up, initial assessment, rapid trauma or focused physical exam and history, detailed exam, and ongoing assessment, and provide appropriate patient care and transportation. pp. 318-326

During your training as a Paramedic you will participate in many classroom practice sessions involving simulated patients. You will also spend some time in the emergency departments of local hospitals as well as in advanced-level ambulances gaining clinical experience. During these times, use your knowledge of abdominal trauma to help you assess and care for the simulated or real patients you attend.

CONTENT SELF-EVALUATION

Multiple Choice

1. Penetrating mechanisms of injury are responsible for what percentage of injuries to the liver?
   - A. 50 percent
   - B. 40 percent
   - C. 30 percent
   - D. 20 percent
   - E. 10 percent

2. Blunt mechanisms of injury are responsible for what percentage of injuries to the liver?
   - A. 50 percent
   - B. 40 percent
   - C. 30 percent
   - D. 20 percent
   - E. 10 percent

3. Which of the following organs is most frequently damaged during blunt abdominal trauma?
   - A. the small bowel
   - B. the liver
   - C. the spleen
   - D. the kidneys
   - E. the pancreas

_____ 4. Penetration of the abdominal wall resulting in protrusion of the abdominal contents is called:
  A. peristalsis.   D. emulsification.
  B. chyme.   E. evisceration.
  C. peritonitis.

_____ 5. The abdominal organs, with deep expiration, move as far up into the thorax as:
  A. the xiphoid process.   D. the seventh intercostal space.
  B. the tips of the floating ribs. E. none of the above
  C. the nipple line.

_____ 6. The term describing frank blood in the stool is:
  A. hematochezia.   D. hematuria.
  B. hematemesis.   E. hematocrit.
  C. hemoptysis.

_____ 7. The organ most likely to be injured by left flank blunt trauma is:
  A. the small bowel.   D. the kidneys.
  B. the liver.   E. the pancreas.
  C. the spleen.

_____ 8. The organ that is likely to be injured in severe deceleration as its ligament restrains, then lacerates it is:

  A. the small bowel.   D. the kidneys.
  B. the liver.   E. the pancreas.
  C. the spleen.

_____ 9. Hemorrhage into the abdomen is of serious concern because it:
  A. quickly puts pressure on internal organs.
  B. limits respirations.
  C. rapidly affects the heart.
  D. may trigger a vagal response, slowing the heart.
  E. none of the above

_____ 10. Blunt injury to the mesentery often occurs at:
  A. the gastric-duodenal juncture. D. the ileocecal juncture.
  B. the duodenal-jejunal juncture. E. both B and C
  C. the jejunal-ileal juncture.

_____ 11. How long does it take bacteria to grow in sufficient numbers to irritate the peritoneum?
  A. 2 to 4 hours   D. 8 to 10 hours
  B. 4 to 6 hours   E. over 12 hours
  C. 6 to 8 hours

_____ 12. The number one killer of pregnant females is:
  A. heart attack.   D. trauma.
  B. ectopic pregnancy.   E. stroke.
  C. allergic reactions.

_____ 13. Unrestrained pregnant occupants in vehicles are how many more times likely to suffer fetal mortality in an auto collision than their belted counterparts?
  A. two   D. five
  B. three   E. six
  C. four

14. Supine positioning of the mother may cause hypotension due to:
  A.   compression of the inferior vena cava.
  B.   increased circulation to the uterus.
  C.   increased intra-abdominal pressure.
  D.   decreased intra-abdominal pressure.
  E.   Kussmaul's respirations.

15. It may take a maternal blood loss of what percentage before the heart rate begins to increase in the late term pregnancy?
  A.   10 to 15 percent   D.   25 to 30 percent
  B.   15 to 20 percent   E.   30 to 35 percent
  C.   20 to 25 percent

16. Due to the flexibility of the pediatric thorax, which injury is more likely to occur with blunt trauma?
  A.   liver injury   D.   all of the above
  B.   splenic injury   E.   none of the above
  C.   kidney injury

17. Children may not show signs of blood loss until they have lost what percentage of their volume?
  A.   25 percent   D.   50 percent
  B.   35 percent   E.   65 percent
  C.   45 percent

18. What percentage of patients with abdominal injury do not present with any signs or symptoms?
  A.   10 percent   D.   40 percent
  B.   20 percent   E.   50 percent
  C.   30 percent

19. Blunt injury to the right flank region is likely to cause which of the following?
  A.   liver injury   D.   bladder injury
  B.   kidney injury   E.   colon injury
  C.   bowel injury

20. Hemorrhage into the abdomen may account for how much blood loss before it becomes noticeable?
  A.   500 mL   D.   1 500 mL
  B.   750 mL   E.   2 500 mL
  C.   1 000 mL

21. The major reason auscultation of bowel and other abdominal sounds is not recommended in the field is because:
  A.   the sounds are not clear.
  B.   the sounds do not rule out injury.
  C.   the lack of sounds does not confirm injury.
  D.   it takes too long to assess bowel sounds adequately.
  E.   B, C, and D.

22. Prehospital administration of IV fluid should be limited to:
  A.   1 000 mL.   D.   4 000 mL.
  B.   2 000 mL.   E.   5 000 mL.
  C.   3 000 mL.

23. Care for the abdominal evisceration includes use of which of the following?
    A.   a dry adherent dressing
    B.   a dry nonadherent dressing
    C.   a sterile dressing moistened with normal saline
    D.   an occlusive dressing
    E.   a sterile cotton gauze dressing

24. At what blood pressure would you consider applying the PASG in the presence of an abdominal evisceration?
    A.   120 mmHg   D.   60 mmHg
    B.   100 mmHg   E.   30 mmHg
    C.   90 mmHg

25. Which position is indicated for the late pregnancy patient?
    A.   supine   D.   Trendelenburg
    B.   left lateral recumbent   E.   with the head elevated 30 degrees
    C.   right lateral recumbent

26. Use of the PASG is contraindicated in:
    A.   geriatric patients.   D.   abdominal evisceration patients.
    B.   patients with low blood pressure.   E.   diabetic patients.
    C.   tuberculosis patients.

27. Penetrating trauma to which of the following may also affect the abdomen and injure its contents.
    A.   the buttocks   D.   the thorax
    B.   the flanks   E.   all of the above
    C.   the back

28. Blood loss from an injured spleen may accumulate against the diaphragm resulting in referred pain to the:
    A.   right shoulder region   D.   left shoulder region
    B.   lower back   E.   periumbilical region
    C.   mid-scapula region

29. By the third trimester, maternal blood volume is increased by what percentage?
    A.   20   D.   25
    B.   35   E.   40
    C.   45

30. Damage to hollow organs results in hemorrhage and in spillage of their contents inot which of the following locations?

    A.   peritoneal spaces   D.   A and B
    B.   retroperitoneal spaces   E.   A, B and C
    C.   pelvic spaces

True/False

31. Due to the anatomy of the abdomen, injury to its contents often presents with limited signs and symptoms.
    A.   True
    B.   False

32. Bullets cause an abdominal wound mortality rate that is about equal to that caused by slow-moving penetrating objects.
    A.   True
    B.   False

_____ **33.** The abdomen is the area for greatest concern when the patient is exposed to severe blast forces.
  A. True
  B. False

_____ **34.** Most abdominal vascular injuries are associated with penetrating trauma.
  A. True
  B. False

_____ **35.** The late-term pregnant female is at increased risk for vomiting and aspiration.
  A. True
  B. False

_____ **36.** The signs of abdominal trauma may become less specific due to the progression of peritonitis.
  A. True
  B. False

_____ **37.** Thirst may be one of the few symptoms of abdominal injury as internal hemorrhage loss draws down the body's blood volume.
  A. True
  B. False

_____ **38.** Aggressive fluid resuscitation may aggravate the relative anemia associated with late term pregnancy.
  A. True
  B. False

_____ **39.** Use of the PASG may be beneficial for the patient in early (first-term) pregnancy.
  A. True
  B. False

_____ **40.** In abdominal trauma, shallow breathing may be due to spilling of the abdominal contents into the thorax.
  A. True
  B. False

Matching

Write the letter of the term in the space provided next to the appropriate description.

A.	evisceration	**F.**	hematuria
B.	hematemesis	**G.**	abruptio placentae
C.	peritonitis	**H.**	rupture
D.	hematochezia	**I.**	sepsis
E.	guarding	**J.**	rebound tenderness

_____ **41.** protective tensing of the abdominal muscles by a patient suffering abdominal pain

_____ **42.** blood in the stool

_____ **43.** pain on release of the paramedic's hands, allowing the patient's abdominal wall to return to its normal position

_____ **44.** fracture

_____ **45.** blood in the urine

_____ **46.** a condition in which the placenta separates from the uterine wall

_____ **47.** a protrusion of organs from a wound

_____ **48.** infection

_____ **49.** the vomiting of blood

_____ **50.** inflammation of the peritoneum caused by chemical or bacterial irritation

Essentials of Paramedic Care

Division 4

Medical Emergencies

Chapter 27

Pulmonology

Review of Chapter Objectives

With each chapter of the Workbook, we identify the objectives and the important elements of the text content. You should review these items and refer to the pages listed if any points are not clear.

After reading this chapter, you should be able to:

1. Discuss the epidemiology of pulmonary diseases and pulmonary conditions. p. 331

Respiratory emergencies are among the most common EMS calls—up to 28 percent, according to one study. Respiratory emergencies lead to over 20 000 deaths per year. Because of the frequency of such calls, it is critical that you be knowledgeable about diseases that affect the respiratory system.

2. Identify and describe the function of the structures located in the upper and lower airway. (see Chapter 12)

The airway is functionally divided into the upper airway and the lower airway. The upper airway is comprised of the nasal cavity, pharynx, and larynx. The lower airway is comprised of the trachea, bronchi, alveoli, and lungs. The ability to take in oxygen and excrete carbon dioxide via the airway is essential to life. Therefore, it is critical that you be able to identify and understand the function of each structure of the airway and of the airway as a whole.

3. Discuss the physiology of ventilation and respiration.   (see Chapter 12)

The major function of the respiratory system is the exchange of gases between the person and the environment. Three processes allow the gas exchange to take place: ventilation, diffusion, and perfusion. Ventilation is the movement of air in and out of the lungs. Diffusion is the movement of gases between the lungs and the pulmonary capillaries (oxygen from the lungs into the bloodstream; waste carbon dioxide from the bloodstream into the lungs) as well as between the systemic capillaries and the body tissues (oxygen from the bloodstream into the cells; waste carbon dioxide from the cells into the bloodstream). Perfusion is the circulation of blood through the capillaries. Adequate perfusion is critical to adequate gas exchange in the lungs and body tissues. These three processes—ventilation, diffusion, and perfusion—together provide for respiration.

4. Identify common pathological events that affect the pulmonary system.   pp. 333-337

Any disease state that affects the pulmonary system will ultimately disrupt ventilation, diffusion, or perfusion, or a combination of these processes. Ventilation may be disrupted by diseases that cause obstruction of any part of the airway, disrupt the normal function of the chest wall, or impair nervous system control of breathing. Diffusion can be disrupted by a change in concentration of atmospheric oxygen or by any disease that affects the structure or patency of alveoli, the thickness of the respiratory membrane, or the permeability of the capillaries. Perfusion will be affected by any disease that limits blood flow through the lungs and the body or reduces the volume of the oxygen-carrying red blood cells or hemoglobin. Understanding how different diseases and conditions may affect the processes of respiration is important to your ability to choose appropriate emergency care for a respiratory emergency.

5. Compare various airway and ventilation techniques used in the management of pulmonary diseases.   pp. 348-369

Two principles govern the overall management of respiratory emergencies. (1) Give first priority to the airway. (2) Always provide oxygen to patients with respiratory distress or the possibility of hypoxia, including those with chronic obstructive pulmonary disease (COPD).

6. Review the use of equipment utilized during the physical examination of patients with complaints associated with respiratory diseases and conditions.   pp. 342-343, 345-347

You should be familiar with the use of equipment that is available for physical examination of patients with respiratory complaints. Equipment includes the stethoscope, the pulse oximeter, hand-held devices for measuring peak expiratory flow rate (PEFR), and end-tidal carbon dioxide detection devices.

7. Identify the epidemiology, anatomy, physiology, pathophysiology, assessment findings, and management (including pre-hospital medications) for the following respiratory diseases and conditions:

a.   Adult respiratory distress syndrome   pp. 349-351

Adult respiratory distress syndrome (ARDS) is characterized by pulmonary edema caused by fluid accumulation in the interstitial spaces in the lungs. The mortality rate is 70 percent. ARDS occurs as a result of increased vascular permeability and decreased fluid removal from the lungs. A variety of lung insults can cause this inability to maintain proper fluid balance, including sepsis, pneumonia, inhalation injuries, emboli, tumors, and others noted in the text chapter. ARDS interferes with diffusion, causing hypoxia. In addition to evaluating the degree of the patient's respiratory distress, assessment is aimed at discovering symptoms and history that point to the underlying condition. Pre-hospital management is supportive (oxygen supplementation is essential to compensate for diffusion defects); in-hospital care is aimed at treatment of the underlying condition.

b.   Bronchial asthma   pp. 351-352, 356-358

Asthma is an obstructive lung disease that causes abnormal ventilation. While deaths from other respiratory diseases are decreasing, deaths from asthma have been on the increase, with 50 percent of those deaths occurring before the patient reaches the hospital. Asthma is thought to be caused by a combination of genetic predisposition and environmental triggers that differ from individual to individual. These include allergens, cold air, exercise, stress, and certain medications. Exposure to a trigger causes release of histamine which, in turn, causes both bronchial constriction and capillary leakage that leads to bronchial edema. The result is a significant decrease in expiratory airflow, which is the essence of an "asthma attack." In the early phase of an attack, inhaled bronchodilator medications such as salbutamol will help. In the late phase, inflammation sets in and anti-inflammatory drugs are required to alleviate the condition. Assessment must focus first on evaluation and support of the airway and breathing. Most patients will report a history of asthma. The physical exam should focus on the chest and neck to assess breathing effort. The respiratory rate is the most critical of the vital signs. EMS systems should also be able to measure the peak expiratory flow rate. Treatment is aimed at correction of hypoxia (oxygen administration) and relief of bronchospasm and inflammation. A special case is status asthmaticus—a severe, prolonged attack that does not respond to bronchodilators. It is a serious emergency requiring prompt recognition, treatment, and transport. Another special case is asthma in children, which is treated much as for adults but with altered medication dosages and some special medications.

c. **Chronic bronchitis** **pp. 351-352, 354-355**

Chronic bronchitis is classified, along with emphysema, as a chronic obstructive pulmonary disease (COPD). COPD affects 25 percent of adults, with chronic bronchitis affecting one in five adult males. Chronic bronchitis reduces ventilation as a result of increased mucus production that blocks airway passages. It is often caused by cigarette smoking but also occurs in nonsmokers. There may be a history of frequent respiratory infections. Chronic bronchitis is usually associated with a productive cough and copious sputum. Patients tend to be overweight and often become cyanotic, so they are sometimes called "blue bloaters." Auscultation of the airway often reveals rhonchi due to mucus occlusion. The goals of treatment are relief of hypoxia and reversal of bronchoconstriction. Because these patients may be dependent on a hypoxic respiratory drive (low oxygen levels stimulate respiration), respiratory effort may become depressed when oxygen is administered. Needed oxygen should not be withheld, but the patient's respirations must be carefully monitored. IV fluids may help loosen mucous congestion. Medical direction may also order administration of a bronchodilator, such as salbutamol, or ipratropium bromide, and may also recommend corticosteroid administration.

d. **Emphysema** **pp. 352-353**

Like chronic bronchitis, emphysema is classified as a chronic obstructive pulmonary disease (COPD). Alveolar walls are destroyed by exposure to noxious substances such as cigarette smoke or other environmental toxins. The disease also causes destruction of the walls of the small bronchioles, which contributes to a trapping of air in the lungs. The result is a decrease in both ventilation and diffusion. Patients tend to breathe through pursed lips, which creates a positive pressure that helps to prevent alveolar collapse. A developing decrease in PaO_2 leads to a compensatory increase in red blood cell production (polycythemia). Emphysema patients are more susceptible to acute respiratory infections and cardiac dysrhythmias. They become dependant on bronchodilators and corticosteroids and, in the final stages, supplemental oxygen. In contrast to chronic bronchitis sufferers, emphysema patients often lose weight and seldom have a cough except early in the morning. Because of the habit of breathing through pursed lips and the color produced by polycythemia, they are sometimes called "pink puffers." Clubbed fingers are common. Auscultation may reveal diminished breath sounds and, at times, wheezes and rhonchi. There may also be signs of right-sided heart disease. As a result of severe respiratory impairment, COPD patients may exhibit confusion, agitation, somnolence, 1-to-2-word dyspnea, and use of accessory muscles to assist respiration.

e. **Pneumonia** **pp. 360-361**

Pneumonia, or lung infection, is a leading cause of death in the elderly and those with HIV infection and is the fifth leading cause of death in Canada overall. It is an infection most commonly caused by bacterial or viral infection, rarely by fungal and other infections. Risk factors center on conditions that cause a defect in mucus production or ciliary action that weaken the body's natural defenses against invaders of the respiratory system. Common signs and symptoms include an ill appearance, fever and shaking chills, a productive cough, and sputum. Many cases involve pleuritic chest pain. Auscultation usually reveals crackles in the involved lung segments, or sometimes wheezes or rhonchi, and occasionally egophony (change in spoken "E" sound to "A"). Percussion produces dullness over the affected areas. Some forms of pneumonia do not produce these distinctive symptoms, presenting instead with systemic complaints such as headache, malaise, fatigue, muscle aches, sore throat, nausea, vomiting, and diarrhea. Diagnosis in the field is unlikely and treatment is supportive. Place the patient in a comfortable position and administer high-flow oxygen. In severe cases, ventilatory assistance and possibly endotracheal intubation may be necessary. Medical direction may recommend administration of a beta agonist. Antipyretics may be given to reduce a high fever.

f. **Pulmonary edema** **pp. 349-350**

Pulmonary edema (fluid in the interstitial spaces of the lungs) is often associated with ineffective cardiac pumping action, as in left-sided ventricular heart disease. (Pulmonary edema associated with heart disease is discussed in Chapter 28, "Cardiology.") Non-cardiogenic pulmonary edema was discussed above under the objective for adult respiratory distress syndrome (ARDS).

g.   Pulmonary thromboembolism   pp. 364-366

A pulmonary embolism is a blood clot (thrombus) that lodges in an artery in the lungs. One in five cases of sudden death is caused by pulmonary thromboembolism. It is a life-threatening condition because it can significantly reduce pulmonary blood flow (perfusion), causing hypoxemia (lack of oxygen in the blood). Immobilization, such as recent surgery, a long bone fracture, or being bedridden, increases the risk of developing an embolism. Other risk factors for clot formation include pregnancy, oral birth control medications, cancer, and sickle cell anemia. The classic symptom of pulmonary embolism is a sudden onset of severe dyspnea, which may or may not be accompanied by pleuritic pain. The physical exam may reveal other signs including labored breathing, tachypnea, and tachycardia. In severe cases, there may be signs of right-sided heart failure, including jugular vein distention and possibly falling blood pressure. Auscultation may reveal no significant findings. In 50 percent of cases, examination of the extremities will reveal signs suggesting deep venous thrombosis (warm, swollen extremity with thick cord palpated along the medial thigh and pain on palpation or when extending the calf). Because a large embolism may cause cardiac arrest, be prepared to perform resuscitation. Primary care is aimed at support of the airway, breathing, and circulation. As necessary, assist ventilations and provide supplemental oxygen. Endotracheal intubation may be required. Establish IV access, monitor vital signs and cardiac rhythms, and transport expeditiously to a facility that can care for the patient's critical needs.

h.   Neoplasms of the lung   pp. 361-362

Lung cancer (neoplasms, literally "new growths" or tumors) is the leading cause of cancer-related death in Canada in both men and women. The primary problems are disruption of diffusion and, if the bronchioles are involved, of ventilation as well. The primary risk factor is cigarette smoking. Inhalation of other environmental toxins is also a risk factor. Less commonly, lung cancer can result from the spread of cancer from another part of the body. EMS calls to patients with lung cancer may involve a variety of complaints related to the disease, including cough, hoarseness, chest pain, and bloody sputum. There may be fever, chills, and chest pain if the patient has developed pneumonia. There can be weakness, numbness of the arm, shoulder pain, and difficulty swallowing. The physical exam may reveal weight loss, crackles, wheezes, rhonchi, and diminished breath sounds in the affected lung. There may be venous distention of the arms and neck. Your primary responsibility is to identify and address signs of respiratory distress. Assist ventilation and administer supplemental oxygen as needed. Establish IV access and consult medical direction about possible administration of bronchodilators and corticosteroids. Transport, but be alert for any DNR (do not resuscitate) orders.

i.   Upper respiratory infections (URI)   pp. 358-360

Infections of the upper airways of the respiratory tract are among the most common infectious conditions for which patients seek medical assistance, and you will see them in the field. Even though these infections are rarely life-threatening, they can produce considerable discomfort. At-home management is usually symptomatic, with treatment for pain and fever, as needed, as well as appropriate antibiotic therapy if the infection is bacterial. However, a URI in a person with pre-existing pulmonary disease can trigger severe problems and you should pay particularly close attention to airway and ventilation in patients with asthma or COPD. Be sure to monitor the condition with pulse oximetry and ECG during transport to a treatment facility.

j.   Spontaneous pneumothorax   pp. 366-367

Spontaneous pneumothorax, which occurs in the absence of trauma, is a relatively common condition, occurring in roughly 18 persons per 100,000 population. It is relatively likely to recur as well (with 50% recurrence rate at two years). Significant risk factors include male gender, age 20 to 40 years, tall, thin stature, and history of cigarette smoking. Presentation is marked by sudden onset pleuritic chest or shoulder pain, often precipitated by a bout of coughing or by heavy lifting. The loss of negative pressure in the affected hemithorax prevents proper chest expansion, and the patient may report dyspnea. In individuals who do NOT have significant underlying pulmonary disease, a pneumothorax of up to 15 to 20% of the chest cavity can be tolerated fairly well. Monitor symptoms and pulse oximetry readings during transport. Be especially attentive in your ongoing assessment of patients who require positive-pressure ventilation. These patients are at higher risk for development of tension pneumothorax, which is marked by increasing resistance to ventilation, along with hypoxia, cyanosis, and possible hypotension. Examination will reveal tracheal deviation away from the affected side of the chest and distention of the jugular vein. Needle decompression of a tension pneumothorax may be required.

k. Hyperventilation syndrome   pp. 367-368

Hyperventilation, with rapid breathing, chest pain, and numbness in the extremities, is often associated with anxiety, and it is called hyperventilation syndrome in this setting. However, you should remember that a number of significant and common medical conditions can cause hyperventilation, including cardiovascular and pulmonary conditions such as acute myocardial infarction and pulmonary thromboembolism, sepsis, pregnancy, liver failure, and several metabolic and neurologic disorders. Be conservative and consider hyperventilation to be a sign of a serious medical problem until proven otherwise. Management centers on reassurance and assisting the patient to consciously decrease the rate and depth of breathing (maneuvers that will increase PCO_2).

8. Given several preprogrammed patients with nontraumatic pulmonary problems, provide the appropriate assessment, pre-hospital care, and transport. pp. 332-369

The airway is functionally divided into the upper airway and the lower airway. The upper airway is comprised of the nasal cavity, pharynx, and larynx. The lower airway is comprised of the trachea, bronchi, alveoli, and lungs. The ability to take in oxygen and excrete carbon dioxide via the airway is essential to life. Therefore, it is critical that you be able to identify and understand the function of each structure of the airway and of the airway as a whole.

9. Describe the anatomy of the airway and the physiology of respiration.   (see Chapter 12)

10. Explain the primary objective of airway maintenance.   p. 370

The primary objective of airway maintenance is to keep the airway open and clear (patent) so that oxygen can be carried to and carbon dioxide carried away from the alveoli and the capillary beds of the pulmonary tissue.

11. Identify commonly neglected pre-hospital skills related to the airway.   p. 380

The manual maintenance of the airway, using the head-tilt/chin-lift or jaw thrust maneuver, is one of the most important but often neglected pre-hospital airway skills. Proper use of these techniques helps ensure an adequate airway early in the care process.

12. Describe assessment of the airway and the respiratory system.   pp. 374-375

Assessment of the airway is an integral part of both the initial assessment and the focused examination. During the initial assessment, the evaluation is directed at detecting any potentially life-threatening airway problems. If the patient is not conscious, alert, and demonstrating articulate speech, the airway and respiration are closely evaluated. The rate, depth, and symmetry of respiration are evaluated, as is the presence of any unusual respiratory sounds. During the focused exam, the emphasis is on the finer details of respiratory evaluation including skin color, auscultation of breath sounds, detection of abnormal breathing sounds, palpation of the thorax, and the use of pulse oximetry and/or capnography.

13. Describe the modified forms of respiration and list the factors that affect respiratory rate and depth.   pp. 374-375

Forms of respiration
• *Coughing*—the forceful exhalation of a large volume of air to expel material from the airway.
• *Sneezing*—sudden, forceful exhalation through the nose usually caused by nasal irritation.
• *Hiccoughing* (hiccups)—sudden diaphragmatic spasm with spasmodic closure of the glottis that

serves no useful purpose.
• *Sighing*—slow, deep involuntary inspiration followed by a prolonged expiration that hyper-inflates the lungs and expands collapsed alveoli.
• *Grunting*—forceful expiration against a partially closed epiglottis, usually an indication of respiratory distress.

Factors affecting respiratory rate and depth
• *Kussmaul's respirations*—deep, slow, or rapid gasping respirations commonly associated with diabetic ketoacidosis.
• *Cheyne-Stokes respirations*—progressively deeper, faster breathing alternating gradually with shallow, slower respirations indicating brainstem injury.
• *Biot's respirations*—irregular breathing pattern with sudden episodes of apnea indicating increased intracranial pressure.
• *Central neurogenic hyperventilation*—deep, rapid respirations indicating increased intracranial pressure.
• *Agonal respirations*—shallow, slow, or infrequent respirations indicating severe brain anoxia.

14. Discuss the methods for measuring oxygen and carbon dioxide in the blood and their pre-hospital use.   pp. 377-380

Pulse oximetry is a non-invasive monitoring of the arterial oxygenation of the skin. It accurately reflects the oxygen delivery to the end organs, giving an ongoing evaluation of circulation and respiration. In pre-hospital care, the oximeter is quick and easy to use and provides an accurate and constant evaluation of the cardiorespiratory system.

Capnography is the measurement of exhaled carbon dioxide concentrations. Devices such as the end-tidal carbon dioxide detectors are commonly used to assess the proper placement of endotracheal tubes. Higher concentrations of carbon dioxide change the color of a sensitive paper or the digital readout of an electronic device.

15. Define and explain the implications of partial airway obstruction with good and poor air exchange and complete airway obstruction.   p. 370

Obstruction of the airway by a foreign object or swelling may range from minor to complete. If the airway obstruction permits speech and coughing and you do not notice skin color changes, respiration is probably adequate and intervention may not be needed. However, if the patient has serious dyspnea, cannot speak or cough, is choking or gagging, and you notice skin color changes, intervention is necessary. Continued inadequate respiration will lead to increasing hypoxia. No air movement due to complete obstruction will rapidly lead to serious hypoxia and death.

16. Describe the common causes of upper airway obstruction, including:

• **tongue p. 371**
  The most common cause of airway obstruction is the tongue. In the unconscious person or the supine patient, the lack of muscle tone allows the tongue to rest against the posterior pharynx and thereby obstruct the airway.

• **foreign body aspiration p. 371**
  Large, poorly chewed lumps of food and objects aspirated by children commonly account for airway obstruction. The victim will often grasp his or her throat, a universal distress signal.

• **laryngeal spasm p. 371**
  The glottis is the smallest part of the airway and may be responsible for obstruction secondary to spasm. Spasm may be caused by stimulation by a foreign object as during endotracheal intubation.

• **laryngeal edema   p. 371**
  As the glottis is the narrowest part of the adult airway, swelling will rapidly reduce the airway lumen size and restrict breathing. Restriction and obstruction may be caused by anaphylaxis, epiglottitis, or the inhalation of toxic substances, superheated steam, or smoke.

- **trauma p. 371**
  Physical injury to the structures of the upper airway may result in loose objects such as the teeth, tissue, or clotted blood obstructing the airway. Further, blunt or penetrating trauma may result in collapse of the airway due to fracture or displacement of the larynx or trachea. Soft-tissue swelling may also restrict the lumen of the airway.

17. Describe complete airway obstruction maneuvers, including:

- **Heimlich maneuver   pp. 422**
  The Heimlich maneuver involves a forceful upward abdominal thrust using the hands placed halfway between the umbilicus and the xiphoid process. The increased abdominal and thoracic pressures help propel an obstruction up and out of the airway.

- **removal with Magill forceps   pp. 422**
  If basic life support measures fail to secure a patent airway, you may introduce a laryngoscope to visualize beyond the oral cavity. If you notice a foreign body obstructing the airway, you may then remove it using the Magill forceps.

18. Describe causes of respiratory distress, including:

- **upper and lower airway obstruction   pp. 370-372**
  Upper and lower airway obstructions range in severity from minor to complete obstructions and may be caused by the tongue, a foreign body, swelling, vomitus, blood, or teeth.

- **inadequate ventilation   p. 372**
  Insufficient minute volume compromises respiratory exchange and may be due to bronchospasm, rib fracture, hemo- or pneumothorax, drug overdose, airway obstruction, renal failure, or central nervous system injury.

- **impairment of respiratory muscles   p. 372**
  The respiratory muscles may be impaired by fatigue, central nervous system depression, or spinal injury.

- **impairment of nervous system   p. 372**
  Respiratory system control, provided by the central nervous system, may be depressed by drugs or by intracranial or spinal injury

19. Explain the risk of infection to EMS providers associated with airway management and ventilation.   pp. 380-440

There are several diseases that can be transmitted by body fluids and airborne droplet transmission. The pocket mask reduces the contact with the patient and, if equipped with a one-way valve, lessens the exposure to droplet contamination.

20. Describe manual airway maneuvers, including:

- **head-tilt/chin-lift maneuver   pp. 380-382**
  To execute the head-tilt/chin-lift airway maneuver, the rescuer places one hand on the patient's forehead, gently tilting the head back, while the other engages the mandible, displacing it anteriorly.

- **jaw-thrust maneuver   p. 382**
  During the jaw-thrust (or the triple-airway maneuver), the rescuer places his fingers on the patient's lateral mandible, displacing it anteriorly while the thumbs displace it inferiorly. The maneuver may rotate the head and extend the neck. If spinal injury is suspected, the head should not be tilted backward (use the modified jaw-thrust).

- **modified jaw-thrust maneuver   p. 382**

The modified jaw-thrust (for the trauma patient) requires that the jaw-thrust maneuver be modified by manually securing the head in a neutral position while the mandible is displaced forward.

21. **Describe the indications, contraindications, advantages, disadvantages, complications, special considerations, equipment, and techniques of the following:**

- **upper airway and tracheobronchial suctioning   pp. 432-433**
Suctioning is the use of pressures that are less than atmospheric to draw fluids and semi-fluids out of the airway. It should be used any time it can effectively remove material from the airway. Continuous suctioning should be avoided because it draws against the patient's ventilation attempts and generally interrupts artificial ventilation of the apneic patient. Suctioning can be provided by an electric or a mechanical device. Tracheobronchial suctioning passes a lubricated soft suction catheter down the endotracheal tube into the trachea or bronchi to remove secretions. Suction is applied for 10 to 15 seconds while the catheter is slowly turned and withdrawn.

- **nasogastric and orogastric tube insertion p. 434**
Nasogastric tube insertion is recommended for the conscious patient, because it permits him or her to talk more easily, while the procedure is to be avoided when there is danger of skull fracture and further injury caused by the tube's placement. Both oral and nasal techniques may be used for gastric decompression when patient ventilation is restricted or there is danger of aspiration. The tube is measured for depth of insertion by measuring from the epigastrium to the angle of the jaw and then to the nares. Use a topical anesthetic spray, and then lubricate the distal tip and insert the tube through the nares and along the nasal floor or through the mouth along the midline. Advance the tube, encourage patient swallowing if possible, and then introduce 30 to 50 mL of air while listening over the epigastrium. The absence of gastric sounds and the inability to speak suggests tracheal placement and the need to re-attempt insertion.

- **oropharyngeal and nasopharyngeal airway   pp. 383-387**
The oropharyngeal airway is designed to maintain an airway by displacing the tongue anteriorly. It should not be used in conscious or semiconscious patients who have an intact gag reflex. Displace the tongue forward with a tongue blade and insert the airway along the base of the tongue. It may also be inserted by placing it, backward, into the oral cavity to the base of the tongue and then rotating it 180 degrees and continuing the insertion. The oral or nasal airway should be used when ventilating the patient using any mechanical device.

The nasopharyngeal airway is inserted into the nasopharynx in the unconscious or semiconscious patient. It is a soft rubber tube that is lubricated and inserted posteriorly in the largest nostril (usually the left). It is indicated in the semiconscious patient or as the oral airway would be used. It should not be used in the patient with possible skull fracture.

- **ventilating a patient by mouth-to-mouth, mouth-to-nose, mouth-to-mask, one/two/three person bag-valve mask, flow-restricted oxygen-powered ventilation device, automatic transport ventilator   pp. 435-441**
Ventilation mouth-to-mouth or mouth-to-nose is an easy technique that requires no equipment, though it risks disease transmission. The rescuer seals his mouth over the patient's mouth or nose (or both with the small child or infant), closes the nostrils or mouth with his fingers, takes a deep breath, and inflates the patient's lungs. The procedure induces air with about 15 percent oxygen that will successfully sustain life. When possible, mouth-to-mask or bag-valve mask ventilation is recommended.

The pocket mask is an adjunct to mouth-to-mouth ventilation that provides some protection against direct contact with the patient and the patient's exhaled air. It is simply sealed to the patient's face with the rescuer's hands and held in place during ventilation. It is recommended for use any time you would otherwise employ direct mouth-to-mouth ventilation. Some masks provide for supplemental oxygen administration that improves the percentage of oxygen provided to the patient. Bag-valve-mask devices are mechanical devices that provide positive-pressure ventilation. The mask is sealed to the patient's face with one hand while the other hand squeezes the bag, pushing air into the patient's lungs. The device is best used for the intubated patient because the volume of air and the pressure delivered to the patient is low. If the patient is not intubated, the air exchange achieved by one person may not be enough to sustain life. With two or more persons, one rescuer seals the mask to the face and maintains head positioning while another uses both hands to squeeze the bag. Since the volume of the bag is limited, it is essential to obtain a good seal on the face when using the BVM. Any time the BVM is used, it should have the oxygen reservoir attached and oxygen flowing at 12 to 15 liters per minute.

Flow-restricted, oxygen-powered ventilation devices, sometimes called demand valve resuscitators, ventilate a patient with a flow of oxygen when a button or bar is pushed. They can be used with a face mask, EOA, EGTA, PtL airway, or endotracheal tube. They provide the patient with 100% oxygen. However, the pressures they use may cause gastric insufflation or lung tissue damage. They are not recommended for intubated or pediatric patients.

Automatic transport ventilators provide a patient with ventilation with 100% oxygen at a rate and volume determined by the user. Recent advances in technology make automatic ventilators compact and dependable for field use. They are not recommended for children under the age of 5 years and are dependent upon a good patient airway.

22. Compare the ventilation techniques used for an adult patient to those used for pediatric patients, and describe special considerations in airway management and ventilation for the pediatric patient.   pp. 410-414, 439

During bag-valve masking, one rescuer seals the mask to the face and thrusts the jaw anteriorly while the other rescuer compresses the bag. The small (450 mL) BVM is used for infants, while the standard pediatric BVM is adequate for children up to 8 years old. Ensure the mask seals well and that ventilation achieves good chest rise and breath sounds.

Endotracheal intubation of the pediatric patient is more difficult than for the adult for the following reasons; the airway structures are smaller and more flexible, the tongue is relatively larger, the epiglottis is floppier and rounder, the vocal folds are more difficult to visualize, and the narrowest part of the airway is the cricoid cartilage. A straight laryngoscope blade and uncuffed endotracheal tube are used for patients under 8 years of age. The tube is only introduced to 2 to 3 cm beyond the vocal cords (place the black glottic mark at the vocal cords). The procedure is more likely to produce vagal stimulation and may require atropine administration.

23. Identify types of oxygen cylinders and pressure regulators and explain safety considerations of oxygen storage and delivery, including steps for delivering oxygen from a cylinder and regulator.   p. 435

Oxygen is commonly available in steel or aluminum cylinders of D (400 L), E (660 L), and M (3,450 L) sizes and is brought to administration pressures by a therapy regulator (50 psi) that allows for the administration of a liter/minute flow rate. Oxygen is a gas that easily supports combustion and should be used with caution near any ignition source or near grease. The pressure in the tank makes rupture an event that may produce serious injury, so tanks must be handled and stored carefully.

24. Describe the indications, contraindications, advantages, disadvantages, complications, liter flow range, and concentration of delivered oxygen for the following supplemental oxygen delivery devices: p. 436

- **nasal cannula**
The nasal cannula is a blind tube with ports to correspond to the patient's nostrils. Oxygen flows into the nares and the patient breathes enriched oxygen when breathing through the nose. The device delivers 24 to 44 percent oxygen with flows of 1 to 6 liters per minute. The nasal cannula is useful for the patient with anxiety regarding oxygen masks and for prolonged oxygen administration. It is of little benefit if the patient is not breathing through the nose unless the prongs are then placed facing into the mouth.

- **simple face mask**
A simple face mask delivers oxygen into the mask in front of the patient's mouth and nose. The patient inhales 40 to 60 percent oxygen when the device receives an oxygen flow of 8 to 12 liters per minute. The simple oxygen face mask is useful for the routine administration of oxygen.

- **partial rebreather mask**

  The partial rebreather mask is indicated for patients needing moderate concentrations of oxygen. One-way disks limit mixing of oxygen with inspired air and help increase the oxygen concentration. Maximum oxygen flow is about 10 liters per minute.

- **nonrebreather mask**

  The nonrebreather mask consists of oxygen tubing and a face mask with a reservoir. Because of valves in the mask, oxygen flows into the reservoir while the patient exhales and into the patient from the input tubing and reservoir when the patient inhales. If the reservoir does not completely collapse (usually 10 to 15 liters per minute flow) on inspiration, oxygen delivery is between 80 percent and 95 percent.

- **Venturi mask**

  The Venturi mask is a high-flow oxygen mask that delivers very precise concentrations of oxygen. The oxygen concentration is generally low, with normal concentrations of 24, 28, 35, and 40 percent. It is often used to treat COPD patients who need supplemental oxygen but who may have respiratory drive problems with high-concentration oxygen.

25. Describe the use, advantages, and disadvantages of an oxygen humidifier. p. 436

Oxygen bubbles through sterile water to obtain humidification. Humidified oxygen administration benefits patients with croup, epiglottitis, or bronchiolitis or patients on long-term oxygen therapy.

26. Describe the indications, contraindications, advantages, disadvantages, complications, equipment, and technique for the following:

- **endotracheal intubation by direct laryngoscopy   pp. 388-400**

  Endotracheal intubation is the method of choice for the patient who is unable to protect his airway. It may also be considered for the patient who is expected to lose the airway due to swelling, as may occur with inhalation injury or with a trauma patient or with one who is in need of assisted ventilation. The only contraindication to endotracheal intubation is the pediatric patient with possible epiglottitis, unless respirations are worsening. The procedure requires an endotracheal tube, a laryngoscope, and tape to secure the tube once in place. Once the patient is hyperventilated, the laryngoscope is inserted into the right side of the oral cavity, then moved to the left, displacing the tongue. It is negotiated down the airway until it engages the epiglottis (straight blade) or is negotiated into the vallecula. As the tongue and pharynx are lifted to visualize the glottic opening, the endotracheal tube is placed through the opening, then advanced 2 to 3 cm beyond. Placement is checked and then the cuff is inflated to seal the trachea.

- **digital endotracheal intubation   pp. 417-419**

  Digital intubation is a blind intubation technique in which the endotracheal tube is guided into the glottis with the fingers of a hand inserted into the oral cavity. One hand is deeply inserted into the oral cavity, and one finger locates the epiglottis while the others direct the tube along its posterior surface and, hopefully, into the trachea. The technique is helpful in the trauma patient whose neck cannot be extended or the patient with a short neck, where visualization of the glottis is very difficult. The fingers of the rescuer must be protected with an oral airway, and great care must be used to ensure the endotracheal tube is correctly placed in the trachea.

- **dual lumen airway   pp. 417-419**

  A dual lumen airway, like the Esophageal Tracheal CombiTube, has two lumens, or tubes. The device is inserted blindly through the mouth, and one lumen enters the trachea and the other enters the esophagus. After determining which tube has entered the trachea, the patient is ventilated through that tube. The dual lumen airway is easy to use and does not require special equipment. The device diminishes gastric distention and regurgitation and can be used on trauma patients because the neck can remain in the neutral position during insertion and ventilation. However, maintaining adequate mask seal is difficult, and the device cannot be used with pediatric patients or those with esophageal disease or caustic ingestions, or in conscious patients or those with a gag reflex.

- **nasotracheal intubation   pp. 414-416**
  Nasotracheal intubation is a blind intubation technique that is recommended for spinal injury, clenched teeth, oral injuries and swelling, and obesity or arthritis preventing patient positioning in the sniffing position. The patient must be breathing and without nasal or basilar skull fractures. The endotracheal tube is inserted blindly into the largest nares and along the floor of the nasal cavity. Listen to the breath sounds, and once the breath sounds are heard clearly, advance the tube during the next inhalation. Carefully confirm proper tube placement. Once inserted, the tube can be secured more easily and the patient cannot bite or compress the tube.

- **rapid sequence intubation   pp. 405-409**
  Rapid sequence intubation is indicated for a patient who has a gag reflex or is likely to fight any intubation attempt but who requires such a procedure. The procedure induces sedation, then muscle paralysis to permit easier intubation. The patient is ventilated while the medications take effect. The procedure requires that care providers continue ventilation during the entire time of paralysis and maintain the airway if endotracheal intubation is unsuccessful. Care must be taken to administer agents that do not cause hypotension and ICP increase in serious trauma patients.

- **endotracheal intubation using sedation   pp. 405-409**
  To perform endotracheal intubation using sedation, the care giver simply medicates the patient without employing a paralytic agent.

- **open cricothyrotomy   pp. 427-430**
  Cricothyrotomy is an incision through the cricothyroid membrane to allow the passage of air. It is employed only when complete airway obstruction makes no other means of effectively ventilating the patient possible. The cricoid membrane is located (the first hard ring moving from the mid-trachea upward), then the membrane between it and the thyroid cartilage. The skin above the membrane is incised vertically with a scalpel and then the membrane is opened with a horizontal incision. A 6- or 7-mm endotracheal tube (or tracheostomy tube) is directed down the trachea, and the cuff is inflated. Complications of the open cricothyrotomy include severe hemorrhage, thyroid gland damage, damage to surrounding airway structures, subcutaneous emphysema, and incorrect tube placement.

- **needle cricothyrotomy (translaryngeal catheter ventilation)   pp. 423-427**
  Percutaneous transtracheal catheter ventilation (or needle cricothyrotomy) is used only for severe, partial airway obstruction above the vocal cords that is not correctable by other methods. An over-the-needle catheter is inserted through the cricothyroid membrane with a syringe attached. Once the membrane is penetrated, air can be inspired into the syringe to confirm proper placement. The catheter is then directed caudally, the needle is withdrawn, and the catheter is attached to a high-pressure, high-volume oxygen line. High-pressure oxygen (50 psi) is passed through the large (14 ga or larger) catheter using special equipment and then is allowed to escape. Expiration should take twice as long as inflation. If the chest does not deflate, a second needle or an open cricothyrotomy may be needed.

- **extubation   p. 416-417**
  Extubation is the removal of the endotracheal tube when a patient awakens and is intolerant of the endotracheal tube. Removal calls for the deflation of the cuff and withdrawal of the tube during expiration or a cough. Laryngospasm may occur with the withdrawal of the endotracheal tube.

27. Describe use of cricoid pressure during intubation.   pp. 382-383, 397

Cricoid pressure or Sellick's maneuver places posteriorly directed pressure on the cricoid cartilage, compressing the esophagus and preventing vomit from entering the pharynx. The procedure also may move the structures of the airway so they may be more easily viewed during intubation attempts. Once applied, Sellick's procedure must be maintained until the endotracheal tube is placed, as early release may permit emesis to enter the pharynx. Do not apply excessive pressure, as doing so may obstruct the trachea.

28. Discuss the precautions that should be taken when intubating the trauma patient.   p. 405

The trauma patient may have sustained spinal injury: all airway care must be provided with limited (if any) movement of the head and neck. In addition to the cervical collar, the head should be held in a neutral position manually by a paramedic while intubation is attempted. Oro- or nasotracheal intubation, lighted stylet intubation, or digital techniques may be attempted.

29. Discuss agents used for sedation and rapid sequence intubation.   pp. 405-407

Midazolam, diazepam, etomidate, ketamine, sodium thiopental, propofol, and fentanyl are used to sedate patients as the first step of rapid sequence intubation. Then paralytics such as succinylcholine, vecuronium, atracurium, and pancuronium are used to relax the skeletal muscles and permit endotracheal intubation. The drugs atropine and lidocaine may also be used as part of the rapid sequence intubation regimen.

30. Discuss methods to confirm correct placement of an endotracheal tube.   pp. 399-400

Verify and document at least three of the following: visualization of the tube passing through the vocal cords, the presence of bilateral breath sounds, absence of breath sounds over the epigastrium, positive end-tidal CO_2 change, verification of placement by an esophageal detector device, condensation in the endotracheal tube, absence of vomitus within the endotracheal tube, and the absence of vocal sounds once the tube is in place. It is highly recommended that the patient's chest be auscultated for bilateral breath sounds to ensure the endotracheal tube has not been introduced too far and into the right mainstem bronchus.

CONTENT SELF-EVALUATION

Multiple Choice

1. Which of the following is considered an intrinsic risk factor for respiratory disease?
   A.   smokestack pollutants
   B.   polluted water
   C.   genetic predisposition
   D.   cigarette smoking
   E.   stress

2. The three processes that allow gas exchange to occur in the lungs and body tissues are:
   A.   ventilation, diffusion, perfusion
   B.   inspiration, expiration, ventilation.
   C.   resistance, compliance, perfusion.
   D.   ventilation, inspiration, expiration.
   E.   inspiration, compliance, diffusion.

3. The mechanical process of moving air in and out of the lungs is:
   A.   ventilation.
   B.   diffusion.
   C.   perfusion.
   D.   inspiration.
   E.   inhalation.

4. The process by which gases move between the alveoli and the pulmonary capillaries is:
   A.   infusion.
   B.   perfusion.
   C.   respiration.
   D.   diffusion.
   E.   permeation.

5. Lung perfusion is dependent on three factors—adequate blood volume, efficient pumping by the heart, and intact:

   A.   alveoli.
         D.   goblet cells.

   B.   respiratory membrane.
         E.   pulmonary capillaries.

   C.   bronchioles.

6. Any of the following can disrupt ventilation EXCEPT:

   A.   obstruction of the upper airway.

   B.   obstruction of the lower airway.

   C.   blockage of the pulmonary arteries.

   D.   impairment of normal function of the chest wall.

   E.   abnormalities of the nervous system's control of breathing.

7. Which of the following abnormal breathing patterns is characterized by long, deep breaths that are stopped during the inspiratory phase and separated by periods of apnea?

   A.   ataxic (Biot's) respirations (seen with increased intracranial pressure)

   B.   central neurogenic hyperventilation (seen with stroke or brainstem injury)

   C.   Kussmaul's respirations (seen with metabolic acidosis)

   D.   apneustic respirations (seen with stroke or severe central nervous system disease)

   E.   Cheyne-Stokes respirations (seen with terminal illness or brain injury)

8. Which of the following is NOT likely to cause hypoxia (a supply of oxygen inadequate to meet the needs of the body's cells)?

   A.   ascension to a high altitude
         D.   left-sided heart failure

   B.   esophageal ulceration
         E.   asbestos inhalation

   C.   black lung disease

9. Pulmonary shunting results from:

   A.   alveolar collapse.
         D.   excess mucus production.

   B.   blockage of pulmonary capillaries.
   E.   airway obstruction.

   C.   bronchoconstriction.

10. The most important action when you arrive on scene and discover that a hazardous material is present is to:

   A.   have supplemental oxygen available.

   B.   remove the patient from the environment.

   C.   search for additional patients.

   D.   put on self-contained breathing apparatus.

   E.   call for a hazardous materials team.

11. You are dispatched to a patient with difficulty breathing. Which of the following should be part of the scene size-up?

   A.   Establish a patent airway.

   B.   Look for clues to the possible cause.

   C.   Evaluate AVPU mental status.

   D.   Determine respiration rate.

   E.   Ready the oxygenation equipment.

12. During the initial assessment, your general impression of the patient's respiratory status should include all of the following elements EXCEPT:

   A.   pulse.
         D.   mental status.

   B.   position.
         E.   ability to speak.

   C.   color.

13. Which of the following is NOT a classic sign of respiratory distress?

   A.   pursed lips
         D.   nasal flaring

   B.   tracheal tugging
         E.   cyanosis

   C.   diaphoresis

14. Which of the following is TRUE with regard to assessing the airway?
    A.   Noisy breathing usually indicates a complete obstruction.
    B.   Obstructed breathing is not always noisy breathing.
    C.   If the airway is blocked, artificial respiration must be started immediately.
    D.   If the airway is blocked, endotracheal intubation must be established.
    E.   If the airway is open, the patient is breathing.

15. Which of the following is the MOST ominous sign of possible life-threatening respiratory distress?
    A.   altered mental status
    D.   tachycardia
    B.   audible stridor
    E.   use of accessory muscles
    C.   1- to 2-word dyspnea

16. Orthopnea is:
    A.   dizziness when rising from a supine position.
    B.   dyspnea that occurs while lying supine.
    C.   short attacks of dyspnea that interrupt sleep.
    D.   apnea that occurs while in an upright position.
    E.   pleuritic pain that occurs during breathing.

17. Many respiratory complaints result from worsening of a long-standing disease the patient knows he has and can tell you about during the history. All of the following are such long-term respiratory diseases EXCEPT:
    A.   pneumonia.
    D.   asthma.
    B.   emphysema.
    E.   lung cancer.
    C.   chronic bronchitis.

18. Which of the following medications would be of LEAST significance if found in the home of a patient with a respiratory complaint?
    A.   oxygen
    D.   corticosteroid
    B.   bronchodilator
    E.   antibiotic
    C.   vitamin C tablets

19. A patient with significant respiratory distress may breathe through pursed lips. Breathing through pursed lips helps to:
    A.   prevent tracheal collapse.
    B.   force air past a bronchial obstruction.
    C.   bring up excess mucus.
    D.   close the epiglottis.
    E.   keep the alveoli open.

20. Pink or bloody sputum is commonly seen with any of the following EXCEPT:
    A.   pulmonary edema.
    D.   allergic reaction.
    B.   lung cancer.
    E.   bronchial infection.
    C.   tuberculosis.

21. Asymmetrical chest movement is most likely to be found during:
    A.   auscultation.
    D.   inspection.
    B.   capnometry.
    E.   percussion.
    C.   oximetry.

22. Subcutaneous emphysema is most likely to be found during:
    A.   oximetry.
    D.   palpation.
    B.   percussion.
    E.   inspection.
    C.   capnometry.

23. Wheezing is most likely to be detected during:
    A.   oximetry.
    D.   capnometry.
    B.   auscultation.
    E.   palpation.
    C.   percussion.

24. Rattling sounds in the larger airways associated with excess mucus are called:

A. stridor.
B. wheezing.
C. crackles.
D. snoring.
E. rhonchi.

25. A harsh, high-pitched sound heard on inspiration, associated with upper airway obstruction, is called:

A. snoring.
B. stridor.
C. crackles.
D. rhonchi.
E. rales.

26. In general, tachycardia is a nonspecific finding seen, for example, with fear, anxiety, or fever. In a patient with a respiratory complaint, however, tachycardia may also indicate:

A. hypothermia.
B. hypertrophy.
C. hypotension.
D. hyperopia.
E. hypoxia.

27. Drugs that may cause an elevation in both heart rate and blood pressure include:

A. diuretics such as furosemide.
B. analgesics such as morphine sulfate.
C. tranqulizers such as diazepam.
D. sympathomimetics such as albuterol.
E. beta blockers such as labetalol.

28. An elevated respiratory rate in a patient with dyspnea is most likely caused by:

A. bradycardia.
B. dysuria.
C. hypoxia.
D. anemia.
E. tachycardia.

29. Which of the following measures end-expiratory carbon dioxide?

A. spirometry
B. sphygmomanometry
C. capnometry
D. oximetry
E. tomography

30. Two conditions in which respiration is frequently dependent on hypoxic respiratory drive and use of supplemental oxygen may induce respiratory depression are:

A. asthma and pneumonia.
B. spontaneous pneumothorax and pneumonia.
C. asthma and emphysema.
D. asthma and adult respiratory distress syndrome.
E. chronic bronchitis and emphysema.

31. The pulmonary edema characteristic of adult respiratory distress syndrome (ARDS) is caused by:

A. left-sided cardiac ventricular failure.
B. right-sided cardiac ventricular failure.
C. accumulation of fluid in the pulmonary interstitial spaces.
D. obstruction of pulmonary capillaries by thrombi.
E. chronic constriction of terminal airways and alveoli.

32. Factors that commonly cause acute aggravation of symptoms due to chronic obstructive pulmonary disease (COPD) include all of the following EXCEPT:

A. progression of lung cancer.
B. exertion, including heavy lifting and exercise.
C. allergens such as foods and dust.
D. tobacco smoke.
E. occupational airborne pollutants such as chemical fumes.

33. Common physical attributes of a person with emphysema include all of the following EXCEPT:
   A. chronic cough.
   B. barrel chest.
   C. clubbing of the fingers.
   D. pinkish tone to skin.
   E. thin build.

34. Common physical attributes of a person with chronic bronchitis include all of the following EXCEPT:
   A. chronic cough.
   B. thin build.
   C. bluish, cyanotic tone to skin.
   D. cough producing large amounts of sputum.
   E. ankle edema.

35. The epidemiology of asthma includes all of the following EXCEPT:
   A. an increase in mortality rate over the past decade.
   B. a death rate in whites that is roughly twice that in blacks.
   C. the fact that it is a common disorder in both males and females.
   D. mortality change seen mostly in persons over age 45 years.
   E. the fact that half of asthma deaths occur in the prehospital setting.

36. Medications commonly used by persons with asthma include all of the following EXCEPT:
   A. beta agonists administered via inhaler.
   B. oral doses of aspirin.
   C. anticholinergics administered via inhaler.
   D. oral doses of corticosteroid.
   E. cromolyn sodium administered via inhaler.

37. The chief management goals for an acute asthma attack involve improvement in:
   A. blood pH (acidosis), hypoxia, and wheezing.
   B. hypoxia, bronchospasm, and wheezing.
   C. blood pH (acidosis), hypoxia, and local inflammation.
   D. hypoxia, bronchospasm, and local inflammation.
   E. hypoxia, wheezing, and local inflammation.

38. Be prepared for which of the following when caring for a patient with status asthmaticus?
   A. respiratory acidosis with electrolyte imbalance
   B. dehydration with early signs of renal failure
   C. respiratory depression when administered supplemental oxygen
   D. respiratory arrest requiring endotracheal intubation
   E. tracheal inflammation causing airway obstruction

39. Upper respiratory infections can affect all of the following EXCEPT:
   A. the sinuses.
   B. the lungs.
   C. the middle ear.
   D. the nose.
   E. the pharynx.

40. Pleuritic chest pain associated with pneumonia is:
   A. dull and aching in character.
   B. sharp or tearing in character.
   C. cramplike and hard to localize.
   D. likely to radiate to the jaw or left arm.
   E. only present on deep inspiration.

41. Standard management of lung cancer includes all of the following EXCEPT:
- **A.** checking for instructions such as DNR (do not resuscitate) orders.
- **B.** placement of ECG leads for cardiac monitoring.
- **C.** administration of supplemental oxygen.
- **D.** airway and ventilatory support as needed.
- **E.** emotional support of patient and family.

42. Risk factors for pulmonary emboli include all of the following EXCEPT:
- **A.** obesity.
- **B.** pregnancy.
- **C.** prolonged immobilization.
- **D.** deep vein thrombophlebitis.
- **E.** use of oral contraceptives, especially in smokers.

43. Common physical findings in pulmonary embolism include all of the following EXCEPT:
- **A.** evidence suggestive of deep venous thrombosis.
- **B.** labored, painful breathing.
- **C.** tachypnea and tachycardia.
- **D.** cardiac dysrythmias.
- **E.** normal chest auscultation.

44. Which of the following statements about spontaneous pneumothorax is FALSE?
- **A.** Most patients have acute onset pain in the chest or shoulder region.
- **B.** Onset of pain often follows coughing or heavy lifting.
- **C.** Spontaneous pneumothorax is much more common in women than in men.
- **D.** Spontaneous pneumothorax is more common among smokers and persons with COPD.
- **E.** Supplemental oxygen is sufficient therapy for the majority of patients with spontaneous pneumothorax.

45. The respiratory alkalosis of hyperventilation syndrome often results in:
- **A.** cramping of the muscles of the hands and feet.
- **B.** slowing of cardiac electrical conduction, causing bradycardia.
- **C.** cramping of facial muscles causing characteristic grimace.
- **D.** one of several cardiac dysrhythmias.
- **E.** altered mental status, specifically, lethargy and depression.

46. The processes of ventilation, diffusion, and perfusion allow gas exchange to occur efficiently in the lungs and other body tissues. The derangement in pulmonary embolism is principally of:
- **A.** ventilation.
- **B.** diffusion.
- **C.** perfusion.
- **D.** a combination of ventilation and diffusion.
- **E.** a combination of diffusion and perfusion.

47. The most common auscultation finding in a patient with pneumonia is:
- **A.** stridor over the involved segment.
- **B.** decreased or absent breath sounds over the involved segment.
- **C.** expiratory wheezing over the involved segment.
- **D.** crackles (rales) over the involved segment.
- **E.** pleural friction rub over the involved segment.

48. Which of the following is the most common cause of upper airway obstruction?
- **A.** the tongue
- **B.** foreign bodies
- **C.** trauma
- **D.** laryngeal swelling
- **E.** aspiration of blood or vomitus

49. All of the following conditions may cause reduced inspiratory volumes EXCEPT:
- **A.** pneumothorax.
- **B.** asthma. **E.** emphysema.
- **C.** high inspired oxygen concentrations.
- **D.** respiratory muscle paralysis.

50. The normal respiratory rate for an adult at rest is:
- **A.** 8 to 12.
- **B.** 12 to 20.
- **C.** 18 to 24.
- **D.** 24 to 32.
- **E.** 40 to 60.

51. Which of the following is a breathing pattern associated with flail chest?
- **A.** abdominal breathing
- **B.** paradoxical breathing
- **C.** diaphragmatic breathing
- **D.** intercostal retraction
- **E.** both A and C

52. Which modified form of respiration is designed to expand alveoli that may have collapsed during periods of inactivity or rest?
- **A.** coughing
- **B.** sneezing
- **C.** hiccoughing
- **D.** grunting
- **E.** sighing

53. The respiratory pattern that presents with deep and rapid respirations is:
- **A.** apneustic respirations.
- **B.** Cheyne-Stokes respirations.
- **C.** Biot's respirations.
- **D.** central neurogenic hyperventilation.
- **E.** agonal respirations.

54. The feeling of flexibility or stiffness associated with the lungs and ventilation is:
- **A.** back pressure.
- **B.** resiliency.
- **C.** compliance.
- **D.** effusion.
- **E.** Hering-Breuer reflex.

55. The absence of CO_2 in exhaled air, as identified by the end-expiratory CO_2 detector, suggests:
- **A.** ventilation is not deep enough.
- **B.** ventilations are not occurring fast enough.
- **C.** the endotracheal tube may be in the esophagus.
- **D.** the oxygen percentage of inspired air is insufficient.
- **E.** all of the above

56. The intent behind employing Sellick's maneuver is to:
- **A.** displace the diaphragm.
- **B.** increase venous return.
- **C.** prevent regurgitation.
- **D.** clear an airway obstruction.
- **E.** increase blood flow to the brain.

57. Which of the following is an advantage of the nasopharyngeal airway over the oropharyngeal airway?
- **A.** It has a larger diameter.
- **B.** It is easier to insert.
- **C.** It is blocked less frequently by vomitus.
- **D.** It does not stimulate the gag reflex as strongly.
- **E.** It can be used with a BVM.

58. Insertion of the nasopharyngeal airway directs the soft rubber tube:
- **A.** directly up and into the nostril.
- **B.** directly along the floor of the nasal cavity.
- **C.** into the left nostril, most frequently.
- **D.** laterally along the side of the nasal cavity.
- **E.** directly into the vallecula space.

59. The airway adjunct that acts primarily by displacing the tongue forward is the:
- **A.** oropharyngeal airway.
- **B.** PtL airway.
- **C.** endotracheal tube.
- **D.** nasopharyngeal airway.
- **E.** esophageal gastric tube airway.

60. The airway technique preferred for use with the patient who is unconscious is:
- **A.** the oropharyngeal airway.
- **B.** the nasopharyngeal airway.
- **C.** endotracheal intubation.
- **D.** nasotracheal intubation.
- **E.** EGTA.

61. The tip of the curve of the Macintosh laryngoscope blade is designed to fit into the:
- **A.** nasopharynx.
- **B.** glottic opening.
- **C.** vallecula.
- **D.** arytenoid fossa.
- **E.** epiglottis.

62. The laryngoscope blade considered to be best designed for intubation of the pediatric patient is:
- **A.** the Macintosh blade.
- **B.** the curved blade.
- **C.** the straight blade.
- **D.** either B or C
- **E.** none of the above

63. The major purpose for using a malleable stylet during endotracheal intubation is to:
- **A.** maintain a pre-set curve in the tube.
- **B.** keep the tube's lumen open.
- **C.** stiffen the tube so it can be pushed through the glottis.
- **D.** prevent foreign matter from entering the tube.
- **E.** all of the above

64. Which of the following is NOT an indication for endotracheal intubation?
- **A.** respiratory arrest
- **B.** cardiac arrest
- **C.** inability to protect the airway
- **D.** obstruction due to foreign object, swelling, or burns
- **E.** severe epiglottitis

65. Which of the following is a likely occurrence when using an endotracheal intubation to secure the airway?
- **A.** Gastric distention is more likely.
- **B.** Complete airway control is achieved.
- **C.** The tracheal suctioning becomes more complicated.
- **D.** Medications can no longer be introduced into the trachea.
- **E.** It makes obtaining a good mask seal more difficult.

66. To reduce the risk of hypoxia, limit attempts at intubation to no more than:
- **A.** 15 seconds.
- **B.** 30 seconds.
- **C.** 45 seconds.
- **D.** 60 seconds.
- **E.** 80 seconds.

67. Which of the following is NOT an indication for esophageal intubation?
    A.   absence of chest rise with ventilation
    B.   gurgling sound over the epigastrium
    C.   a falling pulse oximetry reading
    D.   skin color turning pink
    E.   increasing resistance to ventilatory effort

68. Upon placing the endotracheal tube, you hear very faint breath sounds and some gurgling over the epigastric region. You should next:
    A.   advance the tube slightly.   D.   ventilate more forcibly.
    B.   withdraw the tube slightly.   E.   remove the tube and re-intubate.
    C.   inflate the cuff and auscultate again.

69. Upon placing the endotracheal tube in a patient, you determine that you can only auscultate breath sounds on the right side. You should next:
    A.   withdraw the tube a few centimeters.
    B.   withdraw the tube completely.
    C.   pass the tube a few centimeters further.
    D.   secure the tube and ventilate more aggressively.
    E.   check the mask seal.

70. The purpose of the cuff on the end of the endotracheal tube is to:
    A.   help guide the tube to its proper location.
    B.   prevent dislodging of the tube after it is correctly placed.
    C.   seal the airway.
    D.   center the tube in the trachea.
    E.   widen the opening of the vocal cords.

71. In the intubation of children under 8 years old, it is recommended that the paramedic use:
    A.   a cuffed endotracheal tube and a straight laryngoscope blade.
    B.   an uncuffed endotracheal tube and a straight laryngoscope blade.
    C.   a cuffed endotracheal tube and a curved laryngoscope blade.
    D.   an uncuffed endotracheal tube and a curved laryngoscope blade.
    E.   an uncuffed endotracheal tube and digital technique.

72. Which of the following is NOT required for blind nasotracheal intubation?
    A.   a neutral or slightly extended neck   D.   a patient who is breathing
    B.   a generally quiet environment   E.   a pre-oxygenated patient
    C.   a strong, malleable stylet

73. The primary danger associated with extubation is:
    A.   laryngospasm.   D.   tracheal damage.
    B.   aspiration.   E.   vomiting.
    C.   fasciculations.

74. The major disadvantage to the use of the Esophageal Tracheal CombiTube is that:
    A.   the mask may be difficult to seal.
    B.   the tube must be in the trachea.
    C.   it is associated with gastric distension and vomiting.
    D.   it cannot be used in the trauma patient.
    E.   it is somewhat time-consuming to insert.

75. Which of the following are features of the PtL airway?
    A.   It can be inserted blindly.
    B.   It can seal off the nasal and oral cavities.
    C.   The patient can be ventilated regardless of whether the tube is in the trachea or esophagus.
    D.   It can be inserted without moving the cervical spine.
    E.   All of the above

76. Which of the following is a part of suctioning the stoma patient?
  A. pre-oxygenating with 100 percent oxygen
  B. injecting 3 mL of saline
  C. inserting the catheter until resistance is met
  D. withdrawing the catheter while the patient exhales or coughs
  E. all of the above

77. Which of the following is NOT indicated when suctioning through the endotracheal tube?
  A. Insert the catheter until you meet resistance.
  B. Suction only during insertion.
  C. Pre-oxygenate the patient.
  D. Rotate the suction catheter while suctioning.
  E. Suction no longer than 10 to 15 seconds.

78. Nasogastric tube placement is indicated in a patient:
  A. with facial fractures.
  B. with a possible basilar skull fracture.
  C. who is awake.
  D. for whom a relatively large gastric tube is indicated.
  E. all of the above

79. Which of the devices listed below delivers the highest concentration of oxygen to the patient?
  A. nasal cannula   D. Venturi mask
  B. simple face mask   E. A and D
  C. nonrebreather mask

80. Which of the devices below delivers the most controlled concentration of oxygen to a patient?
  A. nasal cannula   D. Venturi mask
  B. simple face mask   E. B and C
  C. nonrebreather mask

81. The bag-valve mask with an oxygen supply attached and oxygen flowing at 15 L per minute delivers what percentage of oxygen to the patient?
  A. 21 percent   D. 90 to 95 percent
  B. 40 to 60 percent   E. 99.9 percent
  C. 60 to 80 percent

82. One rescuer bag-valve masking is difficult to perform effectively because:
  A. it is difficult to maintain proper airway positioning.
  B. it is difficult to maintain mask seal.
  C. it is difficult to squeeze the bag.
  D. all of the above
  E. none of the above

83. Hazards of using the demand valve to ventilate a patient include all of the following EXCEPT:
  A. oxygen toxicity.   D. pneumothorax.
  B. gastric distention.   E. subcutaneous emphysema.
  C. pulmonary barotrauma.

84. Which of the following is NOT an advantage of automatic ventilators?
  A. They free a rescuer when the patient is not breathing.
  B. They are convenient and easy to use.
  C. They are dependable.
  D. They can be used on children younger than age 5.
  E. They are lightweight and tolerant to temperature extremes.

True/False

85. Allergic reaction to a medication may be the cause of a respiratory complaint.
    A.   True
    B.   False

86. Major risk factors for pneumonia are HIV infection, very young or very old, and immunosuppressive therapy.
    A.   True
    B.   False

87. Roughly one in five cases of sudden death is due to pulmonary emboli.
    A.   True
    B.   False

88. The mortality rate for pulmonary emboli is greater than 50%.
    A.   True
    B.   False

89. The ventilation-perfusion mismatch characteristic of pulmonary embolism is due to loss of blood flow to a ventilated segment of lung tissue.
    A.   True
    B.   False

90. Respiratory emergencies due to central nervous system (CNS) dysfunction are relatively rare.
    A.   True
    B.   False

91. Numerous peripheral nervous system conditions can cause respiratory compromise, including the diseases of polio and amyotrophic lateral sclerosis, as well as Guillian-Barré syndrome.
    A.   True
    B.   False

92. It is unlikely that a patient will have significant hypoxia and not display cyanosis.
    A.   True
    B.   False

93. In the head-tilt/chin-lift maneuver, the fingers under the chin should apply a firm pressure to ensure the jaw remains closed.
    A.   True
    B.   False

94. The preferred technique of insertion for the oropharyngeal airway in pediatric patients calls for inserting the airway using a tongue blade without rotating the device.
    A.   True
    B.   False

95. The light of the laryngoscope should be a bright yellow and flicker slightly when pressure is placed on the blade.
    A.   True
    B.   False

96. The pilot balloon of the endotracheal tube should be very firm to ensure there is a good seal between the tube and the interior of the trachea.
    A.   True
    B.   False

97. When using the laryngoscope to visualize the glottis, it is best to use the teeth as a fulcrum to increase your ability to lift the tissue.
    A.   True
    B.   False

98. Carbon monoxide exposure is potentially life threatening because carbon monoxide displaces oxygen from hemoglobin in red blood cells.
    A.   True
    B.   False

99. If you cannot intubate the patient who has been paralyzed, the patient has no definitive airway.
    A.   True
    B.   False

100. Because of the anterior location of the glottic opening, it is essential to use a stylet with the endotracheal tube during pediatric intubation.
    A.   True
    B.   False

Matching

Match each respiratory emergency with its key prehospital management steps by writing the letter of the steps in the space provided next to the emergency.

101. adult respiratory distress syndrome (ARDS)

102. chronic obstructive pulmonary disease (COPD), either emphysema or chronic

    bronchitis

103. asthma

104. childhood epiglottitis

105. lung cancer

106. inhalation of a toxic substance

107. pulmonary embolism

108. pneumonia

109. Carbon Monoxide posioning

110. Hyperventilation syndrome

A.   correct hypoxia, reverse bronchospasm, and reduce inflammation

B.   ensure safety of rescue personnel, remove patient for transport, maintain open airway, and deliver humidified, high-concentration oxygen

C.   maintain airway and ventilation as needed, deliver oxygen, establish IV access, cardiac monitoring, and pulse oximetry, and transport to facility for care of underlying condition

D.   maintain airway, ventilation, and circulation as needed, deliver oxygen, establish IV access, cardiac monitoring, and pulse oximetry, and check extremities during transport to appropriate facility

E.   maintain airway and ventilation as needed with exception that examination of the throat should be avoided

F.   relieve hypoxia, reverse bronchoconstriction, and assist ventilations as needed

G. deliver oxygen, support ventilation as allowed by orders or advance directive, correct hypoxia as possible, and provide emotional support

H. Administer high concentration oxygen and transport the patient to the hospital knowing that the patient may require treatment in a hyperbaric chamber. Do not rely on oxygen saturation results.

I. primary treatment is antibiotics but pre-hospital should include oxygen therapy, placing a patient in a position of comfort and possibly the use of beta agonists

J. reassurance of the patient and supplemental oxygen while investigating the causes other than anxiety

Chapter 28

Cardiology

Part 1: Cardiovascular Anatomy and Physiology, ECG Monitoring, and Dysrhythmia Analysis

Review of Chapter Objectives

Because Chapter 28 is lengthy, it has been divided into two parts to aid in your study. Read the assigned text pages, then progress through the objectives and self-evaluation materials as you would with other chapters. When you feel secure in your grasp of the content, proceed to the next part.

After reading this part of the chapter, you should be able to:

1. Describe the incidence, morbidity, and mortality of cardiovascular disease. p. 447

The exact number of Canadians who have cardiovascular disease is unknown. It is estimated that one in four Canadians has some form of heart disease-disease of the blood vessels or risk of stroke. If this estimate is accurate, approximately 8 million Canadians have some form of cardiovascular disease. Cardiovascular disease accounts for the death of more Canadians than any other disease. In 1999, cardiovascular disease accounted for 78 942 deaths in Canada.

2. Discuss prevention strategies that may reduce the morbidity and mortality of cardiovascular disease. p. 447

There are two public health prevention strategies. The first is to educate people about the risk factors for CVD and encourage lifestyle modifications to minimize the potential impact of risk factors. The second strategy is to teach signs and symptoms of a heart attack so patients can receive medical intervention as soon as possible. As you will see, the likelihood of success with thrombolytic therapy for a heart attack in evolution (treatment with a clot-buster drug to dissolve the clot causing myocardial ischemia/hypoxia) is highest when care is instituted very early in the course of the attack.

3. Identify the risk factors most predisposing to coronary artery disease.   p. 447

Factors proven to increase the risk of CVD include (1) smoking, (2) older age, (3) family history of cardiac disease, (4) hypertension, (5) hypercholesterolemia, (6) diabetes mellitus, (7) cocaine use, and (8) male gender. Factors that are thought to increase risk include (1) diet, (2) obesity, (3) oral contraceptives, (4) sedentary lifestyle, (5) Type A personality (competitive and aggressive), and (6) psychosocial tension (stress).

4. Describe the anatomy of the heart, including the position in the thoracic cavity, layers of the heart, chambers of the heart, and location and function of the cardiac valves. pp. 448-449; also see Chapter 12

The adult heart is roughly the size of a clenched fist, and it lies in the center of the mediastinum posterior to the sternum and anterior to the spine. Roughly two-thirds of the heart lies to the left of midline, with roughly one-third to the right. The bottom of the heart, the apex, lies just above the diaphragm, whereas the top of the heart, or base, lies at roughly the level of the second rib. The heart's connections with the great vessels are at the base. The heart is made up of three tissue layers: The innermost is the endocardium, which has the same type of cells as the endothelial lining of blood vessels and is continuous with the linings of the vessels entering and leaving the heart. The thickest layer is the middle layer of muscle cells, the myocardium. These unique muscle cells physically resemble skeletal muscle but have electrical properties similar to smooth muscle cells. The outermost layer of the heart is the pericardium, a protective sac made of connective tissue arranged in two layers, the visceral pericardium (also called the epicardium) and the parietal pericardium. Normally, about 25 mL of pericardial fluid is contained between the two layers of pericardium, and the heart moves freely within the pericardial sac.

The heart is made up of two side-by-side pumps, the left side and the right side. Each side has an upper chamber, the atrium, which receives blood, and a lower chamber, the ventricle, which pumps blood into other blood vessels. The atria are separated by an interatrial septum, and the ventricles are separated by an interventricular septum. The atrial walls are thin in contrast with the ventricular walls, and almost all of the heart's pumping force is generated by the ventricles. The left ventricle, which pumps blood into the aorta, has a much thicker wall than the right ventricle, which pumps blood into the pulmonary artery (see Figure 28-1 and Figure 28-2).

The heart contains two sets of valves that help to keep blood flowing properly through the chambers and into the aorta and pulmonary artery: The atrioventricular valves lie between each atrium and ventricle. The left atrioventricular valve is called the mitral valve, and it has two characteristic leaflets. The right atrioventricular valve is called the tricuspid valve, and it has three characteristic leaflets. When the papillary muscles that connect the valves to the walls of the heart relax, the leaflets open and blood flows from the atria into the ventricles. Special fibers called the chordae tendoneae connect the leaflets of a valve to the papillary muscles, and these fibers prevent the leaflets from prolapsing back into the atrium when the valve is open. The semilunar valves lie between the ventricles and the artery into which each empties. The left semilunar valve, or aortic valve, lies between the left ventricle and the aorta. The right semilunar valve, or pulmonic valve, lies between the right ventricle and the pulmonary artery. When these valves open, blood flows in a one-way path from the ventricles into the arteries, and backflow into the ventricles is prevented.

The superior and inferior vena cavae carry deoxygenated blood from the body to the right atrium. Blood flows through the right atrium and ventricle before entering the pulmonary artery, which carries it to the lungs. Oxygenated blood leaves the lungs through the pulmonary veins and enters the left atrium. The left ventricle pumps the blood into the aorta, which feeds the oxygenated blood into peripheral arteries to flow to the rest of the body. Pressure within the heart is markedly higher on the left than on the right because resistance to flow is higher in the peripheral circulation than it is in the pulmonary circulation. Consequently, the myocardium of the left ventricle thickens as an infant ages to the point that the adult left ventricle is markedly thicker than the right.

5. Identify the major structures of the vascular system, the factors affecting venous return, the components of cardiac output, and the phases of the cardiac cycle. pp. 448-449; also see Chapter 12

In the pulmonary circulation, blood enters the lungs via the pulmonary arteries and their smaller branches, the arterioles. It eventually flows through capillaries that form networks over alveoli, and gas exchange (movement of oxygen into the blood and carbon dioxide from the blood) takes place here. The oxygenated blood then flows into the pulmonary venules and larger pulmonary veins and enters the left atrium. The peripheral circulation begins with the aorta, which receives oxygenated blood from the left ventricle. The aorta has numerous branches. These arteries and the smaller arterioles ensure oxygenated blood flows to all parts of the body. Oxygenated blood eventually enters capillary beds and oxygen exchange between blood and tissues occurs. Deoxygenated blood enters smaller venules, which empty into the larger veins that return blood to the right atrium. Gas exchange occurs in capillaries because their walls are only one cell thick. This same cell layer, the endothelium, is the innermost layer of arteries and veins.

Although the heart acts effectively as two side-by-side pumps, the contraction of the myocardium takes place as if the heart is one unit. The two atria contract at the same time, and the ventricles contract together. The atrioventricular valves open and close together, as do the two semilunar valves. The sequence of events that occurs between the end of one ventricular contraction and the next is called the cardiac cycle. Diastole, or relaxation phase, is the first part of the cycle. During diastole, blood enters the ventricles through the mitral and tricuspid valves. The aortic and pulmonic valves are closed, so the ventricles fill and no blood flows into the great vessels. During systole, the second phase, the heart contracts. First, the atria contract quickly, pumping the last of their blood into the ventricles. Then, when the pressure within the ventricles becomes greater than the pressure in the aorta and pulmonary artery, the semilunar valves open, the ventricles contract, and blood is pumped into the great arteries. This same pressure event closes the atrioventricular valves, eliminating backflow through the heart.

Under normal conditions, about two-thirds of the blood in the left ventricle at the end of diastole is pumped into the aorta during systole. This ratio of blood pumped to blood contained is called the cardiac ejection fraction. The amount of blood pumped by the left ventricle in one contraction is called the stroke volume, and it varies between roughly 60 and 100 mL, with an average of 70 mL. Cardiac output is defined as the amount of blood pumped in one minute. It is a function of stroke volume and heart rate: stroke volume (mL/beat) 3 heart rate (beats/minute) = cardiac output (mL/minute). Under average conditions, the heart rate is 60–100 bpm. Thus, average cardiac output = 70 mL 3 70 bpm = 4,900 mL/minute, or almost 5L every minute.

6. Define preload, afterload, and left ventricular end-diastolic pressure and relate each to the pathophysiology of heart failure. (see Chapter 12)

Stroke volume (the volume of blood pumped in one heartbeat) depends on three factors: preload, cardiac contractility, and afterload. The heart can only pump out the blood it receives during diastole. The pressure in the filled ventricle at the end of diastole is termed preload, or end-diastolic volume. Starling's law states that as the stretch on cardiac muscle increases (that is, as preload increases), the greater will be the force of the subsequent contraction. When preload increases, contraction pressure increases. Because the major factor determining preload is venous return from the body (or the lungs), the greater the venous return, the greater the preload and the greater the ventricular contraction pressure. Obviously, this only applies to a range of normal return volumes. If an excessive volume flows into the atrium, the atrium will become overly stretched and eventually weaken. For the left ventricle, which pumps blood to the body (including the vital brain, myocardium, and kidneys), preload is determined by venous return from the lungs. Afterload is the pressure against which the ventricles must contract to pump blood into the aorta and pulmonary arteries. An increase in afterload (peripheral resistance) decreases stroke volume. Conversely, a decrease in afterload eases the work of the ventricles and increases stroke volume.

Cardiac output (the amount of blood pumped into the aorta per minute) depends on left ventricular end-diastolic volume, myocardial contractility, and peripheral vascular resistance as measured at the origin of the aorta. Heart failure, the inability of the left ventricle to pump a physiologically adequate supply of blood, can result from a preload (ventricular end-diastolic volume) that is too low to allow effective pumping (a clinical example is shock), a reduction in cardiac contractility such that effective pumping is impossible (a clinical example is loss of myocardium through one or more MIs), or a significant increase in systemic vascular resistance (hypertension). In many cases, more than one factor (preload, contractility, afterload) may be chronically disturbed.

7. Identify the arterial blood supply to any given area of the myocardium.   (see Chapter 12)

The left coronary artery supplies the left ventricle, the interventricular septum, part of the right ventricle, and the heart's electrical conduction system. It has two main branches, the anterior descending artery and the circumflex artery. The right coronary artery supplies a portion of the right atrium and ventricle and part of the conduction system. It has two main branches, the posterior descending artery and the marginal artery. (Note that anatomic variants do exist.). There are normally numerous anastomoses, or connections, among the coronary arteries and their branches. Most of the blood drains from the coronary circulation through the anterior great cardiac vein and the lateral marginal veins into the coronary sinus. The right coronary artery empties directly into the right atrium via smaller cardiac veins.

8. Compare and contrast the coronary arterial distribution to the major portions of the cardiac conduction system.　　(see Chapter 12)

Objective 7 explains the distribution of blood through the coronary artery system.

The pacemaker cells (those with the highest level of automaticity, and thus the drivers for all of the other conductive cells) are generally in the sinoatrial (SA) node, which is located high in the right atrium (an area supplied by the right coronary artery). One branch of the conduction system leads to the left atrium. Most of the conductive cells run in one of the internodal atrial pathways through the right atrial wall to meet at the atrioventricular (AV) node. The left coronary artery typically supplies these tissues.

The conduction system then passes through the bundle of His into the interventricular septum, where the right and left bundle branches become apparent as feeders of conduction branches into the walls of the right and left ventricles (see Figure 28-3). The right bundle branch delivers the electrical impulse to the apex of the right ventricle. From there, the fibers of the Purkinje system spread it across the myocardium. The interventricular septum is typically supplied by the left coronary artery, as are the conduction fibers in the wall of the left ventricle. Some fibers in the right ventricular wall may be supplied by the right coronary artery.

9. Identify the structure and course of all divisions and subdivisions of the cardiac conduction system. (see Chapter 12)

The cardiac conduction system, which carries the electrical impulse that causes depolarization and contraction of myocardial cells. The pacemaker cells are normally found in the sinoatrial (SA) node, which is located high in the right atrium, and this is the usual origin of the electrical impulse that triggers each heartbeat. Several internodal atrial pathways carry the impulse from the SA node through the wall of the right atrium to the atrioventricular (AV) node. The impulse is carried to the left atrium via another pathway. At the AV junction, the conduction of the impulse is slowed (which allows adequate time for the ventricles to fill). The impulse moves from the AV junction via the AV fibers to the bundle of His, located high in the interventricular septum. The impulse then moves down the right and left bundle branches. The right bundle branch delivers the impulse to the apex of the right ventricle, and the fibers of the Purkinje system deliver it from there across the myocardium. The left bundle branch delivers the impulse to the thicker myocardium of the left ventricle. The left bundle branch does so via the anterior and posterior fascicles, both of which eventually terminate in the Purkinje system. Repolarization, which electrically readies the myocardial cells for the next heartbeat, proceeds in the opposite direction.

10. Identify and describe how the heart's pacemaking control, rate, and rhythm are determined. (see Chapter 12)

The cells with the highest degree of automaticity act as the heart's pacemakers, and these cells are usually found in the SA node, located high in the right atrium. On average, these cells generate impulses at the rate of 60–100 bpm. The cells of the AV node typically generate impulses at the lower rate of 40–60 bpm, and the cells of the Purkinje system, which also demonstrate automaticity, fire at roughly 15–40 bpm. Impulses generated in the SA node and conducted normally through the heart produce the ECG patterns characteristic of normal atrial rhythm.

Heart rate is controlled in part by the nervous system, and this level of control enables heart rate to accommodate the increased body oxygen need characteristic of exertion or stress. Regulation of heart rate by the autonomic nervous system is discussed in detail in objective 17.

11. Explain the physiological basis of conduction delay in the AV node.(see Chapter 12)

Not all fibers within the cardiac conduction system are the same size or absolutely alike in conduction properties. The fibers in the AV junction conduct impulses more slowly than most other conduction fibers, delaying the arrival of the electrical impulse in the AV node. Conduction within the AV node itself is also slower, and the cumulative effect is a delay that allows the ventricles time to fill properly before they contract, pumping blood out of the heart.

12. Define the functional properties of cardiac muscle.   (see Chapter 12)

The heart is made up of three groups of cardiac muscle fibers: atrial, ventricular, and specialized excitatory and conductive fibers. Atrial and ventricular cardiac muscle is striated in the same way that skeletal muscle is structured, and contraction is much the same except for one notable difference. Cardiac muscle has unique structures called intercalated discs that physically connect muscle fibers and enable extremely swift conduction of impulses from fiber to fiber (with a speed approximately 400 times that of a normal cell membrane). This uniquely rapid conduction of an impulse among muscle fibers enables cardiac muscle to function effectively as a single contractile unit. This collective functional unit is termed a syncytium. The heart has two syncytia, the atrial syncytium and the ventricular syncytium. The atria contract together in a superior to inferior direction, expelling blood into the ventricles. The ventricles contract together in an inferior to superior direction, pumping blood into the pulmonary arteries and aorta. The syncytia are separated physically and physiologically by the fibrous structure that supports the atrioventricular valves. The only normal route for impulse conduction from the atria to the ventricles is through the AV node.

Thus, the syncytial myocardial cells have the functional properties of excitability (they can respond to an electrical stimulus), conductivity (they can send an impulse to an adjoining cell), and contractility (they respond to an electrical impulse by contracting).

The even more specialized myocardial cells of the conduction system have the same properties plus an additional one, automaticity. The conductive fibers show excitability and contractility similar to those of other myocardial cells. They have an even higher degree of conductivity, which enables them to transmit an impulse so quickly that it triggers syncytial myocardium to contract in a unified manner. Their unique property is automaticity: They have the ability to depolarize without any external stimulation. This property, which is also called self-excitability, is the basis for electrical initiation of each heartbeat. The conductive cells with the highest degree of automaticity (normally those in the SA node) act as the pacemaker for the whole cardiac unit.

13. Define the events comprising electrical potential.   (see Chapter 12)

Impulse conduction and subsequent muscle fiber contraction are based functionally on depolarization of cells that maintain an electrical resting potential in the unstimulated state. Cardiac muscle cells (atrial, ventricular, and excitatory/conductive) expend energy to maintain a difference between the ion concentrations in the cell and those in the extracellular fluid. Pumps in the cell membrane expel sodium ions (Na^+) from the inside of the cell, making the inside of the cell more negatively charged than the surrounding extracellular fluid. This negative resting potential can be measured, and it is typically about –90 mV for a myocardial cell.

14. List the most important ions involved in myocardial action potential and their primary
**   function in this process. (see Chapter 12)**

The three most important ions in cardiac function are potassium, sodium, and calcium. Proper amounts of potassium in the extracellular fluid and sodium in the internal cellular environment are vital to establish and maintain the resting potential. Extracellular concentration of calcium ions is vital for excitation of the cardiac contractile process.

15. Describe the events involved in the steps from excitation to contraction of cardiac muscle fibers.   (see Chapter 12)

Impulse conduction and subsequent muscle fiber contraction are based functionally on depolarization of cells that maintain an electrical resting potential in the unstimulated state and are described in objective 13 above.

When a myocardial cell is stimulated by an electrical impulse, the membrane opens to ions. As Na^+ ions rush into the cell, the internal charge actually becomes positive relative to the outside environment—with a potential of roughly +20 mV—a change of 110 mV. The rapid influx of Na^+ ions and resultant change of membrane polarity is termed the action potential. During this same period when the membrane is permeable to ions, there is also a slower influx of Ca^{++} ions, which further increases the positive charge within the myocardial cell. After depolarization (the switch from a negative to a positive internal electrical potential) is complete, the syncytial muscle contracts as a unit. Just as rapidly (in a fraction of a second), the membrane pumps become active again, expel the excess ions, and re-establish the resting potential through repolarization of the membrane (re-establishment of the resting, negative potential).

16. Describe the clinical significance of Starling's law.   (see Chapter 12)

Starling's law states that as the stretch on cardiac muscle increases (that is, as preload increases), the greater will be the force of the subsequent contraction. When preload increases, contraction pressure increases. Because the major factor determining preload is venous return from the body (or the lungs), the greater the venous return, the greater the preload and the greater the ventricular contraction pressure. If an excessive volume flows into the atrium, the atrium will become overly stretched and eventually weaken. For the left ventricle, which pumps blood to the body (including the vital brain, myocardium, and kidneys), preload is determined by venous return from the lungs.

17. Identify the structures of the autonomic nervous system and their effect on heart rate, rhythm, and contractility.   (see Chapter 12)

The sympathetic and parasympathetic components of the autonomic nervous system act in opposition to each other, and the balance of their effects regulates heart function. The sympathetic nervous system innervates the heart through the cardiac plexus of nerves, which is located at the base of the heart. Its neurotransmitter, norepinephrine, acts to increase heart rate and cardiac contractility. There are two types of receptors in the sympathetic nervous system. Alpha receptors are found mostly in the peripheral blood vessels, where they modulate vasoconstriction. The $beta_1$ receptors are mostly found within the heart; they are responsible for the increase in heart rate and contractility with sympathetic stimulation. ($Beta_2$ receptors are chiefly in the lungs and peripheral blood vessels, and their stimulation results in bronchodilation and vasodilation.) Parasympathetic innervation of the heart is through the vagus nerve (cranial nerve X). Its neurotransmitter is acetylcholine, and parasympathetic stimulation of the heart (most of the nerve fibers of the vagus end in the atria, although some innervate the upper ventricles) results in slowed heart rate and slowed atrioventricular conduction.

18. Define and give examples of positive and negative inotropism, chronotropism, and dromotropism.   (see Chapter 12)

Inotropy refers to the strength of myocardial contraction. Sympathetic nervous stimulation acts as a positive inotropic agent, one that increases cardiac contractility. Parasympathetic stimulation, by acting as an opposite to sympathetic activity, acts as a negative inotropic agent. Chronotropy refers to heart rate (*chronos* = time). A positive chronotropic agent increases heart rate, whereas a negative chronotropic agent decreases heart rate. Sympathetic nervous stimulation acts as a positive chronotropic agent, whereas parasympathetic stimulation acts as a negative chronotropic agent. Dromotropy refers to the rate of impulse conduction. A positive dromotropic agent increases conduction speed, whereas a negative dromotropic agent slows impulse conduction.

19. Discuss the pathophysiology of cardiac disease and injury. pp. 465-510

Adequate heart function depends on adequate venous return and other vascular factors, as well as the intrinsic factors of myocardial health and function and adequacy of the electrical conduction system. Hypertension, atherosclerosis, and diabetes are risk factors for cardiac disease because they damage blood vessels, including the coronary arteries. Impaired perfusion of the myocardium (particularly the left ventricle responsible for cardiac output to the body) can lead to ischemia or MI. If infarction occurs, the amount of functional myocardium decreases, and this can ultimately lead to a decrease in cardiac output dependent on the area involved and the amount of myocardium lost.

There are innate disorders of the electrical conduction system, including developmental variants such as the accessory pathways that can make dysrhythmias more likely (such as Wolff-Parkinson-White syndrome). In addition, ischemia or infarction of the fibers of the conduction system can also make development of dysrhythmias more likely, including some (such as the tachycardias and the ventricular dysrhythmias) that can impair cardiac output to some degree or be directly life-threatening by precluding any adequacy of cardiac output (namely, ventricular fibrillation).

External agents that can harm cardiac function and possibly damage cardiac tissue include drugs. In some cases, drugs used to treat cardiac dysfunction can cause different cardiac problems.

20. Explain the purpose of ECG monitoring and its limitations.   p. 452

The electrocardiogram (*electro* = electrical, *cardio* = heart, *gram* = record) visualizes the heart's electrical activity as recorded from skin-surface electrodes. The heart is the largest generator of electrical energy in the body, and this is conducted through the body to the skin. An ECG machine records changes in current as a positive impulse (shown on the machine or on a paper printout as an upward deflection), a negative impulse (shown as a downward deflection), or no change (a flat, isoelectric line). The pattern shown over time is a chronological record of the heart's electrical activity, and it is called a rhythm strip.

The ECG in no way assesses the contractility of the myocardium or the pumping ability of the left ventricle, only the electrical activity in the different regions of the heart. There are other limitations of ECG monitoring. Artifacts may occur on the tracing, deflections that do NOT reflect the electrical activity of the heart. Artifacts may be due to a variety of causes, including muscle tremor, shivering, movements by the patient, loose electrodes, interference at the 60-hertz range, and machine malfunction. It is important that you be able to recognize artifacts and try to eliminate them from the tracing.

21. Correlate the electrophysiological and hemodynamic events occurring throughout the entire cardiac cycle with the various ECG wave forms, segments, and intervals.   pp. 456-465

The components of an ECG tracing reflect the electrical changes in the heart with each impulse conducted through the heart (Figure 28-7):
• *P wave.* This first component of the ECG reflects atrial depolarization. On Lead II, it appears as a positive, rounded wave that comes before the QRS complex. Normally, this correlates hemodynamically with the opening of the AV valves and atrial contraction, which completes the filling of the ventricles with blood.
• *QRS complex.* This second component of the ECG reflects ventricular depolarization. The Q wave is the initial negative deflection after the P wave; the R wave is the first positive deflection after the P wave; and the S wave is the first negative deflection after the R wave. You should note that not all three waves need be present, and the shape of the QRS complex can vary among individuals. Normally, this correlates hemodynamically with the opening of the semilunar valves and ventricular contraction, pumping blood into the pulmonary arteries and aorta.

• *T wave.* The T wave, which follows the QRS complex, reflects repolarization of the ventricles. It is normally positive in Lead II, rounded, and moves in the same direction as the QRS complex. This is the correlate of ventricular relaxation after contraction.
• *U wave.* A U wave is an occasional finding; when it occurs, it follows the T wave and is usually positive in deflection. U waves are normal in some individuals. You should note that it reflects electrolyte abnormalities in other patients.

In addition, three time intervals and a segment of the ECG reading also have clinical significance:

• *P-R interval (called PRI or P-Q interval, PQI).* The P-R interval is the distance from the beginning of the P wave (the beginning of atrial depolarization) to the beginning of the QRS complex (the beginning of ventricular depolarization). It represents the time taken to send the impulse from the atria to the ventricles (the delay at the AV junction and node). The R wave is absent in some individuals, and in these patients you will see a P-Q interval instead. The terms PRI and PQI are used interchangeably.

• *QRS interval.* The QRS interval is the distance from the first deflection of the QRS complex to the last, and it represents the time necessary for ventricular depolarization and onset of ventricular contraction.

• *Q-T interval.* This is the distance from the beginning of the Q wave to the beginning of the T wave, and it represents the total duration of ventricular depolarization. The duration of the Q-T interval normally has an inverse relationship with heart rate. At increased heart rates (tachycardia), the Q-T interval is generally shortened. With bradycardia, Q-T interval is generally lengthened.

• *S-T segment.* This is the distance from the S wave to the beginning of the T wave, and generally it is isoelectric. In some states such as myocardial ischemia, this segment may be either elevated or depressed.

22. Identify how heart rates, durations, and amplitudes may be determined from ECG recordings.   pp. 456-463

ECG graph paper is standardized such that paper always moves across the recording stylus at 22 mm/sec. (Each small box represents 0.04 second, and each large box is equivalent to five small boxes, or 0.20 second.) ECG paper also has time interval markings at the top of the paper, with marks placed at 3-second intervals (or 15 large boxes, 15 3 0.20 = 3.0 seconds).

Three methods exist for quickly establishing heart rate. First, if a patient has a regular rhythm, you can take the number of heartbeats in 6 seconds, multiply by 10, and get rate in beats per minute (bpm). Second, you can measure the R-R interval (also in a patient with a regular rhythm) in seconds, divide into 60, and you have heart rate per minute. If the R-R interval is 0.65 second, $60 \div 0.65 = 92$ bpm. (Other methods using the R-R interval are described on text page 96) The triplicate method, also useful only in the case of a regular rhythm, requires you to find an R wave that falls on a dark line bordering a large box. You can then assign numbers corresponding to heart rate to the next six dark lines to the right: This equates to 300, 150, 100, 75, 60, and 50 bpm. The number corresponding to the dark line closest to the peak of the next R wave is a rough estimate of heart rate. Last, you can use a commercial heart rate calculator ruler. If you prefer this method, make sure you are comfortable with at least one alternative method that does not require a physical aid!

The same standardization of time allows you to calculate the durations of the physiologically important intervals in the ECG tracing: Normal P-R interval duration is 0.12–0.20 sec; QRS interval duration is 0.08–0.12 sec; and Q-T interval is 0.33–0.42 sec. A prolonged P-R interval is one that lasts longer than 0.20 second and represents an extended delay in the AV node. A prolonged Q-T interval is one longer than 0.42 second and is thought to be related to an increased risk of certain ventricular dysrhythmias and sudden death.

The amplitude of deflections is also standardized: When a machine is properly calibrated, an amplitude of two large boxes represents 1.0 mV.

23. Relate the cardiac surfaces or areas represented by the ECG leads. p. 453

A pair of electrodes constitutes a lead. In hospital settings, a specific 12-lead configuration is standard for ECGs. In the field, a 3-lead system is often used, although one lead is adequate for detection of life-threatening dysrhythmias.

A 3-lead configuration uses Leads I, II, and III, and it shows three axes of the heart (Figure 28-4):

• Lead I (bipolar placed on a limb: positive = left arm, negative = right arm), axis 0° (parallel to collarbones)

• Lead II (bipolar placed on a limb: positive = left leg, negative = right arm), axis 60° (right atrium downward toward apex)

• Lead III (bipolar placed on a limb: positive = left leg, negative = left arm), axis 120° (left atrium downward toward apex)

Addition of three unipolar (also termed augmented) leads adds additional axes of view:
- aVR (augmented/unipolar on right arm), axis 210°
- aVL (augmented/unipolar on left arm), axis –30°
- aVF (augmented/unipolar on left foot), axis 90°

Normal recordings from the augmented leads are similar to those for Leads I, II, and III except that the deflections for aVR are inverted. The inversion is because the axis is negative, that is, it points upward toward the base of the heart instead of downward toward the apex.

The six precordial (chest) leads permit a view of the horizontal plane of the heart, which makes it possible to distinguish activity in different parts of the left ventricle and in the septum. They are designated V_1–V_6; the letter V identifies them as unipolar leads.

The deflections are primarily downward for Leads V_1 and V_2 because the leads are nearer the base of the heart than the apex, and thus they reflect the direction of electronegativity during depolarization. Deflections are primarily upward for Leads V_4, V_5, and V_6 because they are nearer the apex, and thus they are in the direction of electropositivity during depolarization.

- Leads I and aVL evaluate activity in the left side of the heart in a vertical plane.
- Leads II, III, and aVF evaluate activity in the inferior (diaphragmatic) side of the heart.
- Lead aVR evaluates activity in the right side of the heart in a vertical plane.
- Leads V_1 and V_2 evaluate activity in the right ventricle.
- Leads V_3 and V_4 evaluate activity in the interventricular septum and the anterior wall of the left ventricle.
- Leads V_5 and V_6 evaluate activity in the anterior and lateral walls of the left ventricle.

Overall, Leads V_1–V_4 view the anterior surface of the heart, and Leads I and aVL view the lateral surface of the heart. Leads II, III, and aVF view the inferior surface of the heart. Abnormal activity in a given set of leads, particularly in combination with a clinical picture consistent with acute myocardial infarction, can allow earlier identification and intervention in the ischemia-infarction process.

Lead II gives the best view of the ECG waves, and it best depicts the conduction system's activity. In single-lead systems, the lead used is generally Lead II or a lead called modified chest lead 1 (MCL_1). The chapter, as well as the remainder of the text, uses Lead II as its monitor lead. A monitor lead can provide (1) the rate of heartbeat, (2) the regularity of heartbeat, and (3) the time for conduction of impulse throughout various parts of the heart.

A monitor lead CANNOT provide (1) the presence or location of infarct, (2) the axis deviation or chamber enlargement, (3) the right-to-left differences in conduction or impulse formation, and (4) the quality or presence of pumping action.

24. Differentiate among the primary mechanisms responsible for producing cardiac dysrhythmias. pp. 461-463, 465-510

Major causes of cardiac dysrhythmias include the following: (1) myocardial ischemia, (2) necrosis or infarction, (3) autonomic nervous system imbalance, (4) distention of the heart chambers (especially the atria, secondary to congestive heart failure), (5) blood gas abnormalities, including hypoxia and abnormal pH, (6) electrolyte imbalances (primarily calcium, potassium, and magnesium), (7) trauma to the myocardium (namely, cardiac contusion), (8) drug effects and drug toxicity, (9) electrocution, (10) hypothermia, (11) CNS damage, (12) idiopathic events, (13) normal occurrences.

Note that dysrhythmias in a healthy heart are of little significance.

25. Describe a systematic approach to the analysis and interpretation of cardiac dysrhythmias. pp. 463-465

The following characterize normal sinus rhythm: (1) heart rate between 60 and 100 bpm; (2) regular rhythm, with constant P-P and R-R intervals; (3) P waves that are normal in shape, upright, and appear only before each QRS complex; (4) P-R interval that is constant and lasting 0.12–0.20 second; and (5) QRS complex with normal shape and duration less than 0.12 second. Any deviation from the normal electrical rhythm constitutes a dysrhythmia. The term arrhythmia is properly reserved for states in which there is no cardiac electrical activity.

Dysrhythmias can be approached in a number of ways, including nature of origin (namely, changes in automaticity versus disturbances in conduction), magnitude (major versus minor), severity (life-threatening versus non-life-threatening), and site (or location) of origin. This book classifies dysrhythmias into six categories by origin: (1) dysrhythmias originating in the SA node; (2) dysrhythmias originating in thc atria; (3) dysrhythmias originating within the AV junction; (4) dysrhythmias sustained or originating in the AV junction; (5) dysrhythmias originating in the ventricles; (6) dysrhythmias resulting from disorders of conduction.

26. Describe the dysrhythmias originating in the sinus node, the AV junction, the atria, and the ventricles.   pp. 466-510

Sinus bradycardia results from slowing of impulse generation in the SA node and may be due to increased parasympathetic (vagal) tone, intrinsic disease of the SA node, drug effects (typically digitalis, propranolol [a beta blocker], or quinidine), or it may be found as a normal finding in a healthy, well-conditioned person.

Sinus bradycardia on the ECG: rate less than 60 bpm, rhythm regular, pacemaker site SA node, P waves upright and normal in shape, P-R interval normal in duration and constant, QRS complex normal in duration.

Clinical significance occurs when decreased heart rate causes decreased cardiac output, hypotension, angina, or CNS symptoms; this is especially likely when rate is less than 50 bpm. Slow heart rate may also lead to atrial ectopic or ventricular ectopic rhythms. However, in a healthy athlete, sinus bradycardia may have no clinical significance.

Sinus tachycardia results from an increased rate of SA node discharge, and it may result from any of the following: exercise, fever, anxiety, hypovolemia, anemia, pump failure, increased sympathetic tone, hypoxia, or hyperthyroidism.

Sinus tachycardia on the ECG: rate greater than 100 bpm, rhythm regular, pacemaker site SA node, P waves upright and normal in shape, P-R interval normal, and QRS complex normal in duration.

Clinical significance occurs when sinus tachycardia is a compensatory mechanism for decreased stroke volume. If the rate is greater than 140 bpm, cardiac output may fall because ventricular filling time is inadequate. Very rapid rates increase myocardial oxygen demand and may precipitate ischemia or even infarct in diseased hearts. Prolonged sinus tachycardia accompanying acute myocardial infarction (AMI) is often an ominous finding suggesting cardiogenic shock.

Sinus dysrhythmia often results from a variation of the R-R interval. It may be a normal finding sometimes related to the respiratory cycle and changes in intrathoracic pressure. Pathologically, sinus dysrhythmia can be caused by increased parasympathetic (vagal) tone.

Sinus dysrhythmia on the ECG: rate 60–100 bpm and varying with respiration, rhythm irregular, pacemaker site SA node, P waves upright and normal in shape, P-R interval normal, and QRS complex normal.

Clinical significance is minimal. Sinus dysrhythmia is a normal variant, particularly in the young and the aged.

Sinus arrest occurs when the SA node fails to discharge an impulse, resulting in short periods of cardiac standstill. This standstill can persist until pacemaker cells lower in the conductive system discharge (generating escape beats) or until the sinus node resumes discharge. Sinus arrest can result from ischemia of the SA node, digitalis toxicity, excessive parasympathetic (vagal) tone, or degenerative fibrotic disease.

Sinus arrest on the ECG: rate is normal to slow, depending on the frequency and duration of the arrest, rhythm is irregular, pacemaker site is the SA node, P waves are upright and normal in shape, P-R interval and QRS complex are normal.

Clinical significance is that frequent or prolonged episodes may compromise cardiac output, resulting in syncope or other problems. There is always the danger of complete loss of SA node activity. Usually, an escape rhythm develops; cardiac standstill, however, may result.

Dysrhythmias originating in the atrioventricular (AV) junction may be due to malfunction in the junctional cells themselves or due to a slowing or blockage in conduction of an impulse from the atria to the ventricles through the AV junction. The group of dysrhythmias termed atrioventricular (AV) blocks originate within the AV junction, and they can be due to either pathology within the AV junctional tissue or to a physiological block such as atrial fibrillation.

First-degree AV block actually involves a delay in conduction at the level of the AV node rather than a complete blockage. Thus, first-degree AV block is not a rhythm itself but a condition imposed on an underlying rhythm; you must be able to establish the underlying rhythm. Although first-degree AV block can occur in a healthy heart, it is most commonly due to ischemia at the AV junction.

First-degree AV block on the ECG: rate dependent upon underlying rhythm, rhythm usually regular although it can be slightly irregular, pacemaker site either SA node or atrial, P waves normal, P-R interval longer than 0.20 sec (this is diagnostic), and QRS complex usually less than 0.12 second, but may be bizarre in shape if conductive system disease exists in the ventricles.
Clinical significance lies not in first-degree block, which is usually no danger itself, but rather in the possibility that the observed AV block may precede development of a more advanced block.

Type I second-degree AV block (also termed *second-degree Mobitz I or Wenckebach*) represents an intermittent block at the AV node. The characteristic cyclic pattern features progressively longer P-R intervals followed by a completely blocked impulse. The cycle is repetitive, and the P-P interval remains constant. The ratio of conducted to nonconducted impulses (seen as P waves to QRS complexes) is commonly 5:4, 4:3, 3:2, or 2:1. The pattern may be either constant or variable. Although this type of AV block occurs in healthy hearts, it is most common with ischemia at the AV junction. Additional causes include increased parasympathetic (vagal) tone and drug effect.

Type I second-degree AV block on the ECG: atrial rate is unaffected, whereas ventricular rate may be either normal or slowed. Atrial rhythm is typically regular, whereas ventricular rhythm is irregular because of the nonconducted beats, pacemaker site may be either in SA node or atria, P waves are normal, but the P waves for nonconducted impulses are not followed by QRS complexes. P-R interval becomes progressively longer until QRS complex is dropped, then the cycle repeats. QRS complex is usually shorter than 0.12 second but may be bizarre in shape if conductive system disease exists in the ventricles.

Clinical significance lies in decreased cardiac output if beats are frequently dropped; symptoms include syncope and angina. Note that this block may occur as a transient phenomenon immediately after an inferior wall MI.

Type II second-degree AV block is also called *second-degree Mobitz II* or *infranodal block*. This is also an intermittent block, but it is characterized by P waves that are not conducted to the ventricles without any change in length of the P-R interval before a beat is dropped. The ratio of conduction (P waves to QRS complexes) is commonly 4:1, 3:1, or 2:1, and the ratio may either be constant or vary. A 2:1 Mobitz II block is often indistinguishable from a 2:1 Mobitz I block. Type II second-degree block is usually associated with acute MI and septal necrosis.

Type II second-degree AV block presentation on the ECG: atrial rate is unaffected, whereas ventricular rate is usually bradycardic. Rhythm may be regular or irregular, dependent on whether conduction ratio is constant or variable. Pacemaker site is in the SA node or atria. P waves are normal, although some P waves are not followed by QRS complexes. The P-R interval is constant for conducted beats, but may be longer than 0.21 second. QRS complex may be normal, although it is often longer than 0.12 second because of the abnormal depolarization sequence.

Clinical significance is in the possibility of decreased cardiac output. Because this block is often associated with cell necrosis secondary to MI, it is considered more serious than Mobitz I. Many Mobitz II blocks develop into full AV blocks.

Third-degree AV block, or *complete block,* is characterized by the absence of conduction between the atria and ventricles due to complete electrical block at or below the AV node. In this case, the atria and ventricles pace independently of each other. The sinus node frequently functions normally, depolarizing the atrial syncytium, whereas an escape pacemaker below the atria paces the ventricular syncytium. Third-degree block can occur with acute MI, digitalis toxicity, or degeneration of the conductive system as can occur in the elderly.

Third-degree AV block on the ECG: Atrial rate is unaffected. Ventricular rate is 40–60 bpm if escape pacemaker is junctional, less than 40 bpm if pacemaker is lower in the ventricles. Both the atrial and ventricular rhythms are usually regular. Pacemaker site is typically SA node for atria, AV junction or ventricular for ventricles. P waves are normal but show no relationship to QRS complexes, often falling within the T wave and QRS complex. There is no relationship between the P-R interval and either P waves or R waves. The QRS complex is longer than 0.12 second if the pacemaker is ventricular and less than 0.12 second if pacemaker is junctional.

Clinical significance lies in severe compromise of cardiac output due to decreased ventricular contraction rate and loss of coordinated atrial kick.

A third group of dysrhythmias can originate in the AV junction or AV node, and these include premature junctional contractions, junctional escape complexes and rhythms, accelerated junctional rhythm, and paroxysmal junctional tachycardia. All four of these dysrhythmias share some ECG features: (1) There are inverted P waves on Lead II resulting from the retrograde depolarization of the atria. The P wave's relation to QRS depolarization depends on the relative timing of atrial and ventricular depolarization. The P wave can appear first if the atria depolarize first, or the QRS can come first if the ventricles depolarize first. If all chambers depolarize at the same time, the P wave and QRS complex can be superimposed, which effectively masks the P wave. P-R interval is less than 0.12 second, and there is normal duration of the QRS complex.

Premature junctional contractions (PJCs) result from a single impulse originating in the AV node that occurs before the next expected sinus beat; thus the beat is considered "premature." A PJC causes a compensatory pause when the SA node discharges before the premature impulse reaches it. A PJC is associated with a noncompensatory pause if the premature impulse depolarizes the sinus node and interrupts the heart's normal cadence. PJCs can result from a number of conditions, including use of alcohol, tobacco, or caffeine, sympathomimetic drugs, ischemic heart disease, hypoxia, digitalis toxicity, or from no apparent cause (idiopathic).

PJC presentation on the ECG: Rate and rhythm depend on underlying rhythm, and rhythm is usually regular except for the PJC. Pacemaker site is an ectopic focus in the AV junction. P waves are inverted and may appear before or after the QRS complex. P-R interval is less than 0.12 second if P wave occurs before QRS and is actually an R-P interval if P wave follows QRS complex. QRS complex itself is usually normal, although it may be longer than 0.12 second if the PJC is through the partially refractory ventricles.

Clinical significance of isolated PJCs is minimal. Frequent PJCs suggest organic heart disease and may be precursors of other junctional dysrhythmias.

A *junctional escape beat,* or a *junctional escape rhythm,* is a dysrhythmia that results when the primary pacemaker, usually the SA node, is slower than that of the AV node. The AV node becomes the pacemaker, generally discharging at its typical 40–60 bpm. This is a compensatory mechanism that prevents cardiac standstill. Junctional escape has several etiologies, including increased vagal tone, which can result in SA node slowing, pathological SA node discharge, or heart block.

Junctional escape rhythm presentation on the ECG: Rate typically 40–60 bpm, rhythm irregular in single junctional escape complex or regular in junctional escape rhythm. Pacemaker site is the AV node. P waves are inverted and may have any relationship to the QRS complex. P-R interval is less than 0.12 second if P wave occurs before QRS and is actually an R-P interval if P wave follows QRS complex. QRS complex is generally normal, although it may be greater than 0.12 second.

Clinical significance is decreased cardiac output due to slowed heart rate, with associated risk for precipitation of angina, syncope, or other problems. If rate is fairly rapid, rhythm may be well tolerated.

Accelerated junctional rhythms result from increased automaticity in the AV junction, causing the AV junction to discharge faster than its intrinsic rate. If the rate is fast enough, it will override the SA node. Accelerated junctional rhythm is not fast enough to qualify as tachycardia; however, it is considered accelerated because it is much faster than the typical junctional rate. A common cause is ischemia of the AV junction.

Accelerated junctional rhythm on ECG: Rate is 60–100 bpm, rhythm is regular, and pacemaker site is AV junction. P waves are inverted and may have any relationship with the QRS complex. P-R interval is less than 0.12 second if P wave occurs before QRS and is actually an R-P interval if P wave follows QRS complex. QRS complex is normal.

Clinical significance lies in the possible cause of ischemia, which can precipitate other, much less well-tolerated dysrhythmias.

Paroxysmal junctional tachycardia (PJT) develops when rapid AV junctional depolarization overrides the SA node. It often occurs in paroxysms (sudden episodes), which may last minutes or hours before terminating abruptly. It may be due to increased automaticity of a single AV nodal focus or by a reentry phenomenon at the AV node. PJT is often more appropriately called paroxysmal supraventricular tachycardia (PSVT) because the rapid rate may make it indistinguishable from paroxysmal atrial tachycardia. PJT may occur at any age and may or may not be related to underlying heart disease. Stress, overexertion, tobacco, and caffeine may precipitate it. However, it is frequently associated with underlying atherosclerotic heart disease (ASHD) and rheumatic heart disease. PJT rarely occurs with MI. It can occur with accessory pathway conduction such as Wolff-Parkinson-White syndrome.

PJT on the ECG: Rate 100–180 bpm, with characteristically regular rhythm except at onset and termination of paroxysm. Pacemaker site is AV junction. If present, P waves are inverted and may have any relationship with the QRS complex. Turning up the speed of the ECG recording to 55 mm/sec spreads out the complex and may aid in identifying P waves. P-R interval is less than 0.12 second if P wave occurs before QRS complex and is actually an R-P interval if P wave follows QRS complex. QRS complex is normal.

Clinical significance in younger patients with good cardiac reserve is minimal for a short time, and the patient usually perceives the PJT as palpitations. However, rapid rate decreases ventricular filling time and thus markedly decreases cardiac output. The reduced diastolic phase of the cardiac cycle can also compromise coronary artery perfusion. PJT can precipitate angina, hypotension, or congestive heart failure.

Dysrhythmias can also originate in atrial tissue outside the SA node or in the internodal pathways.

Atrial tachycardia, also called *ectopic tachycardia* or *wandering pacemaker,* is the passive transfer of pacemaker sites from the SA node to other latent sites in the atria or AV junction. Often more than one pacemaker site is present, causing variation in the R-R interval and P wave morphology. Atrial tachycardia can arise as a variant of sinus dysrhythmia, as a normal phenomenon in the very young or aged, or as part of ischemic heart disease or atrial dilation.

Atrial tachycardia on the ECG: Rate is usually normal, and rhythm is slightly irregular. Pacemaker site varies among SA node, atrial tissue, and AV junction. P wave morphology changes from beat to beat (as pacemaker site changes), or there may be no P waves present. P-R interval varies. It may be less than 0.12 second, normal, or longer than 0.20 second. QRS complex is normal.

Clinical significance is minimal because there are usually no detrimental effects. Occasionally, atrial tachycardia may precede other atrial dysrhythmias such as atrial fibrillation, and sometimes it may signal digitalis toxicity.

Multifocal atrial tachycardia (MAT) is usually found in acutely ill patients, and about 60% of them will have significant pulmonary disease. Certain medications used for pulmonary indications (such as theophylline) may worsen the dysrhythmia. At least three different P waves are noted, indicating the various ectopic foci. MAT can result from pulmonary disease, metabolic disorders (namely, hypokalemia), ischemic heart disease, or occur after recent surgery.

Multifocal atrial tachycardia on the ECG: Rate greater than 100 bpm, rhythm irregular. Pacemaker sites are ectopic sites in the atria. There are organized, discrete nonsinus P waves with at least three different forms. P-R interval varies, and the duration of the QRS complex may be less than 0.12 second, normal, or longer than 0.20 second, dependent on the AV node's refractory status when the ectopic impulse reaches it.

Clinical significance lies in the fact most affected patients are acutely ill; this dysrhythmia may inicate a serious underlying medical illness.

Premature atrial contractions (PACs) result from a single electrical impulse originating in the atria outside the SA node, which in turn causes a premature depolarization before the next expected SA impulse. Because the premature impulse depolarizes the atrial syncytium and the SA node, there is a noncompensatory pause in the underlying rhythm. PACs may result from use of caffeine, tobacco, or alcohol, use of sympathomimetic drugs, ischemic heart disease, hypoxia, digitalis toxicity, or no apparent cause (idiopathic).

PACs on the ECG: Rate and rhythm depend on underlying rhythm, with rhythm generally regular except for PAC. Pacemaker site is an ectopic focus in the atria. The P wave of the PAC is different than the P waves of the underlying rhythm. It occurs earlier than the next expected P wave and may be masked by the preceding T wave. The P-R interval is usually normal, although it may vary with the location of the ectopic focus. Foci near the SA node have a P-R interval of 0.12 second or longer, whereas ectopic foci near the AV node have an interval of 0.12 second or less. The QRS complex is usually normal, although duration may exceed 0.12 second if the PAC is abnormally conducted through the partially refractory ventricles. If the ventricles are refractory and do not depolarize, there will not be a QRS complex.

Clinical significance is slight for isolated PACs. However, frequent PACs may indicate organic heart disease and may precede other atrial dysrhythmias.

Paroxysmal supraventricular tachycardia (PSVT) occurs when rapid atrial depolarization overrides the SA node; this often occurs in a sudden onset paroxysm that may last minutes to hours before terminating abruptly. It may be caused by increased automaticity of a single atrial focus or by reentry at the AV node. PSVT may occur at any age and often is not associated with underlying heart disease. It may be precipitated by stress, overexertion, tobacco, or caffeine. It frequently is associated with underlying atherosclerotic cardiovascular disease and rheumatic heart disease. PSVT is rare in patients with MI; it can occur in patients with Wolff-Parkinson-White syndrome.

PSVT on the ECG: Rate 150–250 bpm, rhythm usually regular except at onset and termination of paroxysm. Pacemaker site is in the atria outside the SA node. The atrial P waves vary slightly from the sinus P waves. The atrial P wave may be impossible to see, especially when rate is rapid. Turning up the speed of the machine to 50 mm/sec spreads out the complex and may help in identifying P waves. The P-R interval is usually normal, although it may vary with location of the ectopic focus. Ectopic pacemakers near the SA node have intervals close to 0.12 second, whereas foci near the AV node have intervals of 0.12 second or less. The QRS complex is normal.

Clinical significance is less in younger patients with good cardiac reserve, who may tolerate PSVT well for short periods. Patients often perceive PSVT as palpitations. Rapid rates are associated with decreased cardiac output due to inadequate ventricular filling time. The shortened diastolic phase of the cardiac cycle can compromise coronary artery perfusion. PSVT may precipitate angina, hypotension, or congestive heart failure.

Atrial flutter results from a rapid atrial reentry circuit and an AV node that physiologically cannot conduct all impulses through to the ventricles. The AV junction may allow impulses in a 1:1, 2:1, 3:1, or 4:1 ratio or greater, resulting in a discrepancy between atrial and ventricular rates. AV block may be consistent or variable. Atrial flutter may occur in normal hearts but is usually associated with organic disease. Atrial dilation with congestive heart failure is a cause of atrial flutter. MI is only rarely a cause.

Atrial flutter on the ECG: Atrial rate 250–350 bpm, with ventricular rate dependent on ratio of AV conduction. Atrial rhythm is regular; ventricular rhythm may be regular or irregular if block is variable. Pacemaker sites are in the atria outside the SA node. Rather than a P wave, F (flutter) waves are present, which resemble sawteeth or a picket-fence pattern. This pattern may be difficult to identify in a 2:1 flutter. However, if the ventricular rate is 150 bpm, suspect 2:1 flutter. The P-R interval is usually constant but may vary, and the QRS complex is normal.

Clinical significance depends on ventricular rate. Flutter with normal ventricular rates is generally well tolerated. Rapid ventricular rates may compromise cardiac output and result in symptoms. Atrial flutter often occurs in conjunction with atrial fibrillation and is then termed atrial fib-flutter.

Atrial fibrillation results from multiple areas of reentry within the atria or from multiple ectopic foci bombarding an AV node that physiologically cannot handle all the incoming impulses. AV conduction is random and highly variable. Atrial fibrillation may be chronic and is often associated with underlying heart disease, such as rheumatic or atherosclerotic heart disease or congestive heart failure. Atrial dilation occurs with congestive heart failure and often causes atrial fibrillation.

Atrial fibrillation on the ECG: Atrial rate approximately 350–750 bpm, ventricular rate highly variable depending on conduction through AV node. Rhythm is slightly irregular. Pacemaker sites are numerous ectopic foci in the atria. P waves are not discernible. Fibrillation (f) waves are present, indicating chaotic atrial activity. There is no P-R interval, but the QRS complex is normal.

Clinical significance is in loss of atrial contraction with atrial kick, thus reducing cardiac output 20–25%. There is frequently a pulse deficit between the apical and peripheral pulse rates. If rate of ventricular response is normal, as often occurs in patients on digitalis, the rhythm may be well tolerated. If the ventricular rate is less than 60 bpm, cardiac output may fall. Suspect digitalis toxicity in patients with atrial fibrillation and a ventricular rate less than 60 bpm. If ventricular response is rapid and coupled with loss of atrial kick, cardiovascular decompensation may occur with hypotension, angina, infarct, congestive heart failure, or shock.

Patients with accessory pathways such as those with Wolff-Parkinson-White who develop atrial flutter or atrial fibrillation present special concerns. Verapamil, which decreases conduction through the AV node and may shorten the refractory period of the accessory path, may precipitate either ventricular tachycardia or ventricular fibrillation.

Dysrhythmias originating in the ventricles are associated with many causes, including ischemia, hypoxia, and certain medications. The location of the pacemaker site dictates the shape of the QRS complex.

A *ventricular escape beat (ventricular escape rhythm* or *idioventricular rhythm)* results when impulses from higher pacemakers fail to reach the ventricles or when the discharge rate of higher pacemakers falls to less than that of the ventricles (normally 15–40 bpm). Ventricular escape rhythms are compensatory mechanisms that prevent cardiac standstill. There are several etiologies, including slowing of supraventricular pacemaker sites or high-degree AV block. They are frequently the first organized rhythms seen following successful defibrillation.

Ventricular escape rhythms on ECG: Rate generally 15–40 bpm or less, with irregular rhythm in a single ventricular escape complex. Escape rhythm is usually regular unless the pacemaker site is low in the ventricular conduction system. The pacemaker site is the ventricles, and there are no P waves and no P-R intervals. The QRS complex is longer than 0.12 second and bizarre in shape.

Clinical significance lies in decreased cardiac output secondary to slow heart rate. Ventricular escape rhythms are a safety mechanism that you should NOT suppress. Escape rhythms may be either perfusing or nonperfusing.

Accelerated idioventricular rhythm, a subtype of ventricular escape rhythm, is an abnormally wide ventricular dysrhythmia typically associated with an acute MI. The rate is usually 60–110 bpm, and the patient does not require treatment unless hemodynamic instability is present, in which case the ventricular focus should be treated with atropine or overdrive pacing. The principal goal is treatment of the underlying MI.

Premature ventricular contraction (PVC) is a single ectopic impulse arising in a focus in either ventricle that occurs before the next expected beat in the underlying rhythm. PVCs may result from increased automaticity in the ectopic cell or by a reentry mechanism. The alteration in ventricular depolarization results in a wide and bizarre QRS complex and may, in addition, cause the T wave to deflect in the direction opposite to the QRS complex. Because PVCs normally do not depolarize the SA node and interrupt its rhythm, these ectopic beats lead to a fully compensatory pause. Occasionally, a PVC is interpolated between two sinus beats without causing any disturbance in the underlying rhythm. If more than one PVC is observed, it may be possible to distinguish whether there is one (unifocal) or multiple (multifocal) ectopic foci. PVCs with the same morphology imply the same focus. If the coupling interval (the distance between the preceding beat and the PVC) is constant for multiple PVCs, then the PVCs are probably unifocal. PVCs often occur in cluster patterns, including bigeminy (where every other beat is a PVC), trigeminy (where every third beat is a PVC), and quadrigeminy (where every fourth beat is a PVC). Repetitive PVCs are a pattern of two or more PVCs without a normal (sinus) beat between them, and they typically occur as couplets or triplets. ore than three consecutive PVCs are often considered ventricular tachycardia. Causes of PVCs include myocardial ischemia, increased sympathetic tone, hypoxia, acid-base disturbances, electrolyte imbalances, normal variation, and idiopathic cases.

PVCs on the ECG: Rate depends on underlying rhythm and rate of PVCs, rhythm of PVCs interrupts regularity of underlying rhythm and is occasionally irregular, and pacemaker site is within a ventricle. P waves are absent; however, a normal sinus P wave may appear before a PVC. There is thus no P-R interval. The QRS complex of the PVC is longer than 0.12 second and bizarre in morphology.

Clinical significance may be slight in patients without heart disease, who sense the PVC as a skipped beat. In patients with myocardial ischemia, PVCs may suggest ventricular irritability and may precede lethal ventricular dysrhythmias. PVCs are often classified as benign or malignant. Malignant PVCs show at least one of five traits: (1) more than six PVCs/minute; (2) R on T phenomenon; (3) couplets or runs of ventricular tachycardia; (4) multifocal in nature; and (5) associated chest pain. Because the ventricles do not fill properly with most PVCs, you will usually not feel a pulse during the PVCs themselves. Grades 0–5 on the Lown system equate the combination of malignant PVC traits to a numerical score. Grade 0 has no PVCs, whereas Grade 4 has repetitive PVCs (couplets or triplets) and Grade 5 shows R on T phenomenon.

Treatment is indicated for patients with a prior history of heart disease or symptoms or if the PVCs are malignant.

Ventricular tachycardia (VT) consists of three or more consecutive ventricular complexes at a rate of 100 bpm or higher. This rhythm overrides the heart's normal pacemaker, and thus the atria and ventricles are asynchronous. In monomorphic VT all complexes appear the same, whereas in polymorphic VT the complexes appear in difference sizes and shapes. The causes for VT are the same as for PVCs.

VT on the ECG: Rate roughly 100–250, with regular or slightly irregular rhythm, and pacemaker site in a ventricle. If P waves are present, they are not associated with the QRS complexes. There is no P-R interval, and the QRS complex is longer than 0.12 second and bizarre in morphology.
Clinical significance lies in the poor stroke volume and rapid rate associated with VT, which may cause severe compromise in cardiac output and coronary artery perfusion. Always remember that VT may deteriorate into ventricular fibrillation. Treatment type depends on whether VT is perfusing or nonperfusing.

Ventricular fibrillation is a chaotic ventricular rhythm that usually results from many reentry circuits within the ventricles. There is no ventricular depolarization or contraction. Although many causes have been identified, it is notable that most result from advanced coronary artery disease.

Ventricular fibrillation on ECG: There is no organized rate or rhythm, and P waves are usually absent. P-R interval is absent, as are QRS complexes. The pacemaker sites are numerous ectopic foci within the ventricles.

Clinical significance is the lethal nature of this dysrhythmia due to lack of cardiac output or organized electrical pattern within the heart.

Asystole is cardiac standstill marked by absence of all cardiac electrical activity. Asystole may be the primary event in cardiac arrest; it is usually associated with massive MI, ischemia, and necrosis. It may result from heart block when no escape pacemaker takes over, and asystole is often the final outcome of ventricular fibrillation.

Asystole on the ECG: No electrical activity with complete absence of P waves, QRS complexes, and T waves.

The likelihood of successful resuscitation is very low.

Artificial pacemaker rhythm results from regular cardiac stimulation by an electrode implanted in the heart and connected to a power source. Demand pacemakers represent an escape rhythm. Ventricular pacemakers stimulate only the right ventricle, resulting in an idioventricular-type rhythm. Dual-chambered pacemakers (also called AV sequential pacemakers) stimulate the atria and then the ventricles. Pacemakers are typically implanted in patients who have chronic high-grade heart block or sick sinus syndrome or who have had episodes of severe symptomatic bradycardia.

Pacemakers on the ECG: Rate varies with the preset rate of the pacemaker. Rhythm is regular if the heart is paced constantly, whereas rhythm is irregular if pacing is on demand. Pacemaker site depends on electrode placement. Ventricular pacemakers will not produce a P wave. Any sinus P waves seen are unrelated to the paced QRS complexes. Dual-chambered pacemakers produce a P wave behind each atrial spike. The spike is an artifact caused by each firing of the pacemaker, and it may be an upward or downward deflection. QRS complexes are usually longer than 0.12 second and bizarre in morphology, and they often resemble those of ventricular escape rhythms. A QRS complex should follow each pacemaker spike. When this occurs, the pacemaker is said to be "capturing" the ventricles. With demand pacemakers, some natural QRS complexes may appear, and these will not be associated with any spike.

27. Describe the process and pitfalls of differentiating wide QRS complex tachycardias. pp. 499-500

Ventricular tachycardia (VT) is the paradigm of a tachycardia with a wide, frequently bizarre QRS complex. In the discussion under objective 26, you learned that nonperfusing VT requires immediate treatment in order to restore tissue oxygenation. Drugs that may be useful include lidocaine, procainamide, or amiodarone. Synchronized cardioversion is generally the next alternative treatment. In cases with chest pain, dyspnea, or systolic BP less than 90 mmHg, synchronized cardioversion is indicated as the immediate treatment. *Torsade de pointes,* a subtype of VT, is commonly caused by certain antidysrhythmic drugs, including procainamide and amiodarone. Thus, prompt recognition of *torsade de pointes*—before initiating any treatment—is vital because you do NOT want to use the antidysrhythmics normally used for VT.

When you look at your initial rhythm strip, the QRS complexes of VT are relatively uniform in appearance and amplitude. In contrast, the QRS complexes of *torsade de pointes* characteristically are not uniform in appearance and amplitude. Instead, the QRS complexes are wide and change in amplitude over the span of several complexes. The span of complexes also tends to vary roughly around a central point. Look at Figure 28-41, and draw a line joining the peaks of the upward deflections and another line connecting the lowest points of the downward deflections. You will see that the two lines almost form a "fish" shape that has its ends at a central point and that the strip shows one such large shape after another. This is the twisting about a point that is implicit in the French *torsade de pointes.* Another characteristic on ECG is a Q-T interval lengthened to 600 milliseconds or more during the breaks between the twisting spans of widened QRS complexes.

28. Describe the conditions of pulseless electrical activity. pp. 507-508

Pulseless electrical activity (PEA, also called electrical mechanical dissociation) means that electrical complexes are present on ECG, but there are no accompanying cardiac contractions. This is the paradigm of the situation in which you should treat the patient rather than the monitor. The ECG may show normal sinus rhythm, but your patient will be pulseless. Underlying conditions that can result in PEA and their general treatment (dependent on local protocol) include (1) hypovolemia/fluid resuscitation; (2) cardiac tamponade/pericardiocentesis; (3) tension pneumothorax/needle thoracostomy; (4) hypoxemia/intubation and oxygen; and (5) acidosis/sodium bicarbonate, as well as massive pulmonary embolism and rupture of the ventricular wall.

29. Describe the phenomena of reentry, aberration, and accessory pathways.
pp. 445-446, 446-447, 509-510

Reentry (of an impulse) occurs when two branches of a conduction pathway are altered by a pathologic process such that conduction is slowed in one branch and a unidirectional block is caused in the other. In this case, a normal, anterograde depolarizing impulse travels slowly through the branch with slowed conduction and is blocked in the other. After the impulse travels through the branch with slowed conduction, it enters the branch with the block and is then conducted in the opposite, retrograde direction back toward the source of the impulse. Because this tissue is no longer refractory, it is depolarized by the returning impulse (the one with retrograde directionality). This reentry of an impulse back into the pathway of origin can result in rapid rhythms such as paroxysmal supraventricular tachycardia or atrial fibrillation.

Aberration, or aberrant conduction, reflects conduction of an impulse through the heart's conductive system in abnormal fashion. Aberrant conduction reflects a single supraventricular beat that is conducted through the ventricles in a delayed manner. In bundle branch block (either the right or left bundle can be affected), all supraventricular impulses traveling through the affected branch are delayed. If both branches are affected, third-degree heart block exists. Note that the impulses in these cases arise above the level of the ventricles, unlike the pure ventricular rhythms. In incomplete bundle branch block, the QRS complex will be normal. In complete bundle branch block, there will be a widened QRS complex on the ECG, and this may cause confusion as to whether the rhythm is supraventricular or ventricular in origin. Although there are exceptions, you can use the following guidelines to try to distinguish bundle branch block from a pure ventricular rhythm: (1) a changing bundle branch block suggests SVT with aberrancy; (2) a trial of carotid sinus massage may slow conduction through the AV node and terminate a reentrant SVT or slow conduction of other supraventricular dysrhythmias, whereas it will have no effect on ventricular dysrhythmias; (3) AV block (AV dissociation) indicates ventricular origin; (4) a full compensatory pause, usually seen after a ventricular beat, indicates ventricular tachycardia (VT); (5) fusion beats suggest VT as well; and (6) a QRS duration of longer than 0.14 second usually indicates VT.

An accessory pathway is an extra conduction pathway within the conduction system. In Wolff-Parkinson-White syndrome (WPW), the extra conduction pathway is the bundle of Kent, a pathway that is between the atria and ventricles. The presence of this extra (or accessory) pathway means that the depolarizing impulse effectively bypasses the AV node, shortening the P-R interval and prolonging the QRS complex. Although most patients with the syndrome are asymptomatic, WPW is associated with a high incidence of tachydysrhythmias, usually through a reentry phenomenon. WPW is also referred to as a pre-excitation syndrome because the ventricles are electrically excited before the impulse can arrive via the AV node. Although it is not always present on ECG monitoring, a delta wave (a slur on the upstroke of the QRS complex) is indicative of WPW.

30. Identify the ECG changes characteristically produced by electrolyte imbalances and specify
their clinical implications.   p. 510

You should always suspect hyperkalemia in patients with a history of renal failure who are on dialysis because potassium tends to be retained in the body. On an ECG, an early sign of hyperkalemia is tall, peaked T waves in the precordial leads. As the blood level rises higher, conduction decreases and the P-R and Q-T intervals increase in length. At very high potassium levels, an idioventricular rhythm may develop and eventually become a classic sine wave. In hypokalemia, the opposite ion disturbance, prominent U waves occur. Very low blood potassium levels can cause a widened QRS complex.

Clinically, hyperkalemia causes the heart to dilate and become flaccid and heart rate slows. Elevation of blood potassium to 2–3 times the normal value can cause so much heart weakness and abnormalities in rhythm that death may ensue.

31. Identify patient situations where ECG rhythm analysis is indicated.   pp. 495-510

You will have specific guidelines for ECG monitoring. They will include direct medical cardiac causes such as history of heart disease, MI, or dysrhythmia, as well as any current evidence of dysrhythmia or hemodynamic instability or patient complaints suggestive of angina or acute MI. They will also cover traumatic causes (chest injury that may involve the heart or lungs) and evidence suggesting inadequate oxygenation in the body (such as altered level of consciousness) that may reflect cardiovascular compromise. Last, you may have guidelines recommending monitoring in some metabolic situations (such as hypothermia). Remember that you always treat the patient, not the ECG.

32. Recognize the ECG changes that may reflect evidence of myocardial ischemia and injury and their limitations.   pp. 461-463

Changes in the S-T segment are usually looked for as evidence of myocardial ischemia or acute MI. Ischemic tissue produces abnormalities such as S-T segment depression (the norm is an isoelectric line) or an inverted T wave, with inversion usually symmetrical. Tissue injury, which occurs next in the early phase of an MI, may elevate the S-T segment. Finally, as tissue dies a significant Q wave develops. (Such a Q wave is at least one small square wide, lasting 0.04 second or more, or is more than one-third the height of the QRS complex.) Q waves may also indicate extensive transient ischemia. It is often difficult to interpret an ECG without knowledge of the patient's baseline ECG, and this is particularly true in patients with history of cardiac disease such as prior MI.

33. Correlate abnormal ECG findings with clinical interpretation.   pp. 461-463

See objectives 26–28, 30, 32, and 35. You may also find a J wave (or Osborn wave) on ECG monitoring. This wave is a slow, positive, rounded deflection at the end of the QRS complex that accompanies hypothermia. Other ECG changes seen with hypothermia include T wave inversion, P-R, QRS, or Q-T prolongation, sinus bradycardia, atrial flutter or fibrillation, AV block, PVCs, ventricular fibrillation, or asystole.

34. Identify the major mechanical, pharmacological, and electrical therapeutic objectives in the treatment of the patient with any dysrhythmia.   pp. 465-510

The descriptions of dysrhythmias, their clinical significance, and ECG findings associated with them are given in objective 26 above. Treatments for the conditions are discussed below.

• *Sinus bradycardia.* The overall goal of treatment is satisfactory heart rate, with subsequently adequate cardiac output and blood pressure and decreased risk of more dangerous dysrhythmias. Thus, treatment is based on symptoms, and no treatment may be needed unless hypotension or ventricular irritability is present. If treatment is needed, give a 0.5 mg bolus atropine sulfate, and repeat every 3–5 minutes until rate is satisfactory or you have given 0.04 mg/kg atropine. If atropine fails, consider transcutaneous cardiac pacing (TCP), if available.
• *Sinus tachycardia.* Treatment is directed at the underlying cause. Hypovolemia, fever, anemia, or other cause should be corrected. The overall goal is to reduce heart rate to a level compatible with adequate ventricular filling time, with supports in place to maintain an adequate stroke volume.
• *Sinus dysrhythmia.* Sinus dysrhythmia is a normal variant, particularly in the young and aged. Treatment is thus typically not required.
• *Sinus arrest.* If the patient is extremely bradycardic or symptomatic, give a 0.5 mg bolus atropine sulfate. The goal of pharmacologic therapy is to bring rate up to a level where symptoms are eliminated because cardiac output is adequate.
• *First-degree AV block.* Treatment is generally restricted to observation unless heart rate drops significantly. If possible, avoid administration of any drug that will further slow AV conduction, such as lidocaine and procainamide. The goal of treatment, if needed, is to preserve or improve AV conduction, eliminating the risk of development of a higher degree of heart block. When necessary, treatment may be needed to increase heart rate to a level compatible with adequate cardiac output.
• *Type I second-degree AV block* (also termed *second-degree Mobitz I* or *Wenckebach*). Treatment is generally restricted to observation. If possible, you want to avoid administration of any drug that will further slow AV conduction, such as lidocaine and procainamide. If heart rate falls and the patient

becomes symptomatic, give 0.5 mg atropine IV. Repeat every 3–5 minutes until rate is satisfactory or you have given 0.04 mg/kg of atropine. If atropine fails, consider TCP if available. Overall goal is preservation or improvement of AV conduction and maintenance of a heart rate associated with adequate cardiac output.

• *Type II second-degree AV block* (also called *second-degree Mobitz II* or *infranodal block*). Definitive treatment is pacemaker insertion to preserve a normal rhythm and adequate cardiac output. In the prehospital setting, give medications if needed to stabilize the patient. Use caution in giving atropine to patients with second-degree Mobitz II blocks because the atropine may increase atrial rate but also worsen the AV nodal block. Consider TCP if available. If the patient remains symptomatic, do not delay application of TCP while waiting for IV access or time for atropine to take affect.

• *Third-degree AV block.* Definitive treatment is pacemaker insertion to preserve adequate cardiac output. In the prehospital setting, give medications if needed to stabilize patient. Use caution in giving atropine to patients with third-degree blocks because the atropine may increase atrial rate but also worsen the AV nodal block. Consider TCP if available. If the patient remains symptomatic, do not delay application of TCP while waiting for IV access or time for atropine to take affect. NEVER use lidocaine to treat third-degree block with ventricular escape beats.
• *Premature junctional contractions (PJCs).* Treatment is restricted to observation if the patient is asymptomatic.
• *Junctional escape rhythm.* Treatment in the field is generally restricted to observation (as patients are asymptomatic); however, care is needed if hypotension or ventricular irritability is present. If needed, give 0.5 mg bolus atropine, and repeat every 3–5 minutes until rate is satisfactory or you've given 0.04 mg/kg atropine. If atropine fails, consider TCP if available. Overall goal is preservation of cardiac output and blood pressure and prevention of more dangerous ventricular dysrhythmias.
• *Accelerated junctional rhythm.* Treatment goal is to correct ischemia.
• *Paroxysmal junctional tachycardia (PJT).* Treatment in the patient who is not tolerating PJT, as evidenced by hemodynamic instability, consists of the following sequence of steps. (1) Vagal maneuvers. (2) Therapy with adenosine (Adenocard), followed by verapamil if rate does not respond and there are no contraindications to verapamil. Verapamil should not be used with beta blockers. Verapamil-induced hypotension can often be reversed with 0.5–1.0 gm calcium chloride IV. (3) Electrical therapy with synchronized cardioversion if ventricular rate is higher than 150 bpm or patient is hemodynamically unstable. If time allows, use presedation. Apply synchronized DC countershock of 100 joules. Remember that DC countershock is contraindicated if digitalis toxicity is suspected. The overall goal is to reach a heart rate compatible with adequate ventricular filling time and good cardiac output, as well as to ensure adequate coronary artery perfusion.
• *Atrial tachycardia.* Treatment options for symptomatic patients include consideration of adenosine or verapamil to lower heart rate and prevent other dysrhythmias, including atrial fibrillation.
• *Multifocal atrial tachycardia.* Treatment of the underlying medical condition usually resolves the dysrhythmia. Specific antidysrhythmic therapy is usually not needed.
• *Premature atrial contractions (PACs).* Treatment for the symptomatic patient is oxygen via nonrebreather mask and establishment of IV access, along with consultation with medical direction. Field goal is to maintain tissue oxygenation and prepare for possible development of other, more clinically significant dysrhythmias.
• *Paroxysmal supraventricular tachycardia (PSVT).* Treatment for patients who are not tolerating the rapid heart rate, as evidenced by hemodynamic instability, should consist of the following series of techniques: (1) Vagal maneuvers. Note that carotid sinus massage should not be done in patients with carotid bruits or known cerebrovascular or carotid artery disease. (2) Pharmacological therapy with adenosine IV. If this fails and patient has normal blood pressure and a narrow QRS complex, consider use of verapamil if no contraindications exist. (3) Electrical therapy with synchronized cardioversion. DC countershock is contraindicated when digitalis toxicity is suspected. The overall goal is attainment of heart rate compatible with adequate cardiac output and coronary perfusion.
• *Atrial flutter.* Treatment is indicated for cases with rapid ventricular rates and hemodynamic compromise. Immediate cardioversion is indicated in unstable patients. Occasionally, you may use pharmacological therapy with stable patients, especially if the rapid ventricular rate is causing congestive heart failure. Several medications slow ventricular rate, including diltiazem (Cardizem),

verapamil, digitalis, beta blockers, procainamide, and quinidine. Procainamide and quinidine are often used to convert back to sinus rhythm. Consult local medical direction for protocol specifics.

• *Atrial fibrillation.* Prehospital treatment is necessary when rapid ventricular rates with hemodynamic instability occur. Electrical therapy with immediate cardioversion is required in unstable patients—persons with heart rates greater than 150 bpm and associated chest pain, dyspnea, decreased level of consciousness, or hypotension. Pharmacological therapy may be useful, especially when rapid heart rate is causing congestive heart failure. Drugs that may be used include diltiazem, verapamil, digitalis, beta blockers, procainamide, and quinidine. Atrial fibrillation is a documented risk factor for stroke because atrial dilation allows for stagnation of blood and development of clots. You may wish to consider administration of an anticoagulant. Consult medical direction for specifics of possible pharmacological options. Immediate treatment goal is improvement of cardiac output. (Ultimate goal is adjustment of digitalis level, if toxicity is cause.)

Patients with accessory pathways such as those with Wolff-Parkinson-White who develop atrial flutter or atrial fibrillation present special concerns. Verapamil, which decreases conduction through the AV node and may shorten the refractory period of the accessory path, may precipitate either ventricular tachycardia or ventricular fibrillation.

• *Ventricular escape rhythms.* Treatment depends on whether the rhythm is perfusing or not. If perfusing, the goal is to increase heart rate with atropine or, if it fails, TCP if available. With a nonperfusing rhythm, follow your pulseless electrical activity (PEA) protocol, including airway stabilization and CPR and IV epinephrine. Direct treatment is aimed at the primary problem, such as hypovolemia, hypoxia, cardiac tamponade, acidosis, or other. Consider a fluid challenge.

• *Accelerated idioventricular rhythm.* This is a subtype of ventricular escape rhythm and is an abnormally wide ventricular dysrhythmia typically associated with an acute MI. The rate is usually 60–110 bpm, and the patient does not require treatment unless hemodynamic instability is present, in which case the ventricular focus should be treated with atropine or overdrive pacing. The principal goal is treatment of the underlying MI.

• *Premature ventricular contractions (PVCs).* Treatment is indicated for patients with a prior history of heart disease or symptoms or if the PVCs are malignant. Administer oxygen and establish IV access. If the patient is symptomatic, give lidocaine at a dose of 1.0–1.5 mg/kg body weight. Give an additional bolus of 0.5–0.75 mg/kg every 5–10 minutes as needed until a total of 3.0 mg/kg has been reached. If PVCs are effectively suppressed, start a lidocaine drip at a rate of 2–4 mg/minute. Reduce dose in appropriate patients, and consider procainamide or bretylium if the ceiling dose of lidocaine has been reached or the patient is allergic to lidocaine. Overall goal is adequate ventricular filling and cardiac output and prevention of ventricular tachycardia or ventricular fibrillation.

• *Ventricular tachycardia (VT).* Treatment type depends on whether VT is perfusing or nonperfusing. If there is a pulse (perfusing VT), give oxygen and place an IV line. Give lidocaine IV at 1.0–1.5 mg/kg and additional doses of 0.5–0.75 mg/kg up to a total of 3.0 mg/kg. If unsuccessful, try procainamide or amiodarone as a second-line agent. Instability (namely, chest pain, dyspnea, or systolic BP less than 90 mmHg) calls for synchronized cardioversion. If you note instability at the outset of treatment, such as falling blood pressure or altered level of consciousness, initiate cardioversion immediately after starting oxygen and an IV. If there is no pulse (nonperfusing VT), treat as for ventricular fibrillation. Treatment goals are to maintain adequacy of cardiac output and coronary artery perfusion and to prevent ventricular fibrillation.

• *Ventricular fibrillation.* Treatment of ventricular fibrillation and nonperfusing VT is the same: Initiate CPR and follow with DC countershock at 200 joules. If unsuccessful, repeat at 200–300 joules; if still unsuccessful, try at 360 joules. Subsequent to countershock, control airway and establish IV access. Epinephrine 1:10,000 is the drug of first choice; give every 3–5 minutes as needed. If unsuccessful, consider second-line agents such as lidocaine, amiodarone, procainamide, or even magnesium sulfate.

• *Asystole* (or *cardiac standstill*). Treatment is CPR, airway management, oxygenation, and medication. If there is any doubt of an underlying rhythm, attempt defibrillation.

35. Describe artifacts that may cause confusion when evaluating the ECG of a patient with a pacemaker .   pp.452-453, 505-506

ECG findings for patients with pacemakers are given in objective 26 above.

Note that any patient who has a demand pacemaker may have normal ECG sequences when the pacemaker has not been activated. There will not be any spikes during this time period, only when the pacemaker has been activated. In contrast, patients with a fixed-rate pacemaker will always have spike artifacts because the pacemaker is continually firing at its preset rate.

36. List the possible complications of pacing. p. 505-506

Possible problems with pacemakers include the following: (1) The battery fails. If batteries fail before they are replaced, pacing stops and the patient's underlying rhythm returns. (2) The pacemaker runs away. In this case (rarely seen with newer pacemakers), the pacemaker discharges at a rapid rate rather than the preset rate. In the older pacemakers, this is most likely to be seen when the battery runs low. Newer models avoid this possible problem by gradually increasing rate as the battery runs low. (3) Failure of a demand pacemaker to shut down when the innate rate exceeds the preset rate. When this happens, the heart's pacemaker and the artificial pacemaker compete, with both pacing the myocardium. If a paced beat falls during the absolute or relative refractory period, it can precipitate ventricular fibrillation. (4) Failure to capture. In this instance, battery failure or displacement of the pacemaker lead results in pacemaker discharge (with resultant ECG spike) that does not lead to depolarization of the myocardium (thus there is no QRS complex following the spike). Bradycardia often is seen.

37. List the causes and implications of pacemaker failure.   p. 505-506

As seen in objective 36, battery failure, although unlikely, is probably the most common cause of pacemaker dysfunction or failure. Displacement of the discharge lead can also lead to pacemaker failure. In these cases, the patient's underlying rhythm is usually seen, and it is often bradycardic and sufficiently low in cardiac output to cause symptoms (or the pacemaker would not have been implanted). In other patients, asystole can occur when a fixed-rate pacemaker fails.

The failure of a demand pacemaker to shut down (a different way in which pacemaker function is lost) may lead to ventricular fibrillation if a paced beat occurs while the myocardium is in absolute or relative refractory state.

38. Identify additional hazards that interfere with artificial pacemaker function. pp. 505-506

You should always examine unconscious patients for evidence of a pacemaker: Batteries, for instance, are often palpable under the skin (commonly in the axillary or shoulder region). You can treat bradydysrhythmias, asystole, and ventricular fibrillation in patients with failed pacemakers as you would in other patients, but you must be careful not to discharge defibrillation paddles directly over the battery pack.

39. Recognize the complications of artificial pacemakers as evidenced on an ECG. pp. 505-506

See objective 35.

40. Describe the characteristics of an implanted pacemaking system. pp. 505-506

See objective 32

CONTENT SELF-EVALUATION

Multiple Choice

1. From innermost to outermost, the three tissue layers of the heart are:
   - A.   the endocardium, the pericardium, and the myocardium.
   - B.   the endocardium, the myocardium, and the syncytium.
   - C.   the endocardium, the myocardium, and the pericardium.
   - D.   the myocardium, the epicardium, and the pericardium.
   - E.   the epicardium, the myocardium, and the endocardium.

2. The blood supply to the left ventricle, interventricular septum, part of the right ventricle, and the heart's conduction system comes from the two branches of the left coronary artery, which are the:
   - A.   anterior descending artery and the circumflex artery.
   - B.   anterior descending artery and the posterior descending artery.
   - C.   circumflex artery and the posterior descending artery.
   - D.   circumflex artery and the marginal artery.
   - E.   marginal artery and the posterior descending artery.

3. Stimulation of the heart by the sympathetic nervous system results in:
   - A.   negative inotropic and chronotropic effects.
   - B.   negative chronotropic and dromotropic effects.
   - C.   positive chronotropic and dromotropic effects.
   - D.   positive inotropic and chronotropic effects.
   - E.   positive inotropic and dromotropic effects.

4. The cardiac conductive cells have which of the following properties?
   - A.   excitability
   - B.   conductivity
   - C.   automaticity
   - D.   contractility
   - E.   all of the above

5. All of the following can cause an artifact on ECG EXCEPT:
   - A.   an artificial pacemaker.
   - B.   an enlarged heart.
   - C.   movement by the patient.
   - D.   shivering by the patient.
   - E.   loose electrodes.

6. Common causes of dysrhythmias include all of the following EXCEPT:
   - A.   myocardial ischemia or infarction.
   - B.   electrolyte and pH disturbances.
   - C.   CNS or autonomic nervous system damage.
   - D.   drug effects.
   - E.   hyperthermia.

7. In the bradycardia algorithm, the first drug in the intervention sequence is:
   - A.   procainamide.
   - B.   epinephrine.
   - C.   atropine.
   - D.   isoproterenol.
   - E.   dopamine.

8. Of the atrial dysrhythmias listed below, which is often an indication of serious underlying medical disease?
   - A.   atrial tachycardia
   - B.   atrial flutter
   - C.   premature atrial contractions (PACs)
   - D.   multifocal atrial tachycardia (MAT)
   - E.   paroxysmal supraventricular tachycardia (PSVT)

9. The diagnostic finding for first-degree AV block on ECG is:
   A. the presence of some QRS complexes not preceded by a P wave.
   B. a P-R interval longer than 0.20 second.
   C. a QRS complex widened to longer than 0.12 second.
   D. an R-T interval widened for those beats with an initial P wave.
   E. the presence of some P waves without following QRS complexes.

10. All of the following statements about third-degree AV block are true EXCEPT:
    A. the atrial rate is unaffected, and ventricular rate depends on site of ventricular pacemaker.
    B. P waves are normal but show no relationship to the QRS complex.
    C. there is an absence of conduction between the atria and the ventricles.
    D. both atrial and ventricular rhythms are usually regular.
    E. QRS complexes are normal in length.

11. All of the following statements about ECG findings for dysrhythmias originating in the AV junction are true EXCEPT:
    A. P-R interval is less than 0.12 second.
    B. P waves are inverted in Lead II.
    C. T waves are blunted and widened.
    D. QRS complexes are normal in duration.
    E. P waves are masked if atrial depolarization occurs during ventricular depolarization.

12. Caffeine, tobacco, alcohol, and sympathomimetic drugs are common causes of:
    A. junctional escape rhythms.   D. premature junctional contractions.
    B. accelerated junctional rhythm.   E. junctional bradycardia.
    C. paroxysmal junctional tachycardia.

13. All of the following statements about dysrhythmias originating in the ventricles are true EXCEPT:
    A. ischemia, hypoxia, and drug effects are common causes.
    B. T waves are blunted and widened.
    C. P waves are absent.
    D. the pacemaker site determines QRS morphology.
    E. QRS complexes are 0.12 second or longer in duration.

14. *Torsades de pointes* varies in both cause and ECG appearance from other forms of:
    A. ventricular escape rhythm.   D. premature ventricular contraction.
    B. accelerated idioventricular rhythm. E. ventricular tachycardia.
    C. ventricular fibrillation.

15. Possible characteristics of malignant PVCs include all EXCEPT:
    A. R on T phenomenon.
    B. couplets or longer runs of ventricular tachycardia.
    C. more than eight PVCs per minute.
    D. multifocal origin within the ventricles.
    E. accompanying chest pain.

16. Nonperfusing ventricular tachycardia and ventricular fibrillation are treated identically, including initiation of CPR followed by:
    A. epinephrine 1:10 000 IV bolus.   D. DC countershock at 200 joules.
    B. adenosine IV bolus.   E. atropine IV bolus.
    C. transcutaneous cardiac pacing (TCP).

17. Causes of asystole include all of the following EXCEPT:
    A.   pre-existing alkalosis (respiratory or metabolic).
    B.   hyperkalemia.
    C.   hypokalemia.
    D.   drug overdose.
    E.   hypothermia.

18. The correct bipolar lead placement site for lead two is:
    A.   left arm +, left leg -.
    B.   left leg +, left arm -.
    C.   left leg +, right arm -.
    D.   right arm +, left leg -.
    E.   right arm +, right leg -.

19. One small box on standard ECG graph paper is equivalent to:
    A.   0.04 sec   D.   0.08 sec.
    B.   0.20 sec   E.   0.02 sec.
    C.   0.15 sec.

20. The "P wave" of and ECG corresponds to:
    A.   ventricular depolarization.
    B.   atrial depolarization.
    C.   atrial repolarization.
    D.   ventricular repolarization.
    E.   atrial and ventricular repolarization.

21. Causes of sinus arrest include all of the following EXCEPT:
    A.   digitalis toxicity.   D.   ischemia of the SA node.
    B.   excessive vagal tone.   E.   atrial dilation.
    C.   degenerative fibrotic disease.

22. Which of the following is the appropriate pharmacological treatment for SVT?
    A.   digoxin   D.   metoprolol.
    B.   diltiazem.   E.   morphine sulphate.
    C.   adenosine.

23. Treatment of a third-degree AV block includes:
    A.   lidocaine.
    B.   synchronized cardioversion.
    C.   transcutaneous pacing.
    D.   adenosine.
    E.   metoprolol.

24. Which of the following represents the best order of treatment for asystole?
    A.   epinephrine 1.0 mg IV, intubation, atropine 1.0 mg IV.
    B.   TCP, epinephrine 1.0 mg IV, atropine 1.0 mg IV, intubation.
    C.   intubate, epinephrine 2.0 mg ETT, lidocaine 3.0 mg/kg ETT
    D.   ventilation, TCP, epinephrine 1.0 mg IV, atropine 1.0 mg IV.
    E.   synchronized cardioversion, intubate, epinephrine 1.0 mg IV, atropine 1.0 mg
         IV

25. Which of the following is not a cause of pulseless electrical activity (PEA)?
    A.   hyovolemia
    B.   hyperkalemia.
    C.   hypokalemia.
    D.   hypoglycemia.
    E.   pulmonary embolism

True/False

26. A prolonged QT interval is longer than 0.38 second.
- **A.** True
- **B.** False

27. The chief difference between Type I and Type II second-degree AV block is the pattern of lengthening P-R interval before the blocked impulse in Type I second-degree AV block.
- **A.** True
- **B.** False

28. Never use lidocaine to treat third-degree heart block in patients with ventricular escape beats.
- **A.** True
- **B.** False

29. Sinus tachycardia is often benign.
- **A.** True
- **B.** False

30. The normal P-R interval on an ECG tracing is 0.08-0.12.
- **A.** True
- **B.** False

31. Etiologies of PVCs may include hypoxia, acid-base disturbances, or increased sympathetic tone.
- **A.** True
- **B.** False

32. Ventricular tachycardia consists of four or more ventricular complexes in succession at a rate of 100 or more.
- **A.** True
- **B.** False

33. A second-degree type I AV block produces a cyclic pattern in which the P-R intervals become progressively longer until an impulse is blocked.
- **A.** True
- **B.** False

34. Valsalva maneuvers are the utilized first in the treatment of a patient presenting with a third-degree AV block.
- **A.** True
- **B.** False

35. A PVC does not usually depolarize the SA node and interrupt its rhythm.
- **A.** True
- **B.** False

Matching

Write the letter of the definition or description regarding cardiac function in the space provided next to the term to which it applies. The same description or definition may be used more than once or not at all.

_____**36.** cardiac cycle

_____ **37.** diastole

_____ **38.** systole

_____ **39.** ejection fraction

_____ **40.** preload

_____ **41.** afterload

_____ **42.** cardiac output

_____ **43.** stroke volume

    A. the ratio of blood pumped from the ventricle compared with the amount contained at the end of diastole

    B. the series of events between the end of a cardiac contraction to the end of the next

    C. the resistance against which the heart must pump

    D. the phase of the cardiac cycle during which the heart contracts

    E. the amount of blood pumped by the ventricle during one cardiac contraction

    F. the amount of blood pumped by the ventricle during one minute

    G. the phase of the cardiac cycle during which the heart muscle is relaxed

    H. the end-diastolic volume in the ventricle

    I. the phase of the cardiac cycle during which blood enters the coronary arteries

Write the letter of innate rate of impulse discharge in beats per minute (bpm) in the space provided next to the part of the cardiac conduction system to which it applies.

    A. 60–100 bpm
    B. 15–40 bpm
    C. 40–60 bpm

_____ **44.** Purkinje system

_____ **45.** AV node

Chapter 28

Cardiology

Part 2: Assessment and Management of the Cardiovascular Patient

Review of Chapter Objectives

After reading this part of the chapter, you should be able to:

41. Identify and describe the components of the focused history as it relates to the patient with cardiovascular compromise.   **pp. 512-517**

The focused history for cardiac situations uses the same format you learned for pulmonology, the SAMPLE format: **S**igns/Symptoms, **A**llergies, **M**edications, **P**ast medical history, **L**ast oral intake, and **E**vents preceding the incident.

• *Signs/Symptoms.* The most common symptoms of cardiac disease/compromise include chest pain or discomfort, dyspnea, cough, syncope, and palpitations.

    Use the OPQRST format (also something you encountered with pulmonology) to assess chest pain or discomfort: **O**nset of pain, **P**rovocation/Palliation of pain, **Q**uality of pain, **R**egion where felt/**R**adiation, **S**everity, and **T**iming (duration). (See also objective 54 for full detail.) Questions concerning dyspnea are similar: You want to know how long it has lasted and whether it is continuous or intermittent. Was onset rapid or gradual? Does anything specific either worsen or palliate the dyspnea, and is it exertional or not? Last, be sure to see if orthopnea exists: Does sitting upright give any relief? Questions about cough center on whether it is chronic or acute and whether it suggests congestive heart failure (dry or productive, presence of any wheezing with cough, etc.).

In addition, observe and question for these possible signs/symptoms: level of consciousness, diaphoresis, restlessness/anxiety, feeling of impending doom, nausea/vomiting, fatigue, palpitations, edema of extremities or positional (sacral), headache, syncope, behavioral change, facial expression, limitation of activity, signs of recent trauma. Many signs/symptoms of cardiovascular disease and compromise can be subtle or change (either rapidly or gradually) over time.

• *Allergies.* Check for allergies to medication (prescription and over-the-counter) or X-ray contrast dyes. Try to distinguish between details suggestive of side effect (such as GI upset) and those of allergy (rash, hives, anaphylactic shock).

• *Medications.* Check both for current medications (again, prescription and over-the-counter) and recent medication changes. If there has been a recent change, ask why. Look for use of cardiovascular drugs such as nitroglycerin, propranolol or other beta blockers, digitalis (digoxin, Lanoxin), diuretics (Lasix, Dyazide), antihypertensives (Capoten, Prinivil, Vasotec), antidysrhythmics (Quinaglute, Mexitil, Tambocor), and lipid-lowering agents (Mevacor, Lopid). If possible, check directly (by inspecting med tray, if there is one) or indirectly (by history) about drug compliance and bring containers to the hospital with you.

• *Past medical history.* Ask directed questions about history of heart disease, MI, stroke, high blood pressure, as well as why suggestive drugs are taken. Specific problems you should inquire about include history of rheumatic heart disease (valvular problems), previous cardiac surgery, congenital cardiac anomalies, pericarditis or other inflammatory cardiac disease, or congestive heart failure (CHF). Relevant problems of other organ systems include pulmonary disease/ COPD, diabetes mellitus, renal disease, hypertension, atherosclerosis. Also ask whether there is any family history of illness/death (particularly early deaths before age 50) from cardiovascular disease or other relevant disorders. Last, be sure to ask whether patient smokes or smoked tobacco and whether he/she knows his/her cholesterol level.

• *Last oral intake.* Valuable as a screening question for anyone with a possible surgical condition, this also gives you the chance to ask about most recent caffeine or tobacco use, as well as whether there was a recent fatty meal. (For some patients, this may help steer you to gallbladder disorders.)

• *Events preceding incident.* Ask what the patient was doing just before onset of symptoms. Was there emotional stress or physical exertion? Was there sexual activity? If the patient is male, does he take Viagra? It is often uncomfortable to take a sexual history, but sometimes the information gained is life saving, and you can explain to the patient the possible importance of the answer.

42. Identify and describe the details of inspection, auscultation, and palpation specific to the cardiovascular system.   pp. 517-520

Always do visual inspection first. (1) Look for tracheal position. If isn't in its normal midline position but is toward one side, there may be a pneumothorax. (2) Check neck veins for signs of jugular distention (have the patient elevated about 45° and with head turned to the side). Jugular venous distention (JVD) is evidence of back pressure from causes such as heart (pump) failure or cardiac tamponade. (3) Thorax and chest movement while breathing should be observed with proper exposure so you can see chest shape (barrel chests may indicate COPD) and effort during respiration, such as retractions of the soft tissues between the ribs. Accessory muscles used when breathing is difficult may include those of the neck, back, and abdomen. Always look for surgical scars; a scar over the sternum may indicate prior cardiac surgery. (4) Evaluate the epigastrium while the chest wall is exposed, looking for distention and visible pulsations. Pulsations may signal an aortic aneurysm dissection or rupture. (5) Position-dependent edema may be found in the ankles or sacral area, depending on whether the patient has been sitting or lying in bed. Pitting edema (a depression that persists after you stop applying firm pressure) is significant. (6) Skin changes associated with cardiovascular disease include pallor and diaphoresis (indicating increased sympathetic tone and peripheral vasoconstriction) or a mottled appearance (often an indicator of chronic cardiac failure). (7) Subtle changes associated with cardiovascular disease include not only surgical scars but subcutaneous batteries for a pacemaker or nitroglycerin skin patches.

Auscultation includes listening to the lungs, to the heart, and over the carotid arteries. (1) Assess the lung fields for equality and for sounds such as rales (crackles), rhonchi (whistling or snoring-like sounds), or wheezes, which may signal pulmonary edema or primary pulmonary disease. Note that patients with pulmonary edema may have foamy, blood-tinged sputum evident at the mouth and nose. In advanced cases, you may even hear a gurgling-like sound as the patient breathes. (2) It is difficult to auscultate the heart well in the field because of the number and intensity of background noises. Ideally, you want to listen for heart sounds at four classic sites: aortic, pulmonic, mitral (left AV valve), and tricuspid (right AV valve). The point on the chest wall where heartbeat is loudest or is best felt is called the point of maximum impulse (PMI). (3) Auscultation over the carotid arteries may reveal bruits, murmur sounds due to turbulent flow. A bruit over any artery indicates partial obstruction due to atherosclerosis. Never attempt carotid sinus massage in a patient with a bruit because you might dislodge atherosclerotic material that could lodge in a cerebral artery causing a stroke or other mishap.

Palpation should cover three areas: peripheral pulse, thorax, and epigastrium. (1) Determine rate and regularity of the pulse as well as equality. A pulse deficit (intensity less than expected) may indicate underlying peripheral vascular disease and should be reported to medical direction. (2) Thoracic palpation is extremely important and may reveal crepitus, akin to "bubble wrap" crackling under your fingers, which suggests subcutaneous emphysema. Check for tenderness or possible rib fracture. Remember that at least 15% of MI patients have some associated chest wall tenderness. (3) Abdominal exam may reveal distention or pulsations.

43. Identify and define the heart sounds and relate them to hemodynamic events in the cardiac cycle.   p. 519

Everyone is familiar with the lub-dub of normal heart sounds. The first component, called S_1, is produced by the closing of the AV valves during ventricular systole (at the beginning of the ventricular contraction that expels blood into the aorta and pulmonary artery). The second heart sound (S_2) is produced by the closure of the aortic and pulmonary valves as the ventricles begin to relax and the heart fills with blood again (at early diastole).

44. Describe the differences between normal and abnormal heart sounds.   p. 519

Any extra heart sounds (beyond S_1 and S_2) are abnormal. The sound termed S_3 is associated with congestive heart failure, and it has a cadence like that of the word Kentucky; when it is present, it follows S_2. The fourth heart sound, S_4, appears just before S_1 when it is present, and it is associated with increased effort of atrial contraction. Its cadence resembles that of Tennessee.

45. Define pulse deficit, pulsus paradoxus, and pulsus alternans.   p. 548

A pulse deficit is the less intense of two peripheral pulses that you would expect to be equal, for instance, the right and left carotid or right or left radial pulses. The pulse with the deficit often reflects an artery that is partially blocked by atherosclerosis. Pulsus paradoxus is related to a change in blood pressure with respiration. Specifically, pulsus paradoxus exists when systolic blood pressure decreases by more than 10 mmHg with inspiration, and it is due to compression of either the great vessels or the ventricles. Pulsus alternans exists when the pulse alternates between weak and strong intensity over time. In such cases, pulses may be felt as thready or weak on examination.

46. Identify the normal characteristics of the point of maximal impulse (PMI).   p. 519

The point on the chest wall where heartbeat is loudest on auscultation is usually the point where palpation finds the strongest impulse of the beating heart. This location is called the point of maximum impulse (PMI). You can find additional information about the PMI and cardiac examination in Division 2.

47. Based on field impressions, identify the need for rapid intervention for the patient in cardiovascular compromise.   pp. 511-520

As with any other patient, your first responsibilities are to check airway, breathing, circulation, and the possibility of shock. Only after you have managed life-threatening problems (and if new, life-threatening problems don't develop) can you communicate with and support the patient and family. Note that interventions in the field beyond the absolutely essential are generally limited to administration of analgesia or nitrates for chest pain, treatment of pulmonary edema, and administration of appropriate analgesia for peripheral vascular emergencies. Do be sure, however, to look for the obvious and subtle signs of cardiovascular disease during the focused history and physical. The discovery of an abdominal pulsation that might signal aortic aneurysm dissection or rupture in a patient with some signs of early shock changes the dynamic for intervention and transportation greatly.

48. Describe the incidence, morbidity, and mortality associated with myocardial conduction defects. pp. 541, 542

Remember that dysrhythmias arising from coronary heart disease, or CHD (often part of myocardial ischemia or infarction), cause many of the sudden deaths associated with CHD, and these deaths are too numerous. Many patients have CHD-induced deaths before they can reach a hospital; this amounts to roughly one death per minute. Dysrhythmias are the most common complication of MI and the most common cause of death from an MI. Life-threatening dysrhythmias can develop very early in the course of myocardial ischemia and can cause sudden death (immediate or within one hour of onset of symptoms).

Conduction abnormalities also arise directly from disease or from drug effects or electrolyte abnormalities. Among the forms of AV block, third-degree block is the most serious: In this type, none of the impulses originating in the atria reach the ventricles. Ventricular rate and rhythm are dependent on development of a ventricular escape rhythm. This can lead to morbidity through symptomatic bradycardia and heart failure. In some situations, cardiac arrest and death may result. Bundle branch block can result from age-related deterioration, MI, or transient causes such as drugs and electrolyte abnormalities. Part of your concern with cases of left bundle branch block should lie in the fact that nothing else can be determined from the ECG regarding possible ischemic change. Thus, a patient with left bundle branch block can have a significant MI and ECG changes will not be seen; this can increase the morbidity or mortality from the MI.

49. Identify the clinical indications, components, and the function of transcutaneous and permanent artificial cardiac pacing. pp. 533-535

Permanent artificial pacemakers are generally inserted into patients who have chronic high-grade AV block or sick sinus syndrome or who have had episodes of severe symptomatic bradycardia in the past. The pacemaker (the pulse generator) is implanted near the heart, and its discharge lead is inserted into either the right ventricle or right atrium and ventricle, depending on whether it is a ventricular-type pacemaker or a dual-chambered pacemaker (see Figure 28-45). The battery packs are usually palpable in their subcutaneous position (often in the shoulder or axillary region). Permanent pacemakers are of two functional types: either they can pace continuously or they can pace when the heart's natural rate falls below a preset number of beats per minute. (The two types are called fixed-rate and demand pacemakers.) In all cases, the pacemaker should enable the patient to have a heart rate and rhythm that supports adequate cardiac output.

Transcutaneous cardiac pacing (TCP) allows electrical pacing of the heart through the skin via specially designed thoracic electrodes. You will need to have one of the newer cardiac monitor/defibrillators with an appropriate built-in pacing device. TCP may be highly beneficial for patients with symptomatic bradycardia such as high-degree AV block, atrial fibrillation with slow ventricular response, or other significant bradycardias and asystole. You can use TCP if pharmacological intervention fails and if the patient is hypotensive or hypoperfusing to try to establish a rate and rhythm compatible with adequate cardiac output. You can also use TCP to provide overdrive pacing to suppress recurrent tachycardia or in *torsade de pointes,* a specific form of ventricular tachycardia.

50. Explain what each setting and indicator on a transcutaneous pacing system represents and how the settings may be adjusted. pp. 533-535

One system setting is for heart rate: The range available is typically 60 to 80 bpm, and medical direction will consult with you about setting the appropriate rate. The output setting (in amps) should initially be set to 0 and then gradually increased until you see the pacemaker spike on ECG that shows ventricular capture. Maintenance rate and output are arranged with medical direction. With a patient in asystole, output is generally begun at the maximum setting, with output gradually lowered if ventricular capture occurs.

51. Describe the techniques of applying a transcutaneous pacing system. pp. 533-535

There are eleven steps involved in applying and monitoring TCP. (1) Establish IV access and ECG monitoring and administer oxygen. (2) Place the patient in a supine position. (3) Confirm symptomatic bradycardia (the usual indication) and medical direction's order for TCP. (4) Apply the pacing electrodes according to the manufacturer's directions. Be sure they adhere well to the skin. (5) Connect the electrodes. (6) Set desired heart rate on the pacemaker. (7) Turn output setting to 0. (8) Turn on pacer. (9) Slowly increase output until you see ECG spikes indicating ventricular capture. (10) Check the patient's pulse and blood pressure and adjust rate and amperage (output) per instructions from medical direction. (11) Monitor patient response to treatment.

52. Describe the epidemiology, morbidity, mortality, and pathophysiology of angina pectoris. pp. 537-538

Angina pectoris, or pain in the chest, occurs when the myocardial demand for oxygen exceeds the available supply through the coronary arteries. Myocardial ischemia causes the chest pain. Usually, reduced blood flow through the coronary arteries is correlated with permanent partial obstruction by atherosclerotic lesions. Angina can also result from spasm of the coronary arteries (arterial vasospasm), temporarily reducing the diameter of the lumen and blood flow. About two-thirds of patients with vasospastic angina (commonly called Prinzmetal's angina) have atherosclerosis involving the coronaries. Epidemiologically, though, this still means roughly one-third of patients with Prinzmetal's angina do not have significant coronary atherosclerosis and thus may not fit the risk factor profile for atherosclerosis.

The epidemiology, morbidity, and mortality of cardiovascular disease, including coronary heart disease (CHD, disease of the coronary arteries) are covered in depth in objectives 1 and 3 of Part 1 of this chapter.

53. Describe the assessment and management of a patient with angina pectoris. pp. 537-539

During assessment, remember that weak or absent peripheral pulses (especially when symmetric or global) may signal pending shock, which requires immediate intervention. Pallor and cyanosis of the skin or cold extremities also suggest shock. Because angina is a progressive disorder, a history of angina does not mean that the current episode is "safe." If it is important enough to activate EMS, it is important enough for your full attention and the suspicion of serious underlying problems such as acute MI. Listen to the history of the current event: The chief complaint is usually sudden onset chest pain. Pain may radiate or be localized to the chest. Angina usually lasts 3–5 minutes, although it may last as long as 15 minutes, and it is generally relieved by rest and/or nitroglycerin. Prinzmetal angina is often accompanied by S-T segment elevation on ECG, which may indicate myocardial tissue ischemia. Breathing may or may not be labored, but you should check for lung sounds after ensuring the airway is patent. Listen for congestion, especially at the bases. Although the anginal patient's rate and rhythm may be altered, they may be normal, and peripheral pulses should be equal and normal. Typically, blood pressure rises during the anginal episode and normalizes afterward. Ask the patient for his/her baseline BP, as hypertension may be present. If it is possible without prolonging the time on-scene, get an ECG tracing. A 12-lead ECG provides more information and should be done if possible.

Management includes placing the patient at physical and emotional rest to decrease myocardial oxygen demand: Give oxygen, generally at high-flow rate. Establish IV access on scene or en route to the hospital. Conduct the ECG; do not, however, delay transport to perform it. You can give nitroglycerin sublingually as a tablet or spray. If symptoms persist after 1–2 doses, raise your suspicion for a more serious condition such as acute MI. Nifedipine and other calcium channel blockers can also be used for relief of anginal pain: Morphine may be used for nonresponsive chest pain.

Patients with an initial episode of angina or an episode that does not respond to medication are usually admitted for observation. Immediate transport is indicated if relief does not come after oxygen and nitrates. The absence of relief may signal the beginning of infarction, and in this case reperfusion is crucial. Hypotension may occur, especially if nitroglycerin has been given. It indicates transport as well because it can lead to or worsen hypoperfusion of myocardial tissue. S-T segment changes, particularly elevation, also indicate the need for rapid, efficient transport.

If the patient refuses transport, be sure you clearly explain that immediate evaluation is vital because of the potential for problems such as MI. If you can't reverse the patient's decision, be sure the patient reads and signs the refusal and understands the potential risks. Ask that they contact their cardiologist or other physician for follow-up as soon as possible.

54. Identify what is meant by the OPQRST of chest pain assessment.   p. 513

Use the OPQRST format (also something you encountered with pulmonology) to assess chest pain or discomfort: **O**nset of pain, **P**rovocation/**P**alliation of pain, **Q**uality of pain, **R**egion where felt/**R**adiation, **S**everity, and **T**iming (duration). Questions about onset include when pain began and what was happening at the time. Ask a patient who has had prior episodes of chest pain to compare this one with prior episodes. If it is described as similar to pain that signaled a prior heart attack, you can strongly assume the pain is cardiac in origin. Questions on provocation and palliation of pain also may point to angina or toward another cause. In particular, ask about any relationship to exertion of any type or palliation with rest. If there have been multiple episodes, ask whether it takes less to trigger an episode now than in the past. Ask a general question about the quality of the pain and let the patient describe it. Common words include sharp, tearing, pressured, or heavy. Radiation of chest pain may occur to arm(s), neck, jaw, and/or back. Again, ask if this pattern fits earlier episodes. Ask the patient to evaluate the severity of the pain on a scale of 1–10 (be sure you use the same scale that will be used at the hospital in order to standardize response significance): You can ask the same question later to assess efficacy of therapy. Timing questions get information on how long the pain has lasted (write down the time the patient first noted pain as this may affect decisions later regarding possible thrombolytic therapy) as well as whether pain has been constant or intermittent or has changed with time (Better? Worse?).

55. List other clinical conditions that may mimic signs and symptoms of coronary artery disease and angina pectoris.   pp. 537-538

Causes of chest pain fall into four categories: cardiovascular, respiratory, gastrointestinal, and musculoskeletal. You'll note that the causes range from the troublesome but benign (dyspepsia, or heartburn) to the life threatening (aortic dissection). Cardiovascular causes include coronary artery disease and angina, but also pericarditis and dissection of the thoracic aorta. Respiratory causes include pulmonary embolism, pneumothorax, pneumonia, and pleurisy (pleural inflammation). GI causes are diverse: cholecystitis (gallbladder origin), pancreatitis, hiatal hernia, esophageal disease, gastroesophageal reflux (GERD), peptic ulcer disease, and dyspepsia. Musculoskeletal causes include chest wall syndrome, costochondritis, acromioclavicular disease, herpes zoster (shingles), chest wall trauma, and chest wall tumors. You should always be prepared to treat patients with chest pain as if they may have cardiac ischemia or another major disease process. Only after you have excluded these possibilities should you consider the less critical causes.

56. Identify the ECG findings in patients with angina pectoris.   pp. 538-539

An ECG should be done on-scene; if that would delay transport, it may be done en route. If possible, get a 12-lead ECG because it provides more information. Typical findings in patients with angina include S-T depression and/or T wave inversion. After relief of pain, ECG usually returns to baseline. The most common finding in angina is S-T depression, although Prinzmetal patients typically show S-T elevation. Note that S-T segment changes are not specific, and dysrhythmias and ectopy may not be seen either. Be sure to transmit the ECG to medical direction and discuss as necessary.

57. Based on the pathophysiology and clinical evaluation of the patient with chest pain, list the anticipated clinical problems according to their life-threatening potential.   pp. 537-539

Because angina, whether typical (obstructive) or vasospastic (namely, Prinzmetal's angina), reflects myocardial ischemia, progression to myocardial infarction is always possible. ECG monitoring may pick up signs of ischemia or infarction, as well as related cardiac problems such as dysrhythmia and ectopy, all of which can rapidly develop into life-threatening conditions. Aortic dissection is a life-threatening emergency, as can be pericarditis if pressure on the heart decreases cardiac output to the point of hypoperfusion of the heart (causing angina) or other vital organs such as the brain. Pulmonary embolism may also present as a life-threatening emergency if the embolus is very large or affects flow into both lungs. Pneumothorax and pneumonia are always serious, but they may also be life threatening in a patient with previously compromised cardiopulmonary function. Pleurisy, suspected cholecystitis or pancreatitis, and esophageal disease and peptic ulcer disease are also serious. If any of the GI conditions involve hemorrhage, the patient's condition may become unstable, especially if cardiopulmonary compromise exists. Always carry a degree of suspicion of impending or possible shock. Other causes, including the musculoskeletal causes as well as GI problems such as hiatal hernia, merit medical workup, but these patients are unlikely to be unstable on-scene or during transport. In some cases, such as known GERD, dyspepsia, or costochondritis, a patient with no other signs of a serious condition and no change in condition while you are on-scene may refuse transport. You should always advocate follow-up as quickly as possible with the personal physician because the complaint was severe enough to warrant the call to EMS.

58. Describe the epidemiology, morbidity, mortality, and pathophysiology of myocardial infarction.   pp. 539-541

Myocardial infarction, the death of myocardial tissue, is the result of prolonged oxygen deprivation or when myocardial oxygen demand exceeds oxygen supply for an extended period. MI is most often associated with atherosclerotic heart disease (ASHD, which is the same as atherosclerotic coronary heart disease). The precipitating event is often development of a thrombus in a partially occluded artery, with the thrombus completely occluding the vessel. Other pathophysiologic bases for MI include coronary artery spasm, microemboli as can be seen with cocaine use, acute volume overload, hypotension (causing myocardial hypoperfusion), or acute respiratory failure (leading to acute hypoxia). Trauma can also cause MI, often by loosening atherosclerotic plaque in the coronary artery, blocking it.

The region of the heart affected and the size of the eventual infarcted area depend on the coronary artery involved and the specific site of the obstruction. Most infarctions involve the left ventricle. Obstruction of the left coronary artery or its branches may result in infarction of the anterior or lateral ventricle or the interventricular septum. Right coronary artery occlusions tend to result in infarction of the inferior or posterior wall of the left ventricle or infarction of the right ventricle. The pathophysiologic progression of events starts with ischemia, followed by cell death. The infarcted tissue becomes necrotic and eventually forms scar tissue, if the affected individual survives. Ischemic tissue at the periphery of the infarct will survive but may become the origin of dysrhythmias.

Dysrhythmias are the most common complication of MI and the most common cause of death from an MI.

Infarction of myocardium can cause congestive heart failure. Heart failure implies that the heart is working poorly but adequately. If the heart cannot meet body oxygen demand, cardiogenic shock results. Last, if the damaged portion of the ventricular wall is too weakened, it may form a ventricular aneurysm and rupture, causing death.

Based on pathophysiology, the basic strategies of intervention are pain relief and reperfusion. For reperfusion to be effective, rapid, safe transport is essential.

59. List the mechanisms by which a myocardial infarction may be produced from traumatic and nontraumatic events.   p.540

See objective 58 above.

60. Identify the primary hemodynamic changes produced in myocardial infarction. pp. 540-541

In order for myocardial tissue to become ischemic, there is either hypoperfusion or low blood oxygen. Hypoperfusion is the typical cause of ischemia and eventual infarction. If the affected myocardium includes conductive tissue, dysrhythmias such as ventricular tachycardia or ventricular fibrillation may result. Even if rhythm is preserved, it is possible that infarction can cause pump failure of either the right or left ventricle or both, resulting in heart failure. If the pump failure is severe, cardiogenic shock develops.

61. List and describe the assessment parameters to be evaluated in a patient with a suspected myocardial infarction.   pp. 540-541

Initial size-up, inspection, and vital signs may reveal a lot. Is breathing labored? Is the patient diaphoretic and pale? Are there other signs of shock? Remember that blood pressure usually elevates during an episode of ischemia and then returns to normal. Hypotension more likely suggests cardiac compromise and possible shock. Peripheral pulses should be regular and equal. Irregularities may suggest dysrhythmia.

As you move through the OPQRST mnemonic, look for these signs of MI: sudden onset chest pain that proves to be severe, constant, and unrelenting over a period longer than 30 minutes. Pain may radiate to the arms (usually the left), neck, back, or into the epigastrium. Myocardial ischemia can easily produce pain in the 8–10 range and the pain may be associated with nausea and vomiting. Unlike the situation with angina, neither rest nor nitroglycerin will palliate MI pain. Remember that patients with diabetes mellitus may NOT have this picture even when an MI is in evolution. These patients may minimize the severity of their discomfort or simply complain of feeling unwell. Typically, these patients do not have nausea and vomiting. MIs typically evolve over 48–72 hours, and so the pain seen at 24–48 hours may be very different than if you had seen the patient in the first 12–24 hours after onset of discomfort.

Emotion may suggest MI. Patients with severe chest pain often are very frightened and complain of a sense of doom or fear of death. Denial of emotional upset or severity of pain does not mean a benign episode. Denial may hide severe fear or pain.

Auscultation of the lung fields may show clear fields or congestion in the bases. Other physical findings typical of MI include pallor and diaphoresis, coldness in the extremities, and possible change in body temperature. Heart rate and rhythm may be irregular or not. Blood pressure may be baseline, high, or low.

The ECG should be checked first for underlying rhythm and any sign of dysrhythmia. If you have a 12-lead ECG, look at the S-T segment and QRS complex. Check S-T segment for height, depth, and overall contour. Note any depression or elevation. A pathological Q wave (one deeper than 5 mm and wider than 0.04 sec) can indicate infarcted tissue or extensive transient ischemia. Anticipate dysrhythmias.

Next, assess whether the patient is a likely candidate for rapid transport and reperfusion therapy with thrombolytic agents. The time window for thrombolytic therapy to be effective is generally considered to be the first 6 hours from onset of symptoms. Consult medical direction. Note that some patients will have contraindications to thrombolytic therapy, including bleeding or clotting disorders, possible blood in the stool, uncontrolled hypertension, recent trauma, recent hemorrhagic stroke, or recent surgery. Generally, signs of acute injury or pathological Q waves indicate transport for reperfusion if you are within the 6-hour window. If you are uncertain whether the patient meets criteria for reperfusion therapy, assume that he/she does. Be sure to relay information to medical direction including time of pain onset, any S-T segment change (particularly elevation), and location of ischemia or infarct according to a 12-lead ECG.

62. Identify the anticipated clinical presentation of a patient with a suspected acute myocardial infarction.   pp. 541-542

See objective 61.

63. Differentiate the characteristics of the pain/discomfort occurring in angina pectoris and acute myocardial infarction.   pp. 541-542

Typical picture of angina: The chief complaint is usually sudden onset chest pain. Pain may radiate or be localized to the chest. Angina usually lasts 3–5 minutes, although it may last as long as 15 minutes, and it is generally relieved by rest and/or nitroglycerin. Breathing may or may not be labored, but you should check for lung sounds after ensuring airway is patent.

Typical picture of MI: There is a sudden onset chest pain that proves to be severe, constant, and unrelenting over a period longer than 30 minutes. Pain may radiate to the arms (usually the left), neck, back, or into the epigastrium. An MI can produce pain in the 8–10 range and the pain may be associated with nausea and vomiting. Unlike the situation with angina, neither rest nor nitroglycerin will palliate MI pain. Blood pressure may be high, low, or baseline, but it is unlikely to change solely with decrease in pain.

64. Identify the ECG changes characteristically seen during evolution of an acute myocardial infarction.   p. 542

See objective 61.

65. Identify the most common complications of an acute myocardial infarction. pp. 541-543

Dysrhythmias are the most common complication and one of the most common causes of death associated with MI. Congestive heart failure, or even overt cardiogenic shock, can also occur with an MI, especially when the infarcted area is very large or represents tissue loss on top of previous losses from prior MIs. Rupture of ventricular aneurysms, weakened areas of a ventricular wall due to MI, is another complication and cause of sudden death.

66. List the characteristics of a patient eligible for thrombolytic therapy.   p. 542

The most essential element of eligibility is time from onset of symptoms, as a duration beyond 6 hours from onset is generally correlated with poor success of thrombolytic therapy. In addition, patients who have contraindications to thrombolytic therapy include persons with bleeding or clotting disorders, possible blood in the stool (GI bleeding), uncontrolled hypertension, recent trauma, recent surgery, or recent hemorrhagic stroke.

67. Describe the "window of opportunity" as it pertains to reperfusion of a myocardial injury or infarction.   p. 542

Reperfusion therapy with a thrombolytic agent is most likely to be successful from the onset of symptoms to 6 hours later. Sometimes the window is expanded slightly for a younger patient or one with serious complications.

68. Based on the pathophysiology and clinical evaluation of the patient with a suspected acute myocardial infarction, list the anticipated clinical problems according to their life-threatening potential.   pp. 541-545

Dysrhythmias are the most common complication and one of the most common causes of death associated with myocardial infarction. Cardiogenic shock results from loss of cardiac function such that the minimal oxygen needs of the body are not met. A lesser loss of cardiac function can result in congestive heart failure. An uncommon complication that can result in death is rupture of a ventricular aneurysm.

69. Specify the measures that may be taken to prevent or minimize complications in the patient suspected of myocardial infarction.   p. 543

Act expediently and calmly and keep the patient in as much physical and emotional rest as possible. Provide supplemental oxygen to decrease myocardial oxygen demand and increase available oxygen. Always have good IV access (possibly more than one IV line). Be sure to ask about medication allergies (especially to any that may have been used previously in a cardiac setting) before the patient or family may become unable to give you this information. Transport as rapidly as possible with no lights or sirens if possible. Delay in transport, however, is preferable to a patient's refusal to leave the scene.

70. Describe the most commonly used cardiac drugs in terms of therapeutic effect and dosages, routes of administration, side effects, and toxic effects.   pp. 525-526

The classes of drugs you are most likely to use in the setting of an MI are antidysrhythmics, sympathomimetics, and drugs specific for use in the setting of ischemia (including the thrombolytics), along with less frequently used prehospital medications.

Antidysrhythmics
Antidysrhythmics control or suppress dysrhythmias. Among the most commonly used are atropine, lidocaine, procainamide, bretylium, adenosine, amiodarone, and verapamil.

• Atropine sulfate is a parasympatholytic agent (one that decreases parasympathetic effect by acting as an anticholinergic) used to treat symptomatic bradycardias, especially those arising in the atria, and is sometimes used as part of a treatment regimen for asystole. Dose is 0.5–1.0 mg IV for bradycardia and 1.0 mg for asystole, repeated every 3–5 minutes as needed until a total dose of 0.04 mg/kg is reached. Endotracheal (ET) doses are 2.0–2.5 times the IV doses. Side effects include blurred vision, dilated pupils, dry mouth, tachycardia, and drowsiness. It has no contraindications in the EMS setting.

• Lidocaine is a first-line antidysrhythmic used to treat and prevent life-threatening ventricular dysrhythmias such as ventricular tachycardia. It suppresses abnormal irritability in the ventricles while having little effect on normal myocardial tissue. Dose is 1.0–1.5 mg/kg slow IV push (50 mg/min) for ectopy, or normal IV push in cardiac arrest. An IV drip is prepared by mixing 1 gram into 250 cc D_5W or saline. Typical maintenance dose is 2–4 mg/minute. Maximum bolus dose is 300 mg. The drug can be given IV bolus, IV drip, or through an ET tube. Side effects include drowsiness, seizures, confusion, bradycardia, heart blocks, and nausea and vomiting. Lidocaine is contraindicated by the presence of second- or third-degree AV block.

• Procainamide is a second-line antidysrhythmic to lidocaine, and it is used for ventricular dysrhythmias refractory to lidocaine or for patients who are allergic to lidocaine. It is administered by slow IV bolus or IV drip. IV bolus is 100 mg given over 5 minutes, with a maximum dose of 17 mg/kg. Discontinue when the dysrhythmia is suppressed, hypotension ensues, the QRS complex widens 50%, or the maximum dose is given. Drip rate is the same as for lidocaine. Side effects and contraindications are the same as for lidocaine.

• Adenosine is used to manage supraventricular tachydysrhythmias. It is a naturally occurring nucleoside that acts on the AV node to slow conduction and inhibit reentry pathways. It is given by IV rapid bolus through a venous site as close to the heart as possible. Flush the line with saline immediately after giving adenosine to ensure drug delivery. Initial dose is 6 mg (rapid push) followed by a 15–30 cc saline flush. If the tachydysrhythmia is not eliminated, a second dose of 12 mg and, if needed, a third dose of 12 mg may be given. Maximum dose is 30 mg. Side effects include apprehension, burning sensation, heavy sensation in the arms, hypotension, chest pressure, diaphoresis, numbness or tingling, dyspnea, tightness in the throat and/or groin pressure, headache, and nausea and vomiting. Adenosine is contraindicated in the presence of second- or third-degree AV block or in sick sinus syndrome unless a pacemaker is present.

• Amiodarone (Cordarone) is an antidysrhythmic used in management of recurring ventricular fibrillation and hemodynamically unstable ventricular tachycardia (nonperfusing tachycardia). Amiodarone is also being used more frequently in the prehospital setting of cardiac arrest. Although it is a second-line drug in the United States, it is a first-line agent in several Commonwealth countries. Dosage is 150–300 mg by slow IV infusion. Side effects include hypotension (the most common), bradycardia, and AV blocks. It is contraindicated in cardiogenic shock, marked sinus bradycardia, and second- or third-degree AV block.

• Verapamil is a calcium channel blocker that slows heart rate in symptomatic atrial tachycardias. It is used to terminate paroxysmal supraventricular tachycardia as well as to control the rapid ventricular response often seen with atrial flutter or fibrillation. It is administered by slow IV bolus with a maximum dose of 30 mg.

Sympathomimetic agents

Sympathomimetic agents are similar to the naturally occurring hormones epinephrine ad norepinephrine, and they mimic sympathetic nervous system stimulation on either alpha or beta adrenergic receptors. Alpha receptor stimulation causes peripheral vasoconstriction and beta receptor stimulation increases heart rate and cardiac contractility, causes bronchodilation, and peripheral vasodilation. Stimulation of dopaminergic receptors in the renal and mesenteric vascular beds causes dilation. Commonly used sympathomimetic agents include epinephrine, norepinephrine, isoproterenol, dopamine, and dobutamine.

• Epinephrine, which acts on alpha and beta receptors, is the mainstay of cardiac arrest resuscitation. It is used with ventricular fibrillation, asystole, and pulseless electrical activity. It is also sometimes used for bradycardia refractory to atropine. It is given as IV bolus, subcutaneously, and via ET tube. Dose is 1 mg of 1:10 000 solution given every 3–5 minutes.

• Norepinephrine has alpha agonist properties greater than those of epinephrine. It acts on beta receptors to a lesser degree. It is used occasionally in hemodynamically significant hypotension and cardiogenic shock, although dopamine is the first-line agent for these conditions. Norepinephrine may be effective if total peripheral resistance is low, such as in neurogenic shock. It is administered by IV infusion via drip by placing 4 mg into 1000 cc of D_5W (ONLY) to give a concentration of 4 mcg/cc. Initial loading dose is 8–12 mcg/min to give blood pressure of 80–100 mmHg systolic. Maintenance dose is 2–4 mcg/min. Side effects include anxiety, trembling, headache, dizziness, and nausea and vomiting. It can also cause bradycardia. DO NOT use norepinephrine in patients with hypotension from hypovolemia.

• Isoproterenol is rarely used with the advent of TCP, but it is a potent beta agonist that increases heart rate and cardiac contractility. It is used in bradycardia refractory to atropine and to manage asystole. Isoproterenol is given via IV infusion. Add 1 mg to 250 cc D_5W or saline to give 4 mcg/cc. The drip rate is 2–20 mcg/min. Common procedure is to start with a low dose and titrate upward until a satisfactory rate is achieved. TCP is preferred to use of isoproterenol.

• Dopamine (Intropin) is a vasopressor that increases cardiac output. It stimulates both alpha and beta receptors. It has the advantage over other drugs of preserving renal perfusion at recommended doses. Dose is given via IV drip by mixing 800 mg into 500 cc D_5W or saline to give a concentration of 1 600 mcg/cc (400 mg into 250 cc also works). Dopamine's effects are dose-related: At 1–2 mcg/kg/min, renal artery dilation occurs; at 2–10 mcg/kg/min, beta receptors are primarily stimulated; at 10–15 mcg/kg/min, both beta and alpha receptors are stimulated; and at 15–20 mcg/kg/min, alpha receptors are primarily stimulated. Side effects include nervousness, headache, dysrhythmias, palpitations, chest pain, dyspnea, and nausea and vomiting. Note: Dopamine is contraindicated for hypovolemic shock until fluid resuscitation has been completed.

• Dobutamine (Dobutrex), like dopamine, increases cardiac output and increases stroke volume. It has little effect on heart rate and is occasionally used in isolated left heart failure until medications such as digitalis can take effect. Dobutamine is given by IV infusion by mixing 250 mg into 250 cc D_5W or saline to give a concentration of 1 000 mcg/cc. Dose is 2–10 mcg/kg/min titrated to effect. Its side effects are the same as dopamine's. Do not use dobutamine as the sole agent in hypovolemic shock unless fluid resuscitation is complete. Dopamine is preferred over dobutamine to increase cardiac output in cardiogenic shock.

Drugs used for myocardial ischemia

Drugs used to treat myocardial ischemia and relieve its pain include oxygen, nitrous oxide, nitroglycerin, morphine, and nalbuphine.

• Oxygen is important because it increases the blood's oxygen content and aids oxygenation of peripheral and cardiac tissues. It is indicated in any situation where hypoxia or ischemia is possible.

• Nitrous oxide (Nitronox) is purely an analgesic with no significant hemodynamic effects. However, delivery in fixed combination with 50% oxygen can increase myocardial oxygen supply. Nitrous oxide is self-administered by inhalation via a modified demand valve to the desired effect. Its effects subside within 2–5 minutes. Side effects include CNS depression and potential respiratory depression. Do not give nitrous oxide to patients who cannot comprehend verbal instructions or who are intoxicated with alcohol or other drugs.

• Nitroglycerin is an organic nitrate that dilates peripheral arteries and veins, reducing preload and afterload and myocardial oxygen demand. It may cause some coronary artery dilation, thus increasing blood flow through the collateral circulation. Nitroglycerin use often helps to distinguish the pain of angina from that of an MI. Nitroglycerin does not relieve the pain of an MI, but it should be given before morphine because it works in conjunction with morphine in an MI. Dosage is one tablet sublingually repeated every 5 minutes up to a total of three tablets. Monitor blood pressure before each dose. Its side effects include headache, dizziness, weakness, hypotension, and tachycardia. Note that nitroglycerin loses potency as soon as the bottle is opened to the air. Always use the nitroglycerin provided on the medical intensive care unit and check the date before administration.

• Morphine sulfate is a narcotic drug that is important in managing MI. It reduces myocardial oxygen demand by reducing both preload and afterload. It also acts directly on the CNS to relieve pain, and it reduces sympathetic discharge, which can further decrease myocardial oxygen demand. Dosage is in 1–2 mg increments via slow IV push, titrated to pain relief. Monitor blood pressure before each dose. Side effects include nausea and vomiting, abdominal cramping, respiratory depression, hypotension, and potential altered mental status. Toxic effects are apnea and severe hypotension. Check for drug allergy before administration.

Thrombolytic agents
The use of thrombolytic agents as a definitive treatment for myocardial ischemia is one of the most important recent advances in medicine. In some instances, thrombolytic therapy may even have benefit in the field, and this is especially true in areas with a long transit time to a definitive care facility. Thrombolytic agents are generally very expensive, and their use requires a 12-lead ECG. Alteplase (tPA, Activase) and reteplase (Retavase) are thrombolytic agents. Although aspirin is not a thrombolytic agent, it merits discussion in this section.

• Aspirin is important in treatment of cardiac ischemia because it inhibits platelet aggregation and thus is effective in treating coronary ischemia and stroke secondary to thrombus development. The standard dosage is 160 mg by mouth, although some physicians prefer smaller doses. Baby aspirin may be useful because it can be chewed, thus more quickly reaching a therapeutic blood level. Its most common side effect is GI upset, although bleeding can be a problem in certain patients.

• Alteplase (Activase, tPA). Alteplase, or tPA (tissue plasminogen activator) is a potent thrombolytic agent that is manufactured through recombinant technology, which means it is the same as the biological compound. This minimizes chances of allergic reaction. TPA is effective if given within 6 hours of onset of coronary ischemia. It is given as a bolus dose followed by infusion. The typical dose is 100 mg given over 1.5–2 hours. Complications of tPA include hemorrhage, which can be fatal. Also, when reperfusion occurs, potentially life-threatening dysrhythmias can develop.

• Reteplase (Retavase) is another human plasminogen activator. It functions in a manner similar to tPA and has the same basic side effects and complications. It is administered as a single 10-unit bolus by IV push over 2 minutes. A second 10-unit bolus is given 30 minutes afterward. This dosing regimen makes reteplase attractive for prehospital care.

Other prehospital drugs
Less frequently used agents you may administer in the prehospital setting include furosemide, diazepam, promethazine, and sodium nitroprusside.

• Furosemide (Lasix) is a potent loop diuretic that also relaxes the venous system with effects seen within 5 minutes. Its diuretic effect decreases intravascular fluid volume. Dose is 40 mg slow IV push (40 mg/min). If the patient takes furosemide or another diuretic, you may need to double the dosage. Side effects include hypotension, ECG changes, chest pain, dry mouth, hypokalemia, hypochloremia, hyponatremia, and hyperglycemia. Furosemide should only be used in life-threatening emergencies during pregnancy because it can cause fetal abnormalities.

• Diazepam (Valium) is not an analgesic but rather an anti-anxiety drug, and it may be given to patients who are extremely apprehensive or agitated. Dose is 2–5 mg IV or deep IM.

• Promethazine (Phenergan) has sedative, antihistamine, antiemetic, and anticholinergic properties. It also potentiates narcotics, making it useful in the MI setting by reducing the nausea associated with morphine while enhancing its effects. Dosage is 12.5–25.0 mg given slow IV push or deep IM (25.0 mg/min). Its side effects are drowsiness, sedation, blurred vision, tachycardia, bradycardia, and dizziness. Promethazine is contraindicated in unresponsive patients or those taking large doses of depressants. Extrapyramidal symptoms (namely, dystonia) have been reported with promethazine.

• Sodium nitroprusside (Nipride) is a potent arterial and venous vasodilator, making it popular for use in hypertensive crisis. It is given as an IV infusion, which makes administration more controlled and the patient's response more predictable.

Drugs infrequently used in the prehospital setting
Lastly, certain medications commonly associated with in-hospital use or long-term patient use are included in this discussion. You are most likely to use these often if you work in an emergency department. Drugs in this group include digitalis, beta blockers, calcium channel blockers, and alkalinizing agents.

• Digitalis (digoxin, Lanoxin) is a cardiac glycoside that increases cardiac contractility and cardiac output. It slows impulse conduction through the AV node and decreases the ventricular response to certain supraventricular dysrhythmias such as atrial flutter or fibrillation and paroxysmal supraventricular tachycardia. It is also used long term to treat heart failure. The dose is 8–12 mcg/kg slow IV push over 15–20 minutes. If possible, obtain the patient's digitalis level beforehand (if the patient is on digoxin) before administering any cardiac glycoside. Most patients taking digitalis will remain therapeutic at 10–15 mcg/kg over a 24-hour period. Giving digitalis to patients who already take a cardiac glycoside involves complicated calculations, which makes it impractical for prehospital use in most settings. Its side effects include fatigue, muscle weakness, agitation, hallucinations, headache, malaise, dizziness, vertigo, stupor, blurred vision and yellow-green halo vision, photophobia, diplopia, and nausea and vomiting. Digitalis toxicity, which is not uncommon in some patients, can cause almost any dysrhythmia, including some of the same dysrhythmias it is used to treat, and these will often be refractory to traditional antidysrhythmic drugs. Digitalis is contraindicated in any digitalis-induced toxicity, ventricular fibrillation, or ventricular tachycardia not caused by CHF.

• Beta blockers are frequently used to control dysrhythmias, hypertension, and angina. Many beta blockers such as propranolol (Inderal) are non-selective; other beta blockers such as metoprolol are selective for either B_1 or B_2 receptors. Beta blockers may precipitate CHF, heart block, or asthma in patients predisposed to them. The beta-blocker labetalol (Trandate, Normodyne) effectively decreases blood pressure. It is given by IV bolus and infusion. The IV bolus is 20 mg over 20 minutes and may be repeated at 40–80 mg over 10 minutes. Maximum bolus is 300 mg. Drip is established by mixing 200 mg into 160 cc D_5W, and the drip dose is 2 cc/min.

• Calcium channel blockers are a relatively new class of antihypertensive medication that include verapamil (Isoptin, Calan), diltiazem (Cardizem), and nifedipine (Procardia). Nifedipine is now being used in addition to nitroglycerin to treat angina. Like nitroglycerin, it is a vasodilator but with a different mechanism. It is given orally. Calcium channel blockers are being used increasingly for angina, dysrhythmias, and other cardiovascular problems.

• Alkalinizing agents such as sodium bicarbonate are used late in the management of cardiac arrest, if at all. Occasionally, metabolic acidosis from another disorder may cause pulseless electrical activity, asystole, ventricular tachycardia, or ventricular fibrillation. In these cases, sodium bicarbonate may aid in converting to a perfusing rhythm. Adequate CPR, prompt defibrillation, and appropriate drug administration should always precede the use of bicarbonate. Sodium bicarbonate has few side effects and no contraindications in the emergency setting. Dose is initially 1 mEq/kg followed by 0.5 mEq/kg every 10 minutes. When possible, doses should be based on arterial blood gas (ABG) results.

71. Describe the epidemiology, morbidity, mortality, and physiology associated with heart failure. pp. 545-546

Heart failure is the clinical syndrome in which the heart's pumping capacity is compromised so that cardiac output cannot meet the body's needs. Heart failure can be typed as right ventricle or left ventricle failure or bilateral heart failure. Left ventricular failure occurs when the left ventricle's ability to pump fails, causing back pressure of blood into the pulmonary circulation, which results in pulmonary edema. Right ventricular failure is due to loss of pumping ability in the right ventricle, resulting in back pressure of blood into the systemic venous circulation causing venous congestion. The most common cause of right heart failure is pre-existent left heart failure. Other causes of right ventricular failure include systemic hypertension, pulmonary hypertension due to COPD, or *cor pulmonale.* All of these causes relate to an initial increase in the pressure in the pulmonary arteries, which then results in right ventricular enlargement, and, if untreated, right ventricular failure. Pulmonary embolism causes right ventricular failure if the clot is large enough to block a major pulmonary vessel.

72. Identify the factors that may precipitate or aggravate heart failure.pp. 545-546

There are many causes of heart failure, including valve disorders and coronary or myocardial disease. Dysrhythmias may aggravate heart failure by further decreasing cardiac output, decreasing myocardial perfusion, or both. Other factors that can contribute to heart failure include excess fluid or salt intake, fever (sepsis), hypertension, pulmonary embolism, or excessive alcohol or drug use. Failure can manifest with exertion in a patient who has an underlying disease or who has progressive cardiac disease. Specific causes of left heart failure include MI, valvular disease, chronic hypertension, and dysrhythmias. Because MI is a common cause of left ventricular failure, suspect that all patients with pulmonary edema may have had an MI. Causes of right ventricular failure include initial MI of the left ventricle, systemic hypertension, pulmonary hypertension due to COPD, and *cor pulmonale.* Another major cause of right ventricular failure is pulmonary embolism.

73. Define acute pulmonary edema and describe its relationship to left ventricular failure. p. 546

As the left ventricle's pumping ability falls, it cannot pump out all of the blood delivered to it from the lungs. Consequently, left atrial pressure rises and is transmitted to the pulmonary veins and the pulmonary capillary beds. When pulmonary capillary pressure increases sufficiently, blood plasma is forced into the alveoli and interstitial spaces; this is pulmonary edema (swelling of the lungs). Progressive fluid accumulation in the alveoli decreases the lungs' oxygenation capacity and can cause hypoxia that can be fatal.

74. Differentiate between early and late signs and symptoms of left ventricular failure and those of right ventricular failure.   p.546

For left ventricular failure, the cardinal symptom is dyspnea due to pulmonary edema. Signs include cyanosis, tachycardia, noisy, labored breathing, rales, cough, blood-tinged, frothy sputum, and a gallop rhythm of the heart. The major signs of right ventricular failure: neck veins engorged and pulsating, edema of body and extremities, engorged liver and spleen, abdominal distention with ascites (fluid), as well as tachycardia.

Congestive heart failure (CHF) is a general term for ventricular failure (left, right, or both) that causes excess fluid to accumulate in body tissues (hence, congestion). The excess fluid is manifest as edema, which may be pulmonary, peripheral, sacral, or within the abdomen as ascites. You may find it in the acute setting of MI, pulmonary edema, or pulmonary hypertension. In the chronic setting, it can reflect cardiac enlargement.

75. Define and explain the clinical significance of paroxysmal nocturnal dyspnea, pulmonary edema, and dependent edema.   pp. 545-548

Paroxysmal nocturnal dyspnea (PND) is an episode of waking during the night due to shortness of breath, and it reflects the presence of pulmonary edema. If these episodes become more frequent (more nights or more times/night), it suggests worsening of the underlying pathophysiologic process. Pulmonary edema reflects backup of fluid into the pulmonary alveoli and interstitium, but it does not necessarily imply etiology. Left ventricular failure, however, is probably the best known and most common cause, and you should look for other signs of congestive heart failure in a patient who presents with signs of pulmonary edema. If pulmonary edema seems to be very acute in onset, look for precipitating causes, such as cardiac dysrhythmia or acute MI. Dependent edema represents edema in the gravity-dependent portions of the body. For a bedridden patient, this often manifests as sacral edema. Sometimes edema will be so severe it will eliminate your ability to find a pulse in the affected area (such as a pedal pulse). If edema is severe enough to be pitting edema (a situation in which you press firmly into the affected tissue, lift the finger, and find that the depression caused by your finger persists), you can make a semi-quantitative evaluation by scoring as 0 to 4+.

76. List the interventions prescribed for the patient in acute congestive heart failure.   pp. 545-548

Manage a patient with severe CHF by assessing in an ongoing manner for life-threatening symptoms and intervene promptly while readying the patient for rapid transport. Do not allow the patient to exert in any way, including standing up. Positioning in a seated position with feet dangling promotes venous pooling and, consequently, reduced preload. Administer high-flow oxygen. If necessary, provide positive-pressure ventilations with either a demand valve or a bag-valve-mask device. Establish an IV line at a keep-vein-open rate or place a saline or heparin lock. Place ECG electrodes. If the patient is extremely diaphoretic, apply tincture of Benzoin first so electrodes will be tightly adherent to skin. Record a baseline ECG and continue monitoring.

Medication use will be according to your local protocols or the order of medical direction. Always remember to ask about drug allergies or reactions to any medication.
Transport as a nonemergency unless clinical conditions say otherwise. Indications for emergency transport include hypertension or hypotension, severe respiratory distress or pending respiratory failure, or life-threatening dysrhythmias. If you feel nonemergency transport will compromise the patient's condition, use lights and siren.

77. Describe the most commonly used pharmacological agents in the management of congestive heart failure in terms of therapeutic effect, dosages, routes of administration, side effects, and toxic effects.   pp. 525-526, 548

The drugs most likely to be used in the setting of left ventricular failure and pulmonary edema include morphine sulfate, nitroglycerin, furosemide (Lasix), dopamine (Intropin), dobutamine (Dobutrex), promethazine (Phenergan), and nitrous oxide (Nitronox). Dosages and other information on these medications are given in objective 70 above.

78. Define and describe the incidence, mortality, morbidity, pathophysiology, assessment, and management of the following cardiac related problems: pp. 549-557

Cardiac tamponade
Cardiac tamponade exists when an accumulation of material (air, pus, serum, blood, or a combination) inside the pericardium places pressure on the heart such that diastolic filling is impaired and stroke volume falls. Tamponade may evolve gradually; common progressive causes include pericarditis and benign or malignant neoplasms. Rare medical causes of tamponade include hypothyroidism and renal disease. Acute onset tends to occur when the cause is trauma or MI. Specific traumatic causes include

CPR and penetrating and nonpenetrating chest trauma. Regardless of cause and regardless of gradual or acute onset, cardiac tamponade can lead to death.

During the initial patient assessment, you may suspect cardiac tamponade. If so, limit history taking to questions that might reveal a precipitating cause. Use the OPQRST mnemonic to get information about the patient's symptoms: The most frequent chief complaints in tamponade are chest pain or dyspnea, and pain may be either dull or sharp. On physical exam, cardiac tamponade often presents with a characteristic picture: dyspnea and orthopnea, with clear lung sounds. Typically, peripheral pulses are rapid and weak. In the early stage, venous pressure is often elevated and you may see jugular vein distention. Blood pressure often reveals a decrease in systolic pressure, pulsus paradoxus, and narrowing pulse pressures. Heart sounds may be normal early in tamponade, but they are more likely (especially later) to become muffled or faint because of the presence of the tamponade-producing material in the pericardial sac.

Use of the ECG, whether single monitor lead or 12-lead, is not a diagnostic tool, but it may support your clinical suspicions. ECG findings are generally inconclusive; however, ectopy is usually a late sign due to irritation of the heart's epicardial tissue by the pericardial effusion. QRS and T wave voltages are low, and nonspecific T wave changes occur. S-T segments may elevate. Electrical alternans (weak voltage alternating with normal voltage) may appear in the P, QRS, T, or S-T segments.

Management is primarily supportive except when shock or low perfusion is detected. Maintain airway and deliver high-flow oxygen. If clinically indicated, use endotracheal intubation and maintain circulation with IV support, medications, or CPR. Again, before giving any medication ask about allergies. Medications frequently used in the setting of cardiac tamponade include morphine sulfate, nitrous oxide, furosemide, dopamine, and dobutamine. Rapid transport is indicated.

Hypertensive emergency
Hypertensive emergency occurs when there is a life-threatening elevation of blood pressure. This develops in about 1% of patients with hypertension. Clinically, the emergency is usually characterized by a rapid increase in diastolic pressure (generally, to greater than 130 mmHg) accompanied by restlessness and confusion, blurred vision, and nausea and vomiting. It often occurs with hypertensive encephalopathy, a consequence of severe hypertension marked by severe headache, vomiting, visual changes including transient blindness, paralysis, seizures, and stupor or coma. With modern medications, hypertensive encephalopathy has become rare, although it is still seen in the hospital setting. Both ischemic and hemorrhagic strokes are more common results of severe hypertension and can have devastating consequences. Hypertensive emergency can also cause left ventricular failure and pulmonary edema.

The major causes of hypertensive emergency include noncompliance with antihypertensive drugs or other prescribed medications and lack of treatment for hypertension. Risk factors include age (older age) and race (hypertension is more common in blacks, and morbidity and mortality appear to be higher, too). Among pregnant women, one cause of hypertension is preeclampsia (also called toxemia of pregnancy), which can appear at any point after the 20th week of pregnancy.

Assessment findings on physical exam of a patient with hypertensive emergency commonly include a chief complaint of headache accompanied by any of the following: nausea, vomiting, blurred vision, shortness of breath, epistaxis, and dizziness (vertigo). The patient may be semiconscious or unconscious and seizing. In toxemia of pregnancy, the woman usually has edema of hands or face. Photosensitivity and headache are common complaints in this group. Determine whether there is a documented history of hypertension and to what degree prescribed medications have been taken. Find out whether the patient may have borrowed someone else's medications or taken herbal or over-the-counter drugs. Skin may be pale or flushed, normal, cool, or warm. Look for edema. The patient may confirm PND, orthopnea, vertigo, epistaxis, tinnitus, or visual acuities. Look for possible motor or sensory deficits in parts of the body or on one side. ECG findings are generally inconclusive unless there is an underlying cardiac condition such as angina or MI. If left ventricular failure is present, pulmonary edema may be present. Otherwise, lungs are generally clear. The pulse is strong and may feel bounding. Hypertension is present with systolic pressure greater than 160 mmHg and/or diastolic pressure greater than 90 mmHg. Signs or symptoms of hypertensive encephalopathy in the presence of measured hypertension should be considered hypertensive emergency.

Management centers on positioning for comfort and watching for possible airway compromise if vomiting or stroke occurs. Give oxygen and decide upon transport based on clinical presentation. Attempt supportive IV therapy on-scene or en route. Place pregnant patients on their left sides and transport as smoothly and quietly as possible.

Medications that may be used in the prehospital setting have notably changed recently; know your local protocol. Medications often used include morphine, furosemide, nitroglycerin, sodium nitroprusside, and labetalol (Trandate, Normodyne).

Cardiogenic shock

Cardiogenic shock is the extreme state of heart failure: Cardiac output is so low it cannot sustain minimal physiologic activity. Clinically, you will see it after existing dysrhythmias, hypovolemia, or altered vascular tone have been corrected, leaving only the possibility of endogenous pump failure. This failure of the heart and overwhelming of any compensatory mechanisms usually happens after an extensive MI, often involving more than 40% of the left ventricle, or with diffuse ischemia. Note that cardiogenic shock can occur at any age, but it is most often seen as an end-stage event in geriatric patients with underlying disease. Mortality rate is high for elderly patients following massive MI or septic shock because end-organ damage is so severe that life cannot be sustained.

Numerous mechanisms can lead to cardiogenic shock, and onset may be gradual or acute. Among mechanical causes are tension pneumothorax and cardiac tamponade. Interference with ventricular emptying or afterload (such as pulmonary embolism and prosthetic or natural valve dysfunction) can also cause shock. Impairment in cardiac contractility is also a general cause: examples include MI, myocarditis, and recreational drug use. Trauma is another general cause, either primarily through cardiac damage or secondarily through hypovolemia. Finally, shock can develop secondarily to underlying conditions such as neurologic, GI, renal, or metabolic disorders. Assessment findings depend on whether the patient is in an early phase of shock or a most advanced state. Look for evidence of a possible contributing cause such as hypovolemia, sepsis, or trauma.

Among direct cardiac causes, you will most often see cardiogenic shock in the setting of MI if the MI affects the anterior wall or 40% or more of the left ventricle. Information about the patient's medications may give clues about pre-existing pump compromise. Inquire about the degree of compliance with medication regiments and ask about borrowed or over-the-counter drugs, which might have unpredictable interaction effects.

The altered mental status associated with advancing shock may begin as restlessness and progress through confusion to loss of consciousness. Airway findings include dyspnea, productive cough, or labored breathing. Tachypnea is often present due to pulmonary edema. Also common is a history of paroxysmal nocturnal dyspnea. Typical ECG findings include tachycardia and atrial dysrhythmias such as atrial tachycardia. Ectopy is also common.

MI often precedes cardiogenic shock; symptoms will be compatible with those expected with MI. Expect hypotension to develop as shock progresses. Systolic pressure will often fall to less than 80 mmHg. Try to correct any discovered dysrhythmias.

Management of cardiogenic shock begins by placing the patient in a position of comfort. With pulmonary edema, this may be sitting upright. Treatment consists mostly of caring for underlying conditions (such as MI or CHF) and supportive care. Remember to treat heart rate and rhythm and transport rapidly. Medications that may be used in this setting include the vasopressors dopamine, dobutamine, and norepinephrine. Other medications include morphine, promethazine, nitroglycerin, nitrous oxide, furosemide, digitalis, and sodium bicarbonate.

Cardiac arrest

Cardiac arrest and sudden death account for 60% of all deaths from coronary heart disease. Cardiac arrest is defined as the absence of ventricular contractions that immediately results in systemic circulatory failure. Sudden death is any death that occurs within one hour of the onset of symptoms. At autopsy, signs of MI are not present, and authorities generally believe lethal dysrhythmia secondary to severe atherosclerosis is the most common cause of death. The risk factors for sudden death are similar to those for ASHD and CHD. Other causes of sudden death include drowning, acid-base imbalance, electrocution, drug intoxication, electrolyte imbalance, hypoxia, hypothermia, pulmonary embolism, stroke, hyperkalemia, trauma, and end-stage renal disease.

Assessment for cardiac arrest shows an unresponsive, apneic, pulseless individual. After initiating CPR, place ECG leads and initiate monitoring. Dysrhythmias you may find include ventricular tachycardia or fibrillation, asystole, or PEA. If you find asystole, confirm it in two or more leads. Question bystanders with the goal of finding some specific, prognostic information: Did anyone witness the arrest? If CPR was begun before you arrived, try to learn as precisely as possible the length of time between arrest and initiation of effective CPR. Often, the emergency room physician will also want to know total down time from the beginning of the arrest until arrival at the emergency department. Also, try to get a list of the patient's medications as well as a past history.

Management starts with simultaneous efforts on the ABCs. Ventilate with a bag-valve mask using 100% oxygen. Intubate or insert an airway as quickly as possible. If ECG changes indicate defibrillation or synchronized cardioversion, perform it in conjunction with CPR, stopping CPR only long enough to apply the pads or paddles and deliver the shock. If the patient has an internal pacemaker or defibrillator, be sure not to defibrillate over the device.

After starting CPR and advanced airway management, get IV access with a venous site as close to the heart as possible (for instance, the antecubital area in the arm or the external jugular vein). Follow IV medications with a 30–45 second flush to ensure complete delivery. After each flush, set the line to a keep-vein-open rate. Agents used with cardiac arrest include atropine, lidocaine, procainamide, bretylium, epinephrine, norepinephrine, isoproterenol, dopamine, dobutamine, and sodium bicarbonate.

If blood pressure and pulse return, be aware that the blood pressure itself may be low, normal, or high because of the drugs administered. Pulse may return with a bradycardic, normal, or tachycardic rate. Ventricular ectopy is the most serious concern. If the patient presented in ventricular tachycardia or ventricular fibrillation or if ectopy is seen postarrest, use an antidysrhythmic such as lidocaine. Transport should be done as safely and smoothly as possible and with lights and siren.

79. Identify the limiting factor of pericardial anatomy that determines intrapericardiac pressure.   p. 548

The limitation is in the volume of material that can be held in the pericardial sac without exerting undue pressure on the heart. The normal volume is about 25 cc in an adult. As this volume is exceeded, pressure is exerted on the heart, and it can eventually reach the point of significantly limiting the extent to which the heart can fill during diastole or contract to expel blood during systole. This is cardiac tamponade.

80. Describe how to determine if pulsus paradoxus, pulsus alternans, or electrical alternans is present.   pp. 548

Pulsus paradoxus is determined by measuring blood pressure during respirations. A systolic pressure that falls more than 10 mmHg during inspiration is pulsus paradoxus. Pulsus alternans is an alternation between weak and strong peripheral pulses; this is determined by palpation of the pulse. Electrical alternans is determined by ECG analysis: It consists of an alternating pattern of normal and very low voltage.

81. Explain the essential pathophysiological defect of hypertension in terms of Starling's law of the heart.   pp. 546, 552

Starling's law states that the greater the stretch on myocardial muscle (the preload), the greater will be the force of contraction. This is true until the muscle is overstretched, at which point contraction becomes weaker. Afterload also affects stroke volume. An increase in afterload (peripheral vascular resistance) is an increase in the pressure against which the ventricle must pump, and thus increased afterload decreases stroke volume. Hypertension, or high blood pressure, is a state in which afterload is chronically increased, and thus this represents a chronic stressor on the ventricular myocardium.

82. Rank the clinical problems of patients in hypertensive emergencies according to their sense of urgency.   pp. 550-551

Hypertensive emergency in the general sense is a state in which diastolic blood pressure has risen to dangerous levels (greater than 130 mmHg), mandating a lowering of blood pressure within one hour to minimize or avoid risk for end-organ changes such as hypertensive encephalopathy, renal failure, or blindness. Hypertensive encephalopathy is a life-threatening situation in which stroke, coma, left ventricular failure, or pulmonary edema may occur. A hypertensive emergency in a pregnant patient with preeclampsia poses a high risk of the obstetric complication of abruption of the placenta or progression to eclampsia, with its seizures and risk of death for the woman and unborn fetus.

83. Identify the drugs of choice for hypertensive emergencies, cardiogenic shock, and cardiac arrest, including their indications, contraindications, side effects, route of administration, and dosages.   pp. 525-526, 551, 556

• *Hypertensive emergencies:* Drugs include morphine sulfate, furosemide, nitroglycerin, sodium nitroprusside, and labetalol.
• *Cardiogenic shock:* Drugs include dopamine, dobutamine, norepinephrine, morphine sulfate, promethazine, nitroglycerin, nitrous oxide, furosemide, digitalis, and sodium bicarbonate.
• *Cardiac arrest:* Drugs include atropine, lidocaine, procainamide, , epinephrine, norepinephrine, isoproterenol, dopamine, dobutamine, and sodium bicarbonate.

General descriptions, specific doses, contraindications, and side effects of these medications are given in objective 70 above. Two medications not covered in detail in objective 70 are discussed below.

Labetalol (Trandate, Normodyne). The IV bolus is 20 mg over 20 minutes, and it may be repeated at 40–80 mg over 10 minutes. Maximum bolus is 300 mg. Drip is established by mixing 200 mg into 160 cc D_5W, and the drip dose is 2 cc/min.

Sodium bicarbonate. Sodium bicarbonate is used late in the management of cardiac arrest, if at all.

Occasionally, metabolic acidosis from another disorder may cause pulseless electrical activity, asystole, ventricular tachycardia, or ventricular fibrillation. In these cases, sodium bicarbonate may aid in converting to a perfusing rhythm. Adequate CPR, prompt defibrillation, and appropriate drug administration should always precede the use of bicarbonate. Sodium bicarbonate has few side effects and no contraindications in the emergency setting. Dose is initially 1 mEq/kg followed by 0.5 mEq/kg every 10 minutes. When possible, doses should be based on arterial blood gas (ABG) results.

84. Describe the major systemic effects of reduced tissue perfusion caused by cardiogenic shock. pp. 552-553

A chief effect is CNS compromise, which may manifest early as restlessness or agitation and later as confusion or unconsciousness. Impaired renal function due to poor perfusion may be seen as oliguria or anuria. The decrease in blood flow to the extremities as blood is shunted to core organs is seen as cold, clammy, pale skin.

85. Explain the primary mechanisms by which the heart may compensate for a diminished cardiac output and describe their efficiency in cardiogenic shock.   pp552-553

The three basic mechanisms that increase cardiac output are increase in contractility, increase in preload, or decreasing peripheral resistance. Increased myocardial contractile force will help to increase stroke volume. Increased preload increases the stretch on the myocardium, and, within limits (this is Starling's law), this results in increased contraction force and increased stroke volume. Last, decreasing peripheral resistance (afterload) decreases the force that the ventricles must exert in order to expel blood into the aorta and pulmonary arteries.

86. Identify the clinical criteria and progressive stages of cardiogenic shock.   pp. 552-553

See objective 78.

87. Describe the dysrhythmias seen in cardiac arrest. p. 556

The dysrhythmias seen most frequently in cardiac arrest are ventricular tachycardia, ventricular fibrillation, asystole, and pulseless electrical activity (PEA). Asystole should always be confirmed in two more ECG leads.

88. Explain how to confirm asystole using the 3-lead ECG.   p. 556

An ECG tracing of asystole is shown in Part 1 of this chapter. On each lead, you should see an absence of all cardiac electrical activity: There will be no discernible components of the ECG sequence (no P waves, QRS complexes, or T waves).

89. Define the terms *defibrillation* and *synchronized cardioversion.*   pp. 527, 531

Defibrillation is the process of passing an electrical current through a fibrillating heart in order to depolarize all cells and allow them to repolarize uniformly, thus restoring an organized cardiac rhythm. Synchronized cardioversion is a controlled form of defibrillation for patients who have some organized cardiac activity with a pulse. A synchronizing circuit interprets the QRS cycle and delivers an electrical discharge during the R wave of the QRS complex, reducing the likelihood of delivering the cardioversion during the vulnerable period of the QRS cycle and reducing the likelihood of triggering ventricular fibrillation. Indications for synchronized cardioversion include perfusing ventricular tachycardia, paroxysmal supraventricular tachycardia, rapid atrial fibrillation, and 2:1 atrial flutter.

90. Specify the methods of supporting the patient with a suspected ineffective implanted defibrillation device.   p. 528

When external defibrillation is required, be sure that you do not place paddles over the generator of an implanted automatic defibrillator or pacemaker, because this can damage or disable the implanted device.

91. Describe resuscitation and identify circumstances and situations where resuscitation efforts would not be initiated.   pp. 555-559

Objective 78 covers initial resuscitation procedures as well as care after return of spontaneous pulse. In some situations, the patient will not survive despite resuscitation efforts, and in these cases resuscitation is contraindicated and should not be begun: These settings are rigor mortis, fixed dependent lividity (pooling of blood in gravity-dependent fashion), decapitation, and incineration. Less obvious but equally important settings include those where there is an advance directive to withhold resuscitation.

92. Identify communication and documentation protocols with medical direction and law enforcement used for termination of resuscitation efforts. p. 559

In some settings, resuscitation will begin but criteria for termination of resuscitation may exist. These include (1) age 18 years or older, (2) arrest that is presumed cardiac in origin and not associated with a treatable cause such as hypothermia, overdose, or hypovolemia, (3) successful and maintained endotracheal intubation, (4) ACLS standards having been applied throughout the arrest, (5) on-scene efforts having been sustained for 25 minutes or the patient remaining in asystole through four rounds of ALS drugs, (6) patient rhythm that is asystolic or agonal when the decision to terminate is made and persistence of this rhythm until resuscitation is actually terminated, and (7) victims of blunt trauma who presented in asystole or developed asystole on-scene.

You should be equally familiar with criteria that exclude termination of resuscitation: (1) age under 18 years, (2) cause that might benefit from in-hospital treatment, (3) persistent or recurring ventricular tachycardia or fibrillation, (4) transient return of a pulse, (5) signs of neurologic viability,

(6) arrest witnessed by EMS personnel, (7) and family or other responsible party opposed to termination.

Review local protocols and contact medical direction before attempting to terminate resuscitation. The medical director or other physician may use the following information: (1) medical condition of the patient, (2) known etiologic factors, (3) therapy rendered, (4) family's presence and appraisal of the situation, (5) communication of any resistance or uncertainty on the part of the family, and (6) maintenance of continued documentation including ECG.
Law enforcement regulations will require that all local, state, and federal laws pertaining to death be followed. The officer may also be required to assign the patient to the medical examiner if he/she does not have a physician. Check with your local law enforcement agencies to determine their protocols.

93. Describe the incidence, morbidity, mortality, pathophysiology, assessment, and management of vascular disorders including occlusive disease, phlebitis, aortic aneurysm, and peripheral artery occlusion. pp. 559-562

Conditions discussed in the chapter as peripheral vascular emergencies include atherosclerosis (which is an occlusive disease), aneurysm, acute arterial occlusion, and deep venous thrombosis.

• Atherosclerosis is the progressive degenerative disease affecting medium and large arteries that underlies many cardiovascular emergencies. It is the cause of coronary artery disease and can affect the carotid, aortic, and cerebral arteries, among others. In atherosclerosis, fats are deposited under the inner layer of the artery, causing injury that subsequently damages the middle, muscle-containing tissue layer as well. Progression occurs as calcium is deposited in the fatty material, forming plaques. Small hemorrhages typically occur around atherosclerotic plaques, further damaging the artery. As the disease progresses, the luminal diameter narrows and blood flow may be impaired to the distal tissues. Eventually, the artery may become totally blocked. If tearing occurs in the arterial wall, the vessel may become dilated and frail; this constitutes an atherosclerotic aneurysm. Arteriosclerosis is the related process in which disruption of tissue layers destroys the elasticity of the vessel and contributes to hypertension. You are already familiar with some of the clinical states due to atherosclerosis and arteriosclerosis: angina, MI, carotid bruits, and stroke.

• Aneurysms are dilatations of vessels. There are actually several types of aneurysms, including atherosclerotic, dissecting, infectious, congenital, and traumatic. Most aneurysms are due to atherosclerotic damage and occur in the aorta, the largest artery in the body and the one with the highest blood pressure. Infectious aneurysms are usually syphilitic in nature and are now rare. Congenital aneurysms can occur with several disease states including Marfan's syndrome, a genetic disorder of connective tissue. Aortic aneurysms are not uncommon in individuals with Marfan's syndrome because the aortic wall is relatively weak from birth.
Aneurysms form in the aorta when blood infiltrates the wall through a tear in its innermost layer. An abdominal aortic aneurysm secondary to atherosclerosis is a fairly common finding in persons aged 60 to 70 years and ten times as common in men than in women. Signs and symptoms of an abdominal aneurysm include abdominal, back, or flank pain, hypotension, and an urge to defecate caused by retroperitoneal leakage of blood. Degenerative changes in the smooth muscle and elastic tissue of the aorta cause most dissecting aortic aneurysms. The original tear often results from cystic medial necrosis, a degeneration of connective tissue associated with hypertension and, to some extent, aging. Hypertension is clearly a risk factor; it is present in 75–85% of cases. It occurs most frequently in those older than 40-50 years, although it can occur in younger individuals, especially pregnant women. There can also be a hereditary factor. A dissecting aortic aneurysm is one where a rapid inrushing of blood into the wall causes the layers of the wall to separate and eventually rupture. A dissecting aortic aneurysm is extremely painful, and this is one reason you gently search for pulsating masses during the focused abdominal exam of a patient with back, chest, or abdominal pain.

• Acute arterial occlusion is the sudden blockage of an artery due to trauma, thrombosis, embolus, tumor, or idiopathic means. Emboli are probably most common. They can arise within a chamber of the heart (mural emboli), from a thrombus in the left ventricle, from an atrial thrombus secondary to atrial fibrillation, or from a thrombus caused by abdominal aortic atherosclerosis. Arterial occlusions (from emboli leaving the aorta) most commonly involve vessels in the abdomen or extremities. Emboli leaving the heart via the left ventricle can cause embolic strokes, and emboli leaving the right ventricle (perhaps secondary to atrial fibrillation) can cause pulmonary embolisms.

• Deep venous thrombosis is a blood clot in a vein, usually one in the thigh or calf of the leg. Predisposing factors include recent history of trauma, inactivity, pregnancy, or varicose veins. The patient often complains of gradually increasing pain and tenderness; the affected leg and foot are typically swollen because of occluded venous drainage. Skin may be warm and red. Gentle palpation of the calf and thigh will reveal tenderness, and you may be able to palpate cord-like clotted veins.

Assessment of peripheral vascular disorders starts with the ABCs. Breathing is usually unaffected except in the case of pulmonary emboli. If you find decompensated shock, the cause is most likely to be aneurysm, arterial occlusion, or pulmonary embolus. Circulation is typically compromised distal to the occlusion. Check circulation for the five Ps: pallor, pain, pulselessness, paralysis, and paresthesias. Also check the skin for mottling distal to the affected area. Use the OPQRST acronym to learn more about the patient's pain or other complaint. Find out if this is a new event or a recurrence.

On physical exam, alteration in breathing and heart rate and rhythm are most common, with pulmonary embolus and aortic aneurysm the two conditions most likely to be life threatening. Unequal bilateral blood pressures may indicate a high thoracic aortic aneurysm that affects flow to one arm. Peripheral pulses may be normal, diminished, or absent, dependent on the site of obstruction. Bruits may be audible over a carotid artery partially occluded by atherosclerotic material. ECG findings generally do not contribute to diagnosis or treatment. However, if you find ectopy or dysrhythmias, treat them.

Management of the patient with a peripheral vascular emergency is largely supportive. Place the patient in a position of comfort. Give oxygen by nonrebreather mask if you suspect pulmonary embolus, aortic aneurysm, or acute arterial occlusion or if either hypotension or a hypoperfusion state exists. Ask about drug allergies before giving any medication. Agents you may use in this setting include nitrous oxide and morphine. Transport as soon as possible. Indications for rapid transport with lights and siren include any situation in which medications do not relieve symptoms or in which you suspect pulmonary embolism, aortic aneurysm, or arterial occlusion. Also consider hypotension or hypoperfusion to be an emergency meriting rapid transport.

94. Identify the clinical significance of claudication and presence of arterial bruits in a patient with peripheral vascular disorders.   pp. 559-562

Claudication is severe pain in a calf muscle due to inadequate blood supply. It typically occurs with exertion and subsides with rest. It is, in many respects, a peripheral parallel to cardiac angina. Arterial bruits are another sign of partial arterial blockage, usually due to atherosclerosis. Bruits are soft sounds heard over an artery (often the carotids) and represent the turbulent blood flow due to partial obstruction.

95. Describe the clinical significance of unequal arterial blood pressure readings in the arms.   p. 563

Unequal bilateral blood pressures may indicate an aneurysm high in the thoracic aorta; this is due to unequal flow to the left and right extremities.

96. Recognize and describe the signs and symptoms of dissecting thoracic or abdominal aneurysm.   pp. 560-561

Pain and evolution of shock (including alterations in heart rate and rhythm) are the most common symptom and sign of a dissecting aortic aneurysm. Abdominal aneurysms often present initially with abdominal, back, or flank pain accompanied by development of hypotension. The patient may complain of an urge to defecate if blood leaks into the retroperitoneal space. Thoracic aneurysms also present with pain; look for unequal bilateral blood pressures in the arms as evidence of the dissecting aneurysm.

97. Differentiate between signs and symptoms of cardiac tamponade, hypertensive emergencies, cardiogenic shock, and cardiac arrest.   pp. 549-557

Cardiac tamponade typically presents as dyspnea and chest pain, the latter of which may be either dull or sharp. Onset may be sudden or gradual. Classical physical findings include orthopnea, pulsus paradoxus, and narrowing pulse pressures. (In addition, you may see elevated venous pressures in the early phase represented by jugular venous distention.) The ECG is not a diagnostic tool, but you may well see diminished voltages and electrical alternans.

Hypertensive emergencies often show signs of hypertensive encephalopathy: confusion, headache, vomiting, visual changes, or seizures. The extreme hypertension found on blood pressure measurement (diastolic greater than 130 mmHg) is diagnostic.

Cardiogenic shock presents with the signs typical of shock: tachycardia, hypotension, poor peripheral perfusion. History may reveal evidence of chronic heart disease (medications, surgical scars, PND, or current medication regimen) or an acute event such as an MI as clues to the cardiac origin of shock. The usual heart rhythm is sinus tachycardia, but dysrhythmias are not uncommon. Peripheral edema may be so severe that pulses are not palpable.

Cardiac arrest presents with a completely unresponsive patient with no spontaneous breathing or pulse. ECG may show asystole or PEA or may show a dysrhythmia such as ventricular tachycardia or ventricular fibrillation.

98. Utilize the results of the patient history, assessment findings, and ECG analysis to differentiate between, and provide treatment for, patients with the following conditions: pp. 511-557

• **Cardiovascular disease.** Objectives 93–96 all deal with elements of peripheral vascular disease. Assessment findings are specific to the region of the vascular system affected by occlusion. Central findings such as tachypnea and change in heart rate or rhythm suggest pulmonary embolism or aortic aneurysm. Care is largely supportive unless a life-threatening problem (such as hypotension or dysrhythmia) develops.

• **Chest pain.** Chest pain can have a cardiac (pericarditis, angina, or MI) or vascular (aortic aneurysm) origin, or it can reflect problems of the respiratory system, GI tract, or musculoskeletal system (see objective 55). Look for pain on exertion that is relieved by rest and/or nitroglycerin as a sign of possible angina and pain that is unremitting for an MI. With both you may well see ECG changes including sinus tachycardia, S-T segment depression or elevation, ectopy, or dysrhythmias.

• **In need of a pacemaker.** A patient with a history of high-degree AV block or symptomatic bradycardia or atrial fibrillation has inadequate cardiac output for body needs during the periods of those dysrhythmias. If medications don't convert the dysrhythmia to a rhythm compatible with adequate cardiac output, a pacemaker should be considered. Other patients may have recurrent episodes of life-threatening dysrhythmias such as ventricular tachycardia or ventricular fibrillation, and they may also need a pacemaker.

• **Angina pectoris.** The typical presentation for angina is pain lasting from 3-5 minutes, or perhaps as long as 15 minutes, that is relieved by rest and/or nitroglycerin. Prinzmetal's (vasospastic) angina most often occurs at rest or without a known trigger but has similar duration. Prinzmetal's angina is often accompanied by S-T segment elevation on ECG. A patient with fixed (obstructive) angina may show S-T depression and/or T wave inversion on 12-lead ECG. Relief of pain is generally associated with resolution of ECG disturbances.

• **A suspected myocardial infarction.** The patient with an acute MI has chest pain that is severe, constant, and lasts longer than 30 minutes. Neither rest nor nitroglycerin relieves the pain, and the patient may be fearful or feel a sense of doom. On ECG, check the S-T segment for depression, which suggests ischemia, or elevation, which suggests tissue injury. A pathological Q wave (deeper than 5 mm and longer than 0.04 sec) can indicate either widespread transient ischemia or infarcted tissue. Ectopy and dysrhythmia can appear without warning.

• **Heart failure.** Heart failure, inadequacy of pumping ability to meet the body's oxygen demand, can be left-sided, right-sided, or both. Left-sided ventricular failure typically presents with dyspnea and the following additional signs: cyanosis, tachycardia, noisy, labored breathing, rales, cough, blood-tinged, often frothy sputum, and galloping heart sounds. Decreased lung sounds on exam reflect pulmonary edema. Right-sided ventricular failure typically presents with tachycardia, jugular venous distention, edema of body and extremities, engorged (palpable) liver and spleen, and abdominal distention due to ascites fluid. History will usually reflect past cardiac disease or pulmonary disease (COPD). Paroxysmal nocturnal dyspnea suggests left heart failure.

• **Cardiac tamponade.** Cardiac tamponade may be gradual or acute in onset depending on the origin of the material filling the pericardium and exerting pressure on the heart. Assessment typically finds dyspnea and orthopnea and pulsus paradoxus. ECG is not considered diagnostic, but you may see decreased voltage and electrical alternans in these patients.

• **A hypertensive emergency.** The patient with a hypertensive emergency will have extreme hypertension (diastolic greater than 130 mmHg) and usually will show some signs of hypertensive encephalopathy such as headache, visual change, nausea and vomiting, restlessness, or seizures or coma.

• **Cardiogenic shock.** Cardiogenic shock represents shock of cardiac origin: Exam will show characteristic signs of shock (hyperperfusion to extremities, hypotension, tachycardia) but history and exam will rule out extracardiac causes such as hypovolemia or sepsis. ECG may reveal an underlying acute event such as MI.

• **Cardiac arrest.** Patients in cardiac arrest are unresponsive, apneic, and pulseless. ECG may show asystole, PEA, or ventricular tachycardia or ventricular fibrillation. Confirm arrest in two or more ECG leads before beginning management.

99. Based on the pathophysiology and clinical evaluation of the patient with chest pain, characterize the clinical problems according to their life-threatening potential. 537-538pp.

Among cardiac causes, ischemia and MI are life threatening. Pericarditis becomes immediately life threatening if tamponade develops. Among vascular causes, dissection of the thoracic aorta is also immediately life threatening. Most of the respiratory causes are slightly less urgent (such as pneumonia and pleurisy), although both pulmonary embolism and pneumothorax can be immediately life threatening, especially in an individual with pre-existing respiratory or cardiovascular compromise. The GI causes of chest pain most likely to prove truly urgent are those associated with GI hemorrhage: These may include esophageal disease and peptic ulcer disease. Cholecystitis and pancreatitis are serious medical emergencies, but they are generally slightly less urgent than cases involving active hemorrhage. Hiatal hernia, GERD, and dyspepsia require medical care but are relatively unlikely to require urgent care. Most musculoskeletal causes are not urgent and do not have immediate life-threatening potential, although chest trauma may involve injury to the respiratory and/or cardiovascular systems.

100. Given several preprogrammed patients with cardiac complaints, provide the appropriate assessment, treatment, and transport. pp. 511-557

Because cardiovascular disease is so common and so serious, accounting for considerable morbidity and mortality, you will see patients who have the problems or conditions discussed in this chapter. Review objectives 46, 53, 55, 61–65, 68–70, 76–78, 83, 86, and 96–98 in particular to familiarize yourself with care in the setting of chest pain, angina, and MI, as well as care of heart failure and acute cardiovascular emergencies.

CONTENT SELF-EVALUATION

Multiple Choice

1. Atropine, lidocaine, and adenosine are in which group of drugs?
   - A. sympathomimetics
   - B. sympatholytics
   - C. thrombolytics
   - D. antidysrhythmics
   - E. drugs used for myocardial ischemia and its pain

2. Dopamine, dobutamine, and epinephrine are in which group of drugs?
   - A. sympatholytics
   - B. drugs used for myocardial ischemia and its pain
   - C. antidysrhythmics
   - D. parasympathomimetics
   - E. sympathomimetics

3. Nitrous oxide, nitroglycerin, and morphine are in which group of drugs?
   - A. sympathomimetics
   - B. drugs used for myocardial
   - C. antidysrhythmics
   - D. antiatherosclerotics ischemia and its pain
   - E. sympatholytics

4. Indications for synchronized cardioversion in an unstable patient include all of the following EXCEPT:
   - A. rapid atrial fibrillation.
   - B. nonperfusing ventricular tachycardia.
   - C. paroxysmal supraventricular tachycardia.
   - D. perfusing ventricular tachycardia.
   - E. 2:1 atrial flutter.

5. Potentially urgent noncardiac causes of chest pain include all of the following EXCEPT:
   - A. stroke.
   - B. peptic ulcer disease.
   - C. pneumothorax.
   - D. pulmonary embolism.
   - E. esophageal disease.

6. Always consider the possibility of cardiac tamponade when you encounter a patient:
   - A. with a chest wall tumor.
   - B. with muffled or distant heart and lung sounds.
   - C. with a gallop rhythm (S_1, S_2, S_3, S_4 heart sounds).
   - D. who has just entered ventricular fibrillation.
   - E. who received CPR and later deteriorated.

7. Causes of cardiogenic shock include all of the following EXCEPT:
   - A. subendocardial MI.
   - B. tension pneumothorax.
   - C. pulmonary embolism.
   - D. diffuse myocardial ischemia.
   - E. prosthetic valve malfunction.

8. Which of the following is NOT a possible criteria for termination of resuscitation efforts?
   - A. successful and maintained endotracheal intubation
   - B. patient remains in asystole after four rounds of ALS drugs
   - C. on-scene ALS efforts have been sustained for 25 minutes
   - D. arrest is associated with blunt trauma, hypothermia, or drug overdose
   - E. ACLS standards have been applied throughout the arrest

_____ 9. Which of the following prescription medications may be significant with a patient presenting with chest pain?
- A. Aldactone
- B. propranolol
- C. lanoxin
- D. diphenhydramine
- E. Mevacor

_____ 10. Which of the following is not a typical cause of poor ECG tracing?
- A. excessive hair
- B. diaphoresis
- C. patient size
- D. poor placement
- E. low battery

_____ 11. Without a defibrillator, a precordial thump can be used as an initial treatment for the following rhythm(s).
- A. second degree type II AV block
- B. nonperfusing ventricular tachycardia
- C. PSVT
- D. asystole
- E. normal sinus rhythm

_____ 12. Which of the following is a cardiac glycoside?
- A. metoprolol
- B. nifedipine
- C. nitroprusside
- D. digoxin
- E. dobutamine

_____ 13. For both adults and children in emergency situations, defibrillation pads should be placed with:
- A. one pad to the left of the upper sternum and the other to the right of the right nipple in an anterior axillary line.
- B. each pad placed under the respective clavicles.
- C. one pad under the right clavicle and the other on the back, directly posterior
- D. one pad under the right clavicle and the other on the left lateral chest in an anterior axillary line
- E. one pad directly over the sternum and the other in a mid axillary position on the left lateral chest

_____ 14. The initial defibrillation for a 20 kg patient in ventricular fibrillation is:
- A. 30 joules.
- B. 200 joules.
- C. 80 joules.
- D. 60 joules.
- E. 40 joules.

_____ 15. The initial energy recommendation for defibrillation in an adult patient who is vital signs absent is:
- A. 100 joules.
- B. 200 joules.
- C. 360 joules.
- D. 300 joules.
- E. none of the above.

16. Synchronized cardioversion delivers the electrical discharge during what wave of the ECG complex?
   - **A.** R wave
   - **B.** QRS wave
   - **C.** P wave
   - **D.** S wave
   - **E.** T wave

17. Which of the following energy selections would be used with synchronized cardioversion in the initial electrical treatment of atrial flutter?
   - **A.** 1000 joules
   - **B.** 50 joules
   - **C.** 200 joules
   - **D.** 300 joules
   - **E.** 360 joules

18. Prinzmetal's angina is an atypical angina caused primarily by:
   - **A.** blockage of the left coronary artery
   - **B.** atherosclerosis
   - **C.** pericarditis
   - **D.** abnormal spasm of the coronary arteries
   - **E.** pleural irritation

19. Which of the following may not contribute to heart failure?
   - **A.** excessive salt intake
   - **B.** sepsis
   - **C.** pruritis
   - **D.** excessive alcohol use
   - **E.** hypertension

20. Which pharmacological agent is not used in a cardiac arrest setting:
   - **A.** atropine sulphate
   - **B.** dopamine
   - **C.** vasopressin
   - **D.** labetolol
   - **E.** lidocaine

21. Which of the following medications affect preload and afterload:
   - **A.** NTG; furosemide
   - **B.** morphine; fentanyl
   - **C.** nifedipine; morphine
   - **D.** atenolol; NTG
   - **E.** Levitra; NTG

22. Which of the following is not a sign or symptom of an abdominal aortic aneurysm?
   - **A.** abdominal pain
   - **B.** urge to defecate
   - **C.** bradydcardia
   - **D.** hypotension
   - **E.** back and flank pain

23. During cardiogenic shock the body tries to compensate by:
   - **A.** increasing contractile force, improving preload and increasing PVR.
   - **B.** increasing the contractile force, improving preload and reducing PVR.
   - **C.** decreasing the contractility, improving preload and decreasing PVR.
   - **D.** increasing contractile force, decreasing rate and increasing PVR
   - **E.** increasing rate, decreasing contractility and decreasing PVR

24. All of the following are signs and symptoms of deep venous thrombosis EXCEPT:
   A.   Homan's sign
   B.   warm and red skin to the affected extremity
   C.   edema to the leg and foot
   D.   cool clammy skin to the affected extremity
   E.   cord-like clotted veins

25. Signs and symptoms of hypertensive encephalopathy include all of the following EXCEPT:
   A.   severe headache.   D.   pulmonary edema.
   B.   vomiting.   E.   paralysis.
   C.   angina.

True/False

26. Chest pain is the most common chief complaint among patients with cardiac disease, but not all patients with cardiac disease will have chest pain.
   A.   True
   B.   False

27. Return of spontaneous circulation occurs when resuscitation results in resumption of a pulse; spontaneous breathing may or may not return.
   A.   True
   B.   False

28. A patient complaining of 9/10 chest pain is usually presenting with a greater degree of ischemia in comparison to a patient complaining of 5/10 chest pain.
   A.   True
   B.   False

29. It is important to ask a patient who develops chest pain during sexual intercourse if they take Levitra or Viagara?
   A.   True
   B.   False

30. The S3 heart sound has a cadence like "Tennessee".
   A.   True
   B.   False

31. Failure of TCP is similar to the failure of a permanent pacemaker.
   A.   True
   B.   False

32. In a transmural infarction, the entire thickness of the myocardium is destroyed
   A.   True
   B.   False

33. Carotid sinus massage should not be performed on any patient over 60 years of age.
   A.   True
   B.   False

34. Left ventricular failure is also known as Cor Pulmonale.
   A.   True
   B.   False

35. Fifteen per cent of all patients with acute myocardial infarction will have associated chest wall tenderness.
   A.   True
   B.   False

Matching

Write the letter of the clinical setting in the space provided next to the procedure that should be carried out in that setting.

_____ **36.** defibrillation

_____ **37.** transcutaneous cardiac pacing

_____ **38.** precordial thump

_____ **39.** synchronized cardioversion

_____ **40.** carotid sinus massage

      A.   effort made immediately after onset of ventricular fibrillation or pulseless ventricular tachycardia that may cause conversion to organized rhythm

      B.   passage of electrical current through the heart during a specific part of the cardiac cycle to terminate certain dysrhythmias

      C.   manipulation of an arterial baroreceptor in an effort to increase parasympathetic tone

      D.   electrical pacing of the heart with use of special skin electrodes

      E.   passage of electrical current through a fibrillating heart to depolarize a critical mass of myocardium, resulting in conversion to an organized rhythm

Write the letter of the cardiac condition in the space provided next to the ECG finding that would suggest it.

_____ **41.** pathological Q wave

_____ **42.** S-T segment elevation

_____ **43.** T wave inversion

_____ **44.** S-T segment depression

      A.   infarcted tissue or extensive transient ischemia
      B.   myocardial ischemia
      C.   myocardial injury
      D.   old infarcted tissue that has formed a scar

Write the letter of the probable diagnosis in the space provided next to the appropriate description of the condition. A letter response may be used more than once or not at all.

A.	pulmonary edema	**E.**	right ventricular failure
B.	heart failure	**F.**	cardiac arrest
C.	acute MI	**G.**	cardiac tamponade
D.	left ventricular failure	**H.**	hypertensive encephalopathy

_____ **45.** Constant chest pain that is not relieved by rest or nitroglycerin and lasts longer than 30 minutes

_____ **46.** Dyspnea, tachycardia, noisy, labored breathing, gallop heart rhythm

_____ **47.** Syndrome in which the heart's pumping ability does not meet body needs

_____ **48.** Unresponsiveness with apnea and pulselessness

_____ **49.** Jugular venous distention, engorged liver, edema, tachycardia

_____ **50.** Pulsus paradoxus and pulsus alternans

_____ **51.** Dyspnea, orthopnea, decreased systolic BP with narrowing pulse pressure

_____ **52.** Severe headache, visual disturbance, seizures, stupor, diagnostic vital signs

Write the letter of the definition in the space provided next to the term to which it applies.

_____ **53.** orthopnea

_____ **54.** pulsus alterans

_____ **55.** intermittent claudication

       A. inflammation and clots within a vein
       B. relief of dyspnea on sitting upright
       C. alternation of weak and strong pulse over time

Chapter 29

Neurology

Review of Chapter Objectives

After reading this chapter, you should be able to:

1. Describe the incidence, morbidity, and mortality of neurological emergencies.   **p. 569**

Diseases and conditions of the nervous system affect millions of Canadians: You will see neurological emergencies in the field, and you will also see patients who present with another complaint but who have coexisting neurological conditions. Epilepsy affects 300 000 persons or just less than 1 per cent of the Canadian population. Strokes are a frequent source of considerable morbidity. Recent studies have shown that early recognition and intervention in certain strokes due to thromboembolism may decrease their morbidity and mortality. Strokes afflict approximately 50 000 people every year, of which 60 per cent are women.

Other neurological conditions are extremely common and of variable cause and rate of morbidity/mortality. Headaches of various causes are extremely common, with many people affected by chronic headaches.

2. Identify the risk factors most predisposing to diseases of the nervous system. pp. 585, 589-590, 594, 595, 602-603

Risk factors differ for the various types of neurological conditions. Strokes are vascular in nature (hemorrhagic or occlusive), and the major risk factors for stroke reflect this: atherosclerosis, heart disease, diabetes, abnormal blood lipid levels, hypertension, sickle cell disease, use of oral contraceptives, and the cardiac dysrhythmia atrial fibrillation. Some chronic conditions such as epilepsy reflect different causes and thus have different risk factors. Epilepsy can develop in patients who have had head trauma, brain tumors, or certain vascular disorders such as stroke. Most cases are considered idiopathic, which means the cause is unknown. Syncope is similar in having very different causes. Syncopal episodes can be due to cardiovascular (such as dysrhythmias or mechanical problems) origin or non-cardiovascular (metabolic, neurologic, or psychiatric) origin; indeed, many episodes are considered idiopathic even after workup. Headaches tend to be classified as vascular (such as migraine), tension, or organic (the last including headache due to tumor, infection, or other conditions). Some of the risk factors for low back pain may be gender-related. Symptoms in women over age 60 years, for example, often reflect postmenopausal osteoporosis. Occupations involving exposure to vibrations from vehicles or machinery or jobs requiring repetitive lifting also are associated with risk for low back pain. Other causes include compression or trauma to the sciatic nerve or its roots, as can happen with a herniated intervertebral disk. Most cases, though, are also idiopathic.

3. Discuss the anatomy and physiology of the nervous system.   **(see Chapter 12)**

The nervous system is the body's chief control for virtually every major function. It is divided physically into the central nervous system (CNS) and peripheral nervous system (PNS). The CNS consists of the brain and spinal cord. If the body were visualized as a computer, the CNS would be the central processing unit. Both very basic functions, such as continuance of heartbeat and respiration, and complex functions, such as listening to Mozart and anticipating a musical passage you particularly like, are controlled by cells in the brain. Messages within the CNS, as well as those that connect it with the rest of the body, travel as nerve impulses. The complex network of nerves outside the CNS makes up the peripheral nervous system. The messages that carry information regarding critical body functions such as respiration pass through a part of the PNS called the autonomic nervous system; these functions do not require any conscious effort to maintain them. In contrast, messages that involve voluntary, or conscious, actions and thoughts travel through the other part of the PNS, the somatic nervous system. Both the autonomic and somatic nervous systems have two parallel tracks: one of nerves that carry messages to the brain, and a second that carries messages from the brain. In terms of the computer analogy, the PNS carries the various input and output messages that run between the brain and spinal cord and the rest of the body. The autonomic nervous system is also structurally and functionally broken into two parts: the sympathetic and parasympathetic nervous systems. These two parts work together to make sure the net balance of stimulatory and inhibitory messages from the brain keep body functions such as blood pressure within normal limits.

The basic structural and functional unit is the neuron, or nerve cell. Nerve cells have a body that contains the essential cell machinery of nucleus, mitochondria, etc. Nerve processes (usually there are many) that are capable of receiving impulses from other neurons or body cells are called dendrites. An impulse that is picked up by a dendrite travels toward the cell body. Another process, the axon, carries the impulse away from the cell body. Axons may have multiple tips, which means the neuron has the capacity to send the impulse onward to more than one other nerve or other cell. Dendrites associated with neurons of the major senses organs (such as the eye or ear) convert an environmental stimulus into a nerve impulse that can be forwarded via the axon to other nerves, and eventually the brain. Dendrites associated with neurons that monitor internal conditions such as PaO_2 also convert that information into an impulse and send it to the brain. Eventually all such information is analyzed by neurons in the brain and response impulses travel back through the PNS. These impulses eventually affect a motor neuron, causing a muscle cell to contract, or affect another type of cell such as one in a gland. Messages cannot pass directly from an axon to a dendrite because there is a tiny physical gap, called a synapse, between each pair of neurons. As the wave of electrical depolarization (due to ion fluxes of potassium rapidly leaving the neuron and sodium rapidly entering) reaches the axon tip, it causes a chemical called a neurotransmitter to be released into the synapse. (There are multiple neurotransmitters within the body. Either acetylcholine or norepinephrine is found in the neurons of the PNS. Neurotransmitters within the CNS include dopamine and serotonin.) When the neurotransmitter crosses the synapse and is taken up by the dendrite on the other side, a wave of depolarization is started in that dendrite and the nerve impulse is then carried toward the cell body.

Most of the CNS is protected by the bones of the cranium and spine. The spinal column is made up of 33 vertebrae running from the neck to the junction with the pelvis. There is also an inner shock-absorbing, cushioning protection system. The cells of the brain and spinal cord are bathed in cerebrospinal fluid, and there are three layers of protective membranes between the neural surface and the outer, protective bone. These meninges are called the dura mater, arachnoid membrane, and pia mater (in outer-to-inner sequence).

As you look at a human brain, it has six obvious structural regions: the cerebrum, the diencephalon, the mesencephalon (or midbrain), the pons, the medulla oblongata, and the cerebellum.

Sometimes, the terminology is simplified as follows: the forebrain (cerebrum and diencephalon), the midbrain, and the hindbrain (the brainstem—pons, medulla oblongata—and the cerebellum). The largest part of the brain, with its characteristic folded outer surfaces, is the cerebrum. The cerebrum has left and right sides, or hemispheres, which are connected physically and functionally by tissue called the corpus callosum. The cerebrum is responsible for intelligence, learning, memory, and language, as well as analysis and response to sensory and motor activities. The diencephalon is covered by the cerebrum, and it is made up of a number of vital structures: the thalamus, hypothalamus, and the limbic system. This primal part of the brain is responsible for many involuntary functions such as temperature regulation, sleep, water balance, stress response, and emotion. It also has an important role in regulating the autonomic nervous system. The brainstem consists of the mesencephalon, pons, and medulla oblongata. The mesencephalon is located between the diencephalon and the pons, and it plays a role in motor coordination. It is the major region controlling eye movement. The pons is a major connection point between the upper portions of the brain and the medulla and cerebellum. The medulla oblongata itself marks the division between the brain and the spinal cord. The major centers for control of respiration, cardiac activity, and vasomotor activity are located here. The cerebellum is located in the posterior fossa of the cranium, and it also has two hemispheres, which are closely coordinated to the brainstem and higher centers. The cerebellum coordinates fine motor movement, posture, equilibrium, and muscle tone.

The hemispheres of the cerebrum do not contain identical centers. Rather, the functional responsibilities of the cerebrum have been mapped as a whole. Important centers with clinical implications for you in cases such as stroke or trauma include the following: (1) speech, which is located in the temporal lobe, (2) vision, which is located in the occipital lobe, (3) personality, which is located in the frontal lobes, (4) sensory, which is located in the parietal lobes, and (5) motor, which is located in the frontal lobes. As noted previously, balance and coordination are located in the cerebellum. A last important center is called the reticular activating system (RAS), which operates in the lateral portion of the medulla, pons, and especially the mesencephalon. The RAS sends impulses to and receives messages from the cerebral cortex (the outer portion of the cerebrum). This diffuse system of interlaced cells is responsible for maintaining consciousness and the ability to respond to external stimuli.

The brain receives about 20% of the body's total blood flow per minute. Vascular supply to the brain is provided by two systems, a physical arrangement that provides secondary supply if one system is occluded or severed. The anterior system is the carotid, and the posterior system is the vertebrobasilar. They join at the Circle of Willis before entering the structures of the brain itself. Venous drainage is via the venous sinuses and the internal jugular veins. As previously noted, there is also cerebrospinal fluid (CSF) bathing the tissues of the brain and spinal cord. Most of the intracranial CSF is found in the ventricles.

The spinal cord is 17 to 18 inches long on average in adults. It leaves the brain at the medulla and passes through an opening in the skull called the foramen magnum to enter the spinal canal. The spinal cord, which ends near the level of the first lumbar vertebra (the reason why spinal taps are done below that level), conducts impulses to and from the peripheral nervous system and locally for motor reflexes. Thirty-one pairs of nerves exit the spinal cord between adjacent vertebrae. The dorsal nerve roots carry afferent fibers, ones carrying impulses to the brain. The ventral roots carry efferent fibers, which carry impulses from the brain to the periphery. Each nerve root has a corresponding area of skin called a dermatome, to which it supplies sensation. In the field, you may be able to correlate sensory deficits to the level of a spinal cord problem. The reason why our protective motor reflexes are so fast and effective lies in the fact that the afferent and efferent impulses are coordinated in the spinal cord—they do not travel the whole way to the brain before coming back. However, because they are mediated in the spinal cord, they lack fine motor control.

The peripheral nervous system (PNS) contains 12 pairs of cranial nerves, which extend directly from the lower surface of the brain and exit through small holes in the skull, and the peripheral nerves, which exit from the spinal cord as noted previously. The nerves of the PNS control both voluntary and involuntary activities. The cranial nerves supply nervous control for the head, neck, and certain thoracic and abdominal organs. The peripheral nerves can be divided into four classes: (1) somatic sensory, afferent nerves that carry impulses concerned with touch, pressure, pain, temperature, and position, (2) somatic motor, efferent nerves that carry impulses to the skeletal (voluntary) muscles, (3) visceral (autonomic) sensory, afferent nerves that carry impulses of sensation from the visceral organs (examples being fullness in the bladder or distension of the rectum), and (4) visceral (autonomic) motor, efferent nerves that serve the involuntary cardiac muscle and the smooth muscle of the viscera and the glands.

The involuntary division of the PNS is called the autonomic nervous system, and it has two components: the sympathetic nervous system and the parasympathetic nervous system. The sympathetic system is associated with the primitive "fight or flight" response to sensory stimuli. Its major nerve roots are located near the thoracic and lumbar part of the spinal cord. Stimulation causes increased heart rate and blood pressure, pupillary dilation, rise in blood sugar, as well as bronchodilation, all responses that ready the body for stress. The neurotransmitters norepinephrine and epinephrine mediate its actions, and sympathetic activity is also closely correlated to activity in the adrenal gland medulla, tissue that is of nervous system origin and that also relies on norepinephrine and epinephrine. The parasympathetic nervous system is responsible for controlling vegetative functions such as normal heart rate and blood pressure. It is associated with the cranial nerves and the sacral plexus of nerves, and it is mediated by the neurotransmitter acetylcholine. When stimulated, it causes a decrease in heart rate, an increase in digestive activity, pupillary constriction, and a reduction in blood sugar.

4. Define and discuss the epidemiology (including the morbidity/mortality and preventative strategies), pathophysiology, assessment findings, and management for the following neurologic problems:

a.   Coma and altered mental status   pp. 582-584

Altered mental status is extremely common, as you'll understand when you consider the wide variety of causes. Morbidity and mortality are often correlated to cause. Vigilant assessment and management on your part will optimize your patient's chances, regardless of causes. An alteration in mental status is the hallmark sign of CNS injury or illness; as such, any alteration, be it subtle or as florid as coma, requires evaluation. In coma, the patient cannot be aroused by even powerful external stimuli such as pain. The two mechanisms generally capable of causing altered mental status are structural lesions (such as tumor, trauma, degenerative disease, or another process that destroys or encroaches on the substance of the brain) and toxic-metabolic states (such as the presence of toxins including ammonia or the absence of vital substances such as oxygen, glucose, or thiamine). Causes of toxic-metabolic disturbances include anoxia, diabetic ketoacidosis, hepatic failure, hypoglycemia, renal failure, thiamine deficiency, and toxic exposure (for instance, cyanide). Some of the most common causes you'll see for altered mental status (meaning they can cause a structural lesion or a toxic-metabolic state) are the following: (1) drugs, including depressants such as alcohol, hallucinogens, and narcotics; (2) cardiovascular, including anaphylaxis, cardiac arrest, stroke, dysrhythmias, hypertensive encephalopathy, and shock; (3) respiratory, including chronic obstructive pulmonary disease (COPD), inhalation of a toxic gas such as carbon monoxide, and hypoxia; and (4) infectious, such as AIDS, encephalitis, and meningitis.

During history taking and assessment, remember the mnemonic AEIOU-TIPS, and look for signs of these common causes: A (acidosis or alcohol), E (epilepsy), I (infection), O (overdose), U (uremia, or kidney failure), T (trauma, tumor, or toxin), I (insulin, either hypoglycemia or ketoacidosis), P (psychosis or poison), S (stroke, seizure). During physical assessment, use the AVPU method for determining level of consciousness. Unresponsive patients require especially vigilant monitoring and protection of the airway. Remember that in some cases you will not be able to determine the cause of the problem in the pre-hospital setting.

Management begins with the ABCs. The initial priority is the airway; be sure to immobilize the C-spine in cases of suspected head or neck injury. Then attend to breathing, administering supplemental oxygen and assisting ventilations if needed. An unresponsive patient requires an airway adjunct. As an evaluation of circulation, check heart rate and rhythm and blood pressure.

Then perform the following steps:

• IV of normal saline or lactated Ringer's solution at a keep-vein-open rate; alternatively place a heparin lock.
• Determine blood glucose level with reagent strip or glucometer. If serum glucose is low, give 50% dextrose to mediate the hypoglycemia. Even if the patient is an uncontrolled diabetic, any transient hyperglycemia will do limited harm at most in the short pre-hospital period. In many cases of hypoglycemia, dextrose can be life saving, and you may see an immediate response. Glucose may also be life saving for the alcoholic patient with hypoglycemia.
• Administer naloxone if there is suspicion of narcotic overdose. (See Chapter 34, "Toxicology and Substance Abuse," for details).

In chronic alcoholism, intake, absorption, and use of thiamine is impaired. Among these patients, you may see Wernicke's syndrome, a condition marked by loss of memory and disorientation that is associated with a diet deficient in thiamine. Of even greater concern is Korsakoff's psychosis, marked by memory disorder, because it may be irreversible. Thus, the administration of thiamine as per local protocols and the judgment of medical direction may be important.

If increased intracranial pressure is possible, as in a closed head injury, hyperoxygenate the patient at 20 breaths per minute. The decrease in carbon dioxide causes cerebral vasoconstriction and reduces brain swelling. DO NOT overoxygenate, as this can decrease CO_2 to dangerously low levels.

b.   Seizures   pp. 589-594

A seizure is a temporary alteration in behavior due to a massive discharge of one or more groups of neurons in the brain. Seizures can be induced in anyone under certain stressful conditions such as hypoxia or rapidly decreasing blood glucose. Febrile seizures often occur in young children with a sudden increase in body temperature. Structural diseases of the brain such as tumors, head trauma, toxic eclampsia, and vascular disorders can also cause a seizure. Recurrent seizures without such a known cause are termed epilepsy. Most cases of epilepsy are idiopathic, that is, without known cause, whereas others arise secondary to damage from strokes, head trauma, tumor surgery or radiation, etc.

Assessment begins with history according to the patient or bystanders, as well as physical impression. Remember that many people think the only kind of seizure is a "grand mal," so a bystander who does not know the patient may suggest he is on drugs, or that he fainted, or give other information that is misleading. In addition, other medical conditions can present similarly to a seizure: Examples are migraine headaches, cardiac dysrhythmias, hypoglycemia, or orthostatic hypotension. Hyperventilation, as well as a number of CNS conditions, can cause stiffness in the extremities. Decerebrate movements can be caused by increased intracranial pressure. Thus, there is often more potential harm than good in administering an anticonvulsant.

The patient history should include an attempt to ascertain the following information: (1) history of seizures, and, if so, particulars of type, nature, and frequency, (2) recent history of head trauma, (3) possibility of alcohol or other drug use, (4) recent history of fever, headache, or stiff neck, (5) history of diabetes, heart disease, or stroke, and (6) current medications. During physical exam, look for evidence of head injury or injury to the tongue and for evidence of alcohol or drug abuse. Be sure to document any dysrhythmias.

Active management may not be needed for many types of seizures, including short generalized tonic-clonic seizures that have ended before you arrive. Management for most generalized seizures in process is supportive: Manage the airway, make sure the patient does not injure him- or herself, and monitor for possible hyper- or hypothermia, depending on environmental conditions. General procedures include the following: (1) assurance of scene safety, (2) maintenance of airway (DO NOT force objects between the patient's teeth or push objects into the mouth that may initiate vomiting), (3) administration of high-flow oxygen, (4) establishment of IV access, running normal saline or lactated Ringer's solution at keep-vein-open rate, (5) determination of blood glucose level, with 50% glucose given in hypoglycemia, (6) physical protection of patient from surroundings, (7) maintenance of temperature, (8) postictal positioning on left side with suction if required, (9) monitoring of cardiac rhythm, (10) consideration of an anticonvulsant if seizure is prolonged (greater than 5 minutes), (11) transport the patient in supine or lateral recumbent position in quiet, reassuring atmosphere.

Status epilepticus, two or more generalized seizures without intervening return of consciousness, can be a life-threatening emergency. The most common cause in adults with epilepsy is failure to comply with medication regimen. Status is a major emergency because it involves a prolonged period of apnea with the possibility of CNS hypoxia. The most valuable intervention is to protect the airway and to deliver 100% oxygen, preferably by BVM device. After airway and breathing have been addressed, start an IV with normal saline at keep-vein-open rate, monitor cardiac rhythm, give 25 g 50% dextrose IV push if hypoglycemia is present, give 5–10 mg diazepam IV push for an adult, and continue to monitor airway. Note that some patients will require large doses of diazepam, and this may cause respiratory depression.

c.   Syncope   pp. 594-596

Syncope, or fainting, is characterized by a sudden, temporary loss of consciousness caused by insufficient blood flow to the brain, with recovery almost immediate upon supine positioning. Syncope is very common, with nearly half of all Canadians experiencing at least one episode of syncope during their lifetime. It can occur at any age and symptoms may include prior feelings of dizziness or lightheadedness or there may be no warning at all. By definition, if return of consciousness does not occur within a few moments, the event is NOT syncope, it is something more serious. (Review Table 29-2, text page 592, for help in distinguishing between syncope and seizure.)

There are three pathophysiologic mechanisms for syncope: cardiovascular, non-cardiovascular, and idiopathic. Cardiovascular causes include dysrhythmias or mechanical problems such as an abnormally functioning heart valve. Non-cardiovascular causes include metabolic, neurological, or psychiatric conditions. For instance, hypoglycemia, a transient ischemic attack (TIA), or an anxiety attack my all precipitate syncope. Idiopathic, as always, means there is no known cause even after careful evaluation. Management begins with an attempt to find and treat the underlying cause. If no cause is established, the patient should be transported to an appropriate emergency department for evaluation. Field management is somewhat similar to that for seizure: assure scene safety, maintain open airway, administer high-flow oxygen and assist ventilations as needed, check circulatory status (heart rate and rhythm, blood pressure), check and continue monitoring mental status, start IV with normal saline or lactated Ringer's at keep-vein-open rate, determine blood glucose level, monitor cardiac rhythm, and transport in reassuring environment.

d.   Headache   pp. 595-596

Headaches, either acute or chronic, are a tremendously common complaint: You've probably had problems with a headache at least once. There three general categories of headache: vascular, tension, and organic. Headaches of vascular origin include migraines and cluster headaches. Migraines occur more commonly in women, whereas cluster headaches occur more commonly in men. Nearly 3 million Canadians suffer migraine headaches. Migraines are typically characterized by intense, throbbing pain, sensitivity to light or sound, nausea, vomiting, and sweating. Migraines may last from several minutes to several days. They typically present as one-sided headaches and they may be preceded by an aura. Cluster headaches usually occur as a series of one-sided headaches that are sudden in onset, intense, and continue for roughly 15 minutes to 4 hours. Symptoms may include nasal congestion, drooping eyelid, and an irritated eye. Tension headaches account for a significant percentage of headaches. Most personnel in emergency medicine, have, or will, have a tension headache. Some people experience them on a daily basis. These persons may wake with a headache that worsens over the course of the day. The typical tension headache has a dull, achy pain that feels as if forceful pressure is being applied to the neck or head. The last class of headache, organic headaches, is less common. They occur in association with tumor, infection, or other diseases of the brain, eye, or other body system.

Because headaches can herald serious illness or precede a catastrophic event such as a ruptured aneurysm, it is always important to keep these possible underlying causes in mind when you speak with a patient complaining of headache. A continuous throbbing headache, particularly if over the occiput, accompanied by fever, confusion, and stiffness of the neck is classic for meningitis. Sudden onset pain, often described as "the worst pain of my life," or changes in pain pattern should all be considered possible signs of conditions as grave as intracranial hemorrhage. In general, any headache of acute onset or of changing pattern demands immediate attention on your part.

A complete and thorough history is important in evaluating the patient with headache. Questions that may evoke valuable information include the following: What were you doing when the pain started? Does anything make the pain worse (such as light, sound, or movement)? What is the quality of the pain, throbbing, crushing, tension? Does pain radiate to the neck, arm, back, or jaw? What is the severity of the pain on a scale of 1–10 and has severity changed? How long has the headache been present (is it acute or chronic)? You will see that the same line of questioning about pain is used in other settings, too, as with patients who complain of abdominal pain (Chapter 32, "Gastroenterology").

Management is supportive and generally includes the following: (1) assurance of scene safety, (2) protection of airway, (3) placement of patient in position of comfort (often accomplished by patients themselves), (4) high-flow oxygen with ventilation assistance as needed, (5) IV with normal saline or lactated Ringer's at keep-vein-open rate, determination of blood glucose, monitoring of cardiac rhythm, (6) transport with reassurance in an environment that is calm and quiet.

e. Neoplasms   pp. 597-598

Neoplasm is a general term for "new growth," and it is used to describe tumors that arise after birth. Neoplasms that affect the CNS have a mortality rate of 188 per 100 000 in Canada per year. These neoplasms can be divided into benign and malignant tumors based on several characteristics. The cells of a benign tumor generally resemble normal cells, grow relatively slowly, and tend to remain confined to one location. In contrast, malignant tumors of the CNS often have cells that are primitive in appearance and don't resemble normal cells, grow quickly, and may invade adjacent, healthy tissue or spread within the CNS. Both kinds of CNS tumors can be dangerous because any tumor growth can place pressure on other tissues and impair their function and because the pressure cannot be relieved by expansion of the cranial space. In adults, the cranium is rigid and fixed. Pressure exerted by a tumor causes increased intracranial pressure. There are numerous types of brain tumors, and the cause is unknown for most of them.

CNS tumors present with many signs and symptoms dependent on the size, type, and location of the tumor. It isn't your role in the field to diagnose new tumors; rather, you are more likely to have patients with previously diagnosed tumors or patients who present with problems that may reflect a CNS tumor. Common complaints among persons with undiagnosed brain tumors include the following: headache (often severe and recurrent), new onset seizures, nausea and vomiting, behavioral or cognitive changes, weakness or paralysis of one or more limbs or one side of the face, change in sensation in one or more limbs or one side of the face, new onset uncoordination, difficulty walking or unsteady gait, dizziness, double vision. Be alert for any of these signs and be sure to obtain a thorough history. In addition to the SAMPLE questions, ask the following: (1) What is the state of your general health? (2) Have you had any seizure activity, headache, or nosebleed? (3) Have you ever had surgery for removal of a brain tumor, chemotherapy, radiation therapy, holistic therapy, or any form of experimental treatment?

Management is largely supportive, with the goal of reducing anxiety and palliating symptoms. The general steps of field management have much in common with those for seizures and headaches. Assure scene safety, and protect airway. Position the patient for comfort, generally with head elevated. Use high-flow oxygen and assist ventilations as needed. Start an IV with normal saline or lactated Ringer's at keep-vein-open rate or use a saline or heparin lock. Monitor cardiac rhythm and consider narcotic analgesia if approved by medical direction or consider diazepam if seizures are present. Last, transport in a calm, quiet environment while reassuring the patient.

f. Abscess p. 589

A brain abscess is a pocket of pus localized to one area of the brain. They are uncommon, accounting for 2% of intracranial masses. Signs and symptoms are similar to those of a neoplasm and include headache, lethargy, hemiparesis (weakness on one side of the body), seizures, rigidity of the neck, nausea and vomiting. Fever is frequently present, suggesting an infectious cause. Your field management is supportive and similar to that for neoplasm or meningitis.

g. Stroke pp. 584-589

Stroke is a general term for injury or death of brain tissue, usually due to interruption of blood flow to that region of the cerebrum. The term "brain attack" is being used more frequently because of some similarities between stroke and heart attack, the latter also being due to oxygen deprivation. You should also realize that there are more treatment similarities to heart attacks. Strokes due to thromboembolic causes may be aborted or minimized with use of thrombolytic agents now used with heart attack (such as tissue plasminogen activator, tPA). The importance to you is that prompt recognition and transport of stroke patients is greater than ever. Stroke patients who may be candidates for thrombolytic therapy must receive definitive treatment within 3 hours of onset.

Strokes are the third most common cause of death and a frequent cause of considerable disability among middle-aged and elderly persons. Major risk factors include atherosclerosis, heart disease, hypertension, diabetes, abnormal blood lipid levels, use of oral contraceptives, and sickle cell disease. Strokes can be caused either by occlusion of an artery or by hemorrhage. Both interrupt blood flow to distal tissues. An occlusive stroke is any caused by blockage of the artery, resulting in ischemia to brain tissue that may progress to infarction if oxygen deprivation continues long enough. Infarcted brain tissue swells, further damaging nearby tissue that might have only a marginal blood supply itself. If swelling is sufficiently severe, herniation (protrusion of tissue through the foramen magnum, the opening at the base of the skull through which the spinal cord emerges from the cranium) can occur. Occlusive strokes are either thrombotic or embolic in origin.

Thrombotic strokes are due to a thrombus, or blood clot, that forms in and then obstructs a cerebral artery. Thrombosis is often related to atherosclerotic change in the artery. Unsurprisingly, the signs and symptoms of a thrombotic stroke are often gradual in onset. The stroke often occurs at night and is characterized by the patient waking with altered mental status and/or loss of speech, sensation, or motor function. An embolic stroke is caused by a solid, liquid, or gaseous mass that is carried to the site of obstruction from a remote site. The most common brain emboli are blood clots that often arise from diseased blood vessels in the neck (namely, the carotid artery) or from abnormal cardiac contraction. Atrial fibrillation often results in atrial dilation, a precursor to clot formation. Other types of emobli include air, tumor tissue, and fat. Typically, embolic strokes present with sudden onset of severe headaches. Hemorrhagic strokes are due to bleeding within brain tissue, and they can be categorized as intracerebral or subarachnoid (see Figure 29-7, text page 586). They are discussed in detail below under intracranial hemorrhage.

Prompt and proper assessment of a stroke in progress is very important. Signs and symptoms will depend on the type of stroke and the area of the brain affected by it. Onset of symptoms may be acute, and the patient may be unconscious. You may observe stertorous breathing due to paralysis of part of the soft palate. Respiratory expirations may be puffs of air out of the cheeks and mouth. The patient's pupils may be unequal. If so, the larger pupil will be on the side of the hemorrhage. Paralysis, when present, usually involves one side of the face, one arm, or one leg. Speech disturbances may be noted, and the patient's skin may be cool and clammy.

In list form, common signs and symptoms of stroke include the following: one-sided facial drooping, headache, confusion and agitation, dysphasia (difficulty in speech), aphasia (inability to speak), dysarthria (impairment of tongue and muscles making speech difficult), vision problems such as blindness in one eye or double vision, hemiparesis (one-sided weakness), hemiplegia (one-sided paralysis), paresthesias, inability to recognize by touch, gait disturbances or uncoordinated motor movements, dizziness, incontinence, or coma.

Management of stroke emphasizes early recognition, supportive measures, prompt, rapid transport, and notification of the emergency department (see algorithm in Figure 29-8 of the textbook). Remember that aggressive airway management is vital in these patients. Other field measures include the following: (1) assurance of scene safety, including body substance isolation, (2) airway management including suction as needed, (3) ventilation assistance as needed: If the patient is apneic or breathing is inadequate, provide positive-pressure ventilation at 16-20/minute. Hyperoxygenation eliminates excessive CO_2 levels. Avoid overzealous hyperoxygenation because excessively low CO_2 levels can cause profound cerebral vasoconstriction. If breathing is adequate, give oxygen via nonrebreather mask at 15 L/minute, (4) complete a detailed patient history, (5) keep patient supine or in recovery position. If the patient has congestive heart failure, place patient in semi-upright position as needed. If patient has altered mental status and you suspect potential for airway compromise, keep him or her in left lateral recumbent, or recovery position, (6) determine blood glucose level; if hypoglycemia is present, consider 50% dextrose by IV push, (7) start an IV of normal saline or lactated Ringer's at a keep-vein-open rate or place a saline or heparin lock (avoiding dextrose solutions, which may increase intracranial pressure due to osmotic effect), (8) monitor cardiac rhythm, (9) protect paralyzed extremities, (10) reassure patient and explain all procedures as patient may be able to understand even if he or she cannot respond, and (11) transport without excessive movement or noise.

h.   Intracranial hemorrhage   pp. 585-586

Hemorrhagic strokes are due to blood within brain tissue, and they can be categorized as intracerebral or subarachnoid. These intracranial hemorrhages often occur with sudden onset of a severe headache. Most intracranial hemorrhages occur in a hypertensive patient when a small vessel deep within brain tissue ruptures. Subarachnoid hemorrhages most commonly result from either congenital blood vessel anomalies or from head trauma. Congenital anomalies include aneurysms and arteriovenous malformations. Aneurysms tend to be on the brain's surface and may either hemorrhage into brain tissue or into the subarachnoid space. Hemorrhage within brain tissue may tear and separate normal brain tissue. Release of blood into the ventricles containing CSF may paralyze vital centers. If blood impairs drainage of CSF, the resultant increase in intracranial pressure may cause herniation of brain tissue.

i. Transient ischemic attack   pp. 587-588

A transient ischemic attack (TIA) is a temporary manifestation of the signs and/or symptoms of stroke that is due to temporary interference with blood supply to the affected part of the brain. These symptoms may persist for a few minutes or for hours, but they almost always resolve within 24 hours. After the attack (because it reflects ischemia, not infarction), there is no evidence of brain or neurological damage. The most common cause is carotid artery disease (provoking an embolic event). Other causes can be small emboli of different origin, decreased cardiac output, hypotension, overmedication with antihypertensive medications, or cerebrovascular spasm. Part of the importance of recognizing TIAs is that they may be the precursor to a stroke. One third of TIA patients suffer a stroke soon afterward. A TIA is typically sudden in onset, with specific signs and symptoms depending on the part of the brain involved.

In the pre-hospital setting, it is virtually impossible to distinguish a TIA from a stroke. While taking the history, try to get the following information: previous neurological symptoms, if any; initial symptoms and their progression; changes in mental status; precipitating factors, if any; dizziness; palpitations; history of hypertension, cardiac disease, sickle cell disease, or previous TIA or stroke. Because TIAs and strokes are generally indistinguishable in the field, the management is the same. (See Stroke above.)

j. Degenerative neurological diseases   pp. 598-602

The term "degenerative neurological disease" characterizes diseases that selectively affect one or more functional systems of the CNS. Generally, they produce symmetrical and progressive involvement of the CNS, affect similar areas of the brain, and produce similar clinical signs and symptoms. Examples discussed in the text include Alzheimer's disease, muscular dystrophy, multiple sclerosis, dystonias, Parkinson's disease, central pain syndrome, Bell's palsy, amyotrophic lateral sclerosis, myoclonus, spina bifida, and poliomyelitis. Alzheimer's disease is perhaps the most important of the degenerative disorders because of its frequency and its devastating nature. It is the most common cause of dementia in the elderly. Alzheimer's results from neuronal cell death and disappearance in the cerebral cortex, causing marked atrophy of the brain. Initially, patients have problems with short-term memory, and this usually progresses to problems with thought and intellect. Patients also develop a shuffling gait and have stiffness of body muscles. As the disease progresses, the patient develops aphasia and psychiatric problems. In its final stages, the patient may become virtually decorticate, losing all ability to think, speak, and move. Muscular dystrophy (MD) actually refers to a group of genetic diseases characterized by progressive muscle weakness and degeneration of skeletal muscle fibers. The heart and other involuntary muscles are affected in some types of MD. The most common form is Duchenne's MD. Some forms begin in childhood whereas others do not appear until midlife. Prognosis depends on the type and individual progression of the disorder. Multiple sclerosis (MS) is another common and potentially devastating degenerative disorder. It involves inflammation of certain nerve cells followed by demyelination (loss of the fatty insulation surrounding nerve fibers in the CNS). Prevalence in Canada is approximately 50 000 persons. Most are women who first developed symptoms between ages 20–40 years. The pathophysiology of MS involves autoimmune attack against myelin. Signs and symptoms include weakness of one or more limbs, sensory loss, paresthesias, and changes in vision. Symptoms may wax and wane over years, and they may range from mild to severe. Severe cases leave the patient so debilitated she may not be able to care for herself.

The dystonias are characterized by muscle contractions that cause twisting, repetitive movements, abnormal postures, or freezing in the middle of an action. Early symptoms include deterioration in handwriting, foot cramps, or tendency of one foot to drag after walking or running. In some cases, symptoms become more noticeable and widespread over time. In other individuals, there is little or no progression over time. Parkinson's disease is a motor system disorder also called a "shaking palsy." Parkinson's is characterized chemically by a deficiency of dopamine in the CNS, and treatment is generally aimed at increasing levels in the brain. Parkinson's is common, and you will see it. Roughly 100 000 Canadians are affected, with many new cases reported annually. It affects men and women equally and has an average age at onset of 60 years. It usually does not develop in persons under 40. Parkinson's is chronic and progressive, and its signs fall into four categories: tremor (which usually begins in the hand and may progress to involve the arm, a foot, or the jaw), rigidity (resistance to movement among muscles in opposing pairs), bradykinesia (slowing or loss of normal, spontaneous movement), and postural instability (with development of a forward or backward lean, stooped posture, or tendency to fall easily).

Central pain syndrome results from damage or injury to the brain, brainstem, or spinal cord, and it is marked by intense, steady pain that may be described as burning, aching, tingling, or "pins and needles." It occurs in patients who, at some point in the past, have had strokes, multiple sclerosis, limb amputation, or spinal cord injury. Pain medications generally do not provide relief, and patients often rely on sedatives or other means of keeping the CNS free from stress. One example is trigeminal neuralgia, which is caused by abnormal impulse conduction along the trigeminal nerve (cranial nerve V). It often has brief episodes of intense facial pain. The fear of a possible attack may be debilitating. Medications including carbamazepine (Tegretol) may be helpful, and surgery may be indicated for select cases.

Bell's palsy is the most common form of facial paralysis, affecting roughly 6 000 Canadians yearly. It results from inflammation of the facial nerve (cranial nerve VII) and is marked by one-sided facial paralysis, inability to close the eye on the affected side, pain, tearing of that eye, drooling, hypersensitivity to sound, and impaired taste. Multiple causes exist, among them head trauma, herpes simplex virus, and Lyme disease. Treatment is usually aimed at protecting the eye. Corticosteroids may be used for inflammation when pain is severe. Most patients recover within 3 months. Amyotrophic lateral sclerosis (ALS, or Lou Gehrig's disease) affects 1 500-2 000 Canadians with 2-3 deaths a day due to it. ALS involves progressive degeneration of the nerve cells that control voluntary movement. It is marked by weakness, loss of motor control, difficulty speaking, and cramping. Eventually a weakened diaphragm and intercostal muscles lead to breathing problems. There is currently no effective therapy and no cure, and prognosis continues to be poor, with death within 3–5 years of diagnosis (often as a result of pulmonary infection). Myoclonus refers to temporary involuntary twitching or spasm of a muscle or muscle group. It is generally considered not a disorder, but a symptom. It occurs with a variety of disorders including multiple sclerosis, Parkinson's, and Alzheimer's. Pathologic myoclonus may limit a person's ability to eat, walk, and talk. Treatment consists of medication that reduces symptoms, often antiepileptic drugs such as clonazepam, phenytoin, and sodium valproate.

Spina bifida (SB) is a congenital neural defect due to failure of one or more fetal vertebrae to close properly during development, leaving a portion of the spinal cord unprotected. Long-term effects include impairment in physical mobility, and most individuals have some form of learning disability. The three most common types are myelomeningocele, the most severe form, in which the spinal cord and meninges protrude from the opening in the spine, meningocele, in which the meninges only protrude through the spinal opening, and SB occulta, the mildest form, in which one or more vertebrae are malformed and covered only by a layer of skin. Treatment includes surgery, medication, and physiotherapy appropriate for the extent of deformity. Poliomyelitis (polio) is an infectious disease that sometimes results in permanent paralysis. The acute disease is marked by fatigue, headache, fever, vomiting, stiffness of the neck, and pain in the hands and feet. New cases in the North America are rare due to routine childhood vaccination. However, thousands of pre-vaccine polio survivors are alive today and you may see them as patients. Many of these individuals require supportive care.

Assessment of any of the degenerative disorders requires your personal impressions and history taking to determine the chief complaint. The patient may be having a flare-up of a problem or they may have an unrelated complaint. In all cases, make your assessment, intervene for any life-threatening problems, and learn exactly what prompted a call for EMS. Management relies on treating the chief complaint. You don't want to overlook the underlying condition, but you also don't want it to get in the way of recognizing and treating a more immediately serious problem. While providing care, you should keep in mind these general aspects of patients who have a disorder in this group: Mobility may be affected, and the patient may need assistance to move. Communication may be difficult. Take the time to ensure open communication with patient, family, caregivers, or bystanders. Respiratory compromise may be a concern, particularly in exacerbations of ALS or some other conditions. Any breathing problem is a priority. Last, recognize the anxiety attendant with these disorders. Approach the patient and family with compassion. The following specific guidelines may be useful for a number of patients: Determine blood glucose; this may help you detect whether altered mental status is due to hypoglycemia. Establish an IV with normal saline or lactated Ringer's at a keep-vein-open rate. Monitor cardiac rhythm during transport.

5. Describe and differentiate the major types of seizures pp. 590-591

Seizures can be clinically grouped as generalized or partial on a pathophysiologic basis. Generalized seizures begin with an electrical discharge in a small part of the brain but the abnormal activity spreads to involve the entire cerebral cortex. In contrast, partial seizures may remain confined to a small area, causing localized malfunction, or they may spread and become secondarily generalized seizures.

Generalized seizures include tonic-clonic (also commonly called grand mal) and absence seizures. A tonic-clonic seizure is a generalized motor seizure that produces a temporary loss of consciousness. Usually, it includes a tonic phase (in which muscle tone is increased) and a clonic phase (in which muscles in the extremities jerk rhythmically). In some cases, temporary paralysis of the intercostal muscles causes an interruption in breathing and cyanosis may become evident. When respirations resume, you may see copious amounts of frothy oral secretions. Incontinence is also common during a seizure, and you may note agitation or confusion, drowsiness, or even coma following a seizure, depending on the norm for that patient. Absence seizures present very differently. They are characterized by a sudden onset of a brief (typically 10- to 30-second) loss of consciousness or awareness. Loss of consciousness may be so brief that the casual observer misses it altogether. These idiopathic seizures of childhood rarely occur after age 20 years. Note that absence seizures may not respond to your normal treatment modalities.

Pseudoseizures, also called hysterical seizures, are not true electrical seizures. Rather, they represent psychiatric phenomena. The patient typically presents with sharp, bizarre movements that may be interrupted with a terse command such as "Stop it!"

Partial seizures may be either simple or complex. Simple seizures involve local motor, sensory, or autonomic dysfunction in one area of the body; there is no loss of consciousness. You should remember, however, that they may spread in area of involvement and progress to a generalized, tonic-clonic seizure. Complex seizures, which usually originate in the temporal lobe, are often characterized by an aura and focal findings such as alterations in mental status or mood. Patients in the midst of such a seizure may appear intoxicated or mentally unstable: They may be confused, stagger, have purposeless movements, or show sudden personality changes. These seizures typically last 1–2 minutes, and the patient will slowly come back to baseline after that period.

6. Describe the phases of a generalized seizure. p. 590

Although patients are individuals with their own seizure patterns, many tonic-clonic seizures progress through seven phases: (1) aura, a subjective sensation that serves as a warning to those patients who experience it, (2) loss of consciousness, during the aura sensation, if there is one, (3) tonic phase, (4) hypertonic phase, during which you will see extreme muscular rigidity, including hyperextension of the back, (5) clonic phase of muscle spasms (often including the jaws) marked by rhythmic movements, (6) post-seizure, during which the patient is in a coma, and (7) postictal, during which the patient awakens.

7. Define the following:

The degenerative neurological diseases are discussed in some detail in objective 4j above, and you may wish to check that section for review on any or all of these disorders.

a. Muscular dystrophy p. 599
Muscular dystrophy (MD) is actually a group of genetic diseases characterized by progressive muscle weakness and degeneration of the skeletal or voluntary muscle fibers.

b.   Multiple sclerosis   p. 599
Multiple sclerosis (MS) is a disease that involves inflammation of certain nerve cells followed by demyelination; the destruction of the insulating myelin sheath is due to autoimmune activity.

c.   Dystonia   p. 599
The dystonias are a group of disorders characterized by muscle contractions that cause twisting and repetitive movements, abnormal posturing, or freezing in the middle of an action.

d.   Parkinson's disease   pp. 599-600
Parkinson's disease is a chronic and progressive disorder of the motor system within the CNS and is characterized by tremor, rigidity, bradykinesia, and postural instability.

e.   Trigeminal neuralgia   p. 600
Trigeminal neuralgia is due to abnormal conduction of impulses along the trigeminal nerve (cranial nerve V). The condition is an example of a central pain syndrome.

f.   Bell's palsy   p. 600
Bell's palsy, the most common form of facial paralysis, is a one-sided phenomenon with unknown cause, marked by inability to close the eye, pain, tearing of the eye, drooling, hypersensitivity to sound, and impairment of taste.

g.   Amyotrophic lateral sclerosis   p. 601
Amyotrophic lateral sclerosis (ALS), or Lou Gehrig's disease, is a progressive degenerative condition of specific nerve cells that control voluntary movement; it is marked by weakness, loss of motor control, difficulty speaking, and cramping.

h.   Peripheral neuropathy   pp. 571-572
Peripheral neuropathy is not considered a degenerative neurological condition; rather, it is a descriptive term that includes any malfunction or damage of the peripheral nerves. Results may include muscle weakness, loss of sensation, impaired reflexes, and malfunction of internal organs. Diabetes is one of the major causes of peripheral neuropathy involving multiple nerves (also called a polyneuropathy).

i.   Myoclonus   p. 601
Myoclonus is a temporary, involuntary twitching or spasm of a muscle or group of muscles. It is actually a symptom rather than a disorder. A very benign example of myoclonus is hiccups. Pathological myoclonus may be part of disorders including Alzheimer's, Parkinson's, and multiple sclerosis.

j.   Spina bifida   p. 601
Spina bifida (SB) is a congenital neural defect that results from failure of one or more vertebrae to close properly during fetal development. The defect may range from the asymptomatic (vertebral malformation covered by skin) to the severe (protrusion of spinal cord and meninges through an opening in the spine).

k.   Poliomyelitis   pp. 601
Poliomyelitis (polio) is a viral infectious disease characterized by inflammation of the CNS, which sometimes results in permanent paralysis.

8.   Define and discuss the pathophysiology, assessment findings, and management for nontraumatic spinal injury, including:

a.   Low back pain   pp. 602-603
Low back pain, defined as pain felt between the lower rib cage and the gluteal muscles, often radiating to the thighs, is an extremely common complaint but only occasionally the reason for an EMS call. Men and women are equally affected, but you should keep in mind that back pain in women over 60 years may represent the first sign of osteoporosis, an important medical condition. Vertebral fractures from causes other than osteoporosis are also possible causes. Other causes of low back pain include sciatica, which is reflected as severe pain along the path of the sciatic nerve down the back of the thigh and inner leg. Sciatica may be due to compression or trauma to the sciatic nerve or its roots, perhaps from a herniated intervertebral disk or an osteoarthritic

lumbosacral vertebral bone. Sciatica may also be due to inflammation of the nerve secondary to metabolic, toxic, or infectious causes. Pain at the level of L-3, L-4, L-5, and S-1 may be due to inflammation of interspinous bursae. External to the spine are other causes of low back pain: inflammation or sprain of muscles and ligaments that attach to the spine. Most low back pain, though, is found to be idiopathic.

Assessment of back pain is based on chief complaint, history, and physical exam. When the complaint is low back pain, a precise diagnosis is likely to be difficult. Preliminary diagnosis may focus on occupational risk from repetitive lifting or exposure to machinery vibrations. Listen for clues in the history about the nature and timing of the pain and whether the current complaint is acute pain or exacerbation of a chronic condition. Your priorities in the field are to determine whether pain is due to a life-threatening or non-life-threatening condition. Note: The presence of any identifiable neurological deficit may point to a serious underlying cause, as may a gradual onset of pain consistent with degenerative disk disease or tumor growth. The location of the injury may be revealed on exam by a limited range of motion in the lumbar spine, point tenderness on palpation, alterations in sensation, pain, and temperature at a localized point, or pain or paresthesia below a point of injury. Always keep in mind that you are unlikely to be able to determine the cause of the pain in the field. Your primary goal is to look for signs of life-threatening problems and to gather historical and exam information that will be useful to the receiving physician. You will also need to decide, perhaps after consultation with medical direction, whether immobilization (and, if so, to what degree) is necessary during transport.

If there are no clear life-threatening problems requiring intervention, management is primarily aimed at minimizing pain and immobilizing as per local protocol. If there is no historical reason to suspect injury in the past or an underlying condition such as osteoporosis (which makes patients vulnerable to pathologic fracture), C-spine immobilization may still be recommended as a comfort measure during transport. Also remember that some patients will require parenteral analgesia and diazepam before they can lie on a stretcher. Consult medical direction if you feel your patient might fit into this category. Last, remember to provide ongoing assessment en route with special attention to the ABCs, vitals, and the possible presence or development of motor or sensory deficits that might indicate a critical condition capable of compromising ventilatory efforts.

b.   Herniated intervertebral disk   p. 603

Intervertebral disks may rupture due to injury or due to degeneration associated with aging. Degenerative disk disease is most common in patients over 50 years of age. A herniated disk occurs when the gelatinous center of the disk extrudes through a tear in the tough outer capsule, and the resulting pain is due to pressure on the spinal cord or to muscle spasm at the site. The disks themselves are not innervated. Non-injury-related herniation may also be caused by improper lifting. Men aged 30 to 50 years are more prone to herniated disks than are women. Herniation is most common at levels L-4, L-5, and S-1, but it also may occur at C-5, C-6, and C-7. Assessment and management are discussed under low back pain in objective 8a.

c.   Spinal cord tumors   p. 604

A cyst or tumor along the spine or intruding into the spinal canal may cause pain by pressing on the spinal cord, causing degenerative changes in bone, or interrupting blood supply. The specific manifestations depend on location and type of tumor or cyst. Assessment and management are discussed under low back pain in objective 8a.

9. Differentiate between neurologic emergencies based on assessment findings. pp. 572-581

Because many signs and symptoms of neurologic dysfunction are subtle, you should use the observations made during scene size-up and formation of general impressions to look for evidence suggesting focus on the neurological system. Environmental clues may include medical equipment, medication bottles, Medic-Alert identification, alcohol bottles, etc. Note, for instance, if the patient is conscious, and, if so, is he confused or lucid? Is his posture or gait normal? Speech can give many clues, particularly if either the patient or a bystander can tell you if the speech you hear is normal for the patient. Skin color, temperature, and moisture are valuable, as is any evidence of facial drooping or muscle spasm. Mental status can then be quickly ascertained through the AVPU method.

Assessment of higher cerebral functioning includes assessment of emotional status. Try to evaluate the patient's affect, thought patterns, perceptions, judgments, and memory and attention. ANY alteration from the patient's normal mental status or mood is considered significant and warrants further assessment. After that level of assessment is done, evaluate for the ABCs, including respiration pattern, effort of breathing, heart rate, rhythm, and ECG pattern. An unresponsive patient can be evaluated further with use of the Glasgow Coma Scale. Be aware that a midlevel GCS score (such as 5, 6, or 7) that drops on reevaluation has grim implications.

Scene size-up and initial history will usually make clear whether trauma is involved or not. Regardless of whether trauma is a factor, try to get information on the presence or severity of medical conditions that are risk factors for neurologic conditions, hypertension, heart disease, diabetes, atherosclerosis, as well as any chronic neurologic conditions such as epilepsy. In addition, history should try to establish whether current complaint is acute, an exacerbation of a chronic problem, or a chronic state.

Physical exam of a patient with a neurologic emergency includes the standard head-to-toe exam as well as a more detailed neurological evaluation. Look closely at the patient's face. The ability to smile, frown, or wrinkle the forehead gives information about the status of the facial nerve. Although slight pupillary asymmetry is normal, abnormal pupils can be an early indicator of increasing intracranial pressure. If both pupils are dilated and don't react to light, suspect brainstem injury or serious anoxia. If the pupils are dilated but still react, injury may be reversible. Most of all, remember that any patient with altered mental status and a unilaterally dilated pupil is in the "immediate transport" category. When you check the pupils, look for contact lenses. If present, they should be removed, placed in their container or saline solution, and transported with the patient.

Respiratory derangements are common with CNS illness or injury. Five abnormal breathing patterns may be commonly observed in this setting: Cheyne-Stokes respiration is a pattern marked by apnea lasting 10–60 seconds followed by gradually increasing depth and frequency of respiration. It can be seen with brain damage due to trauma or cerebral hemorrhage and with chronic hypoxia. Kussmaul's respirations are deep, rapid breaths caused by severe metabolic or CNS problems. Central neurogenic hyperventilation is caused by a lesion in the CNS and is marked by rapid, deep, noisy respirations. Ataxic respirations are poor breaths due to CNS damage causing ineffective thoracic muscular coordination. Apneustic respiration is breathing marked by prolonged inspiration unrelieved by expiration attempts and it is due to damage in the upper pons. Always remember that CO_2 has a critical effect on cerebral vessels: Increased levels cause vascular dilation, whereas low levels cause vasoconstriction. This is the basis for controlled hyperventilation in settings where some degree of vasoconstriction might minimize brain swelling.

Cardiovascular status is always important. Even if a primary cardiovascular problem is not present, CNS events are likely to cause changes to the cardiovascular system. In particular, assess heart rate, ECG rhythm, bruits over the carotid arteries, and possible presence of jugular venous distension, a sign of ineffective cardiac pumping. You should be aware that vital signs and changes in them are crucial in following the course of a neurological emergency. Note Cushing's reflex, a grouping of four characteristics in vital signs that signals increased intracranial pressure: increased blood pressure, decreased pulse, decreased respirations, and increased temperature. The earliest signs are the decrease in pulse rate and an increase in blood pressure and temperature.

The exam for neurologic system status is covered in detail on text pages 577-579. Note that the components of the exam include sensorimotor evaluation (if posture is abnormal, consider whether it might be decorticate or decerebrate in nature), motor system status, and cranial nerve status.

Last, be particularly aware with elderly patients and with patients with a chronic neurological condition (such as the degenerative disorders) that it is vital to know the patient's baseline values in all areas before you can put your current findings into the context of acute changes or not. Interviewing family members or caregivers may be very helpful.

10. Given several preprogrammed nontraumatic neurological emergency patients, provide the appropriate assessment, management, and transport.   pp. 572-605

The priorities for someone who is unconscious or clearly in urgent distress with neurologic difficulties are the same as for a patient who is affected by a potentially life-threatening emergency of another origin: Ensure adequate airway, breathing (ventilation), and circulation. This is particularly important for someone whose emergency may be originating in, or affecting, the CNS: The brain requires a constant supply of oxygen, glucose, and vitamins. After 10–20 seconds without blood flow, unconsciousness will occur. Significant deprivation of oxygen (anoxia) or glucose (hypoglycemia) can cause seizures or coma. You should always give high-flow oxygen to a patient with a neurologic emergency and give glucose to any one found to be hypoglycemic.

Neurologic injuries and illnesses usually require treatment as soon as possible to prevent progressive damage. In the case of thromboembolic stroke, this may be particularly true because therapies are coming into use that can minimize the region of brain tissue infarcted in the stroke or even prevent the progression of tissue ischemia to tissue infarction. Patients who show altered mental status and/or any clear neurologic impairment (pupillary dilation, especially unilateral, facial drooping, slurred speech, abnormal posturing—if these appear to be new or progressing findings) that may suggest TIA or stroke need immediate intervention and transport. Management of seizures and syncope often mandates prompt intervention and care, as well.

You will see many calls for complaints such as low back pain and headache. These conditions may be relatively minor or the signal of a serious underlying disorder. History suggesting new onset, severe pain, or clearly progressive pain indicates the need for aggressive assessment and management, whereas other patients with chronic pain of either origin also require full assessment but may need only supportive care.

Patients with known CNS neoplasms or degenerative neurological conditions may present with a complaint related to their underlying disease or a problem of completely different origin. Be aware that these persons are always more vulnerable to oxygen or glucose deprivation from another source (for example, cardiac disease or diabetes, respectively); in addition, remember that some patients will have airways vulnerable to compromise secondary to muscle paralysis or other neurologic causes.

CONTENT SELF-EVALUATION

Multiple Choice

1. The two mechanisms that generally cause altered mental status are:
   A. occlusive and hemorrhagic strokes.
   B. systemic diseases and drugs or toxic agents.
   C. structural lesions and toxic-metabolic states.
   D. head trauma and CNS disease.
   E. toxic-metabolic states and brain tumors.

2. If the patient is able to smile, frown, and wrinkle forehead muscles, which cranial nerve is intact?
   A. I   D. XI
   B. V   E. XII
   C. VII

3. The Glasgow Coma Scale assesses eye opening, verbal response, and motor response. Which correlation of score and likely outcome is incorrect?
   A. score or 3 or 4, 10% favorable outcome
   B. score of 8 or higher, 94% favorable outcome
   C. score of 5–7 that increases to 8 or higher, 80% favorable outcome
   D. score of 5–7, 50% favorable outcome in adults and 90% in children
   E. score of 5–7 that decreases by one point, 10% favorable outcome

4. Three interventions that may be indicated in treatment of a patient with altered mental status of unknown cause are:
   A. hyperventilation, 50% dextrose, and naloxone.
   B. mannitol (Osmotrol), 50% dextrose, and naloxone.
   C. 50% dextrose, thiamine, and naloxone.
   D. mannitol (Osmotrol), hyperventilation, and 50% dextrose.
   E. mannitol (Osmotrol), thiamine, and naloxone.

5. A condition characterized by a loss of memory and disorientation and often associated with chronic alcoholism and a diet deficient in thiamine is:
   A. Korsakoff's psychosis.
   B. Wernicke's syndrome.
   C. Lein's psychosis.
   D. Esselstyne's syndrome.
   E. Makynen seizure.

6. The type of stroke caused by a ruptures cerebral artery is a(n) _____ stroke.
   A. occlusive
   B. embolic
   C. thrombotic
   D. hemorrhagic
   E. aneural

7. If a stroke patient is apneic or breathing inadequately, controlled positive-pressure hyperoxygenation may be beneficial because it:
   A. causes cerebral vasoconstriction, decreasing cerebral swelling.
   B. causes a reflex increase in respiration rate.
   C. eliminates excess CO_2 levels.
   D. increases CO_2 levels toward normal range.
   E. increases the ability of brain cells to take up any available oxygen.

8. Among the many types of epileptic seizures, the most likely to require intervention on your part are:
   A. absence seizures.
   B. tonic-clonic seizures.
   C. petit mal seizures.
   D. simple partial seizures.
   E. complex partial seizures.

9. The phase of a seizure in which a patient experiences alternating contraction and relaxation of the muscles is the _____ phase.
   A. tonic
   B. clonic
   C. aural
   D. hypertonic
   E. postictal

10. All of the following are characteristics of a complex partial seizure EXCEPT:
    A. auditory hallucinations.
    B. a sense of deja vu.
    C. localized tonic-clonic movement of one extremity.
    D. unusual odors.
    E. strange tastes.

11. The two most common causes of headache are:
    A. vascular and organic.
    B. vascular and neurogenic.
    C. tension and vascular.
    D. tension and organic.
    E. tension and neurogenic.

12. A disease that is chronic and is characterized by progressive motor disorder with tremor, rigidity, bradykinesia, and postural instability is:

    A. Alzheimer's.
    B. Reed-Sternberg's.
    C. Parkinson's.
    D. Lou Gehrig's.
    E. Bell's palsy.

13. Which one of the following is NOT a degenerative neurological disorder?
    A. multiple sclerosis (MS)
    B. Parkinson's disease
    C. Bell's palsy
    D. muscular dystrophy
    E. vertebral disk disease

14. Examples of structural lesions capable of producing alterations in mental status include all BUT which of the following:

A. neoplasm
B. parasites
C. trauma
D. degenerative disease
E. toxic-metabolic states

15. Which of the following is considered a toxic-metabolic state with the ability of altering mental status and progressing to coma?

A. diabetic ketoacidosis
B. thiamine dificiency
C. organophosphate poisoning
D. hepatic failure
E. all of the above

16. Which of the following is an example of polyneuropathy?

A. ALS
B. ataxia
C. athromatorus simplex
D. Guillian Barre syndrome
E. degenerative neurological disorder

17. Which cranial nerves influence the "cardinal rules of gaze"?

A. II, III, and VI
B. III, IV, and VI
C. IV, V, and VI
D. IV, V, VI, and VII
E. II and III

18. Which of the following respiratory patterns is characterized by prolonged inspiration unrelieved by expiration attempts?

A. ataxic respirations
B. Kussmaul's respirations
C. Cheyne-Stokes respiration
D. apneustic respiration
E. central neurogenic hyperventilation

19. A patient with decorticate posturing will have:

A. arms and legs extended
B. arms and legs flexed
C. one arm flexed and one arm extended
D. arms flexed, legs extended
E. arms extended, legs flexed

20. During your assessment of a 20-year-old male involved in a motor vehicle collision you observe that he opens his eyes to pain, is mumbling and moves his hands away when he is palpated. His GCS is:

A. 6.
B. 7.
C. 11.
D. 8.
E. 9.

21. Increased intracranial pressure is characterized by which of the following changes in vital signs, referred to as Cushing's reflex.

A. increased temperature, decreased pulse, increased respirations and increased BP
B. increased BP, decreased respirations, decreased pulse and increased temperature
C. increased BP, increased pulse, decreased respirations and increased temperature
D. decreased respirations, decreased temperature, increased pulse and increased BP
E. increased pulse, decreased BP, decreased respirations and increased temperature

22. Which of the following can cause stiffness of extremities?

A. tranquilizers
B. hyperventilation
C. intracranial hemorrhage
D. meningitis
E. all of the above

23. Syncope caused by unknown reasons can be classified as:
  A.   noncardiovascular.
  B.   idiopathic.
  C.   localized .
  D.   cardiovascular.
  E.   hypoxic.

24. Respiratory arrest, increased intracranial pressure, necrosis of the cardiac muscle, metabolic and respiratory acidosis can be adverse results of:
  A.   myoclonus   .   D.   CVA.
  B.   dystonias   .   E.   status epilepticus.
  C.   hypoglycemia.

25. Bell's Palsy is the most common form of facial paralysis, resulting in an inflammatory reaction of which cranial nerve?
  A.   VII   .   D.   X
  B.   VI   E.   IV
  C.   V

True/False

26. Peripheral neuropathy can affect muscle activity, sensation, and reflexes, but not internal organ function.
  A.   True
  B.   False

27. If a patient with suspected syncope does not regain consciousness within a few moments, the event is NOT syncope, but something more serious.
  A.   True
  B.   False

28. The most common cause of a TIA is carotid artery disease.
  A.   True
  B.   False

29. During the hypertonic phase of a seizure the patient experiences extreme muscular rigidity and hyperflexion of the back..
  A.   True
  B.   False

30. Trigeminal neuralgia or tic douloureux is primarily a psychosomatic disorder.
  A.   True
  B.   False

31. A blood glucose level should be checked on all patients experiencing syncope regardless of their medical history.
  A.   True
  B.   False

32. Myelomeningocele, meningocele, and occulta are the three most common types of spina bifida.
  A.   True
  B.   False

33. A seizing patient's airway should be maintained by placing a padded tongue blade between their teeth.
  A.   True
  B.   False

_____ **34.** Herniated discs in the back commonly occur at T-2, T-3, and L-1.
     A. True
     B. False

_____ **35.** Normal ventilatory mechanisms of a seizing patient are seriously impaired and air exchange is generally ineffective.
     A. True
     B. False

Matching

Write the letter of the term in the space provided next to the appropriate description.

A.	dystonias	**F.**	spina bifida
B.	GCS	**G.**	transient ischemic attack
C.	myoclonus	**H.**	neoplasm
D.	decorticate posture	**I.**	clonic phase
E.	brain abscess	**J.**	tonic phase

_____ **36.** a new or abnormal formation

_____ **37.** temporary, involuntary twitching or spasm of a muscle

_____ **38.** phase of a seizure characterized by alternating contraction and relaxation of muscles

_____ **39.** characterized posture associated with a lesion at or above the upper brainstem

_____ **40.** a group of disorders characterized by muscle contractions that cause twisting and repetitive movements

_____ **41.** a collection of pus localized in the area of the brain

_____ **42.** temporary interruption of blood supply to the brain

_____ **43.** a neural defect effecting the fetal vertebrae closure

_____ **44.** phase of a seizure characterized by tension or contraction of muscles

_____ **45.** Glascow Coma Scale

Chapter 30

Endocrinology

Review of Chapter Objectives

After reading this chapter, you should be able to:

1. Describe the incidence, morbidity, and mortality of endocrinologic emergencies.
   pp. 608-609, 611-612, 616-617

Many people have endocrine disorders that involve excessive or deficient hormone production or function. The incidence of such disorders is widely variable. Some disorders are readily controlled by hormone replacement therapy; others are more complex and thus more difficult to manage. The most common of all of the endocrine disorders is diabetes mellitus, affecting about 1.2-1.4 million Canadians.

2. Identify the risk factors that predispose a person to endocrinologic disease.
   pp. 611, 616-617, 619, 620

Diabetes mellitus is the most commonly encountered endocrine disorder. Among the predisposing factors that have been identified for this condition are heredity, viral infection, autoimmune antibodies, and obesity.

Heredity is thought to be the key factor in the predisposition for Graves' disease, although autoimmune antibodies are known to trigger the excess production of thyroid hormone. Severe physiologic stress has been found to be a common triggering factor for thyrotoxicosis (thyroid storm). On the other hand, hypothyroidism or myxedema may be either congenital or acquired.
The risk of adrenal gland disorders is increased by the administration of glucocorticoids or may be a consequence of abnormalities of the anterior pituitary gland or the adrenal cortex. Approximately half of all adrenal gland disorders are due to autoimmune disorders or may be aggravated by acute physiologic stress.

3. Discuss the anatomy and physiology of the endocrinologic diseases. (see Chapter 12)

There are eight major structures associated with the endocrine system located throughout the body: the hypothalamus, pituitary gland, thyroid gland, parathyroid glands, thymus, pancreas, adrenal glands, and gonads. The pineal gland is also part of the endocrine system.
The hypothalamus, located deep within the cerebrum of the brain, is the junction between the endocrine system and the central nervous system. About the size of a pea, the pituitary gland is located adjacent to the hypothalamus within the cerebrum. The pineal gland is also located adjacent to the hypothalamus. The double-lobed thyroid gland is located in the neck anterior to and just below the cartilage of the larynx. The parathyroid glands are very small and are found on the posterior lateral surface of the thyroid gland. The thymus is located in the mediastinum just behind the sternum. The pancreas is located in the upper abdomen behind the stomach and between the duodenum and the spleen. The adrenal glands are somewhat triangular in shape and are located on the superior surface of the kidneys. Gonads can be found in the lower pelvis in women, with each ovary resembling an almond in size and shape. In men, the gonads are located in the scrotum.

The endocrine system is closely linked to the nervous system and plays a critical role in our ability to maintain life by regulating many bodily functions through chemical substances called hormones. The endocrine system is made up of ductless glands, which manufacture and secrete hormones that act in adjacent tissues or travel via the bloodstream to target organs or other endocrine glands to produce specific or generalized effects. Hormones regulate metabolic activity, growth and development, as well as mediate chemical reactions, maintain homeostatic balance, and initiate our adaptive response to stress.

4. Discuss the pathophysiology, assessment findings, need for rapid intervention and transport, and management of endocrinologic emergencies.   pp. 608-621

As you review the anatomy and physiology of the endocrine system, it is clearly evident that the endocrine system is closely linked to the nervous system and controls a variety of physiologic processes that are essential for survival. The causes of endocrine disorders are variable and include heredity, congenital anomalies, viral infection, and autoimmune disease processes. The most commonly encountered endocrine emergencies in the prehospital setting are related to diabetes mellitus and disorders of the thyroid or adrenal glands. You should review the sections of the text which clarify the differences in clinical presentation, assessment, and management of these disorders.

5. Describe osmotic diuresis and its relationship to diabetes mellitus. p. 611

Osmosis is the tendency for water molecules to migrate across a semi-permeable membrane so that the concentrations of particles approach equivalence on both sides. When blood glucose levels rise above 180 mg/dL, no more glucose can be reabsorbed through the renal tubules and glucose begins to be lost (or "spill") into the urine. This causes the osmotic pressure, or concentration of particulates, to rise inside the kidney tubule to a level higher than that of the blood. Water follows glucose into the urine to cause a marked water loss termed osmotic diuresis that is the basis for the polyuria (excessive urination) associated with untreated diabetes.

6. Describe the pathophysiology of adult and juvenile onset diabetes mellitus. pp. 611-612

Juvenile onset or Type I diabetes mellitus is a serious disease characterized by very low production of insulin by the beta cells of the pancreas. In many cases, there is no insulin being produced. It is called juvenile onset diabetes because of the average age of the patient at the time of diagnosis. Type I diabetes is also known as insulin-dependent diabetes because patients require regular injections of insulin to control their disease. Heredity appears to be an important factor in determining which people will develop Type I diabetes. The cause of Type I diabetes is not clear. Other factors attributed to triggering juvenile onset diabetes are viral infection, an autoimmune response, or genetically determined premature deterioration of beta cells. The immediate cause of Type I diabetes is the destruction of pancreatic beta cells.

Type II diabetes mellitus, also known as non-insulin-dependent diabetes, is responsible for almost 90 percent of all cases of diabetes. Type II diabetes usually begins in later life and is often associated with obesity, so it is known as adult onset diabetes. Type II diabetes is associated with a moderate decline in insulin production accompanied by a marked decrease in the utilization of the insulin within the body. The cause is not clearly understood, although obesity is believed to play a role in its development. Increased weight, along with the increased size of fat cells, causes a relative deficiency in the number of insulin receptors, thus making the fat cells less responsive to insulin. Type II diabetes is usually managed through a combination of diet, exercise, and the administration of medications to reduce either blood glucose or enhance the efficiency of insulin. Occasionally insulin administration is required.

7. Differentiate between the pathophysiology of normal glucose metabolism and diabetic glucose metabolism.   pp. 609-611

Metabolism, which means "to change," is a term used to refer to all of the chemical and energy transformations within the body. Two kinds of change take place in the cell. One kind builds complex molecules from simple ones (anabolism), such as the synthesis of glycogen from glucose. The other kind breaks down complex molecules into simpler ones (catabolism), such as occurs with the breakdown of glucose into carbon dioxide, water, and energy (in the form of ATP). When materials are abundant after meals and the glucose is high, insulin enables cells to use glucose directly and to store energy as glycogen, protein, and fat. Insulin stimulates glucose pathways. In contrast, glucagon, the dominant hormone during periods of low blood glucose, stimulates catabolic pathways to produce usable energy from the body's stores.

The rate at which glucose can enter the cell is dependent upon insulin levels. Insulin combines with insulin receptors on the surface of the cell membrane, allowing glucose to enter the cell by increasing the permeability of the cell membrane. The rate at which glucose can be transported into the cells can be accelerated tenfold by insulin.

Sometimes the body cannot use glucose as its primary energy source, as is the case in patients with diabetes mellitus. Without insulin, the amount of glucose that can be transported into the cells is far too small to meet the body's energy demands. Without insulin, the glucose remains in the bloodstream, resulting in hyperglycemia. Carbohydrate depletion is also seen in other conditions, such as a high-fat, low-carbohydrate diet or starvation (which can be associated with some eating disorders). Under these conditions, the body slowly switches from glucose to fat as the primary energy source. Adipose cells break down fats into their component free fatty acids, and the blood concentration of these acids rises considerably.

Most of the fatty acids are used directly by the body's cells as an energy source. The liver takes in some, where the catabolism of fatty acids produces acetoacetic acid. When more acetoacetic acid is released by the liver than can be effectively utilized by body cells, it accumulates in the bloodstream along with two other closely related substances, acetone and b-hydroxybutyric acid. The three substances are collectively called ketone bodies. Their presence in excessive quantities is called ketosis.

8. Describe the mechanism of ketone body formation and its relationship to ketoacidosis. pp. 610, 612-614

When the body's carbohydrate stores begin to become depleted, small amounts of glucose can be formed by the breakdown of protein and fat through the process of gluconeogenesis. The byproducts of amino acid breakdown include carbon dioxide and water and the formation of urea. The breakdown of fat results in the formation of carbon dioxide, water, and ketone bodies.

The normal blood ketone level in humans is low because ketones are usually metabolized as rapidly as they are formed. If there are low levels of glucose stored in the cells, the ability of the body to oxidize the ketones is soon exceeded and ketones begin to build up in the bloodstream, resulting in a condition known as ketosis. This results in an increased amount of acid in the body fluids. The resulting metabolic acidosis is often severe and can be fatal.

9. Discuss the physiology of the excretion of potassium and ketone bodies by the kidneys. pp. 610-611

Whenever the flow rate of fluid inside the tubules of the kidney rises, as in osmotic diuresis, an increase in excretion of potassium occurs. This leads to the potential for significant hypokalemia and its effects, such as potentially life-threatening cardiac dysrhythmias. In ketotic states, ketone bodies are excreted through respiration and will also spill into the urine.

10. Describe the relationship of insulin to serum glucose levels. pp. 608-616

Insulin is a glucagon antagonist and lowers the blood glucose level by promoting energy storage. Insulin increases the rate at which various body cells take up glucose by changing the permeability of the cell membranes. These changes also make the cell more permeable to potassium, magnesium, and phosphate ions, as well as many amino acids. Because the liver rapidly breaks down insulin, the hormone must be secreted constantly.

Homeostasis of blood glucose is remarkably effective. In non-diabetics, when blood glucose is high, as after a meal, the beta cells of the pancreas release insulin. Insulin enables cells to use glucose directly as well as to store energy as glycogen, protein, and fat. If you were to draw a venous blood sample to measure fasting blood glucose levels, you'd find the level in healthy individuals is usually between 4.4-5.0 mmol/L blood. In the first 60–90 minutes after a meal the level will increase to approximately 6.6-7.7 mmom/L before dropping off to near-fasting levels as insulin is released to move the glucose from the bloodstream into the cells. Conversely, when blood glucose levels are low, the alpha cells of the pancreas release glucagon to raise the blood glucose level.

11. Describe the effects of decreased levels of insulin on the body.　　pp. 611-615

Insulin deficiency contributes to the development of hyperglycemia. Without insulin to facilitate the movement of large glucose molecules across cell membranes, the blood glucose level rises even as the intracellular level of glucose plummets. At the same time, the alpha cells of the pancreas release glucagon to increase blood glucose by stimulating the breakdown of glycogen, as well as stimulating the breakdown of body proteins and fats with subsequent chemical conversion to glucose (gluconeogenesis).

12. Describe the effects of increased serum glucose levels on the body.　pp. 615-616

With a rise in blood glucose levels, as is the case in Type I diabetes, the body's cells cannot take up circulating glucose. Glucose then spills into urine, leading to a large water loss, via osmotic diuresis, and significant dehydration. This can lead to significant loss of potassium and hypokalemia.

13. Discuss the pathophysiology, assessment findings, and management of the following endocrine emergencies:

a.　　nonketotic hyperosmolar coma　　pp. 612-613, 614-615
This condition is a complication of Type II diabetes due to inadequate insulin activity and is marked by high blood glucose, marked dehydration, and decreased mental function.

Development of the coma is slower than with ketoacidosis. Early signs include increased urination and thirst. Later signs may include orthostatic hypotension, dry skin, and tachycardia. This condition is difficult to distinguish from ketoacidosis in the field. Field management focuses on maintaining ABCs and fluid resuscitation.

b.　　diabetic ketoacidosis　　pp. 612-614
Diabetic ketoacidosis is a serious, potentially life-threatening complication of diabetes mellitus. It occurs when profound insulin deficiency is coupled with increased glucagon activity.

The onset is slow, lasting from 12 to 24 hours. In its early stages, the signs and symptoms include increased thirst, excessive hunger, urination, and malaise. Increased urination results from the osmotic diuresis accompanying glucose spillage into the urine. Intensified thirst is caused by the body's attempt to replace the fluids lost by increased urination. Nausea, vomiting, marked dehydration, tachycardia, and weakness characterize diabetic ketoacidosis. The skin is usually warm and dry. Coma is not uncommon. The breath may have a sweet or acetone-like character due to the increased ketones in the blood. Very deep, rapid respirations, called Kussmaul's respirations, also occur. Kussmaul's respirations represent the body's attempt to compensate for the metabolic acidosis produced by the ketones and organic acids present in the blood. It may be complicated by several electrolyte imbalances. The most significant is decreased potassium. Decreased potassium (hypokalemia) can lead to serious dysrhythmias or even death.

The approach used with the patient suffering from diabetic ketoacidosis is essentially the same as with any unconscious patient. You should first complete your initial assessment of airway, breathing, and circulation. You will then complete your focused history and physical exam. Pay particular attention to the presence of a Medic-Alert bracelet and/or insulin in the refrigerator. Also, obtain a history from bystanders. The fruity odor of ketones occasionally can be detected on the breath. If possible, complete the rapid test for blood glucose.

It is not uncommon for patients in ketoacidosis to have blood glucose levels well in excess of 16 mmol/L. The field management of such cases is focused on maintenance of ABCs and fluid resuscitation to counteract the patient's dehydration.

If the blood glucose level cannot be quickly determined, draw a red top tube of blood for analysis and start an IV of normal saline. Following this, administer 50 ml (25 grams) of 50 percent dextrose solution. This additional glucose load will not adversely affect the ketoacidotic patient because it is negligible compared to the total quantity present in the body. If the patient is alcoholic, consider administering 100 mg of thiamine. Transportation to an appropriate facility should be expedited.

c.   hypoglycemia   pp. 615-616

Hypoglycemia, or low blood glucose, is a potentially life-threatening medical emergency. Sometimes called insulin shock, it can occur if a patient accidentally or intentionally injects too much insulin, eats an inadequate amount of food after taking insulin, or has overexercised and burned up all available glucose. Untreated, the insulin will cause the blood glucose to drop to a very low level. The longer the period of hypoglycemia persists, the greater the risk that the brain cells will be permanently damaged or even killed.

The signs and symptoms of hypoglycemia are many and varied. An abnormal mental status is the most important and often the earliest sign. In the earliest stages of hypoglycemia, the patient may appear restless or impatient or complain of hunger. As the blood sugar falls lower, he or she may display inappropriate anger or display a variety of bizarre behaviors. Physical signs may include diaphoresis and tachycardia. If the blood sugar falls to a critically low level, the patient may sustain a hypoglycemic seizure or become comatose. In contrast to diabetic ketoacidosis, hypoglycemia can develop quickly. When encountering a patient behaving bizarrely, you should always consider hypoglycemia.

In suspected cases of hypoglycemia, perform the initial assessment quickly. Inspect the patient for a Medic-Alert bracelet. If possible, determine the blood glucose level. If the blood glucose level is noted to be less than 4.0 mmol/L, start an IV of normal saline. Next, administer 50–100 milliliters (25–50 grams) of 50 percent dextrose intravenously. If the patient is conscious and able to swallow, complete glucose administration with orange juice, sodas, or commercially available glucose pastes.

d.   hyperglycemia   pp. 614-615

Diabetes mellitus results from either inadequate amounts of circulating insulin or inadequate utilization of insulin. This means that there is an excess of blood glucose while there is an intracellular deficit. In diabetes, glucose builds up in the bloodstream, especially after meals. The blood glucose level rises higher and returns to normal more slowly in the diabetic than in the non-diabetic. An oral glucose tolerance test uses this phenomenon in the diagnosis of diabetes. The diabetic's inadequate insulin level and impaired glucose tolerance are partly due to the decreased entry of glucose into the cells, thus leaving more glucose in the bloodstream.

The second cause of hyperglycemia in the diabetic results from difficulties with the function of the liver. When blood glucose levels are high, insulin secretion is normally increased and the breakdown of glycogen is decreased. In the diabetic, however, insulin secretion is decreased, and the alpha cells secrete glucagon to stimulate glycogenolysis by the liver, thus raising the blood glucose level.

In Type I diabetes the decreased insulin secretion is accompanied by a steady accumulation of glucose in the blood. Hyperglycemia acts like an osmotic diuretic and glucose "spills over" into the urine (glycosuria) pulling large amounts of water with it (polyuria). The body's attempt to dilute the concentration of glucose in the bloodstream results in intracellular dehydration and stimulates thirst (polydipsia). As the cells become glucose-depleted, they begin to use proteins and fats as an energy source resulting in weight loss and the formation of harmful byproducts, such as ketones and organic free fatty acids. The body's response to this state of cellular starvation is to trigger hunger in the patient (polyphagia). If the acids and ketones continue to collect in the blood, severe metabolic acidosis occurs and coma ensues, resulting in serious brain damage or death.

Type II diabetes does not usually result in diabetic ketoacidosis. It can, however, develop into a life-threatening emergency termed hyperglycemic hyperosmolar nonketotic (HHNK) coma. In Type II diabetes, when blood glucose levels exceed 55 mmol/L, the high osmolality of the blood causes an osmotic diuresis and marked dehydration of body cells. However, sufficient insulin is produced to prevent the manufacture of ketones and the complications of metabolic acidosis. In this respect, the condition differs from diabetic ketoacidosis.

e.   thyrotoxicosis   pp. 616-617

Thyrotoxic crisis, more commonly known as "thyroid storm," is a life-threatening medical emergency which can be fatal within as little as 48 hours if not treated. It is usually associated with severe physiologic (trauma, infection, uncontrolled diabetes mellitus, etc.) or psychological stress. You will also encounter thyroid storm from an accidental or intentional overdose of thyroid hormone. Many patients with thyrotoxicosis have underlying Graves' disease (hyperthyroidism).

The signs and symptoms associated with thyroid storm reflect the patient's profound hypermetabolic state and increased adrenergic response. The patient may be hyperthermic and tachycardic (especially common are atrial tachydysrhythmias), with a high pulse pressure and dyspnea. Mental status changes range from agitation and restlessness to delirium and coma. Nausea, vomiting, and diarrhea are also often present. Death often follows heart failure and profound cardiovascular collapse.

Field management is focused on supportive care with oxygenation, ventilatory assistance, fluid resuscitation, and cardiac monitoring, along with expedited transport for definitive care to block the high circulating levels of thyroid hormones.

f.   myxedema   pp. 618-619

Inadequate levels of the thyroid hormones in adults produce hypothyroidism or myxedema, which results in a generalized decrease in metabolism. While it may occur in males or females of any age, it is most commonly seen among middle-aged females or as a consequence when surgery or radiation is used to treat hyperthyroidism.

This disorder tends to have a gradual onset, and the initial signs and symptoms tend to be quite subtle and include hoarse voice and slow speech, facial bloating, weakness, cold intolerance, lethargy, and fatigue as well as altered mental states, particularly depression. Additionally, the skin and hair are quite dry and coarse in texture. Patients with hypothyroidism are treated with replacement thyroid hormone, usually synthetic T_4 agents such as levothyroxine (Synthroid). Rarely do these patients require emergency treatment for their hypothyroidism unless it progresses to myxedema coma; however, you will encounter many patients who take thyroid replacement hormones.

Myxedema coma, a life-threatening complication of hypothyroidism, is not uncommon in colder climates but is unusual in warm ones. It is most often seen in older patients who have pulmonary or vascular disease. Other contributing factors include a history of thyroid disease, exposure to cold, infection, trauma, or drugs that suppress the central nervous system such as sedatives and hypnotics. The mortality rate associated with myxedema coma is high.

Myxedema coma usually has a gradual onset, with lethargy and depression that progresses to coma. Other signs and symptoms include extreme hypothermia, low amplitude bradycardia, carbon dioxide retention, and profound respiratory depression.

Emergency management of myxedema coma is focused on maintenance of the ABCs and, as always, careful monitoring of the patient's cardiac and oxygenation status; most patients will require intubation and ventilatory assistance. Active rewarming is contraindicated due to the risk of cardiac dysrhythmias and the potential to cause vasodilatation, which may contribute to cardiovascular collapse. Although it is appropriate to initiate intravenous access, care must be taken to limit fluids since fluid and electrolyte imbalance is common. Follow local protocols or contact medical direction for specific orders based on your patient's presentation.

g.   Cushing's syndrome   pp. 619-620

Chronic high levels of glucocorticoids result in the development of Cushing's syndrome or hyperadrenalism. Cushing's syndrome may occur as a result of long-term glucocorticoid (steroid) therapy, or by abnormalities of the adrenal glands, or by a pituitary tumor triggering excessive secretion of adrenocorticotropic hormone (ACTH), which stimulates the adrenals to produce excessive amounts of glucocorticoids.

Presenting signs and symptoms include: weight gain, particularly through the trunk of the body, face, and neck, with a typical "moon-faced" appearance and often a "buffalo hump" due to the fat deposits in these areas; skin changes, such as the thinning of the skin to an almost transparent appearance, a tendency to bruise easily, delayed healing from even minor wounds, and the development of facial hair among women; increased vascular sensitivity; hypertension; mood swings and memory impairment or decreased ability to concentrate.

Treatment involves removing the cause, such as the surgical removal of a tumor, or adjusting the dosage of glucocorticoids. While it is unlikely that you would encounter a patient with an acute hyperadrenal crisis, you are very likely to encounter patients who exhibit signs and symptoms of Cushing's syndrome. These patients have a higher incidence of cardiovascular disease, hypertension, and stroke than the general population and are prone to infection. When performing your assessment, be alert for the signs mentioned above which are associated with high glucocorticoid levels. Pay particular attention to skin preparation when starting intravenous lines, due to the fragility of these patients' skin and their susceptibility to infection. Your observations noted in your patient care report and relayed to the receiving hospital staff may contribute to the early diagnosis and treatment of this disorder, especially in those patients who do not have a primary care provider whom they see on a regular basis.

h.   adrenal insufficiency, or Addison's disease   p.620

Most commonly, adrenal insufficiency, or Addison's disease, is an idiopathic autoimmune disorder causing atrophy of the adrenal glands and resulting in the inadequate production of the adrenal hormones, such as cortisol, aldosterone, and androgens. Other causes include pituitary or hypothalamic dysfunction, adrenal hemorrhage, infections, such as tuberculosis, acquired immunodeficiency syndrome (AIDS), or sudden cessation of long-term or high-dose therapy with synthetic glucocorticoids.

Chronic adrenal insufficiency is characterized by progressive weakness, fatigue, decreased appetite, and weight loss. Hyperpigmentation of the skin and mucous membranes is one of the earliest signs. The hyperpigmentation tends to be most significant in sun-exposed areas, joints, and pressure points. Patients with Addison's disease are prone to hypotension, hypoglycemia, hyponatremia, and hyperkalemia. About half of the patients will have gastrointestinal problems such as nausea, vomiting, or diarrhea, which will exacerbate the electrolyte imbalances and increase the potential for cardiac dysrhythmias.

Acute adrenal insufficiency, known as Addisonian crisis, is a life-threatening medical emergency characterized by profound hypotension and shock, which can be rapidly fatal. It is most commonly seen in those patients with Addison's disease who've been exposed to stress such as acute infection, trauma, dehydration, or emotional duress. It has been suggested that adrenal insufficiency should be considered in any patient with unexplained cardiovascular collapse. Vomiting and diarrhea tend to increase the volume depletion and subsequent hypotension. It is not uncommon for patients to report abdominal pain, which tends to mimic an acute abdomen. Fever, weakness, and confusion are also common.

Lifelong replacement hormone therapy and careful monitoring of electrolyte levels are used to treat chronic adrenal insufficiency. Most of this is provided by the primary care physician. Patient education is critical to maintenance of well-being. All patients with Addison's disease are advised to wear a Medic-Alert tag in addition to carrying an identification card detailing their current medication regimen and physician's phone number.

Emergency management is focused on maintenance of the ABCs and, as always, careful monitoring of the patient's cardiac and oxygenation status as well as blood glucose level. Hypoglycemia poses its own threat to the patient's well-being, so blood glucose levels should be assessed and 25–50 grams of 50% dextrose should be administered to patients with levels less than 4.0 mmol/L or those with altered mental status. Obtaining a baseline 12-lead EKG is important due to the potential for dysrhythmias related to electrolyte imbalance. Fluid resuscitation should be aggressive. Follow your local protocol or contact medical direction for specific orders based on your patient's presentation. Immediate transport to an appropriate facility is imperative since definitive treatment includes the administration of glucocorticoids and/or mineralocorticoids in conjunction with correcting other electrolyte or hormonal abnormalities.

14. Describe the actions of epinephrine as it relates to the pathophysiology of hypoglycemia.
p. 615

Hypoglycemia, or low blood sugar, reflects high insulin and low glucose levels. Regardless of the cause, when insulin levels are high, glucagon may be ineffective in raising blood glucose levels. In prolonged fasts, almost half the glucose normally produced through gluconeogenesis is of renal origin. This activity is stimulated by epinephrine.

15. Describe the compensatory mechanisms utilized by the body to promote homeostasis when hypoglycemia is present. pp. 608, 615

When blood glucose levels fall, the alpha cells of the pancreas secrete glucagon. Glucagon stimulates the breakdown of glycogen into glucose for release into the bloodstream. This process, called glycogenolysis, takes place throughout the body but occurs primarily in the liver. In addition to stimulating the breakdown of glycogen, glucagon also stimulates the breakdown of proteins and fats with subsequent conversion to glucose. This process of producing sugar from nonsugar sources is called gluconeogenesis. Both of these processes contribute to the maintenance of homeostasis by raising blood glucose levels.

16. Differentiate among different endocrine emergencies based on assessment and history. pp. 608-621

As you proceed through your course, you will encounter a variety of real and simulated patients with endocrinologic disorders and emergencies. Use the information provided in this chapter of your text, as well as the application of this information as demonstrated by your instructors, preceptors, and mentors to enhance your own ability to differentiate endocrinologic emergencies.

17. Given several scenarios involving endocrine emergency patients, provide the appropriate assessment, management, and transportation.   pp. 608-621

Throughout your classroom, clinical, and field training, you will encounter a variety of real and simulated patients with endocrinologic emergencies. Use the information provided in this chapter of your text, as well as the application of this information as demonstrated by your instructors, preceptors, and mentors to enhance your ability to assess, manage, and transport patients with endocrinologic emergencies.

CONTENT SELF-EVALUATION

Multiple Choice

_____ 1. Which of the following is an exocrine gland?
   A.   pineal   D.   parathyroid
   B.   thymus   E.   adrenal
   C.   salivary

_____ 2. The term describing the sum of cellular processes that produce energy and molecules needed for growth and repair is:
   A.   anabolism.   D.   homeostasis.
   B.   catabolism.   E.   physiology.
   C.   metabolism.

_____ 3. Insulin's primary function is to:
   A.   metabolize glucose at the cellular level.
   B.   free glucose from muscle storage sites.
   C.   transport glucose across the cell membrane.
   D.   store glucose at the cellular level.
   E.   enhance the function of glucagon.

_____ 4. Diabetes mellitus is caused by the inadequate production or activity of:
   A.   polypeptide.   D.   cortisol.
   B.   glucagon.   E.   insulin.
   C.   somatostatin.

5. Osmotic diuresis, a characteristic of untreated diabetes, contributes to the development of:
   A. polydipsia and polyphagia.   D. polyuria.
   B. polydipsia and polyuria.   E. polyphagia.
   C. polyuria and polyphagia.

6. All of the following are signs and symptoms of diabetic ketoacidosis EXCEPT:
   A. abdominal pain.   D. cold, clammy skin.
   B. deep rapid respirations.   E. tachycardia.
   C. decreased mental function.

7. Diabetic ketoacidosis, characterized by high blood glucose and metabolic acidosis, occurs as a result of all of the following EXCEPT:
   A. profound insulin deficiency.   D. physiologic stress.
   B. increased glucagon activity.   E. overexertion.
   C. cessation of insulin injections.

8. Which of the following signs or symptoms will be present in the patient experiencing diabetic ketoacidosis?
   A. acetone breath odor   D. drooling
   B. apathy   E. diaphoresis
   C. diplopia

9. Kussmaul's respirations are seen in which of the following conditions?
   A. diabetic ketoacidosis
   B. hyperglycemic hyperosmolar nonketotic coma
   C. hypoglycemia
   D. insulin shock
   E. thyrotoxicosis

10. The most important sign or symptom associated with hypoglycemia is:
    A. tachycardia.   D. polydipsia.
    B. cool, clammy skin.   E. polyphagia.
    C. altered mental status.

11. Hyperglycemic hyperosmolar nonketotic acidosis differs from diabetic ketoacidosis because significant production of ketone bodies is prevented by the action of:
    A. polypeptide.   D. cortisol.
    B. glucagon.   E. insulin.
    C. somatostatin.

12. All of the following are signs and symptoms associated with thyrotoxic crisis EXCEPT:
    A. high fever.   D. delirium.
    B. bradycardia.   E. vomiting.
    C. hypotension.

13. Potential causes for myxedema coma include all of the following EXCEPT:
    A. excessive thyroid medication. D. cold environment.
    B. infection.   E. CNS depressants.
    C. trauma.

14. Signs and symptoms associated with myxedema coma include all of the following EXCEPT:
    A. hypothermia.   D. CO_2 retention.
    B. decreased mental status.   E. seizures.
    C. low amplitude bradycardia.

15. Which disorder exhibits prominent weight gain in the trunk, face, and neck, with accumulation of fat on the upper back and easily bruised, translucent skin?

   A. Addison's disease
   B. Cushing's syndrome
   C. Graves' disease
   D. myxedema
   E. "thyroid storm"

16. Which disorder exhibits progressive weakness, fatigue, decreased appetite, and weight loss?

   A. Addison's disease
   B. Cushing's syndrome
   C. Graves' disease
   D. myxedema
   E. "thyroid storm"

17. A high fever 41 C or greater may be associated with:

   A. thyrotoxic crisis
   B. Graves disease
   C. Myxedema
   D. hypoglycemia
   E. ketoacidosis

18. Which body hormone is dominant when the blood glucose level is low?

   A. insulin.
   B. levothyroxine.
   C. ATP
   D. glucagon.
   E. glucose.

19. During glucose metabolism, in order for anabolic pathways to proceed, _____ must first exert its stimulatory effects.

   A. epinephrine.
   B. glucagon.
   C. levothyroxin.
   D. cortisol.
   E. insulin.

20. The baseline reflecting hypoglycemia is less than:

   A. 4.0 mmol/L
   B. 6.3 mmol/L.
   C. 6.3 gmol/L.
   D. 7.7 mmol/L.
   E. 10 mmol/L.

21. In the first hour or so after a meal, it is normal for a blood glucose to increase to:

   A. 15-18 mmol/L.
   B. less than 4.0 mmol/L.
   C. 4.0-5.5 mmol/L.
   D. 6.6-7.7 mmol/L.
   E. 3.6-6.3 mmol/L.

22. Signs and symptoms of Hyperglycemic Hyperosmolar Nonketotic Coma (HHNK) include all of the following EXCEPT:

   A. dry mouth.
   B. tremors.
   C. tachycardia.
   D. normal respirations.
   E. normal vision.

23. You are presented with a 25-year-old female complaining of weight loss despite increased appetite, weakness, dyspnea, tachycardia and new-onset atrial fibrillation. These are all signs and symptoms of which disorder?

   A. Grave's Disease
   B. thyroid storm
   C. hypoglycemia
   D. thyrotoxicosis
   E. HHNK Coma

24. What diagnostic sign should be included in all assessments with a patient presenting with unexplained changes in mental status?

   A. deep tendon reflexes
   B. blood glucose
   C. gag reflex
   D. Babinski reflex
   E. bulbous cavernosum reflex

25. Which glands tend to have localized effects?

    A.   exocrine   **D.**   ductless

    B.   endocine   **E.**   volvulus

    C.   mixed

True/False

26. Kussmaul's respirations are a primary compensatory mechanism for reducing acidosis in the patient with diabetic ketoacidosis.

    A.   True

    B.   False

27. Even in the absence of a blood glucose level, altered mental status in a known diabetic should always be treated with 50 percent dextrose.

    A.   True

    B.   False

28. Long-term exposure to excess glucocorticoids or abnormalities to either the adrenal cortex or pituitary gland may cause hyperadrenalism.

    A.   True

    B.   False

29. Addison's disease is characterized by high corticosteroid activity that causes major disturbances in water and electrolyte balance.

    A.   True

    B.   False

30. Graves disease is more common in males than females.

    A.   True

    B.   False

31. Glucose is the only substance that brain cells can use as an energy source.

    A.   True

    B.   False

32. In the body, insulin is the dominant hormone when the blood glucose level is high.

    A.   True

    B.   False

33. For insulin to be effective, it must be able to bind to body cells in such a way that adequate levels of stimulation occur.

    A.   True

    B.   False

34. Type II diabetes is commonly referred to as juvenile-onset diabetes.

    A.   True

    B.   False

35. The pancreas is an example of an exocrine gland.

    A.   True

    B.   False

Matching

Write the letter of the term in the space provided next to the appropriate description.

A.	catabolism	**F.**	metabolism
B.	hyperglycemia	**G.**	hypoglycemia
C.	myxedema	**H.**	ketosis
D.	hormone	**I.**	glucosuria
E.	diuresis	**J.**	anabolism

_____ **36.** the sum of cellular processes that produce the energy needed for growth and repair

_____ **37.** excessive blood glucose

_____ **38.** the constructive phase of metabolism

_____ **39.** formation and secretion of large quantities of urine

_____ **40.** condition reflecting long-term exposure to inadequate levels of thyroid hormones

_____ **41.** chemical substance released by a gland that controls or effects processes in other glands or body systems

_____ **42.** deficiency of blood glucose

_____ **43.** glucose in urine

_____ **44.** the destructive phase of metabolism

_____ **45.** the presence of significant quantities of ketone bodies in the blood

Chapter 31

Allergies and Anaphylaxis

Review of Chapter Objectives

After reading this chapter, you should be able to:

1. Describe the incidence, morbidity, and mortality of anaphylaxis.   p. 623

Anaphylaxis results from an exposure to a particular substance that sets off a chain of biochemical events that can ultimately lead to shock and death. While the exact incidence is unknown, an estimated 1-2 per cent of Canadians live with the risk of an allergic reaction. Two of the most common fatal causes of anaphylaxis are attributed to injected penicillin and stings from bees and wasps (*Hymenoptera*). Fewer than five deaths per year are attributed to *Hymenoptera* stings. Overall, the incidence of anaphylaxis seems to be declining due to better recognition and treatment, particularly the availability of numerous potent antihistamines.

2. Identify the risk factors most predisposing to anaphylaxis. p. 623

Anaphylaxis is the fastest and most severe form of immediate hypersenstivity reaction. Some persons have an allergic tendency. This allergic tendency is genetically passed from parent to child and is characterized by the presence of large quantities of IgE antibodies.

3. Discuss the anatomy and physiology of the organs and structures related to anaphylaxis.   pp. 624-626

The immune system is a complex system responsible for combating infection. Components of the immune system can be found in the blood, the bone marrow, and the lymphatic system. The immune response is a complex cascade of events that occurs following activation by an invading substance.

   Following exposure to a particular antigen, large quantities of IgE antibodies are released. These antibodies attach to the membranes of basophils and mast cells, causing them to release histamine, heparin, and other chemicals into the surrounding tissue. The release of these chemical mediators causes a response in the cardiovascular, respiratory, and gastrointestinal systems as well as in the skin.

4. Discuss the pathophysiology of allergy and anaphylaxis.   pp. 624-627

The signs and symptoms associated with allergy and anaphylaxis are due to the physiologic changes triggered by the chemical mediators of the immune response that are released from the basophils and mast cells. Histamine is the primary mediator of all allergic reactions. It is a potent substance that causes bronchoconstriction, vasodilation and increased vascular permeability, and increased intestinal motility. Other chemical substances are also released that have effects similar to or synergistic with histamine, such as SRS-A (slow-reacting substance of anaphylaxis), which results in an asthma-like attack or asphyxia.

5. Describe the common routes of substance entry into the body.   pp. 626-627

Allergens can enter the body through various routes including oral ingestion, inhalation, topically, and through injection or envenomation. The vast majority of anaphylactic reactions result from injection or envenomation.

6. Define allergic reaction, anaphylaxis, antigen, antibody, and natural and acquired immunity. pp. 624-627

An allergic reaction is an exaggerated immune response to a foreign protein or other substance, while anaphylaxis is an unusual or exaggerated allergic reaction to a foreign protein or other substance.

An antigen is any substance that is capable, under appropriate conditions, of inducing a specific immune response. An antibody is a member of a unique class of chemicals that are manufactured by specialized cells of the immune system. The antibody is the principle agent of a chemical attack on an invading substance. Following exposure to an antigen, antibodies are released from cells of the immune system. The antibodies attach themselves to the invading substance so it can be removed from the body by other cells of the immune system.

Natural immunity refers to the immunity that is present at birth; also called innate immunity, it is genetically determined. Acquired immunity is immunity that develops over time and results from exposure to an antigen.

7. List common antigens most frequently associated with anaphylaxis. pp. 624-625

Any substance that is capable, under appropriate conditions, of inducing a specific immune response is known as an antigen. Most antigens are proteins. The following agents are among those that commonly trigger anaphylaxis: antibiotics, foods, or insect stings. Refer to Table 31-1 on text page 624 for a more complete list.

8. Discuss human antibody formation.   pp. 624-626

Antibodies are a unique class of chemicals that are manufactured by specialized cells of the immune system, called B cells. Another name for antibodies is immunoglobulins (Igs), and there are five different classes: IgA, IgD, IgE, IgG, and IgM. Following exposure to an antigen, antibodies are released from cells of the immune system. The antibodies attach themselves to the invading substance to facilitate removal of the substance from the body by other cells of the immune system. This response is known as humoral immunity.

If the body has never been exposed to a particular antigen, the response of the immune system is different than if it has been previously exposed. The initial response to an antigen is called the primary response. Following exposure to a new antigen, several days pass before both the cellular and humoral components of the immune system respond. Generalized antibodies (IgG and IgM) are released first. Simultaneously other components of the immune system begin to develop antibodies specific to the new antigen. The cells also develop a memory of the particular antigen and, if there is a subsequent exposure to this same substance, the immune system response is much faster. This is known as the secondary response. As part of this secondary response, antibodies specific for the offending antigen are released. Antigen-specific antibodies are much more effective in facilitating removal of the offending antigen than the generalized antibodies released during the primary response.

9. Describe the physical manifestations of anaphylaxis.   pp. 627-629, 631-632

The signs and symptoms of anaphylaxis begin within 30 to 60 seconds following exposure for the vast majority of patients. The more rapid the onset, the more severe the patient presentation. Respiratory manifestations of anaphylaxis include laryngeal edema and bronchoconstriction. Cardiovascular symptoms include tachycardia plus massive vasodilation resulting in profound hypotension. The combination of respiratory and cardiovascular signs will lead to a rapid deterioration of the patient's mental status. Generalized flushing and urticaria are common, as is angioedema about the head, face, and neck. Nausea, vomiting, and diarrhea may accompany hypermotility of the gastrointestinal tract.

10. Identify and differentiate between the signs and symptoms of allergic reaction and anaphylaxis.   pp. 631-632

Allergic reactions can range from a mild skin rash to a severe life-threatening multisystem response. Allergic reaction, also known as hypersensitivity, takes two forms, delayed or immediate. Delayed hypersensitivity is the result of cellular immunity and does not involve antibodies. It may occur hours to days after exposure and is very common. Delayed hypersensitivity usually presents as a skin rash and is often due to exposure to certain drugs and chemicals, for instance, poison ivy. Other signs and symptoms may include mild bronchoconstriction, mild intestinal cramps, or diarrhea, while the patient's mental status and vital signs will remain normal.

Immediate hypersensitivity is antibody-mediated immunity and often has a genetic link. The range of clinical presentation is widely variable. Examples of these reactions include hay fever, drug and food allergies, eczema, and asthma. Allergens can enter the body by various routes, but as a rule, those that enter by injection tend to have more rapid and more severe effects. Immediate hypersensitivities may be merely annoying, like the itching eyes and runny nose of hay fever, or may pose a real and immediate life threat, as seen in the anaphylactic reaction described in the case study at the beginning of this chapter.

The signs and symptoms of anaphylaxis begin within seconds following exposure. The more rapid the onset of symptoms, the more severe the patient presentation. Respiratory manifestations of anaphylaxis include laryngeal edema and bronchoconstriction. Cardiovascular symptoms include tachycardia plus massive vasodilation resulting in profound hypotension. A rapid deterioration of the patient's mental status accompanies the cardiovascular collapse. Generalized flushing and urticaria are common, as is angioedema about the head, face, and neck. Nausea, vomiting, and diarrhea may accompany hypermotility of the gastrointestinal tract. Refer to Table 31-2 on text page 631 for a comparison of signs and symptoms of mild allergic reactions and severe allergic reactions or anaphylaxis.

11. Explain the various treatments and pharmacological interventions used in the management of allergic reactions and anaphylaxis.   pp. 629-632

The first priority in the management of allergic reactions and anaphylaxis is to establish and maintain the patient's airway. Administer oxygen immediately along with ventilatory support as needed. You should be prepared to intubate, recognizing that laryngeal edema may change the size and appearance of the airway.

Establish vascular access as soon as possible and be prepared to run crystalloid solutions wide open if the patient is hypotensive. Epinephrine is the drug of choice for severe allergic reaction and anaphylaxis. In severe cases, administer 0.3–0.5 mg of 1:1,000 epinephrine subcutaneously. Remember that the effects of epinephrine wear off quickly, so be prepared to repeat administration in 3 to 5 minutes. Antihistamines, such as diphenhydramine, are widely used for the management of allergic reactions due to their ability to block histamine receptors. The usual dosage is 25–50 mg given either intravenously or intramuscularly. It may also be helpful to administer beta agonist agents via hand-held nebulizer to help reverse bronchospasm. Adult patients should receive 5 mg of salbutamol.

As is always the case, your management approach should always be dictated by local protocols. Other medications that may be used to manage severe anaphylaxis include corticosteroids, such as SoluMedrol, to suppress the inflammatory response or vasopressors, such as dopamine, to enhance cardiac output. You'll recall that adequate fluid resuscitation prior to initiating vasopressor therapy is important.

12. Correlate abnormal findings in assessment with the clinical significance in the patient with an allergic reaction or anaphylaxis.   pp. 627-629, 631-632

The central physiological action in severe allergic reaction and anaphylaxis is the massive release of histamine and other chemical mediators of the immune system. The resultant bronchospasm, airway edema, peripheral vasodilation, and increased capillary permeability can take a patient from his or her usual state of health to the brink of death in mere seconds. This chemically caused transformation is readily evident in the patient's clinical presentation: air hunger, dyspnea, angioedema, tachycardia, and hypotension. Your timely intervention is imperative to your patient's survival.

13. Given several preprogrammed and moulaged patients, provide the appropriate assessment, care, and transport for the allergic reaction and anaphylaxis patient. pp. 623-632

Throughout your classroom, clinical, and field training, you will encounter a variety of real and simulated patients with allergic reactions or anaphylaxis emergencies. Use the information provided in this chapter of your text, as well as the application of this information as demonstrated by your instructors, preceptors, and mentors to enhance your ability to assess, manage, and transport these patients.

CONTENT SELF-EVALUATION

Multiple Choice

1. The type of immunity resulting from a direct attack of a foreign substance by specialized cells of the immune system is known as:
   A. humoral.   D. acquired.
   B. cellular.   E. genetic.
   C. natural.

2. The unique class of chemicals that are manufactured by specialized cells of the immune system to attack invading foreign proteins is:
   A. allergens.   D. antibodies.
   B. antigens.   E. pathogens.
   C. toxins.

3. Any substance that is capable, under appropriate conditions, of inducing a specific immune response is a(n):
   A. immunoglobulin.   D. antibody.
   B. antigen.   E. pathogen.
   C. toxin.

4. The type of immunity that is present at birth and has no relation to a previous exposure to a particular antigen is:
   A. humoral.   D. acquired.
   B. cellular.   E. genetic.
   C. natural.

5. The type of immunity that develops over time as a result of exposure to an antigen is:
   A. humoral.   D. acquired.
   B. cellular.   E. genetic.
   C. natural.

6. All of the following are common allergens EXCEPT:
   A. insect stings.   D. seafood.
   B. drugs.   E. radiology contrast materials.
   C. antibodies.

7. The vast majority of anaphylactic reactions occur as a result of:
   A. inhalation.   D. topical exposure.
   B. ingestion.   E. genetics.
   C. injection.

8. The antibody most commonly associated with hypersensitivity reactions is:
   - **A.** IgA.
   - **B.** IgD.
   - **C.** IgE.
   - **D.** IgG.
   - **E.** IgM.

9. The primary chemical mediator of an allergic reaction is:
   - **A.** heparin.
   - **B.** histamine.
   - **C.** SRS-A.
   - **D.** basophil.
   - **E.** the mast cell.

10. All of the following are physiologic effects associated with the release of the chemical mediators of anaphylaxis EXCEPT:
    - **A.** bronchodilation.
    - **B.** vasodilation.
    - **C.** increased intestinal motility.
    - **D.** increased vascular permeability.
    - **E.** secretion of gastric acids.

11. Urticaria, a wheal and flare reaction characterized by red raised bumps that appear on the skin, is due to:
    - **A.** bronchodilation.
    - **B.** vasodilation.
    - **C.** increased intestinal motility.
    - **D.** decreased vascular permeability.
    - **E.** secretion of gastric acids.

12. The first line parenteral drug for the management of anaphylaxis is:
    - **A.** oxygen.
    - **B.** diphenhydramine.
    - **C.** epinephrine.
    - **D.** methylprednisolone.
    - **E.** albuterol.

13. The first priority when responding to a patient with an anaphylactic reaction is to:
    - **A.** protect the airway.
    - **B.** administer diphenhydramine.
    - **C.** stabilize the cervical spine.
    - **D.** ensure scene safety.
    - **E.** establish vascular access.

14. Hypotension that is seen in severe anaphylaxis is due to:
    - **A.** internal hemorrhage.
    - **B.** inadequate oxygenation.
    - **C.** bradycardia.
    - **D.** vasodilation.
    - **E.** gastrointestinal hypermotility.

15. A hoarse voice and eventually stridor is caused by which of the following during an anaphylaxis emergency?
    - **A.** urticaria.
    - **B.** laryngeal edema
    - **C.** cyanosis
    - **D.** delayed hypersensitivity
    - **E.** branchilian response

True/False

16. An allergic reaction is best defined as an exaggerated, sometimes potentially life-threatening response by the immune system to a foreign substance.
    - **A.** True
    - **B.** False

17. Anaphylaxis is seldom a life-threatening emergency that requires prompt recognition and specific treatments by paramedics.
    - **A.** True
    - **B.** False

18. Hymenoptera is one of the two most common causes of fatal anaphylaxis in Canada.
    - **A.** True
    - **B.** False

19. Acquired immunity develops rapidly after an exposure to an antigen.
- **A.** True
- **B.** False

20. A Diptheria/Pertussis/Tetanus (DPT) vaccine is an example of induced active immunity.
- **A.** True
- **B.** False

21. During anaphylaxis, H2 receptors, when stimulated cause bronchoconstriction and contraction of the intestines.
- **A.** True
- **B.** False

22. People sustaining anaphylaxis can actually die from circulatory shock if not treated.
- **A.** True
- **B.** False

23. Patients suffering from anaphylaxis are volume depleted due to histamine-mediated third spacing of fluids.
- **A.** True
- **B.** False

24. The primary treatment for anaphylaxis is pharmacological.
- **A.** True
- **B.** False

25. Inhaled beta agonists are useful in cases of severe bronchospasm and airway involvement.
- **A.** True
- **B.** False

Matching

Write the letter of the term in the space provided next to the appropriate description.

A.	antigen	**F.**	mast cell
B.	natural immunity	**G.**	sensitization
C.	pathogen	**H.**	urticaria
D.	allergy	**I.**	hypersensitivity
E.	antibody	**J.**	hymenoptera

26. specialized cell of the immune system that contains chemicals that assist in the immune system

27. any of an order of highly specialized insects, such as bees and wasps

28. principal agent of a chemical attack of an invading substance

29. innate immunity

30. initial exposure of a person to an antigen that results in an immune response

31. any substance that is capable, under appropriate conditions, of inducing a specific immune response

32. an unexpected and exaggerated reaction to a particular antigen

33. a disease-producing agent or invading substance

34. a hypersensitive state acquired through exposure to a particular allergen

35. the raised areas or hives that occur on the skin, associated with vasodilation due to histamine release

Chapter 32

Gastroenterology

Review of Chapter Objectives

After reading this chapter, you should be able to:

1. Describe the incidence, morbidity, and mortality of gastrointestinal emergencies.   **p. 634**

Gastrointestinal (GI) emergencies account for over 500 000 emergency visits and hospitalizations annually in the United States. Of that total, more than 300 000 are due to GI bleeding. While statistics are not available for Canadian hospitals, we would expect a similar percentage of visits to Canadian hospitals for this reason. These numbers are expected to increase over time due to the aging society and the trend of delaying treatment until over-the-counter medications no longer control symptoms. You will see GI emergencies in your practice, and it is likely that a large proportion will involve older persons. The number of patients over age 60 years in this patient population has risen from roughly 3% to over 45% in only a few years.

2. Identify the risk factors most predisposing to gastrointestinal emergencies. pp. 634–635

Many of the most common risk factors are self-induced by patients. They include excessive alcohol and tobacco consumption, stress, ingestion of caustic substances, and poor bowel habits. Because of the various risk factors and possible causes of GI emergencies, it is particularly important that you know how to complete a thorough focused history and examination before making a field diagnosis and how to assess the seriousness of the emergency and possible prevention strategies to minimize organ damage.

3. Discuss the anatomy and physiology of the organs and structures related to gastrointestinal diseases.   **(see Chapter 12)**

The GI tract is a long tube that extends from the mouth to the anus and is divided structurally and functionally into different parts. In general, the GI system is divided into the upper and lower GI tracts. The upper GI tract includes the mouth, esophagus, stomach, and duodenum, whereas the lower GI tract includes the remainder of the small intestine and the large intestine, rectum, and anus. In the upper GI tract, food is ingested and preliminary physical and chemical digestion is begun. In the lower GI tract, digestion of food is completed, nutrients are absorbed into the body, and remaining fiber, intestinal bacteria, and other materials are eliminated through the anus as feces. In addition, three additional organs—the liver, gallbladder, and pancreas—are intimately associated with the GI system both structurally (through connections with the duodenum) and functionally. The vermiform appendix, a blind sac found at the junction of the small and large intestines, does not have any apparent physiologic role in GI function but is important to you because of the inflammatory condition called appendicitis, which you will see in patients in the field.

4. Discuss the pathophysiology of abdominal inflammation and its relationship to acute pain. pp. 635-636

Sudden onset, or acute, pain can be caused by a variety of mechanisms, one of which is inflammation. Inflammation of hollow organs such as the appendix or gallbladder produces pain that is characteristically poorly localized and crampy in nature (visceral pain). When inflammation is widespread within the abdomen, as happens after an inflamed appendix ruptures, inflammation of the peritoneal membrane (peritonitis) results in pain that is usually localized and sharp in nature (somatic pain). It is important for you to become familiar with the different types of pain because they often represent progressive stages in an inflammatory condition—for example, appendiceal pain that changes from visceral to somatic pain over time.

5. Define somatic, visceral, and referred pain as they relate to gastroenterology. pp. 635-636

Somatic pain is characteristically sharp and localized, and it originates in the peritoneal membrane or within elements of the wall of the abdominal cavity, such as skeletal muscle. Bacterial irritation, which is common after perforation of the gut or rupture of the appendix or gallbladder, causes somatic pain where the degree of extension of irritation through the abdominal cavity is often paralleled in the physical extent of the abdomen in which pain is perceived. Visceral pain is typically crampy and vague in character and poorly localized; it is commonly due to inflammation, distention, or ischemia in the walls of the GI tract (which is hollow) or in the capsule of a solid organ such as the liver. Referred pain is not a type of pain; rather, it is the term applied to any pain that is felt in a site other than the site of origin. Appendicitis is often first felt as periumbilical pain.

6. Differentiate between hemorrhagic and nonhemorrhagic abdominal pain. pp. 636, 638

Recall that many GI emergencies are hemorrhagic. If hemorrhage results from perforation or rupture of an organ, pain will often be sudden in onset, somatic in nature, and extend in location as blood spreads through the abdominal cavity. Hemorrhage within the GI tract may initially produce visceral pain that is more characteristic of a nonhemorrhagic process such as inflammation or ischemia. Hemorrhage that is extensive enough to cause abdominal distention implies serious volume loss and will also be reflected in altered vital signs. Finally, pain from a dissecting aortic aneurysm (a grave, non-GI surgical emergency) is often felt between the shoulder blades.

7. Discuss the signs and symptoms and differentiate between local, general, and peritoneal inflammation relative to acute abdominal pain. pp. 635-636

Local inflammation within the GI tract often produces visceral pain associated with sympathetic nervous system stimulation (which typically results in nausea, vomiting, diaphoresis, and tachycardia). General inflammation within the abdomen often includes bacterial or chemical irritation of the peritoneum (the origins of peritonitis) and is thus associated with increasingly widespread somatic pain. Peritonitis (inflammation of the peritoneum) often represents the end stage of a generalized inflammatory or hemorrhagic process; as such, it is often associated with the most significant physical signs including altered vitals or overt shock. Because pain associated with peritonitis is often very severe, it is typical to find the patient lying with knees to chest as this position minimizes stretch on the already inflamed peritoneum.

8. Describe the questioning technique and specific questions when gathering a focused history in a patient with abdominal pain. pp. 636-637

Questioning is done with the SAMPLE technique (Symptoms, Allergies, Medication, Past medical history, Last oral intake, and Events leading to the current complaint). Specific questions about the present illness typically use the OPQRST-ASPN mnemonic to gather information about the abdominal pain:

- **O**nset of pain (sudden or slow)
- **P**rovocation or palliation of pain in terms of position or activity such as walking
- **Q**uality (or nature) of the pain
- **R**egion where pain is felt, along with any radiation of pain (For instance, radiation of pain among different locations implies similar neural pathways as referred pain and may give clues to origin of problem.)
- **S**everity of pain at the moment and over time
- **T**ime over which pain has been felt (Note that any patient with pain lasting over 6 hours is considered a surgical emergency and requires transport to an appropriate facility for evaluation.)
- **A**ssociated Symptoms, such as vomiting (if yes, ask about appearance of vomitus), change in bowel habits (if "diarrheal," inquire whether stool may suggest hemorrhage via foul-smelling, tarry appearance or obvious blood), or lost appetite
- **P**ertinent Negatives such as absence of change in GI tract function associated with positives such as pelvic pain, change in urinary habits, or positive cardiovascular history. (Remember that diaphragmatic irritation with pain felt in neck or shoulder may reflect inferior myocardial infarction.)

9. Describe the technique for performing a comprehensive physical examination on a patient complaining of abdominal pain. p. 638

Always start with the least invasive step, visual inspection. This includes checking patient appearance and positioning as well as visually inspecting the abdomen for signs of distention or discoloration. Be sure to get a complete set of baseline vital signs early in the process. Changes in vitals along with alterations in mental status may indicate early shock due to hemorrhage or other processes. Auscultation and percussion often do NOT provide useful information in the field; however, if you do auscultate, be sure to do so before palpating in order to avoid perturbation in abdominal sounds. Palpation with gentle pressure should start in the LEAST affected area and move toward the point of greatest pain. Remember to immediate stop palpation if you feel any pulsation. Further palpation may cause rupture of the affected blood vessel or organ.

10. Discuss the pathophysiology, assessment findings, and management of the following gastroenterological problems:

Upper gastrointestinal bleeding   pp. 639-641
The six most common causes of hemorrhage in the upper GI tract are (in descending order) peptic ulcer disease, gastritis, variceal rupture, Mallory-Weiss syndrome (esophageal laceration, generally secondary to vomiting), esophagitis, and duodenitis. Note that ulcers and gastritis account for 75% of cases (with 50% due to ulcers). Irritation and erosion of the GI lining is the most common pathophysiologic basis for bleeding, and involvement of the stomach lining underlies 75% of upper GI bleeds. Because most such cases involve chronic, low-level hemorrhage, many patients can be cared for on an outpatient basis. However, brisk upper GI bleeds may be life threatening. Assessment findings that can help to distinguish the severity of the bleed include presence and severity of hematemesis (vomiting of blood) and/or melena (passage of partially digested blood represented as dark, tarry stools). Look for subtle signs of shock and manage accordingly. Besides shock, another potentially grave complication of some bleeds is airway compromise due to aspiration of vomitus (when vomiting is present). Be sure to support the airway, and beware of vomiting in patients who are lying in a supine position. A patient with pain characteristic of peritonitis, especially with discoloration or bulging of the abdomen, may have a life-threatening blood loss. General management centers on airway, oxygenation, and circulatory status. Position to minimize risk of aspiration, provide high-flow oxygen, and start two large-bore IV lines (one with blood tubing and one for volume replacement with normal saline). Base fluid resuscitation on patient condition and response to treatment.

Lower gastrointestinal bleeding   pp. 646-647
Hemorrhage from the lower GI tract is most commonly associated with chronic medical conditions and the anatomic changes of advancing age. Typical causes include diverticulosis, colorectal lesions, and inflammatory bowel disease. Remember that lower GI bleeds rarely result in the massive hemorrhage that can be associated with esophageal or stomach pathology. Assessment should

establish whether the problem is new in onset or chronic (be sure to look for scars from previous surgical procedures). Questions about stool or inspection of stool may show melena, which usually indicates a slow lower GI bleed, or bright red blood, which indicates severe hemorrhage with rapid passage through the intestines or a source in the distal colon. Distal GI causes include hemorrhoids and rectal fissures. Be sure to assess for abdominal signs such as discoloration or bulging and maintain ongoing check for signs of early shock. General management centers on the patient's physiologic status. Watch airway and oxygenation closely, and use oxygen if necessary. Establish IV access and fluid resuscitation based on patient's findings or shift in findings over time. If there are any signs of significant blood loss, be sure one IV line is capable of use for blood transfusion.

Acute gastroenteritis   pp. 642-643

Acute gastroenteritis involves inflammation of the stomach and intestines associated with sudden onset vomiting, diarrhea, or both. It is very common; the underlying inflammation causes erosion of the mucosal and submucosal layers of the GI tract with blood loss and damage to the intestinal villi. Triggers can include alcohol or tobacco use, use of nonsteroidal anti-inflammatory agents, stress, and GI or systemic infection. The most common and striking finding is copious volumes of watery diarrhea secondary to damage to the intestinal lining. Diarrhea may contain blood. In general, patients are often febrile and suffering from general malaise as well as nausea and vomiting. Watch for any signs of early shock such as altered mental status, development of pale, clammy skin, or changes in vitals. Abdominal tenderness is common; distention is uncommon unless significant amounts of gas are in the intestines. In cases of severe dehydration, watch for problems such as cardiac arrhythmia secondary to electrolyte disturbance. Management is supportive and palliative, with any needed support for airway (position to minimize odds of aspiration), oxygenation, or circulation. Fluid resuscitation via oral or IV route may be indicated. Be sure you take appropriate precautions during patient care to prevent spread of any possible infectious disease.

Colitis   pp. 647-648

Colitis is a general term for inflammation of the large intestine. Ulcerative colitis, which you may see in the field, is an inflammatory bowel disease that frequently affects relatively young people (with average age of 20 to 40 years at onset). Mild disease may only affect the distal colon, and it may present in the field with bloody diarrhea and discomfort. More severe disease may affect the entire colon, and this may present with severe, bloody diarrhea, electrolyte disturbances, or even hypovolemic shock. Management is tied to the patient's condition and includes appropriate support of oxygenation and circulation. If the patient has bouts of nausea and vomiting, beware of possible aspiration and airway compromise. Any patient who presents with a lower GI bleed or colicky, visceral-type pain should be transported for diagnostic evaluation.

Gastroenteritis   pp. 642-644

Gastroenteritis, inflammation of the stomach and intestines, is characterized by longer-term changes in the mucosa, thus distinguishing it from acute gastroenteritis. Gastroenteritis is usually due to microbial infection, with viral infection most common. However, patients with bacterial infection are usually the sickest. Common findings are fever, nausea, vomiting, diarrhea, lethargy, and, in the most severe cases, shock. Infection with *H. pylori* (the most common infectious cause in the U.S.) commonly presents with heartburn, abdominal pain, and the presence of gastric ulcers. Management includes appropriate infection precautions and patient care centered on monitoring of ABCs and transport. When outbreaks are associated with natural disaster or other possible contamination of water supply, be sure to protect yourself by use of proper sanitation and protection of water and food supplies.

Diverticulitis   p. 649

Diverticulitis represents inflammation secondary to infection of diverticula, the outpouchings of intestinal mucosa and submucosa common in older Americans. Diverticulitis frequently starts with occlusion of a diverticulum by fecal material followed by bacterial infection. Complications include colonic hemorrhage or perforation. Common presenting signs of diverticulitis include low-grade fever, nausea and vomiting, and point tenderness on palpation. Because roughly 95% of cases involve the sigmoid colon, another name for this condition is "left-sided appendicitis." Management is supportive, with attention to the ABCs. Signs of shock suggest significant hemorrhage.

Appendicitis   pp. 652-653

Appendicitis is inflammation of the vermiform appendix. You will encounter acute appendicitis in the field, most commonly in older children and young adults. Untreated appendicitis can result in rupture with subsequent peritonitis. The pathophysiology has parallels to that of diverticulitis: The appendix becomes obstructed with fecal material, and the resultant inflammation and infection cause the characteristic discomfort, which may present initially as periumbilical, visceral pain, but later becomes the well-known somatic, right lower quadrant pain. Somatic pain or signs of peritonitis suggest significant inflammation with ischemia or infarction of the appendix or appendiceal rupture, respectively. Other findings such as fever, anorexia, and nausea or vomiting relate to the stage of appendiceal inflammation. Exam findings range from vague abdominal discomfort on palpation (in early cases) to clear peritonitis. Management during transport centers on positioning for comfort, managing airway to avoid aspiration, and establishing IV access. Monitor as you would for bowel obstruction and be aware of any early signs of shock.

Ulcer disease   pp. 644-646

Peptic ulcers, created secondary to mucosal erosion by gastric acid, can occur anywhere in the GI tract and are particularly common in the duodenum and stomach. You will see ulcer cases and GI problems complicated by the presence of peptic ulcers. Pathophysiology includes genetic predisposition (seen as positive family history) as well as risk factors such as stress, use of nonsteroidal anti-inflammatory drugs, acid-stimulating products such as alcohol and nicotine, and chronic infection with *H. pylori*. The common mechanism is a breach of the mucous layer that protects the mucosa from the acid secreted in the stomach. Findings can vary widely. Chronic pain is typically worst when the stomach is empty and is relieved by eating or drinking coating liquids such as milk. Acute pain, particularly when somatic in character, may suggest rupture of the ulcer with hemorrhage into the abdomen. Bleeds manifest similarly to other upper GI hemorrhages and are handled similarly. In severely ill patients, appearance suggests severity of distress (such as lying still with knees drawn to chest), and there are often signs of shock. Management depends on physiologic status and involves monitoring of ABCs with appropriate intervention for possible or overt shock.

Bowel obstruction   pp. 650-652

Bowel obstruction involves partial or complete blockage of a portion of the small or large intestine. Rapid diagnosis and treatment are essential to avoid complications such as bowel infarction. The four most common causes are hernias, intussusception, volvulus, and adhesions. The most common site is the small intestine due to smaller diameter and greater length and motility of intestinal loops. Chronic obstruction is often due to a progressive process such as tumor growth or adhesions. Acute obstruction may be due to ingestion of a foreign body or incarceration and strangulation of a hernia or loop of intussuscepted bowel. Findings suggestive of obstruction include pain (which is often diffuse and visceral in nature) and vomiting. The character of the vomitus (for example, feces-like material) may suggest the approximate site of the obstruction. Significant ischemia or infarction is suggested by findings of early or overt shock. Visual inspection may reveal distention, peritonitis, or free air within the abdomen. Ask about scars that indicate prior surgery and look for discoloration that may indicate the presence of free blood in the abdominal cavity. Palpation may be useful in localizing discomfort but beware of any but light pressure because heavier pressure may cause rupture of the obstructed segment. Treatment depends on the patient's physiologic status, with attention and support of the ABCs. Remember to place one IV line capable of blood transfusion if there are any indications of significant hemorrhage.

Crohn's disease   p. 648

Crohn's disease, like ulcerative colitis, is an inflammatory bowel disease. However, the pathologic inflammation can occur anywhere in the GI tract from the mouth to the rectum. After inflammation damages the mucosa and submucosa, granulomas form that further damage the wall of the GI tract. Patients with Crohn's frequently have narrowing of damaged segments, occasionally to the point of complete obstruction. Other findings include diarrhea and intestinal or perianal abscesses or fistulas. Because of the variety of sites involved in different patients, as well as the variety of complications due to progressive damage, prehospital diagnosis is nearly impossible. You should remember that an acute flare-up of symptoms accompanied by absence of bowel sounds suggests intestinal obstruction, which is a surgical emergency. Because significant hemorrhage is unusual, however, hypovolemic shock is infrequent among these patients. Prehospital management is largely palliative, with specific monitoring and support of the ABCs. Evidence of obstruction or shock calls for high-flow oxygen and circulatory support including IV access and fluid resuscitation.

Pancreatitis   pp. 654-655

Pancreatitis is inflammation of the pancreas. The four main pathologic types are metabolic, mechanical, vascular, and infectious. Metabolic causes (specifically alcoholism) account for over 80% of cases. Alcohol causes deposition of platelet plugs in the acini. As flow of digestive secretions from the pancreas is impaired, digestive enzymes become activated while within the pancreas, damaging pancreatic tissue. Progression of this chronic damage can lead to hemorrhage, which presents as sudden onset nausea, vomiting, and severe pain that is in the left upper quadrant and may radiate to the back or the epigastric region. Mechanical pancreatitis is due to gallstones or elevated serum lipids. As digestive secretions accumulate behind the obstruction, pancreatic tissue damage occurs, edema develops, and blood flow is secondarily impaired, causing further damage due to ischemia. Mechanical pancreatitis is often acute in onset. Vascular causes of pancreatitis include thromboembolism and ischemia secondary to shock. Findings of mild pancreatitis include visceral pain, often epigastric in location, abdominal distension, nausea and vomiting, and elevated blood amylase and lipase. Findings in severe pancreatitis include refractory hypotensive shock, blood loss, and respiratory failure. As with other conditions involving hemorrhage, management of severe pancreatitis centers on support of ABCs including use of high-flow oxygen and appropriate IV access.

Esophageal varices pp. 641-642

A varix is a swollen vein, and esophageal varices (plural) are usually due to hypertension in the portal system. Varices are subject to rupture and hemorrhage, and mortality in these cases exceeds 35%. The most common cause is liver damage secondary to alcohol consumption (via cirrhosis of the liver and portal hypertension). The other common cause is ingestion of caustic substances, which damage the esophagus directly and eventually cause rupture of an esophageal vein. Initial presentation of rupture features painless bleeding with evolution of signs of hemodynamic instability. Hematemesis can be both forceful and large in volume. Clotting time increases as high portal pressure backs up blood into the spleen, destroying platelets. Because tamponade isn't possible in the prehospital setting, management centers on rapid transport with care focusing on aggressive airway management (including orotracheal intubation if needed), use of high-flow oxygen, and IV fluid resuscitation.

Hemorrhoids   pp. 649-650

Hemorrhoids are small masses of swollen veins in the rectum or anus (internal and external hemorrhoids, respectively). Most are of unknown origin and occur in midlife, although some result from recognizable causes such as pregnancy or portal hypertension. In addition, external hemorrhoids can be caused by heavy lifting with straining. Although hemorrhoids frequently bleed during defecation, particularly in the setting of constipation, significant hemorrhage is rare. The typical cause for your call will be distress over the presence of bright red blood with defecation. The physical findings are usually benign, with hemodynamic stability and absence of signs of shock (skin is warm and dry, tachycardia is consistent with anxiety). Emotional assurance and monitoring for continued physiologic stability (due to possibility that bleeding is first sign of a lower GI bleed) is usually sufficient during transport. Either signs of significant bleeding or bleeding hemorrhoids in an alcoholic patient warrant closer monitoring and transport for immediate care.

Cholecystitis   pp. 653-654

Roughly 90% of cases of cholecystitis, inflammation of the gallbladder, are due to gallstones. Cholecystitis caused by stones can be acute or chronic. In both cases, the basic pathophysiology involves obstruction of the flow of bile by gallstones, with resultant inflammation of the gallbladder. Bacterial infection can also cause chronic cholecystitis. An acute attack is characterized by right upper quadrant pain, often with referred pain in the right shoulder. The right subcostal region may be tender due to muscle spasm. Sympathetic nervous stimulation may cause pale, cool, clammy skin. Prehospital care centers on palliation of distress and monitoring of ABCs with use of oxygen if needed and with establishment of IV access.

Acute hepatitis   pp. 655-656

Acute hepatitis, inflammation of the liver, can result from any injury to liver cells associated with an infectious or inflammatory process. Viral hepatitis is most common, and alcoholic hepatitis secondary to cirrhosis is also common. Symptoms range from mild manifestations to overt liver failure and death, and mortality is high due to the wide range of potential causes. You will find that presentation often parallels severity of hepatitis: Common complaints include right upper quadrant tenderness not relieved by eating or antacids and development of clay-colored stools (this secondary to decreased bile production). If bilirubin retention exists, scleral icterus and jaundice may be present. Palpation may reveal liver enlargement, and fever may be due to infection or tissue necrosis. Presence of cool, clammy, diaphoretic skin suggests hemorrhage of a hepatic lesion. Secure ABCs and establish IV access. Be particularly careful in consideration of use of any pharmacologic agent because liver failure may impair drug metabolism. Never forget to use personal protective equipment and to use body substance isolation precautions.

11. Differentiate between gastrointestinal emergencies based on assessment findings. pp. 636-638

Assessment includes initial size-up, SAMPLE focused history with attention to current complaint, personal medical and family history, and physical examination. History of present illness will reveal whether condition is acute, chronic, or an acute flare-up of a chronic problem. The relation of pain (if any) with last oral intake may suggest ulcers (in which eating typically relieves pain) or, in contrast, cholecystitis (where pain may worsen after eating, particularly a fatty meal). The presence of chest pain rather than abdominal pain (or in addition to abdominal pain) may mean a condition has generated referred pain: Examples include gastroesophageal reflux (heartburn), gastric or duodenal ulcers, or cholecystitis. A change in nature of pain from visceral to somatic may infer a progression of abdominal pathology. Always remember before starting the physical exam that the majority of GI emergencies entail bleeding from the upper or lower GI tract: Watch for signs of hemorrhage in vitals (and changes in vitals) and on visual inspection of the abdomen, as well as examination of any vomitus or stool.

12. Given several preprogrammed patients with abdominal pain and symptoms, provide the appropriate assessment, treatment, and transport. pp. 634-656

Care of any hemorrhagic case entails close monitoring of ABCs with attention to airway (minimizing risk of aspiration of any vomitus), breathing (high-flow oxygen is often indicated), and circulation (establishment of one or two IV lines with ability for blood transfusion where appropriate, and fluid resuscitation as needed). Although there are some conditions such as Crohn's disease in which bleeding rarely leads to hypovolemic shock, you should always be prepared to treat shock. Cases that seem to represent progressive, nonhemorrhagic conditions such as appendicitis, cholecystitis, or diverticulitis should also be monitored for stability and signs of acute events such as rupture or hemorrhage. Last, be aware that GI emergencies often present in older patients with coexisting morbid conditions and monitor cardiopulmonary status and other organ function carefully. Take close note of conditions such as alcoholism, consider GI problems associated with them (such as hepatitis, pancreatitis, or esophageal varices), and adjust assessment and treatment accordingly.

CONTENT SELF-EVALUATION

Multiple Choice

_____ 1. Which of the following statements about gastrointestinal (GI) emergencies is NOT true?

    A. GI emergencies account for about 5% of all annual visits to the emergency department.

    B. The majority of GI emergencies entail GI hemorrhage

    C. The number of GI emergencies is expected to rise, in part due to aging of the population.

    D. The risk factors for GI emergencies are well known, and most (such as familial predisposition to GI conditions) are out of control of the patient.

    E. The number of GI emergencies is expected to rise, in part due to delays in seeking treatment by patients who treat themselves as long as symptoms allow.

_____ 2. All of the following statements about physical examination of the abdomen are true EXCEPT:

    A. Visual inspection should always be done first.

    B. Palpation should always precede auscultation.

    C. Of auscultation, percussion, palpation, and visual inspection, palpation may be most likely to produce a lot of useful information.

    D. Discoloration of the skin (specifically, ecchymosis) may indicate where hemorrhage has occurred into the abdominal cavity.

    E. Abdominal distension may be an ominous sign, suggesting either free air in the abdomen or loss of a large amount of circulating volume.

_____ 3. Three organs intimately associated with the GI tract are the:

    A. teeth, tongue, and epiglottis.

    B. appendix, gallbladder, and parotid gland.

    C. cystic duct, the bile duct, and the common bile duct.

    D. appendix, the rectum, and the anus.

    E. liver, pancreas, and gallbladder.

_____ 4. Major causes of upper GI hemorrhage include all of the following EXCEPT:

    A. gastritis.   **D.** peptic ulcers.

    B. rupture of an esophageal varix.   **E.** Mallory-Weiss syndrome.

    C. gastroenteritis.

_____ 5. Severe, potentially life-threatening upper GI hemorrhage is common with:

    A. variceal and hemorrhoidal rupture and bleeding.

    B. peptic ulcer disease and Crohn's disease.

    C. esophageal varices and hepatic cirrhosis.

    D. esophageal varix rupture and esophageal Mallory-Weiss tears.

    E. eroded gastric ulcers and eroded ulcerative colitis lesions.

_____ 6. Conditions that routinely call for the paramedic to take infectious precautions include:

    A. hepatitis and cirrhosis.

    B. peptic ulcer disease and gastroenteritis.

    C. cholecystitis and pancreatitis.

    D. gastroenteritis and appendicitis.

    E. hepatitis and gastroenteritis.

7. Conditions that typically have lesions in the rectum and anus include:
   A. diverticulosis and hemorrhoids.
   B. ulcerative colitis and Crohn's disease.
   C. ulcerative colitis and hemorrhoids.
   D. volvulus and intussusception.
   E. hernias and hemorrhoids.

8. Among the most common causes of bowel obstruction are:
   A. intestinal tumors, volvulus, and hernias.
   B. intussusception, volvulus, and hemorrhoids.
   C. adhesions, hernias, and intestinal tumors.
   D. hernias, volvulus, and adhesions.
   E. appendicitis, volvulus, and diverticulitis.

9. Acute pancreatitis is most commonly caused by:
   A. excessive use of alcohol and tobacco.
   B. gallstones and excessive use of alcohol.
   C. infectious GI disease and gallstones.
   D. drug toxicity and excessive use of alcohol.
   E. vascular disease causing ischemia and gallstones causing obstruction of the pancreatic duct.

10. Appendicitis may initially present with visceral pain located:
    A. in the right lower quadrant of the abdomen.
    B. at McBurney's point.
    C. in the right shoulder blade.
    D. periumbilically.
    E. in the right flank.

11. Chronic gastroenteritis is primarily due to microbial infection with the prevalent being:
    A. Giardia lamblia.
    B. Helicobacter pylori.
    C. Glasofinis fluorini
    D. Cyclosporidium cayetenis.
    E. Peritoni deventia

12. A patient presenting with clay coloured stools, photophobia, pharyngitis, general malaise and jaundice is likely to be suffering from:
    A. meningitis.
    B. Crohn's Disease.
    C. hepatitis.
    D. colloidal occlusion.
    E. pancreatitis.

13. Since the circulatory system's oxygen-carrying capabilities are intact with a patient with chronic gastroenteritis and no significant blood loss, oxygen administration should be:
    A. delivered at 12 Lpm via a non-rebreather mask.
    B. avoided completely.
    C. delivered via nasal cannula at 2-4 Lpm.
    D. delivered via Venturi mask at 60%.
    E. delivered via a partil-rebreather at 10 Lpm.

14. Sudden onsets of sharp abdominal pain is usually an indication of:
    A. ischemia.
    B. perforations of abdominal organs or capsules.
    C. referred pain.
    D. blockage of hollow organs.
    E. obstructions.

15. To help breakdown food boluses, the stomach secretes hydrochloric acid. One of the enzymes that control this secretion is::
   A.   cokinogen.
   B.   pepsinogen.
   C.   gastonigen.
   D.   sulfaside.
   E.   shellison

16. Cullen's sign is described as:
   A.   vomiting of frank blood.
   B.   periumbilical ecchymosis.
   C.   a buildup of free air in the abdomen.
   D.   an absence of bowel sounds.
   E.   ecchymosis in the flank area.

17. After traveling down the common bile duct, bile enters the small intestine at:
   A.   the circle of Frodo.
   B.   the pyloric sphincter.
   C.   the sphincter of Weiss
   D.   the sphincter of Oddi.
   E.   the Avalon Pass

18. All of the following are located in the lower GI tract EXCEPT the:
   A.   anus.
   B.   ileum.
   C.   jejunum.
   D.   rectum.
   E.   pancreas.

19. Alcohol liver cirrhosis and an increase in portal hypertension usually results in:
   A.   a pulmonary embolism.
   B.   right sided heart failure.
   C.   esophagheal varices.
   D.   gross hematuria.
   E.   erosion of the mucosal layers of the GI tract.

20. The overall mortality rate of acute pancreatitis is relatively high, approximately:
   A.   80-90%.
   B.   20-40%.
   C.   30-40%
   D.   60-70%.
   E.   70-80%.

21. When the stomach's mucosal barrier is damaged, which locally acting hormone decreases the stimulation of blood flow through the gastric mucosa, allowing its further destruction?
   A.   Helicobacter pylori
   B.   testosterone
   C.   quinifibrine
   D.   prostaglandin
   E.   estrogen

22. Which of the following medications can lead to the breakdown of the mucosal surfaces of the stomach and GI tract?
   A.   calcium channel blockers   D.   NSAIDs
   B.   antacids   E.   hypnotics
   C.   nitrates

23. Bloody diarrhea, stools containing mucus, colicky abdominal pain, nausea, vomiting, and occasionally weight loss and fever are typical signs and symptoms of:
   A.   bowel obstruction.
   B.   esophageal varices.
   C.   peptic ulcer.
   D.   Chrohn's Disease.
   E.   Ulcerative Colitis.

24. The most common cause of lower gastrointestinal bleeding is:
   A.   hemorrhoids.
   B.   diverticulosis.
   C.   anal fissures.
   D.   Crohn's disease.
   E.   benign polyps.

25. What type of ulcer generally presents with pain at night or when the stomach is empty?
   A.   duodenal ulcers
   B.   peptic ulcers
   C.   gastric ulcers
   D.   colonal ulcers
   E.   pyloric ulcers

True/False

26. Risk factors for GI disease include excessive use of alcohol and tobacco, stress, ingestion of caustic substances, and poor bowel habits.
   A.   True
   B.   False

27. The chief function of the upper GI tract is digestion, whereas the chief functions of the lower GI tract are absorption of nutrients and excretion of wastes.
   A.   True
   B.   False

28. Blood is indicated by melena, stool containing small or large amounts of bright red blood, and hematochezia, dark, tarry, foul-smelling stool.
   A.   True
   B.   False

29. A common difference between acute gastroenteritis and gastroenteritis is that gastroenteritis is more likely to be caused by microbial infection.
   A.   True
   B.   False

30. Any patient who presents with lower GI bleeding or colicky abdominal pain should be transported to the emergency department for evaluation.
   A.   True
   B.   False

31. Patients with peptic ulcer disease typically have worsening of pain after eating, whereas patients with cholecystitis typically have relief of pain after eating.
   A.   True
   B.   False

32. Somatic pain is described as achy or vague.
   A.   True
   B.   False

_____ **33.** In your history of the present illness pneumonic OPQRST-ASPN, the PN stands for per nocte, referring to pain at night.
    A.   True
    B.   False

_____ **34.** Zollinger-Ellison syndrome is a condition that causes the stomach to secrete more bile in an attempt to combat the effects of increased hydrochloric acid.
    A.   True
    B.   False

_____ **35.** Hepatitis B is also known as "serum hepatitis".
    A.   True
    B.   False

Matching

Write the letter of the term in the space provided next to the appropriate description.

A.	melena	**F.**	Mallory-Weiss tear
B.	proctitis	**G.**	hematochezia
C.	portal	**H.**	volvulus
D.	hemorrhoid	**I.**	esophageal varix
E.	hematemesis	**J.**	pancolitis

_____ **36.** pertaining to the flow of blood into the liver

_____ **37.** twisting of the intestines on itself

_____ **38.** bloody vomitus

_____ **39.** ulcerative colitis limited to the rectum

_____ **40.** bright red blood in the stool

_____ **41.** small mass of swollen veins in the anus or rectum

_____ **42.** swollen vein of the esophagus

_____ **43.** ulcerative colitis spread throughout the entire colon

_____ **44.** esophageal lasceration

_____ **45.** dark, tarry, foul smelling stool

Chapter 33

Urology and Nephrology

Review of Chapter Objectives

After reading this chapter, you should be able to:

1. **Describe the incidence, morbidity, mortality, and risk factors predisposing to urologic and nephrologic emergencies.**   pp. 659-660, 665-666, 669-670, 675-677

Renal (kidney) and urologic (urinary tract) disorders are very common, affecting about 20 million Americans, so you will definitely see emergencies related to these disorders in the field. The seriousness of these disorders is demonstrated by two statistics: Roughly 4 000 Canadians have the most severe form of long-term kidney failure (end-stage failure) and require either dialysis or transplantation to live. Every day an average of 10 Canadians learns that their kidneys have failed and their lives depend on dialysis. Some emergencies are not necessarily life threatening but are very painful to experience and common in the population: The two risk factors most significant for end-stage renal failure are hypertension and diabetes, which account for more than half of all cases. The risk factors for kidney stones are very different. Some kinds of stones follow a familial pattern, suggesting genetic predisposition. Other risk factors include physical immobilization, use of certain medications (anesthetics, opiates, and psychotropic drugs), and metabolic disorders such as gout. Finally, urinary tract infection, which accounts for many office visits yearly, has identified risk factors: female gender, paraplegic persons and others (notably some persons with diabetes) with nerve disruption to the bladder, pregnancy, and regular use of instrumentation such as catheters.

2. **Discuss the anatomy and physiology of the organs and structures related to urologic and nephrologic diseases.**   (see Chapter 12)

The two major organs of the urinary system are the kidneys and the urinary bladder. Two major structures are the ureters and the urethra. The kidney is the critical organ of the urinary system: The kidneys perform the vital functions of the urinary system, which include:

- Maintenance of blood volume with proper balance of water, electrolytes, and pH
- Retention of key substances such as glucose and removal of toxic wastes such as urea
- Major role in regulation of arterial blood pressure
- Control of the development of red blood cells

The first two roles are achieved through the production of urine in the kidneys. The kidneys' role in regulation of blood pressure is achieved in part through control of the body's fluid volume. In addition, they produce an enzyme called renin, which acts to activate a hormone (chemical messenger) called angiotensin, which is part of a hormonal pathway that acts to retain water in the body (increase blood pressure).

The structural and functional unit within the kidney is the nephron, and each kidney contains about 1 million nephrons, establishing the functional reserve that most people take for granted. Blood is filtered into the first part of the nephron, the glomerulus, and then moves through a length of specialized tubule. As the fluid moves through the parts of the tubule, movement of water and some materials out of the tubule and into the blood occurs (reabsorption), as does movement of some materials out of blood and into the tubule (secretion). The kidneys can maintain an exquisitely fine control over the relative activity of reabsorption and secretion for virtually every substance that is filtered into the glomerulus. The ability of the kidney to retain glucose, excrete wastes such as urea, and thus perform all of its vital roles is extraordinary, and life depends upon it. When kidney function is too low or nonexistent, an individual will die unless the function is replaced through artificial dialysis or through kidney transplantation. The final role of the kidney, control over development of red blood cells, is achieved through production and release of a hormone called erythropoietin, which stimulates red blood cell synthesis in the bone marrow.

Each ureter runs from a kidney to the bladder, and urine moves out of the kidney through them to reach the bladder. Because ureters are very small in internal diameter, they can become blocked by internal objects such as kidney stones. The bladder is a muscular sac that expands to hold urine. During urination, stored urine is eliminated from the bladder (and the body) through the tube called the urethra.

In women, the structures of the urinary system and the reproductive system are completely separate. In men, however, reproductive fluid (semen) is also eliminated from the body through the urethra. Thus, consideration of symptoms of urinary tract trouble in men is sometimes more complex than consideration of the same problem in women. For instance, infection in a man's urethra can come directly through sexual activity.

The genitourinary systems of men include some specifically reproductive organs and structures: the testes (the primary male reproductive organs, which produce testosterone and sperm cells) and tubing called the epididymis and vas deferens, through which sperm cells leave the testes and move toward the urethra. Sperm leaves the vas deferens to enter the urethra as it passes through the substance of the other male reproductive organ, the prostate gland, which produces fluid that mixes with sperm to produce semen, the male reproductive fluid. The prostate will be important to you in field work because it surrounds the first part of the male urethra. Prostate enlargement, which occurs routinely with age, can compress the urethra to the point of closure. This can result in retention of urine and a medical emergency call.

3. Define referred pain and visceral pain as they relate to urology.   p. 661

Visceral pain and referred pain have the same underlying pathophysiology as they do in the setting of GI emergencies. In the setting of urology, visceral pain usually arises in the walls of hollow structures such as the ureters, bladder, and urethra or the male vas deferens or epididymis. Visceral pain is characteristically described as aching or crampy and feels deeply internal within the body and poorly localized. Visceral pain can mark the first presentation of both kidney stones and urinary tract infection (although both are better known for somatic pain patterns that arise later). Referred pain, which is felt in a location other than the one of origin, has some notable urologic examples. Pyelonephritis, inflammation within the kidney, is often referred to the neck or shoulder.

4. Describe the questioning technique and specific questions the paramedic should use when gathering a focused history in a patient with abdominal pain.   pp. 661-663

Recall Chapter 32, "Gastroenterology," where you learned about the focused history relating to abdominal pain that might be GI in origin. The technique is similar when the GI system is not the focus of attention. For instance, initial questioning still follows the OPQRST format (shown below with some specific questions in parentheses):

• Onset of pain (Sudden or slow? Activity at the time?)
• Provocation or palliation of pain (Pain on urination, inability to void or void normally, and palliation with walking all may suggest urinary tract origin.)
• Quality of the pain (Visceral pain is common with urinary emergencies; a change to somatic pain, particularly flank pain, may suggest ureteral obstruction by a stone.)

• Region where pain is felt, along with any radiation of pain (Listen for suggestions of referred/radiated pain; in postpubertal women, be sure to get menstrual history and follow-up comments suggesting OB/GYN problems)

• Severity of pain currently and over time (Most urinary conditions don't cause the abrupt switch to somatic pain—with increase in severity—seen with a ruptured appendix, for instance.)

• Time over which pain has been felt. (Note that any patient with pain lasting over 6 hours is considered a surgical emergency and requires transport to an appropriate facility for evaluation.) When in doubt, consider case a potential surgical emergency and treat/transport as such.

Additional questions center on:

• Previous history of similar event (Note that kidney stones and infections may be recurrent problems; family history may also be helpful.)

• Nausea/vomiting (Because nausea and vomiting can be caused purely by autonomic nervous system discharge, this is not necessarily a sign localizing to GI system; nausea and vomiting is common with severe pain associated with kidney stones.)

• Changes in bowel habits (Diarrhea may suggest a GI condition; constipation may be less helpful as a clue to the origin of a problem.)

• Weight loss (Loss over hours to days suggests dehydration, whereas longer-term loss suggests chronic illness of GI dysfunction.)

• Last oral intake, include beverages (Learning this is necessary for possible surgical cases; timing of a meal may also suggest acute onset problem or aggravation of an existing one.)

• Chest pain (Consider MI but also consider referred pain; note that diabetic persons may not have typical pain pattern during MI due to neuropathy.)

5. Describe the technique for performing a comprehensive physical examination of a patient complaining of abdominal pain.   pp. 663-665

The physical exam includes overall impressions as well as examination of the abdomen. Elements include both patient appearance and posture/activity. Walking often suggests urinary origin: Walking that relieves pain may suggest a kidney stone, and walking hunched up in a febrile person complaining of back pain may suggest kidney infection. Additionally, altered level of consciousness in the absence of fever may suggest hemorrhage and evolution of hypovolemic shock. Hemorrhage should lead you to consider GI or reproductive (OB) emergencies. Patients undergoing dialysis may have chronic changes in mental status during dialysis; try to discern whether the level you see is the norm for that person or represents an acute or subacute change. Also consider the apparent state of the patient's health and his or her personal appearance, which can often give leads to a chronic condition or one of acute onset. Skin color and appearance can suggest chronic anemia (pale, cool, dry skin), shock (pale, clammy skin), or fever (dry, flushed).

Examination of the abdomen was covered in Chapter 32. Percussion may be very useful in the setting of urology. Pain on percussion of the flanks may suggest kidney inflammation and infection, and pain on percussion of the pelvic rim may suggest problems in the bladder. Remember that pregnancy may also be found during physical examination as you palpate above the pelvic rim. A ruptured ectopic pregnancy may be suggested by lower quadrant pain that increases with palpation and evidence of hemorrhage. In older men, palpation above the pelvic rim may reveal the enlarged, fluctuant mass of an obstructed bladder due to prostatic hypertrophy. In all men, exam includes examination of the scrotum and penis. Urethral discharge may suggest infection. Scrotal masses may be painful (such as infectious epididymitis) or nonpainful (testicular cancer, which is most common in young men, or a varicocele). Ask questions about acute or longer-term presence of any mass. For men with an apparently obstructed bladder, find out when they last urinated and whether there had been any change in pattern.

Generally, nephrologic and urologic emergencies don't produce acute abnormalities on exam, unlike GI emergencies. However, pain from an inflamed or infected kidney may be felt in the flank, and pelvic pain may suggest bladder origin or a reproductive problem in either a man or woman. Always consider possible miscarriage from either an ectopic pregnancy or an intrauterine one in girls and women of childbearing age.

6. Define acute renal failure. pp. 665-666

Acute renal failure is defined as a sudden (over a period of a day or days) drop in urine output to less than 400–500 ml per day. Low urine output is oliguria, whereas no urine output is anuria.

7. Discuss the pathophysiology of acute renal failure. pp. 665-668

There are three types of acute renal failure (ARF) based on pathophysiology: prerenal, renal, and postrenal. You may see all three types in the field. Remember that acute renal failure may be reversible if recognized and treated early enough.

• Prerenal ARF is due to insufficient blood flow to the kidneys. This type accounts for 40–80% of cases, and it is the most likely to be reversible if perfusion is restored. Common causes in the field include cardiac failure (often an MI), hemorrhage, dehydration, shock, and sepsis, as well as anomalies of a renal artery or vein.
• Renal ARF is due to a pathologic process within the kidney tissue itself. The three general causes are damage to small vessels and/or glomeruli, tubular cell damage, and interstitial damage. In each type, nephron function is lost.
• Postrenal ARF is due to obstruction at some point distal to the kidneys: both ureters, the bladder outlet, or the urethra. Postrenal ARF may be reversible if the obstruction is identified and removed before permanent kidney damage occurs.

8. Recognize the signs and symptoms related to acute renal failure. pp. 667-669

Timing of voiding difficulty can provide vital information: A normal history with sudden onset inability to void may suggest distal obstruction, whereas feeling ill over a number of days with some decrease in voiding may suggest chronic renal problems with an acute aggravation: Ask for renal history. Some triggers of acute renal failure may be obvious: dehydration secondary to diarrhea, hemorrhage, shock, sepsis. Visual inspection may reveal cool, pale, moist skin (which suggests shunting of blood to core, including kidneys, if shock is absent) and edema in hands, feet, or face. Physical findings may reveal the trigger for the failure: A distended, discolored abdomen may suggest severe intra-abdominal hemorrhage with hypoperfusion to kidneys.

9. Describe the management of acute renal failure. pp. 668-670

Because acute renal failure can cause life-threatening metabolic complications (consider the key role of the kidneys in regulation of fluid volume, electrolytes, and pH), provide close monitoring and support of the ABCs. High-flow oxygen should be used, and patient positioning and IV fluid resuscitation are important. In general, you want to protect fluid volume and cardiovascular function to minimize damage due to renal hypoperfusion and eliminate or reduce exposure to any potentially nephrotoxic drug.

Drug information may be available from medical direction; likewise, specific advice for care of dialysis patients may also be obtained before or during transit.

10. Integrate pathophysiological principles and assessment findings to formulate a field impression and implement a treatment plan for the patient with acute renal failure.
   pp. 665-670

If onset is acute and without evidence of distal obstruction, prerenal ARF may be suggested. Be sure to treat any identifiable potential trigger condition and aggressively protect fluid volume and oxygenation. Always remember that prerenal ARF may be reversible if you act quickly and correctly; this is still true in patients with chronic renal failure. Quick action may also preserve remaining function if renal causes are suspected. Renal causes may require the hospital setting for definitive treatment, but the treatment staples are the same as for prerenal. If history or exam suggests postrenal obstruction, be sure to get as much information as possible for use by hospital staff. For instance, known cancer in the abdomen or pelvis may suggest bilateral ureteral obstruction. Advanced age in men may suggest acute renal retention secondary to prostate enlargement, and history in boys or men of recent sexual activity, recreational drugs, or parties may suggest the possible presence of a foreign body in the urethra.

11. Define chronic renal failure.   p. 669-670

Chronic renal failure is inadequate kidney function due to the permanent loss of nephrons (usually representing a loss of at least 70–80% of total nephrons). When metabolic instability sets in (around 80% loss), the condition is termed end-stage renal failure, and either dialysis or kidney transplantation is required to survive.

12. Discuss the pathophysiology of chronic renal failure.   pp. 669-670

The three processes that can underlie chronic renal failure are the same as those producing acute renal failure: damage to small blood vessels or glomeruli, tubular cell injury, and damage to interstitial tissue. In each case, surviving nephrons adapt by structural changes that increase function, but these changes damage the nephrons themselves over time, leading to greater loss of nephron numbers. Common causes of damage to blood vessels and glomeruli include systemic hypertension, atherosclerosis, diabetes, and systemic lupus erythematosus, an autoimmune disease. Causes of tubular cell injury include nephrotoxic drugs and heavy metals and distal obstruction with backup of urine into the kidney. Finally, interstitial damage can be caused by infections including pyelonephritis and tuberculosis.

13. Recognize the signs and symptoms related to chronic renal failure. pp. 670-672

All of the kidney's major functions are deranged or lost in chronic renal failure. The general syndrome of signs and symptoms associated with chronic failure is termed uremia or uremic syndrome, so-called for the characteristic buildup of the waste urea. Clinical elements of uremia are found in Table 33-3 on text page 671. They include peripheral and pulmonary edema, hypertension, hyperkalemia and acidosis, congestive heart failure and accelerated atherosclerosis, headache, impaired mental status, seizures, muscle irritability, anorexia/nausea/vomiting, ulcers and GI bleeding, glucose intolerance due to cellular resistance to insulin, jaundice, uremic frost, pruritus, easy bleeding, chronic anemia, and vulnerability to infection. In addition, children and young adults may show poor growth and development, including delayed sexual maturation.

14. Describe the management of chronic renal failure.   pp. 672-675

Long-term management will focus on dialysis (either hemodialysis or peritoneal dialysis, dependent on individual circumstances) or transplantation.

15. Integrate pathophysiological principles and assessment findings to formulate a field impression and implement a treatment plan for the patient with chronic renal failure.   pp.

Immediate management is similar to that for acute renal failure. Focus on close monitoring and support of the ABCs with high-flow oxygen, positioning to support blood flow to internal organs and brain, and administration of IV fluid if hypovolemia is suggested. Chief prevention strategies are protection of fluid volume and cardiovascular function with correction of major electrolyte disturbances as merited by individual findings and the philosophy of erring on the side of conservative treatment. Close monitoring of the ECG may give you time to adjust and respond to cardiac problems caused by fluid overload or electrolyte disturbances. Life-threatening conditions should always be treated and lesser conditions or complications noted for consideration by the receiving staff. Where possible, be sure your impressions clearly note which conditions have been chronic (or the norm) for the patient and which findings represent acute changes. As indicated and allowed by medical direction, fluid lavage may be considered for patients who use peritoneal dialysis.

16. Define renal dialysis.   pp. 672-675

Renal dialysis is artificial replacement of some of the kidneys' vital functions. Two different technologies, hemodialysis and peritoneal dialysis, are widely used. Both rely on the physiologic principles of osmosis and equalization of osmolarity across a semipermeable membrane. As blood flows over such a membrane, many critical substances such as urea and sodium, potassium, and hydrogen ions move from blood into the hypo-osmolar solution, the dialysate, thus reducing the concentrations in blood. The overall effect is to lessen or eliminate temporarily volume overload and toxically high blood concentrations of electrolytes, urea, and other substances.

In hemodialysis, the patient's blood is passed through a machine containing a semipermeable membrane. Vascular access is established through a permanent anastamosis of an artery and vein in the forearm. If such a fistula is not possible, an indwelling catheter may be placed in the internal jugular vein. In peritoneal dialysis, the peritoneal membrane is used as the semipermeable membrane and dialysate solution is introduced into, and then removed from, the abdominal cavity via an indwelling catheter.

17. Discuss the common complications of renal dialysis.   pp. 673-674

Complications common to both forms of dialysis include physiologically destabilizing shifts in blood volume and composition and blood pressure during and shortly after dialysis. Other complications common to both forms include shortness of breath or dizziness and neurologic abnormalities ranging from headache to seizure or coma. Hypotension may represent dehydration, hemorrhage, or infection. Shortness of breath or chest pain may reflect cardiac dysrhythmias, ischemia, or even MI. In many cases the neurologic abnormalities represent shifts in the chemical milieu of the brain. Seizures are usually responsive to benzodiazepines.

Complications specific to hemodialysis include bleeding at the needle puncture site, local infection, and stenosis or obstruction of the internal fistula. Under normal flow conditions, you will hear or feel a bruit or thrill. Leading complications requiring hospitalization include thrombosis, infection, and development of an aneurysm. The latter are particularly common in patients in whom artificial graft material was used to construct the fistula. The most common complications in patients undergoing peritoneal dialysis include infection in the catheter or tunnel containing the catheter, or in the peritoneum itself. Because the incidence of peritonitis is roughly one episode per year, you may find the signs of peritonitis in this patient group.

18. Define renal calculi.   p. 675

Renal calculi (calculus, singular) are crystal aggregations in the kidney's urine collecting system. The same condition is referred to as nephrolithiasis. Although overall morbidity and mortality are low, brief hospitalizations are common for patients because of the severity of the pain as stones move through the renal pelvis, ureter, bladder, and urethra.

19. Discuss the pathophysiology of renal calculi.   p. 676

Some kinds of stones form as part of a systemic metabolic disorder such as gout (excess uric acid) or primary hyperparathyroidism (excess calcium). Most stones, however, form due to a more general imbalance between the amount of water flowing through the kidney tubing and the mineral ions, uric acid, and other relatively insoluble substances that are dissolved in that water. Trigger events for stone formation include change in diet, activity, or climate, all of which can alter water conservation or the amount of one or more such substances in the blood and, thus, the filtrate. Calcium stones are the most common and are most frequently seen in men aged 20 to 30 years. This type of stone is likely to recur and is likely to be found in a family history. Struvite stones are also common; their formation is often related to chronic urinary tract infection or frequent bladder catheterization. Perhaps because of the tie to infection, these stones are more common in women. Struvite stones can grow to fill the renal pelvis; in such cases, they present a "staghorn" appearance on X-rays. The less common stones are made of uric acid or cystine. Uric acid stones can occur in the presence of gout (about 50% of cases); they are also more common men and tend to occur in families. Cystine stones are the least common, and they are associated with excess cystine in filtrate. There is probably at least a partial genetic predisposition, and they are known to occur in families.

20. Recognize the signs and symptoms of renal calculi. **p. 676**

The assessment almost always focuses on pain as the chief complaint; the pain associated with kidney stones is generally conceded to be among the most severe known, ranking up there with labor pain. Typical history is a vague onset of discomfort in the flank progressing within an hour or so to an extremely sharp pain that may remain in the flank or radiate downward toward the pelvis or scrotum in men. Migrating pain suggests that the stone is in the lowest third of the involved ureter. Stones that lodge low in the ureter or within the bladder wall characteristically cause bladder symptoms such as frequency, urgency, and painful urination. In women these symptoms may make it difficult to distinguish stones from an infection. Physical exam will almost always reveal someone in considerable distress, often agitated and walking restlessly. High blood pressure and tachycardia may correlate with the degree of pain. Skin is typically cool, clammy, and pale due to autonomic discharge. Abdominal exam may be difficult to perform or assess given patient restlessness and muscle guarding secondary to pain.

21. Describe the management of renal calculi. **p. 677**

Management, as always, begins with the ABCs. Position for comfort, but be ready for vomiting, particularly if pain is severe or last oral intake recent. IV access may be needed for analgesic administration (if needed and appropriate per local protocol) or fluid to promote urine formation and movement of the stone through the urinary tract.

22. Integrate pathophysiological principles and assessment findings to formulate a field impression and implement a treatment plan for the patient with renal calculi.
   pp. 675-677

The common pathophysiology for all types of stones rests on an imbalance of water and relatively insoluble substances in the kidney filtrate. The type and size of stone, as well as current site in the urinary tract, may be discerned from personal and family history, as well as physical examination. Assessment for treatment (prior to and during transport) focuses on nature, site, and severity of pain. A urine sample may reveal blood in the presence of any type of stone. A urine sample may be particularly valuable from a woman patient because of inclusion of infection in the differential diagnosis, especially when bladder symptoms are present. Because passage of the stone is the ultimate goal, IV fluid may be beneficial as soon as it can be started as it promotes urine formation. Analgesia may be necessary, dependent on the individual patient and local protocol.

23. Define urinary tract infection. **p. 677**

Infection of the urinary tract implies infection in the urethra, bladder, or kidney, or the prostate gland in men. Urinary tract infections (UTI) are extremely common, accounting for about 6 million office visits per year, and you will see them in the field.

24. Discuss the pathophysiology of urinary tract infection. **pp. 677-678**

Because bacteria usually enter via the urethra, infections are more common in women (who have a much shorter urethra), paraplegic patients or others who require catheterization, and diabetic persons who have neuropathy involving the bladder. UTIs are generally divided into those affecting the lower urinary tract (namely, urethritis, cystitis, and prostatitis) and those of the upper urinary tract (pyelonephritis). Lower UTIs are much more common because of bacterial entrance via the urethra and NOT commonly via the bloodstream. Sexually active females may be at higher risk due to indirect factors (use of contraceptives vaginally and unintentional introduction of enteric flora into the urethra), and direct sexual transmission of infection can occur in males. Pyelonephritis usually occurs due to an infection that ascends through the urinary tract. The infectious inflammation can affect the interstitium, nephrons, or both. Incidence is highest during pregnancy and among the sexually active, paralleling the epidemiology of lower UTIs. Intrarenal abscesses can result, and rupture with spillage of contents into adjacent perirenal fat can cause formation of a perinephric abscess. Note that the likely pathogens are distinctly different in community-acquired and nosocomial infections.

25. Recognize the signs and symptoms related to urinary tract infection.   pp. 678-679

The typical triad of a lower UTI consists of painful urination, frequent urge to urinate, and difficulty in beginning and continuing flow. Pain frequently is visceral in character before voiding, progresses to severe, burning pain during and after urination, and then receding to visceral pain again. Many women will have a past medical history of such episodes, which may or may not have been diagnosed and treated. Vitals generally reflect those of someone in pain, with slight tachycardia and an increase in blood pressure. Exam will probably show tenderness over the pubis and cool, clammy skin. Patients with pyelonephritis typically have a fever and feel more generally ill. Their pain is typically in the flank or lower back with occasional reference to the neck or shoulder. Pain tends to be somewhat more somatic in character: moderately severe or severe and constant. The triad of lower urinary tract symptoms may or may not be present. (If not, ask whether they have been present recently.) The exam of a patient with pyelonephritis will be more striking, with a restless and ill appearance, warm, dry skin if fever is present, and possible tenderness over the flank. Lloyd's sign, tenderness on percussion of the lower back at the costovertebral angle, indicates pyelonephritis.

26. Describe the management of a urinary tract infection.   pp. 678-679

Management centers on monitoring and support of the ABCs. Positioning may help the patient with severe pain; be prepared in case the patient vomits. Analgesics are usually unnecessary; severely painful cases of pyelonephritis may be the exception. As with renal stones, hydration to increase and dilute urine flow is generally helpful. Use of IV fluid eliminates the risk of vomiting and satisfies treatment guidelines for possible surgical cases.

27. Integrate pathophysiological principles and assessment findings to formulate a field impression and implement a treatment plan for the patient with a urinary tract infection. pp. 677-679

Lower UTIs typically arise from infection that has entered via the urethra and has damaged tissue in the lower urinary tract. Hydration increases urine formation and promotes a more dilute urine (in a patient with normal renal function), and so it may help ease the symptoms of urgency, frequency, and pain in the patient with a lower UTI. Lack of systemic signs indicates that normal monitoring of ABCs is probably sufficient before and during transport. Patients with pyelonephritis (upper UTI) are more likely to show fever and other signs of systemic infection. IV hydration is also indicated for the same reasons and because IV access may be needed if physiologic instability develops or the patient is deemed later to be a surgical case. Transport for diagnosis and definitive treatment (appropriate antibiotic therapy) provides the link to long-term care.

28. Apply epidemiology to develop prevention strategies for urologic and nephrologic emergencies.   pp. 660, 670

Urinary tract infections, which include genitourinary infections in men, are the most typical urologic emergency. IV hydration promotes formation of a dilute urine that will help to eliminate bacteria within the urinary tract and decrease the triad of symptoms typically associated with lower UTIs: pain, frequency, and urgency. In elderly men, pain or poor urination may frequently be due to obstruction by an enlarged prostate: In these cases, the enlarged bladder will be felt on exam. Hydration is also useful for patients with pyelonephritis. ABCs should always be supported. Because UTIs, particularly lower UTIs, are more common among diabetic patients with neuropathy, it is also wise to assess diabetic status for signs of instability while monitoring ABCs as in all other patients. Remember to relay all relevant information on fetal age, presence of any complications, etc., in pregnant women presenting with UTIs to the receiving facility so they can arrange appropriate OB support.

Prevention strategies are probably most critical for the nephrologic emergencies directly involving kidney function (acute and chronic renal failure) and indirectly involving function (renal calculi with possible obstruction of the distal urinary tract). Prevention strategies in patients with acute renal failure (ARF), particularly cases that may be prerenal in origin, center on protection of fluid volume (usually through IV fluid) and support of cardiovascular function. Close monitoring of the ABCs is critical because of the possibility of metabolic derangements secondary to renal failure. Although reversibility is less likely with renal and postrenal ARF, the same strategies are important.

Avoidance of nephrotoxic drugs is important, as is alleviation of postrenal obstruction as soon as possible.

29. Integrate pathophysiological principles to the assessment of a patient with abdominal pain. pp. 660-665

Abdominal pain is questioned in similar ways whether or not the system of origin (GI, urinary tract, reproductive) is suspected from the initial size-up or complaint. The distinction of visceral and somatic pain may be useful in discerning cause, as is any referred pain pattern. For instance, most urologic/nephrologic emergencies typically feature visceral pain. However, renal stones are notorious for severe, somatic pain when they lodge somewhere in the distal urinary tract. Although the presence of nausea and vomiting is generally not helpful (if not due to GI disturbance, it is frequently due to autonomic discharge), presence of diarrhea suggests GI origin. Similarly, pain associated with urination suggests urinary tract origin.

30. Synthesize assessment findings and patient history information to accurately differentiate between pain of a urologic or nephrologic emergency and that of another origin. pp. 660-665

As noted in Chapter 32, many GI emergencies feature hemorrhage, and discernment through vital signs and physical exam of likely hemorrhage is an important first step in looking for system of origin. Examination of vomitus or diarrhea is also helpful. Gross examination of urine may not be helpful; however, gross blood is consistent with kidney stone in an otherwise appropriate presentation, and cloudiness of urine may represent the large numbers of white cells that may be present in pyelonephritis. Remember the typical pain patterns: GI emergencies often start with visceral pain (frequently located higher than in urinary tract conditions) and progress to somatic pain if an inflamed or damaged structure ruptures; postrupture peritonitis is not unusual. In contrast, most urologic/nephrologic emergencies feature visceral pain felt in the pelvis or male scrotum. Somatic-like pain felt in the flank, shoulder, or neck may suggest a kidney stone. Tenderness in the lower back at the costovertebral angle may suggest pyelonephritis, particularly if systemic signs of infection are present. If the urinary system appears likely, be sure to address the issue of renal function. Prevention strategies to prevent further loss of nephrons are vital to implement expediently.

31. Develop, execute, and evaluate a treatment plan based on the field impression made in the assessment. pp. 659-679

Because acute renal failure can cause life-threatening metabolic complications (consider the key role of the kidneys in regulation of fluid volume, electrolytes, and pH), close monitoring and support of the ABCs are essential. High-flow oxygen should be used, and positioning and IV fluid resuscitation are important. In general, you want to protect fluid volume and cardiovascular function to minimize damage due to renal hypoperfusion and eliminate or reduce exposure to any potentially nephrotoxic drug. The same applies to an acute problem in a patient with chronic renal failure. It is always important to prevent nephron loss, even in patients who already have compromise. In patients with renal calculi, it is important to promote urine formation and flow in an effort to move the stone through the distal urinary tract. In urinary tract infections (either lower or upper), IV hydration may promote formation of dilute urine that will flush some microbes from the urinary tract and relieve some of the pain, frequency, and urgency that might be present. Monitoring of the ABCs and support of any acute complications is always mandated.

CONTENT SELF-EVALUATION

Multiple Choice

1. The major functions of the urinary system include all EXCEPT:
   - A. maintenance of blood volume.
   - B. control of development of white blood cells.
   - C. regulation of arterial blood pressure.
   - D. maintenance of the balance of electrolytes and blood pH.
   - E. removal of many toxic wastes from the blood.

2. From which of these diseases do more than 25 000 Canadians suffer?
   - A. colitis
   - B. diabetes
   - C. kidney failure
   - D. pancreatitis
   - E. prostatic hypertrophy

3. Pain arising in hollow organs such as the ureter and bladder is know as:
   - A. parietal pain.
   - B. referred pain.
   - C. somatic pain.
   - D. visceral pain.
   - E. parenteral pain.

4. Pain that occurs when afferent nerve fibers carrying the pain message merge with other pain-carrying fibers at the spinal cord junction is called:
   - A. parietal pain.
   - B. referred pain.
   - C. somatic pain.
   - D. visceral pain.
   - E. parenteral pain.

5. Typical questions to ask when obtaining a focused history related to abdominal pain include all of the following EXCEPT:
   - A. previous history of similar event?
   - B. sudden or gradual unintended weight loss?
   - C. presence of chest pain?
   - D. last oral intake?
   - E. last date of sexual activity, if sexually active?

6. Indications that a woman's abdominal pain might be of obstetric (pregnancy-related) origin include all of the following EXCEPT:
   - A. known pregnancy or last menstrual period not in immediate past.
   - B. frequency and urgency of urination.
   - C. indications of intra-abdominal hemorrhage.
   - D. presence of blood in the vagina and on the vulva.
   - E. palpation of the uterus above the pelvic rim.

7. Lloyd's sign, which is an indication of pyelonephritis, is associated with:
   - A. pain on percussion of the costovertebral angle.
   - B. pain on palpation of the anterior costal margin.
   - C. periumbilical tenderness.
   - D. rebound pain at the level of the umbilicus.
   - E. pain on inhalation.

8. The two factors responsible for more than half of all cases of end-stage renal failure are:
   - A. damage due to nephrotoxic drugs and other substances and hypertension.
   - B. pyelonephritis and diabetes mellitus.
   - C. diabetes mellitus and hypertension.
   - D. infections and glomerulonephritis.
   - E. atherosclerosis and hypertension.

9. Common elements of uremic syndrome include all of the following EXCEPT:
    A. peptic ulcer.
    B. hyperkalemia and metabolic acidosis.
    C. easy bleeding and bruising.
    D. hypoglycemia.
    E. chronic anemia.

10. All of the following may be complications related to hemodialysis or peritoneal dialysis EXCEPT:
    A. chest pain.   **D.** seizure.
    B. dyspnea.   **E.** infection.
    C. hypertension.

11. All of the following statements about kidney stones are true EXCEPT:
    A. Renal calculi and nephrolithiasis are synonymous terms for kidney stones.
    B. Brief hospitalization for kidney stones is common because of the severity of pain while a stone is being passed.
    C. Immobilization and use of opiates and psychotropic drugs are risk factors for stones.
    D. Calcium and uric acid stones tend to run in families, suggesting a genetic link.
    E. Calcium stones are associated with chronic urinary tract infection or frequent bladder catheterization.

12. Which of the following types of renal calculi is found more often in women than in men?
    A. calcium stones   **D.** uric acid stones
    B. cystines stones   **E.** oxalate stones
    C. struvite stones

13. Risk factors for urinary tract infection include all of the following EXCEPT:
    A. female gender.
    B. pregnancy.
    C. advanced age.
    D. persons requiring routine bladder catheterization.
    E. persons with conditions causing urinary stasis.

14. The pathophysiology of urinary tract infections is due primarily to:
    A. bacterial infections.
    B. decreases in sexual intercourse.
    C. sexually transmitted disease infections.
    D. urinary tract lesions.
    E. viral infections.

15. Which of the following is not a problem triggering prerenal ARF?
    A. sepsis
    B. renal calculi
    C. heart failure
    D. hemorrhage
    E. shock

16. Atypical dermatological presentations of uremic syndrome include which of the following:
    A. pale, warm skin   **D.** uremic frost
    B. jaundice   **E.** pruritis
    C. ecchymoses

17. Which of the following is not a complication related to vascular access in dialysis?
    A. hypertension   **D.** headache
    B. shortness of breath   **E.** seizure
    C. chest pain

18. Which of the following DOES NOT occur during the attempted maintenance of blood volume with proper balance of water, electrolytes, and pH in a chronic renal failure patient?

A. retention of Na   D. metabolic acidosis
B. hypercalcemia   E. hypocalcemia
C. hyperkalemia

19. In dialysis , the patient's blood flows over a semi-permeable membrane to a special cleansing fluid that is hypo-osmolar to blood for a number of impurities EXCEPT:

A. urea.
B. sodium.
C. potassium.
D. calcium.
E. all of the above

20. The urinary system:

A. maintains blood volume.
B. enables blood to retain key substances.
C. removes a variety of toxic wastes from the blood.
D. controls maturation of red blood cells.
E. all of the above.

21. Palpable nontesticular masses which are painful may indicate:

A. prostatitis.
B. infectious epididymitis.
C. ectopic pregnancy.
D. pyelonephritis.
E. cystitis.

22. Which of the following is rarely the cause of urinary tract infections?

A. Candida   D. Klebsiella
B. Chlamydia   E. Pseudomonas
C. Proteus

23. As the GFR drops in prerenal failure, it results in:

A. retained phosphorous
B. metabolic alkalosis
C. respiratory acidosis
D. the formation of more urine
E. hyperkalemia

24. Which of the following is not a cause of renal ARF?

A. acute glomerulonephritis
B. acute tubular necrosis
C. pyelonephritis
D. embolism of the renal vein
E. malignant hypertension

25. Pain induced by palpation of the flanks, especially when accompanied by fever strongly suggests:

A. cystitis.
B. epididymitis.
C. pyelonephritis.
D. prostatitis.
E. a STD.

True/False

_____ 26. Patients most at risk for kidney disorders are the elderly, persons with diabetes mellitus, hypertension, or both, and patients with more than one risk factor.
   A. True
   B. False

_____ 27. Oliguria is defined as low urine output (roughly 400–500 ml daily or less), whereas anuria is complete absence of urine output.
   A. True
   B. False

_____ 28. In its earliest phase, postrenal ARF is reversible.
   A. True
   B. False

_____ 29. Always be alert for development of physiologic instability in patients with chronic renal failure, regardless of initial presentation.
   A. True
   B. False

_____ 30. Male patients with kidney stones rarely have referred pain in the testicle on the affected side.
   A. True
   B. False

_____ 31. Prostatis is the inflammation of the prostate gland.
   A. True
   B. False

_____ 32. Testicular cancer is more common in younger men.
   A. True
   B. False

_____ 33. A common element of uremic syndrome includes an increased vulnerability to infection.
   A. True
   B. False

_____ 34. The kidneys receive 30-35 per cent of cardiac output.
   A. True
   B. False

_____ 35. Auscultation of the abdomen is rarely helpful in renal and urological emergencies.
   A. True
   B. False

Matching

Write the letter of the term in the space provided next to the appropriate description.

   A. anuria   F. urinary stasis
   B. isothenuria   G. dialysis
   C. urethritis   H. perinephric abscess
   D. oliguria   I. cystitis
   E. pyelonephritis J. renal calculi

_____ 36. an infection and inflammation of the urinary bladder

_____ 37. kidney stones

_____ 38. decreased urine elimination to 400-500 mL or less per day

_____ **39.** the inability to concentrate or dilute urine relative to the osmolarity of blood

_____ **40.** a procedure that replaces some lost kidney function

_____ **41.** a pocket of infection in the layer of fat surrounding the kidney

_____ **42.** an infection and inflammation of the urethra

_____ **43.** an infection and inflammation of the kidney

_____ **44.** a condition in which the bladder empties incompletely during urination

_____ **45.** no elimination of urine

Chapter 34

Toxicology and Substance Abuse

Review of Chapter Objectives

After reading this chapter, you should be able to:

1. Describe the incidence, morbidity, and mortality of toxic and drug abuse emergencies. pp. 681-682

Toxicological emergencies are defined as those relating to exposure to a toxin, which is a chemical substance that causes adverse effects within the exposed individual. The term toxin includes drugs and poisons. Over the years, both the number and severity of toxicological emergencies has increased, so this is an area with which you must become familiar and must take steps to remain current in your knowledge. Roughly 10% of all EMS calls involve toxic exposures. About half of all accidental poisonings involve children under the age of 6 years; however, these poisonings tend to be relatively mild, accounting for only 5% of fatalities. Adult poisonings and drug overdoses are less frequent but they account for over 90% of hospital admissions for toxic exposures and 95% of the fatalities in this category.

2. Identify the risk factors most predisposing to toxic emergencies. pp. 681-682

Age is an important risk factor: About half of all accidental poisonings involve children under the age of 6 years. Intentional exposure as a form of drug experimentation or suicide is common in older children and young adults. Although adult poisonings and overdoses are less frequent, they account for 90% of hospital admissions for exposure to a toxic substance and 95% of fatalities. Among adults, most poisonings and drug overdoses are intentional. Interpersonal violence is a second risk factor: Poisoning in an older child can be the result of an intentional act by a parent or caregiver. Third, specific settings and situations make accidental poisoning more likely: Exposure in an industrial workplace or on a farm is increasingly common. Finally, use of medications is itself a risk factor. Most often, accidental exposures among older children and adults represent hypersensitivity reactions or dosage errors when taking prescribed medications.

3. Discuss the anatomy and physiology of the organs and structures related to toxic emergencies. pp. 682-684

Agents that are ingested through the mouth are exposed to the teeth, tongue, and mucous membranes of the mouth, as well as the throat and esophagus, before entering the stomach. As with intentionally ingested foods, agents remain in the stomach for a period of time before they pass into the small intestine (length of time depends on amount of stomach contents, whether contents are liquid or solid, etc.). Most absorption into the bloodstream takes place during passage of the agent through the small intestine.

Agents that are inhaled pass through the nose (possibly also the mouth), pharynx, trachea, and other, increasingly small airways before reaching the alveoli of the lungs. Absorption is largely at the distal end of the respiratory tree, the alveolar-capillary interface, which is the normal site for gas exchange (typically oxygen and carbon dioxide). Because the epithelial lining of the airways is relatively delicate, local effects can occur through tissue irritation in these medial structures. With surface absorption, the agent must pass through the skin or mucous membranes to which it has been applied in order to enter the body and cause local or systemic effects (the latter if agent is absorbed into bloodstream).

In cases of injection, the needle passes through the skin and subcutaneous tissues to reach a vein. The amount and depth of skin and subcutaneous tissue varies widely on different body sites. Typically, skin is thin and there is little subcutaneous tissue at sites with easy venous access such as the forearms and hands, as well as the comparable sites on the lower extremities. Be aware that drug addicts who have sclerosed readily available veins may have the ability to inject substances successfully into very small and usually inaccessible vessels.

4. Describe the routes of entry of toxic substances into the body.   pp. 682-684

There are four routes of entry into the body: ingestion, inhalation, surface absorption, and injection. Ingestion via the mouth is the most common route of entry for toxic exposure. Inhalation of a poison into the lungs results in rapid absorption from the alveolar air into the blood. Causative agents are in the form of gases, vapors, fumes, or aerosols. Surface absorption applies to cases in which entry is through the skin or mucous membranes. Injection applies when the toxic agent is injected under the skin, into muscle, or directly into the bloodstream.

5. Discuss the role of Poison Control Centers in the United States.   P. 682

Poison Control Centers of Canada assist in the treatment of poison victims and provide information on new products and new treatment recommendations. They are usually based in major medical centers serving large populations, and many have computer systems that allow staff to rapidly and accurately access information. Centers are available to you 24 hours a day, 7 days a week: Take the time to memorize the telephone number of the Center serving your area. Your Center can help you determine the potential toxicity for your patient when you give them the following information: type of agent, amount and time of exposure, and physical condition of the patient. With this information, you may be able to start the current, definitive treatment in the field. The Center can notify the receiving facility before you get the patient there.

6. Discuss the pathophysiology, assessment findings, need for rapid intervention and transport, and management of toxic emergencies.   pp. 681-722

• *Pathophysiology:* With each route of entry, there is a general pattern of possible toxic effects depending on the type and amount of agent involved: Immediate effects involve the tissues exposed to the toxic agent during entry. Delayed, systemic effects are related to absorption into the bloodstream and circulation throughout the body. In ingestion, corrosive agents can cause immediate injury through burns of the lips, oral mucous membranes, tongue, throat, and esophagus. Delayed effects can arise from absorption via the small intestine into the blood with effects on distant organs and tissues. In inhalation, immediate injury can occur from irritation of the airways resulting in extensive edema and damaged tissue. Delayed, systemic effects occur when the agent travels through the bloodstream and interacts with distant organs and tissues. In surface absorption, immediate injury can occur in the involved skin or mucous membranes. Delayed effects again relate to absorption into the bloodstream. With injection, immediate injury is seen as irritation at the injection site, usually visible as red, irritated, edematous skin. Delayed, systemic effects are again due to distribution throughout the body via the bloodstream.

• *Assessment:* Certain basic principles of assessment apply to most toxicological emergencies. For instance, maintain a high index of suspicion that a poisoning or drug overdose may have occurred. During scene size-up, look for potential dangers to yourself and other rescuers, such as a threat of violence from suicidal patients and the threat of accidental injection from used needles that may be hidden on the patient's person or at the scene. In cases with chemicals and hazardous materials, it is crucial that you use the proper clothing and equipment. Be sure that such articles are distributed to team members who have been trained in their use.

Assessment of the patient begins with a history if the patient appears to be able to give one. Critical questions include what kind of toxin the patient was exposed to and when exposure occurred (so you have clues for likelihood of immediate or delayed effects or both). Physical involves a rapid head-to-toe exam with full vital signs.

• *Time needs:* In accordance with your local protocols, relay information to Poison Control. Generally speaking, you never want to delay initiation of supportive or definitive care or transport because of delays in sending information to, or receiving information from, Poison Control. Time is of the essence, literally. Ongoing assessment is particularly important for this group of patients because they can deteriorate rapidly. Repeat initial assessment and vitals every five minutes for critical or unstable patients and every fifteen minutes for stable patients. Specific assessment findings are given for each type of agent.

• *General management:* The preliminary steps of management include securing rescuer safety and removing the patient from any toxic environment. Support ABCs as you would with any other patient, keeping in mind that damage may have occurred to the mouth, pharynx, and/or airway in inhalation injury, and to the mouth and pharynx in ingestion incidents. The direct access to the cardiovascular system that occurs with injection cases may also complicate support of the ABCs.

The first management step specific to toxicological emergencies is decontamination, that is, minimization of toxicity by reducing the amount of toxin absorbed into the body. Decontamination involves three steps: The first is reduction of intake of toxin (steps will be route-specific, such as removal from fume-filled atmosphere in inhalation, removal of clothes and cleansing of skin in surface absorption, removal of stinger in injection, etc.).

The second step is reduction of absorption after toxin is in the body, and this usually applies to ingestion incidents. The most common method entails use of activated charcoal to bind molecules of the toxin to it and prevent absorption into the bloodstream. Gastric lavage (stomach pumping) is of limited use as a step to reduce absorption. Lavage must be done within about one hour of exposure to be effective, and its possible complications (aspiration and perforation) are significant. Lavage is uncommon except in specific circumstances, for example, when the toxin doesn't bind to activated charcoal or when the toxin has no antidote. The third step in decontamination is enhanced elimination of toxin from the body. Cathartics enhance gastric mobility and thus may shorten the time the toxin is in the GI tract. Know the limitations in use of cathartics in your area, especially among pediatric patients, in whom they can induce severe electrolyte disturbances. Whole bowel irrigation with use of a gastric tube seems to be effective and carries few potential complications; however, its use is limited to only a few centers.

The third management step specific to toxicological emergencies is use of an antidote, a substance that neutralizes the specific toxin and counteracts its effects in the body. As you can see in Table 34-1 on text page 1461, there are not many antidotes, and few are 100% effective. Your best guide is to be thoroughly knowledgeable with your local protocols, the directions given by the Poison Control Center, and by counsel given by medical direction.

7. List the most common poisonings, pathophysiology, assessment findings, and management of poisoning by ingestion, inhalation, absorption, injection, and overdose.   pp. 682-722

Ingestion is the most common route of poisoning that you will see. Frequently ingested poisons include household products, petroleum-based agents such as gasoline and paint, cleaning agents such as alkalis and soaps, cosmetics, drugs (prescription, non-prescription, and illicit), plants, and foods. Some poisons can remain in the stomach for several hours, which may permit removal of the poison from the stomach and the body before systemic absorption can occur via passage through the small intestine. In at least one case, ingestion of aspirin, removal from the stomach is difficult because the ingested tablets bind together to form one large bolus. Useful questions for historical assessment include: (1) What did you ingest? (Obtain samples or containers whenever possible) (2) When did you ingest the substance? (3) How much did you ingest? (4) Did you drink any alcohol? (5) Have you attempted to treat yourself? (including induction of vomiting) (6) Have you been under mental health care, and, if so, why? (answer may indicate potential for suicide) (7) What is your weight? Physical exam is especially important because history may be unavailable or unreliable. Your exam should provide physical evidence of intoxication and discover co-morbid conditions that may affect treatment or response. Pay particular attention to skin, eyes, mouth, chest, circulation status, and abdomen. Be aware that a patient may have ingested multiple substances. Management centers on prevention of aspiration, intubation where necessary (RSI may be required to avoid patient's clamping down on tube), use of high-flow oxygen, and IV access for volume replacement and possible IV drug administration. Remember that it is always important to have ongoing cardiac monitoring and reassessment of vital signs.

Toxic inhalations can be self-induced or due to accidental exposure. Commonly inhaled poisons include toxic gases, carbon monoxide, ammonia, chlorine, freon, toxic vapors, fumes, or aerosols (from products such as paint and other hydrocarbons, glue, etc.), carbon tetrachloride, methyl chloride, tear gas, mustard gas, amyl nitrite, butyl nitrite, and nitrous oxide. Inhaled toxins primarily cause direct injury in the respiratory system, and these problems may be most severe in patients who inhaled a chemical or propellant concentrated in either a paper or plastic bag.

Given the pathophysiology of inhaled toxins, you should look for signs/symptoms related to three major systems: the central nervous system (dizziness, headache, confusion, hallucinations, seizures, or coma), the respiratory system (tachypnea, cough, hoarseness, stridor, dyspnea, retractions, wheezing, chest pain or tightness, rales or rhonchi), and the heart (dysrhythmias). Management starts with protecting yourself from any toxins in the atmosphere and removal of the patient from the injurious environment. Follow these guidelines: Wear protective clothing, use appropriate respiratory protection, and remove the patient's contaminated clothing. Then you can perform the initial assessment, history, and physical examination focusing on the central nervous system, respiratory, and cardiac systems. Support ABCs as you would with any other patient, keeping in mind that damage may have occurred to the mouth, pharynx, and/or airway as a direct, immediate injury. Contact medical direction and your Poison Control Center according to your particular protocols.

For **surface absorption,** the most common contacts are with poisonous plants such as poison ivy, poison sumac, and poison oak. Many toxic chemicals can be absorbed through the skin. Organophosphates, which are used as pesticides, are easily absorbed through the skin and mucous membranes, as is cyanide. The signs and symptoms vary widely depending on the toxin involved. Whenever you suspect surface absorption, take the following general steps: (1) wear protective clothing; (2) use appropriate respiratory protection; (3) remove the patient's contaminated clothing; (4) perform initial assessment, history, and physical exam; (5) initiate supportive measures; and (6) contact Poison Control Center and medical direction.

Females in the insect class *Hymenoptera,* honeybees, hornets, yellow jackets, wasps, and fire ants, are common causes of **injection injury.** In addition, spiders, ticks, snakes, and certain marine animals are known causes of toxic exposure by injection. In addition to intentional injections, most poisonings by injection involve bites and stings from insects and animals. Be alert for the possibility of allergic reactions or anaphylaxis. Over time, beware of delayed systemic reactions. General principles of field management include the following: (1) protection of all rescue personnel because the culprit organism may still be in the area; (2) removal of the patient from danger of repeated injection (particularly in the case of yellow jackets, wasps, or hornets); (3) whenever possible and safe, obtain the injury-causing organism and bring it to the emergency department; (4) perform initial assessment and rapid physical exam; (5) prevent or delay further absorption of the poison; (6) initiate supportive measures as needed; (7) watch for anaphylaxis; (8) transport as rapidly as possible; and (9) contact Poison Control Center and medical direction per protocols.

8. Define the following terms:

a.   Substance or drug abuse p. 715
Substance or drug abuse is use of a pharmacological product for purposes other than medically defined reasons.

b.   Substance or drug dependence   p. 715

Substance or drug dependence is the same thing as addiction: Physiological dependence exists if discontinuance of the drug would cause adverse physical reactions. Psychological dependence exists if discontinuance of the drug would cause the presence or increase in tension or emotional stress.

c.   Tolerance   p. 715

Tolerance is a phenomenon associated with continued use of a drug; it implies that the user must take increasingly large doses of the drug in order to achieve the same effect.

d.   Withdrawal   p. 715

Withdrawal refers to alcohol or drug discontinuance in which the patient's body reacts severely when deprived of the abused substance.

e.   Addiction   p. 715

Addiction is the same thing as dependence: Addiction can have a physiological or psychological component or both.

9.   List the most commonly abused drugs (both by chemical name and by street names). pp. 717-718

The most commonly abused drugs include: (1) alcohol in its fermented and distilled forms; (2) barbiturates such as phenobarbital and thiopental; (3) cocaine (both crack and rock forms); (4) narcotics/opiates such as heroin, codeine, meperidine, morphine, hydromorphone, pentazocine, methadone, Darvon, and Darvocet; (5) marijuana and hashish (also called grass or weed on the street); (6) amphetamines such as Benzedrine, Dexedrine, and Ritalin (called speed on the street); (7) hallucinogens including LSD, STP, mescaline, psilocybin, and PCP (also called angel dust); (8) sedatives from different chemical families such as Seconal, Valium, Librium, Xanax, Halcion, Restoril, Dalmane, and phenobarbital; and (9) the benzodiazepines, Valium, Librium, Xanax, Halcion, Restoril, Dalmane, Centrax, Ativan, and Serax.

10. Describe the pathophysiology, assessment findings, and management of commonly used drugs.   pp. 715-722

In addition to the specific drugs discussed in objective 11 below, it is notable that many groups of drugs produce definable toxic syndromes. Knowledge of these syndromes is useful because it helps you cluster information for compounds that produce similar clinical pictures. (1) Anticholinergic toxidrome is caused by belladonna alkaloids, atropine, scopolamine, synthetic anticholinergics, and incidental anticholinergics such as antihistamines, tricyclic antidepressants, and phenothiazines. Signs and symptoms include dry skin/mucous membranes, blurred near vision, fixed dilated pupils, tachycardia, hyperthermia and flushing, lethargy, and CNS signs, respiratory failure, and cardiovascular collapse. Management is as described for the tricyclics in objective 11. (2) Narcotic toxidrome is due to illicit drugs such as heroin and opium, prescription narcotics such as meperidine and methadone, and combination medications including narcotic agents such as hydromorphone, diphenoxylate (Lomotil), and oxycodone. Assessment findings include CNS depression, pinpoint pupils, slowed respirations, hypotension, positive response to naloxone. Note that pupils may be dilated and excitement may predominate the clinical picture. Management is described in objective 11 below. (3) The sympathomimetic toxidrome is caused by aminophylline, amphetamines, caffeine, cocaine, ephedrine, dopamine, methylphenidate (Ritalin), and phencyclidine. Features include CNS excitation, hypertension, seizures, tachycardia (hypotension with caffeine). Management is discussed in objective 11.

11. List the clinical uses, street names, pharmacology, assessment findings, and management for patients who have taken the following drugs or been exposed to the following substances:

a.   Cocaine pp. 693, 716-717

Cocaine has sympathomimetic effects, and assessment findings include CNS excitation, dilated pupils, hyperactivity, hypertension, seizures, tachycardia, and hypotension if taken with caffeine. Benzodiazepines may be required for seizures or diazepam 5–10 mg can be given as a seizure precaution; beta blockers are contraindicated because their unopposed alpha receptor stimulation can cause cardiac ischemia, increased hypertension, and hyperthermia. General measures include ABCs, respiratory support and oxygenation, ECG monitoring, IV access, and treatment of any life-threatening dysrhythmia.

b.   Marijuana and cannabis compounds   p. 718

Marijuana and related compounds can be smoked (inhaled) or taken orally, and pertinent signs and symptoms include euphoria, dry mouth, dilated pupils, and altered sensation. Management centers on ABCs, reassurance and speaking in a quiet voice, and ECG monitoring if indicated.

c.   Amphetamines and amphetamine-like drugs   pp. 716, 718

Amphetamines are CNS stimulants that can be taken orally or injected. Assessment findings include exhilaration, hyperactivity, dilated pupils, hypertension, psychosis, tremors, and seizures. Management centers on ABCs, oxygenation and ECG monitoring, IV access, treatment of any life-threatening dysrhythmia, and diazepam 5–10 mg as a seizure precaution. Diazepam and haloperidol in combination may be useful in controlling hyperactivity.

d.   Barbiturates   pp. 716, 718

The barbiturates, which are CNS depressants, can be taken orally or injected. Signs and symptoms include lethargy, emotional lability, incoordination, slurred speech, nystagmus, coma, hypotension, and respiratory depression. Management focuses on ABCs and respiratory support with oxygenation, IV access, ECG monitoring, and contact with Poison Control. Alkalinization of urine and diuresis may improve elimination of barbiturates from the body.

e.   Sedative-hypnotics   p. 718

Sedative-hypnotics are generally taken orally, and they are also CNS depressants. Assessment findings include altered mental status, hypotension, slurred speech, respiratory depression, shock, bradycardia, and seizures. Management centers on ABCs with respiratory support and oxygenation, IV access, ECG monitoring, and possible use of naloxone dependent on agent taken and advice of medical direction.

f.   Cyanide   p. 694

Cyanide can enter the body by different routes dependent on the product in which it is found. It is present in household items such as rodenticides and silver polish, as well as in foods such as fruit pits and seeds. It can be liberated into inhalable form through burning of nitrogen-containing products such as plastics, silks, or synthetic carpets. Cyanide also forms in patients on long-term therapy with nitroprusside. Regardless of entry, cyanide acts extremely quickly as a cellular asphyxiant, inhibiting the vital process of cellular respiration. Signs and symptoms include a burning sensation in mouth and throat, headache, confusion, combative behavior, hypertension, and tachycardia, followed by hypotension and further dysrhythmias, seizures and coma, and pulmonary edema. Management relies on removal from the source, immediate supportive measures, and treatment with a cyanide antidote kit containing amyl nitrite ampules, a sodium nitrite, and a sodium thiosulfate solution. Adding nitrites to blood converts some hemoglobin to methemoglobin, which binds cyanide, removing it from its free form in the blood. Thiosulfate binds with cyanide to form a soluble nontoxic compound. Note: Cyanide is rapidly toxic, so it is crucial you be familiar with a cyanide antidote kit if your unit carries one.

g.   Narcotics/opiates   p. 716

The narcotics can be taken orally or by injection. Pertinent assessment findings include CNS depression, constricted pupils, respiratory depression, hypotension, bradycardia, pulmonary edema, and coma. General management centers on ABCs with respiratory support and oxygenation, IV access, and ECG monitoring. You may use the antidote naloxone, which can be titrated to relieve symptoms of toxicity without provoking withdrawal symptoms in addicts. General instructions involve use of 1–2 mg naloxone IV or endotracheally per medical direction until respiration improves. Larger doses (2–5 mg) may be required in the management of Darvon overdose and alcoholic coma.

### h.	Cardiac medications	pp. 696

The number of available cardiac medications grows continually, and many classes exist, including antidysrhythmics, beta blockers, calcium channel blockers, glycosides, ACE inhibitors, etc. General pharmacology includes regulation of heart function by reducing heart rate, suppressing automaticity, reducing vascular tone, or some combination of these. Although overdose can be intentional, it often is due to an error in dosage. At the level of overdose, signs and symptoms include (1) nausea and vomiting, (2) headache, dizziness, and confusion, (3) profound hypotension, (4) cardiac dysrhythmias (usually bradycardic), (5) cardiac conduction blocks, and (6) bronchospasm and pulmonary edema (especially with beta blockers). Management centers on initiating standard toxicological emergency assessment and treatment immediately. Severe bradycardia may not respond well to atropine, so you should have an external pacing device at hand. Some cardiac medications have antidotes; these include calcium for calcium channel blockers, glucagon for beta blockers, and digoxin-specific Fab (Digibind) for digoxin. Contact medical direction before giving any of these antidotes.

### i.	Caustics	pp. 696-698

Caustic substances can either be acids or alkalis, and such substances are common at home and in the industrial workplace. Strong caustics can cause severe burns at the site of contact; if ingested, they can cause tissue destruction at the lips, mouth, esophagus, and more distal regions of the GI tract. Strong acids by definition have a pH less than 2; they are found in plumbing solutions and bathroom cleaners. Contact usually produces immediate, severe pain due to tissue coagulation and necrosis. Often this type of burn produces an eschar over the site, which may act as a shield to protect deeper tissues from damage. Because the substance is in the stomach much longer than the esophagus, the stomach is the more likely to sustain damage. Immediate or delayed hemorrhage is possible, as is perforation. Absorption of acids into the bloodstream produces acidemia, which needs to be managed along with the local, direct effects. Strong alkaline agents by definition have a pH greater than 12.5; they are present in solid or liquid form in household products such as drain cleaners.

These agents cause local injury through liquefaction necrosis. Because of a delay in pain sensation, these agents are often present longer at the site of contact, allowing for greater tissue damage and deeper tissue injury. Solid products can stick to the oropharynx or esophagus, causing bleeding, perforation, and inflammation of central chest structures. Liquid alkalis are more likely to injure the stomach because, like the liquid strong acids, they pass quickly through the esophagus. Within 1–2 days of exposure to a strong alkali, complete loss of mucosal tissue can occur, followed either by gradual healing or further bleeding, necrosis, and stricture formation.

Assessment findings include facial burns, pain in the lips, tongue, throat and/or gums, drooling and trouble swallowing, hoarseness, stridor, or shortness of breath, and shock from bleeding and vomiting. Both assessment and initiation of management must be rapid and aggressive to avoid significant morbidity and mortality. As with other toxicological situations, protect yourself and initiate standard toxicological assessment and treatment: Pay particular attention to the airway. Injury to the oropharynx and/or larynx may make airway control and ventilation very difficult and may go so far as to require cricothyrotomy. Because caustic substances do not adhere to activated charcoal, there is no indication for it. It is controversial whether ingestion of milk or water acts effectively to coat the stomach lining or dilute the caustic. It is clear that rapid transport is essential. Hydrofluoric acid, which is used to clean glass in laboratory settings and in etching glass in art work, is a specific example of a strong acid that can be lethal in even small exposure doses. Management specific to this agent is immersion of the exposed limb in iced water with magnesium sulfate, calcium salts, or benzethonium chloride.

### j.	Common household substances	p. 708

Many of these substances contain caustic agents (either strong acids or strong alkalis) as major ingredients; see objective i above for details.

### k.	Drugs abused for sexual purposes/sexual gratification	p. 716

This group includes a number of miscellaneous agents that are used to stimulate and enhance sexual experience but do not have medically approved indications for such use. MDMA, popularly known as Ecstasy, is an example. Ecstasy is a modified form of methamphetamine and has similar, although milder, effects. Look for its use on college campuses and in nightclub settings. Initial signs and symptoms of use include anxiety, tachycardia, nausea, and hypertension, followed by relaxation, euphoria, and feelings of enhanced emotional insight. Studies indicate prolonged use may cause brain damage. Cases that can lead to death have the following assessment findings: confusion, agitation, tremor, high temperature, and diarrhea. No specific treatment exists, so supportive measures should be taken. Flunitrazepam, or Rohypnol, is illegal in Canada. but has been used as a "date rape drug" when slipped into a woman's drink. The drug is a strong benzodiazepine that causes sedation and amnesia. When this drug is suspected, treat as for other benzodiazepines but remember to look for consequences of sexual assault and be sure to treat them as well.

l.   Carbon monoxide   pp. 695
Carbon monoxide is a tasteless, odorless gas that is often created by incomplete combustion. Because of its chemical structure, it has an affinity for hemoglobin over 200 times greater than that of oxygen. Once carbon monoxide has bound to hemoglobin, it is very difficult to displace and it causes an effective hypoxia. Because of the variability of signs and symptoms (depending on dose and duration of exposure), many people ignore poisoning until toxic levels are in the blood. Early symptoms resemble those of the flu. Combining likely causes of carbon monoxide generation with early symptoms raises this red flag: Beware carbon monoxide poisoning in multiple patients living together in a poorly heated and ventilated space who have "flu-like" symptoms. Specific signs and symptoms include headache, nausea and vomiting, confusion or other manifestation of altered mental status, and tachypnea. Because of the difficulty of displacing carbon monoxide from hemoglobin, definitive treatment may require use of a hyperbaric chamber (in which oxygen is present at greater than atmospheric pressure). In the field, take these steps: Ensure safety of rescuing personnel, remove the patient(s) from contaminated area, begin immediate ventilation of affected area, and initiate supportive measures including high-flow oxygen via nonrebreather device (this last is critical).

m.   Alcohols   pp. 719-722
Ethyl alcohol is the form of alcohol in beverages, and it is the single most common substance of abuse among Canadians. Alcoholism, dependence on alcohol, progresses in much the same way as drug dependence discussed earlier in the chapter. The early symptoms of alcohol use, especially at low doses, include loss of inhibitions and emotionally excitatory effects, which can cause some of the aberrant behaviors associated with alcohol intoxication. Once ingested, alcohol is completely absorbed from the stomach and intestinal tract within approximately 30–120 minutes. After absorption, it is widely distributed in blood to all body tissues, and concentrations of alcohol in the brain rapidly approach the level in the blood. Alcohol's major physiologic effects are as a CNS depressant: toxicity, can include stupor, coma, and death. Because the liver is the major site of detoxification within the body, compromise of liver function increases the course and severity of alcohol intoxication.

Another significant health effect is peripheral vasodilation, which results in flushing of the skin and a feeling of warmth. In cold conditions, this can increase loss of body heat and help to produce hypothermia. Alcohol-related diuresis is due to inhibition of vasopressin, a hormone responsible for homeostasis of water balance. The dry mouth associated with hangovers may in part be due to the alcohol-induced dehydration. Methanol, wood alcohol, is so toxic it is not safe for human consumption. However, methanol toxicity can occur either as an accident or because an alcoholic individual could not obtain ethyl alcohol. Methanol causes visual disturbances, abdominal pain, and nausea and vomiting even at low doses. Occasionally, methanol toxic patients complain of headache or dizziness or present with seizures and obtundation. Ethylene glycol, a related compound, can also be involved in toxic emergencies. It produces similar symptoms, but its CNS effects, including hallucinations, coma, and seizures, present at even earlier stages.

Assessment findings in an individual with chronic alcoholism include poor nutrition, alcoholic hepatitis, liver cirrhosis with subsequent esophageal varices, loss of sensation in hands and feet, loss of cerebellar function shown as poor balance and coordination, pancreatitis, upper GI hemorrhage (which is often fatal), hypoglycemia, subdural hematoma secondary to falls, and rib and extremity fractures, also secondary to falls. When you are in the field, keep in mind that conditions such as a subdural hematoma, sepsis, and diabetic ketoacidosis can, along with other conditions, mimic alcohol intoxication. For instance, the breath odor of ketoacidosis can resemble that of alcohol.

Abrupt discontinuance of alcohol by a dependent individual may provoke a withdrawal syndrome that can prove to be potentially lethal. Withdrawal symptoms can occur several hours after sudden abstinence and last up to 5–7 days. Common signs and symptoms include a coarse tremor of hands, tongue, and eyelids, nausea and vomiting, general weakness, increased sympathetic tone, tachycardia, sweating, hypertension, orthostatic hypotension, anxiety, irritability or depressed mood, and poor sleep. Seizures may occur, as can delirium tremens (DTs). DTs usually develop on the second or third day of withdrawal and are characterized by a decreased level of consciousness associated with hallucinations and misinterpretation of nearby events. Both seizures and delirium tremens are ominous signs.

Alcohol intoxication, whether acute or chronic, should not be underestimated as a toxic emergency. In cases of suspected alcohol abuse, manage as follows: (1) Establish and maintain the airway, (2) determine if other drugs or substances are involved, (3) start an IV with lactated Ringer's solution or normal saline, (4) complete blood glucometry and give 25 g $D_{50}W$ if the patient is hypoglycemic, (5) administer 100 mg thiamine IV or IM, (6) maintain a sympathetic and supportive attitude with the patient, and (7) transport to emergency department for further care. Note: Medical direction may suggest diazepam in severe cases of seizure or hallucination.

n.   Hydrocarbons   p. 698
Numerous household substances contain hydrocarbons, organic compounds composed primarily of carbon and hydrogen. Hydrocarbons include kerosene, naphtha, turpentine, mineral oil, chloroform, toluene, and benzene, and they are found in lighter fluid, paint, glue, lubricants, solvents, and aerosol propellants. Exposure can be via ingestion, inhalation, or surface absorption. Signs and symptoms of hydrocarbon exposure vary according to agent, dose, and route of exposure, but common problems include burns due to local contact, respiratory signs (wheezing, dyspnea, hypoxia, or pneumonitis from aspiration or inhalation), CNS signs (headache, dizziness, slurred speech, ataxia, and obtundation), foot and wrist drop with numbness and tingling, and cardiac dysrhythmias. Research has shown that fewer than 1% of hydrocarbon poisonings require physician care. In cases where you know the agent in question and in which the patient is asymptomatic, medical direction may permit the patient to stay at home. On the other hand, hydrocarbon poisonings can be very serious. If the patient is symptomatic, does not know the causative agent, or has taken a specific agent (such as halogenated or aromatic hydrocarbon compounds) that requires GI decontamination, standard toxicological emergency procedures and prompt transport are indicated.

o.   Psychiatric medications   pp. 698-701
The tricyclic antidepressants were standard therapy for depression for years, despite concerns that their generally narrow therapeutic window made accidental toxic-level exposure, as well as intentional overdose, potentially common. Despite the introduction of newer, safer antidepressants, a number of tricyclics are still in use for depression, as well as chronic pain syndromes and migraine prophylaxis. Agents still in use include amitriptyline (Elavil), amoxapine, clomipramine, doxepin, imipramine, and nortriptyline. Signs and symptoms on assessment include dry mouth, blurred vision, urinary retention, and constipation. Late into overdose, you may find confusion and hallucinations, hyperthermia, respiratory depression, seizures, tachycardia and hypotension, and cardiac dysrhythmias (such as heart block, wide QRS complex, and *torsade de pointes*.) In addition to standard toxicological procedures, cardiac monitoring is critical because dysrhythmias are the most common cause of death. If you suspect a mixed overdose with a benzodiazepine, DO NOT use Flumazenil because it might precipitate a seizure. If significant cardiac toxicity is evident, sodium bicarbonate may be used as an additional therapy; contact medical direction as needed.

p.   Newer anti-depressants and serotonin syndromes   pp. 700-701
In the recent past, a number of new antidepressants that are not related to the tricyclics have been introduced. Because of their high safety profile in both therapeutic and overdose amounts, these drugs have virtually replaced the tricyclics in clinical practice. This group includes trazodone

(Desyrel), bupropion (Wellbutrin), and the large group of drugs known as selective serotonin reuptake inhibitors (SSRIs). Drugs in this group include Prozac, Luvox, Paxil, and Zoloft. Their pharmacology, as indicated by group name, centers on prevention of reuptake of serotonin from neural synapses in the brain, theoretically raising the amount of serotonin available to modulate brain function. The usual signs and symptoms in overdose cases are generally mild, including drowsiness, tremor, nausea and vomiting, and sinus tachycardia. Occasionally trazodone and bupropion cause CNS depression and seizures, but deaths are rare, and they have been reported in situations with mixed overdoses and multiple ingestions.

You should know that the SSRIs have been associated with serotonin syndrome, a constellation of signs/symptoms correlated with increased serotonin level and triggered by increasing the dose of SSRI or adding a second drug such as a narcotic or another antidepressant. Serotonin syndrome is marked by the following: (1) agitation, anxiety, confusion, and insomnia, (2) headache, drowsiness, and coma, (3) nausea, salivation, diarrhea, and abdominal cramps, (4) cutaneous piloerection and flushed skin, (5) hyperthermia and tachycardia, and (6) rigidity, shivering, incoordination, and myoclonic jerks. Because of the lower morbidity and mortality in these drugs compared with overdoses with the older antidepressants, standard toxicological emergency procedures suffice. The patient should discontinue all serotonergic drugs and you should institute supportive measures. Benzodiazepines or beta blockers are occasionally used to improve patient comfort, but they are rarely given in the field.

q. Lithium   p. 701

Lithium is the most effective drug used in the treatment of bipolar disorder (a psychiatric disorder also known as manic depression). Pharmacology is unclear. However, it is known that lithium has a narrow therapeutic index, making toxicity relatively common during normal use and in overdose situations. Assessment findings of toxicity include thirst and dry mouth, tremor, muscle twitching, increased reflexes, confusion, stupor, seizures, coma, nausea, vomiting, diarrhea, and bradycardia and dysrhythmias. Lithium overdose should be treated primarily with supportive measures. Use standard toxicological procedures but remember that activated charcoal does not bind lithium and should not be used. Alkalinization of the urine with sodium bicarbonate and diuresis with mannitol may increase elimination of lithium, but severe toxicity requires hemodialysis.

r. MAO inhibitors pp. 699-700

Monoamine oxidase inhibitors (MAO inhibitors) have been used historically as psychiatric agents, primarily as antidepressants. Recently they have found limited use as treatment for obsessive-compulsive disorder. These drugs have always had relatively limited usage for several reasons: They have a narrow therapeutic index, multiple drug interactions, potentially serious interactions with foods rich in tyramine (for instance, red wine and cheese), and high morbidity and mortality in overdose incidents. The pharmacology of MAO inhibitors directly affects CNS neurotransmitters: The drugs inhibit the breakdown of norepinephrine and dopamine while increasing the molecular components necessary to produce more. Remember that overdose with this group of drugs is very serious, even though symptoms may not appear for up to 6 hours.

Assessment findings include headache, agitation, restlessness, tremor, nausea, palpitations, tachycardia, severe hypertension, hyperthermia, and eventually bradycardia, hypotension, coma, and death. Newer MAO inhibitors have been introduced into the marketplace; they appear to be less toxic and avoid the food interactions that involved the older generation of MAO inhibitors. They are reversible in effect; however, overdose outcome data are not yet available for these drugs. Management includes reversal if the drug is in the newer class of reversible MAO inhibitors, prompt institution of standard toxicological procedures, and, if needed, symptomatic support for seizures and hyperthermia with use of benzodiazepines. If a vasopressor is needed, use norepinephrine.

s. Non-prescription pain medications: (1) nonsteroidal anti-inflammatory agents (2) salicylates (3) acetaminophen   pp. 702-703

(1) Nonsteroidal anti-inflammatory agents (called NSAIDs) are a large, commonly used group of drugs such as naproxen sodium, indomethacin, ibuprofen, and ketorolac (Toradol). Overdose is common, and assessment findings include headache, ringing in the ears (tinnitus), nausea, vomiting, abdominal pain, swelling of the extremities, mild drowsiness, dyspnea, wheezing,

pulmonary edema, and rash and itching. There is no specific antidote for NSAID toxicity, so use general overdose procedures including supportive care and transport to the emergency department for evaluation and any necessary symptomatic treatment.

(2) Salicylates are some of the most common over-the-counter drugs taken and among the most common taken in overdose. They include aspirin, oil of wintergreen, and some prescription combination medications. About 300 mg/kg aspirin can cause toxicity. In these amounts, the salicylate inhibits normal energy production and acid buffering in the body, resulting in metabolic acidosis that further injures other organ systems. Assessment findings include tachypnea, hyperthermia, confusion, lethargy and coma, cardiac failure and dysrhythmias, abdominal pain and vomiting, and non-cardiogenic (inflammatory) pulmonary edema and adult respiratory distress syndrome. The findings of chronic overdose are somewhat less severe and tend not to include abdominal complaints. It is thus difficult to distinguish chronic overdose from early acute overdose or acute overdose that has progressed past the initial abdominal irritation stage. In all cases, management of salicylate poisoning should be treated with use of standard toxicological emergency procedures. Activated charcoal definitely reduces drug absorption and should be used. If possible, learn the time of ingestion because blood levels measured at the right interval can be indicative of the expected degree of injury. Most symptomatic patients require generous IV fluids and may need urine alkalinization with sodium bicarbonate. Severe cases may require dialysis.

(3) Acetaminophen (Tylenol) has few side effects in normal dosage, and it is one of the most commonly used drugs in America for fever/pain. It is also a common ingredient in combination medications and is found in some prescription combination medications. In large doses, acetaminophen can be very dangerous: A dose of 150 mg/kg is considered toxic and may result in death secondary to liver damage. A highly reactive metabolite is responsible for most adverse effects, but this is avoided in most cases by detoxification. When large amounts enter the body in overdose, this detoxification system is overloaded and gradually depleted, leaving the metabolite in the circulation to cause liver necrosis. It is important for you to learn and remember that the signs and symptoms of toxicity appear in four stages: Stage 1—0.5 to 24 hours after ingestion, marked by nausea, vomiting, weakness, and fatigue; Stage 2—24 to 48 hours, marked by abdominal pain, decreased urine, elevated liver enzymes; Stage 3—72 to 96 hours, marked by liver function disruption; and Stage 4—4 to 14 days, marked by gradual recovery or progressive liver failure. Field management relies on standard toxicological procedures. Again, it is important to find time of ingestion because this may allow blood levels to be drawn at a time appropriate to predict potential injury. An antidote (N-acetylcysteine, or NAC, Mucomyst) is available and highly effective. However, NAC is usually given based on clinical and lab studies and in the hospital setting.

t.   Theophylline   p. 703
Theophylline is a member of the group of drugs called xanthines. It is generally used by patients with asthma or COPD because it has moderate bronchodilation and mild anti-inflammatory effects. It has a narrow therapeutic index and high toxicity, so it has been used less frequently recently. Thus, it is not a factor as often as it once was in overdose injuries. Assessment findings include agitation, tremors, seizures, cardiac dysrhythmias, and nausea and vomiting. Theophylline can cause significant morbidity and mortality. In an overdose setting, you must start toxicological emergency procedures immediately. Theophylline is on a short list of drugs that have significant entero-hepatic circulation. Thus, activated charcoal in multiple doses over time will continuously remove more and more theophylline from the body. Dysrhythmias should be treated according to ACLS procedures.

u.   Metals   pp. 703-704
With the exception of iron, heavy metal overdose is rare. Metals that can cause toxicity include lead, arsenic, and mercury, all of which affect numerous enzyme systems in the body and thus cause a variety of symptoms. Some also have direct local effects when ingested and they accumulate in various organs.

• *Iron:* The body needs only small daily amounts of iron; excess amounts are easily obtained through non-prescription supplements and multivitamins. Children have the tendency to overdose on iron by taking too many candy-flavored chewable vitamins containing iron. Symptoms occur when more than 20 mg/kg of elemental iron are ingested. Excess iron causes GI injury and possible hemorrhagic shock, especially if it forms concretions (lumps formed when tablets fuse together). Patients with significant iron ingestions may have visible tablets or concretions in the stomach or small intestine on X-ray. Other signs and symptoms include vomiting (often hematemesis) and diarrhea, abdominal pain, shock, liver failure, metabolic acidosis with tachypnea, and eventual bowel scarring and possible obstruction. It is essential to start standard toxicological procedures promptly. Because iron inhibits GI motility, tablets remain in the stomach for a long time and may possibly be easier to remove via gastric lavage (especially if concretions are not present). Because activated charcoal does not bind metals, it should not be used for iron overdose or for any other metal overdose. Deferoxamine, a chelating agent, may be used in iron overdose as an antidote because it binds iron such that less enters cells to cause damage.

• *Lead and mercury:* Both metals are found in varying amounts in the environment. Lead was often used in glazes and paints before its toxic potential was realized. Mercury is a contaminant from industrial processing and is also found in some thermometers and temperature-control switches in homes. Both acute and chronic overdose are possible with both metals. Signs and symptoms of heavy metal toxicity include headache, irritability, confusion, coma, memory disturbance, tremor, weakness, agitation, and abdominal pain. Chronic poisoning can result in permanent neurological injury, which makes it crucial that heavy metal levels be monitored in the environment of a patient with toxicity. You need to remember the signs and symptoms of heavy metal poisoning and promptly institute standard procedures. Although activated charcoal is not helpful, various chelating agents (such as DMSA, BAL, and CDE) are available and may be used in definitive management in the hospital.

v. Plants and mushrooms pp. 705-706

Plants, trees, and mushrooms are common contributors to accidental toxic ingestions. You should know that many decorative home plants can present a toxic danger to children. Most Poison Control Centers distribute pamphlets that list relevant household plants. In nature, it is impossible to identify all toxic plants and mushrooms. A general approach for you to take is to obtain a sample of the offending plant if possible, trying to find a complete leaf, stem, or flower. Mushrooms are very difficult to identify from small pieces. Because many ornamental plants contain irritating material, be sure to examine the patient's mouth and throat for redness, blistering, or edema. Identify other findings during the focused physical exam. Mushroom poisonings generally involve a mistake in identification of edible mushrooms or accidental ingestion by children. Mushrooms in the class *Amanita* account for over 90% of deaths; they produce a poison that is extremely toxic to the liver and carry a mortality rate of about 50%. Signs and symptoms of poisonous plant ingestion include excessive salivation, lacrimation, diaphoresis, abdominal cramps, nausea, vomiting, and diarrhea, as well as decreasing levels of consciousness, eventually progressing to coma. Contact Poison Control if at all possible for guidance on management. If contact isn't possible, follow the procedures outlined under food poisoning.

12. Discuss common causative agents or offending organisms, pharmacology, assessment findings, and management for a patient with food poisoning, a bite, or a sting. pp. 704-714

Food poisoning can be due to a variety of causes including bacteria, viruses, and bacterial-associated chemical toxins. All notoriously produce varying degrees of gastrointestinal distress. Bacterial food poisonings range in severity. Bacterial exotoxins (secreted by bacteria) and enterotoxins (exotoxins associated with GI diseases) cause nausea, vomiting, diarrhea, and abdominal pain. Food contaminated with the bacteria *Shigella, Salmonella,* or *E. coli* can produce more severe reactions, often leading to electrolyte imbalance and hypovolemia. The world's most toxic poison is produced by *Clostridium botulinum,* and exposure presents as severe respiratory distress or even arrest. Fortunately, botulism rarely occurs except in cases of improper food storage procedures such as canning. A variety of seafood poisonings result from toxins produced by dinoflagellate-contaminated shellfish such as clams, mussels, oysters, and scallops. This exposure syndrome is called paralytic shellfish poisoning and can lead to respiratory arrest in addition to the GI symptoms. Toxicological emergencies can also arise from toxins found within commonly eaten fish. Bony fish poisoning (Ciguatera poisoning) is most frequent in fish caught in the Pacific Ocean or along the tropical reefs of Florida and the West Indies. Ciguatera may have an incubation period of 2–6 hours before producing myalgia and paresthesia. Scombroid (histamine) poisoning results from bacterial contamination of mackerel, tuna, bonitos, and albacore. Both Ciguatera and scombroid poisoning cause the standard GI symptoms; scombroid poisoning also produces immediate facial flushing due to histamine-induced vasodilation.

Except for botulism, food poisoning is rarely life threatening and treatment is largely supportive. In cases of suspected food poisoning, contact Poison Control and medical direction, and take the following steps: (1) perform necessary assessment, (2) collect samples of suspected food source, (3) support ABCs with airway maintenance, high-flow oxygen, intubation or assisted ventilation as needed, and establish IV access. In addition, consider administration of antihistamines (especially in seafood poisonings) and antiemetics.

Spider and snake bites can be common and significant toxicological emergencies in certain parts of the country. The brown recluse spider lives in southern and midwestern states. It is found in large numbers in Tennessee, Arkansas, Oklahoma, and Texas. It has also been reported in Hawaii and California. The brown recluse is about 15 mm in length, generally lives in dark, dry locations, and can often be found in or around a house. The bites themselves are usually painless, and bites often occur at night while the victim is asleep. The initial, local reaction occurs within minutes and consists of a small erythematous macule surrounded by a white ring. Over the next 8 hours or so localized pain, redness, and swelling develop. Tissue necrosis develops over days to weeks. Other symptoms include fever, chills, nausea, vomiting, joint pain, and in severe cases, bleeding disorders (namely, disseminated intravascular coagulation, DIC). Treatment is largely supportive, and there is no antivenin. Antihistamines may reduce systemic reactions and surgical excision may be required for necrotic tissue. Black widow spiders live in all parts of the continental U.S. and are often found in woodpiles or brush. The female spider bites, and the venom is very potent, causing excessive neurotransmitter release at the synaptic junctions. Immediate, local reaction includes pain, redness, and swelling. Progressive muscle spasms of all large muscles can develop and are usually associated with severe pain. Other systemic symptoms are nausea, vomiting, sweating, seizures, paralysis, and decreased level of consciousness. Field treatment is largely supportive, with reassurance an important factor. IV muscle relaxants may be needed for severe spasms. If medical direction orders it, you may use diazepam or calcium gluconate. Calcium chloride is ineffective and should not be used. Because hypertensive crisis is possible, monitor BP carefully. Transport as rapidly as possible so antivenin can be given in the hospital.

There are hundreds of snake bites annually in North America., but few deaths. The assessment findings depend on snake, location of the bite, and the type and amount of venom injected. Two families of poisonous snakes are native to North America.: the pit vipers (cottonmouths, rattlesnakes, and copperheads) and the coral snake, a distant relative of the cobra. Pit viper venom contains hydrolytic enzymes capable of destroying most tissue components. They can produce hemolysis, destroy of other tissue elements, and may affect the clotting ability of the blood. They produce tissue infarction and necrosis, especially at the site of the bite. A severe pit viper bite can produce death within 30 minutes. However, most fatalities occur from 6 to 30 hours after the bite, with 90% within the first 48 hours. Assessment findings for pit viper bites include fang marks (often little more than a scratch or abrasion), swelling and pain at wound site, continued oozing from wound, weakness, dizziness, or faintness, sweating and/or chills, thirst, nausea and vomiting, diarrhea, tachycardia and hypotension, bloody urine and GI hemorrhage (these are late), ecchymosis, necrosis, shallow respirations progressing to respiratory failure, and numbness and tingling around face and head. The first goal in treatment is to slow absorption of venom; remember that about 25% of bites are dry, that is, no venom is injected. Antivenin is available but should only be considered for severe cases as evidence by marked systemic signs and symptoms. Routine treatment involves keeping the patient supine, immobilizing the affected limb with a splint, maintaining the extremity in a neutral position without any constricting bands, and giving supportive care with high-flow oxygen, IV with crystalloid fluid, and rapid transport. Note: DO NOT apply ice, cold pack, or freon spray to wound, DO NOT apply an arterial tourniquet, and DO NOT apply electrical stimulation from any source in an attempt to retard or reverse venom spread.

Coral snakes, which are small and with small fangs, are primarily found in the southwest. A mnemonic that you should remember is "Red touch yellow, kill a fellow; red touch black, venom lack." This indicates the stripe pattern of the coral snake: red-yellow-black-yellow-red. Coral snake venom contains some of the same enzymes as pit viper venom, but it additionally has a neurotoxin that will result in respiratory and skeletal muscle paralysis. Assessment findings include the following (noting that there may be no local or systemic effects for as long as 12–24 hours): localized numbness, weakness, and drowsiness, ataxia, slurred speech and excessive salivation, paralysis of tongue and larynx producing difficulty in swallowing and breathing, drooping of eyelids, double vision, dilated pupils, abdominal pain, nausea and vomiting, loss of consciousness, seizures, respiratory failure, and hypotension. Treatment includes the following steps: (1) wash the wound with lots of water, (2) apply a compression bandage and keep extremity at the level of the heart, (3) immobilize the limb with a splint, (4) start an IV with crystalloid fluid, and (5) transport to the emergency department for antivenin. Note: DO NOT apply ice, cold pack, or freon spray to the wound; DO NOT incise the wound; and DO NOT apply electrical stimulation from any device in an attempt to retard or reverse venom spread.

Stings (injection injuries) can come from insects and marine animals. Many people die from allergic reactions to insect stings, particularly wasps, bees, hornets, and fire ants. Only the common honeybee leaves a stinger. Wasps, hornets, yellow jackets, and fire ants sting repeatedly until removed from contact. Assessment findings include localized pain, redness, swelling, and a skin wheal. Idiosyncratic reactions are not considered allergic if they respond well to antihistamines. Signs and symptoms of an allergic reaction include localized pain, swelling, redness, and skin wheal, itching or flushing of skin or rash, tachycardia, hypotension, bronchospasm, or laryngeal edema, facial edema, and uvular swelling.

General management includes washing of the sting area, gentle removal of stinger, if present (scrape, do not squeeze), application of cool compresses, and observation for allergic reaction or anaphylactic shock. Marine animal injection injuries are a threat in some coastal areas, especially in warmer, tropical waters. Toxin injection can be from jellyfish or coral stings or from punctures by the bony spines of animals such as sea urchins and stingrays. All marine venoms contain substances that produce pain that is disproportionate to the size of the injury. These toxins are unstable and heat sensitive, and heat will relieve the pain and inactivate the venom. Signs and symptoms of marine animal injection include intense local pain and swelling, weakness, nausea and vomiting, dyspnea, tachycardia, and hypotension or shock (in severe cases). In any case of suspected injection, treat by establishing and maintaining airway, application of a constriction bandage between the wound and the heart no tighter than a watchband (to occlude lymphatic flow only), application of heat or hot water, and inactivation or removal or any stingers. Because both fresh and salt water contain considerable bacterial and viral pollution, you should always be alert to possible secondary infection of a wound. In cases of marine-acquired infections, be sure to consider *Vibrio* species.

13. Given several scenarios of poisoning or overdose, provide the appropriate assessment, treatment, and transport.   pp. 681-722

Remember that the basic assessment of a patient with a toxicological emergency includes careful scene size-up, protection of rescue personnel, and rapid response to any needs to support the ABCs. Treatment includes decontamination and use of antidotes, where available. Rapid transport is standard. Detailed specifics for many drugs, toxic substances, and animal bites and stings are given in other objectives for this chapter.

CONTENT SELF-EVALUATION

Multiple Choice

_____ 1. Which of the following statements about the epidemiology of toxicological emergencies is NOT true?
- A. The frequency of toxicological emergencies continues to increase both in number and severity.
- B. About 70% of accidental poisonings occur among children aged 6 years or younger.
- C. Toxicological emergencies account for about 5% of emergency department visits and EMS responses.
- D. More serious poisonings, especially in older children, may represent intentional poisoning by a parent or caregiver.
- E. Adult poisonings and overdoses account for 95% of the fatalities in this category.

_____ 2. Many inhalation exposures are accidental, and leading agents include the following:
- A. carbon dioxide, carbon tetrachloride, and ammonia.
- B. toxic vapors, plants, and chlorine.
- C. carbon monoxide, nitrous oxide, and petroleum-based products such as gasoline.
- D. carbon monoxide, ammonia, and toxic vapors.
- E. chlorine, cleaners (soaps and alkalis), and carbon monoxide.

_____ 3. All of the following are guidelines to follow in cases of toxicological emergencies EXCEPT:
- A. maintaining a high index of suspicion for possible poisonings.
- B. recording everything you see or smell at the scene that might help determine cause.
- C. taking appropriate measures to protect all rescue personnel and any bystanders.
- D. centering general management on support of ABCs, decontamination of patient, and use of antidote, if there is one.
- E. removing the patient from a toxic environment as promptly as possible.

_____ 4. The most common route of entry for toxic substances is:
- A. inhalation.
- B. ingestion.
- C. surface absorption.
- D. injection.
- E. adsorption.

_____ 5. The three principles of decontamination are:
- A. removal of patient from toxic environment, reduction in intake of toxin, and increase in elimination of toxin from body.
- B. removal of patient from toxic environment, removal of patient's clothing and washing of patient's body, increase in elimination of toxin from body.
- C. removal of patient from toxic environment, reduction in intake of toxin, and use of antidote, if one.
- D. removal of patient's clothing and washing of body, reduction in intake of toxin, and reduction in absorption of toxin already in body.
- E. reduction in intake of toxin into the body, reduction of absorption of toxin already in the body, and increase in elimination of toxin from the body.

_____ 6. The most widely used means of reducing absorption of toxins in the body is:
- A. gastric lavage (stomach pumping).
- B. activated charcoal.
- C. syrup of ipecac.
- D. whole bowel irrigation.
- E. chelating agents.

7. Flumazenil is an antidote for which of the following ingested substances?
   - **A.** arsenic
   - **B.** benzodiazepines
   - **C.** cyanide
   - **D.** ethylene glycol
   - **E.** methyl alcohol

8. Which of the following is not a question commonly asked of a poisoning patient during the focused history?
   - **A.** How much of the agent(s) did you ingest?
   - **B.** How long ago did you ingest the agent(s)?
   - **C.** Were any people with you when you ingested the agent(s)?
   - **D.** What is your weight?
   - **E.** Have you attempted to treat yourself in any way?

9. All of the following statements are correct when treating ingestion emergencies EXCEPT:
   - **A.** Maintaining the ABCs is the top priority along with monitoring of all vitals.
   - **B.** Prevention of aspiration is a major objective, and intubation may be necessary.
   - **C.** An IV at keep-vein-open rate is recommended for all potentially dangerous ingestion incidents.
   - **D.** Induce vomiting unless it is against local protocol or you are told not to do so by Poison Control.
   - **E.** Follow general treatment guidelines with decontamination procedures.

10. All of the following are respiratory signs or symptoms of a toxic inhalation exposure EXCEPT:
    - **A.** bradycardia.
    - **B.** chest tightness.
    - **C.** cough.
    - **D.** tachypnea.
    - **E.** dizziness.

11. The typical signs and symptoms of carbon monoxide poisoning include:
    - **A.** a burning sensation in mouth and throat, headache, and confusion.
    - **B.** headache, seizure or coma, tachypnea.
    - **C.** tachypnea, pulmonary edema, a burning sensation in mouth and throat.
    - **D.** tachypnea, tachycardia, headache, and confusion.
    - **E.** headache, nausea and vomiting, confusion or other altered mental status.

12. Response to poisoning with one of the cardiac medications often involves bradycardia, which may require use of:
    - **A.** atropine.
    - **B.** an external pacing device.
    - **C.** a beta blocker.
    - **D.** digoxin.
    - **E.** calcium.

13. Common assessment findings for ingestion with a caustic include all of the following EXCEPT:
    - **A.** chest and abdominal pain.
    - **B.** drooling and trouble swallowing.
    - **C.** facial burns.
    - **D.** hoarseness and/or stridor
    - **E.** pain in the lips, tongue, throat, or gums.

14. A patient has spilled a large quantity of an unknown acid on his skin. Treatment should consist of:
    - **A.** contacting poison control for instructions.
    - **B.** covering the area with activated charcoal.
    - **C.** diluting the acid with bicarbonate.
    - **D.** irrigation with copius amounts of water.
    - **E.** irrigation with copius amounts of milk.

15. Ingestion of alkalis usually results in:
  A.   immediate and intense pain.
  B.   bradycardia.
  C.   local burns to the mouth and throat.
  D.   ulceration and perforation of the stomach lining.
  E.   liquefaction necrosis.

16. Drugs with narrow therapeutic indexes are more likely to be involved in accidental toxicological emergencies. Two such drugs are:
  A.   lithium and the selective serotonin reuptake inhibitors (SSRIs).
  B.   tricyclic antidepressants and salicylates.
  C.   tricyclic antidepressants and lithium.
  D.   tricyclic antidepressants and SSRIs.
  E.   salicylates and lithium.

17. It is particularly important to know time of ingestion when a blood test (timed properly) can predict degree of damage. Two drugs to which this statement especially applies are:
  A.   acetaminophen and tricyclics.
  B.   SSRIs and tricyclics.
  C.   acetaminophen and non-steroidal anti-inflammatory drugs.
  D.   salicylates and non-steroidal anti-inflammatory drugs.
  E.   salicylates and acetaminophen.

18. Serotonin syndrome includes all of the following signs and symptoms EXCEPT:
  A.   nausea, diarrhea, abdominal cramps.
  B.   hypotension.
  C.   agitation and confusion.
  D.   hyperthermia.
  E.   rigidity, incoordination, myoclonic jerks.

19. Chelating agents are often useful in cases of toxicity due to:
  A.   lithium.   D.   heavy metals.
  B.   theophylline.   E.   salicylates.
  C.   some cardiac medications.

20. All of the following statements are true about MAO inhibitors EXCEPT:
  A.   Overdose cases may be very serious, even though initial signs/symptoms may appear hours after ingestion.
  B.   MAO inhibitors have been used to treat depression and obsessive-compulsive disorder.
  C.   MAO inhibitors as a group have a narrow therapeutic index.
  D.   MAO inhibitors may interact negatively with foods containing tyramine, such as cheese and wine.
  E.   In overdose, death usually follows the eventual signs of tachycardia, hypertension, and coma.

21. In common toxic drug ingestions, the use of benzodiazepines is frequently recommended with:
  A.   alcohol, narcotics, and barbiturates.
  B.   alcohol, hallucinogens, and barbiturates.
  C.   cocaine, amphetamines, and hallucinogens.
  D.   cocaine, alcohol, and amphetamines.
  E.   cocaine, amphetamines, and barbiturates.

22. Alcohol is a(n):
  A.   depressant.   D.   stimulant.
  B.   narcotic.   E.   oxidant.
  C.   opiate.

23. Signs and symptoms associated with amphetamine usage include all of the following EXCEPT:
   A. constricted pupils.   D. psychosis.
   B. exhilaration.   E. tremors.
   C. hypertension.

24. Which of the following statements about delirium tremens is NOT true?
   A. They usually develop 2–3 days after withdrawal of alcohol.
   B. They can occur in individuals who have experienced recent binge drinking.
   C. DTs are marked by decreased level of consciousness with hallucinations.
   D. Seizures and delirium tremens are ominous signs.
   E. DTs are associated with a significant mortality rate.

25. Which of the following statements is NOT a sign or symptom of heavy metal toxicity?
   A. headache, irritability, confusion
   B. memory disturbance
   C. hallucinations.
   D. tremor, weakness, agitation.
   E. abdominal pain

True/False

26. Immediate effects of toxins are often localized to the site of entry, whereas delayed effects are often systemic in nature.
   A. True
   B. False

27. Never delay supportive measures or transport due to a delay in contacting Poison Control Center.
   A. True
   B. False

28. Do not involve law enforcement in a possible suicide case until it is clear that suicide was intended.
   A. True
   B. False

29. The physical exam is crucial in toxicological emergencies, and it has two purposes: (1) documenting physical evidence of intoxication and (2) detecting any underlying illness or condition that might affect either patient's symptoms or outcome of exposure.
   A. True
   B. False

30. The first priorities, in proper order, with surface-absorption exposures are to remove the patient from the toxic environment, perform the initial assessment, and then ensure your safety.
   A. True
   B. False

31. The narcotic toxidrome is characterized by CNS depression, whereas the sympathomimetic toxidrome is characterized by CNS excitation.
   A. True
   B. False

32. If you suspect mixed ingestion with tricyclics and benzodiazepines, do NOT use Flumazenil because it may precipitate seizures.
   A. True
   B. False

33. In cases of suspected food poisoning or poisoning involving plants and mushrooms, it is important to bring samples along with the patient if possible.
  A.   True
  B.   False

34. In cases involving bites or stings, fatalities are most likely among patients who have an allergic reaction or anaphylaxis to insect stings.
  A.   True
  B.   False

35. Altered mental status and slurred speech are signs/symptoms of Xanax overdose.
  A.   True
  B.   False

Matching

Write the letter of the definition in the space provided next to the term to which it applies.

_____	**36.** injection	_____	**41.**	therapeutic index
_____	**37.** tolerance	_____	**42.**	ingestion
_____	**38.** toxin	_____	**43.**	delirium tremens (DTs)
_____	**39.** inhalation	_____	**44.**	enterotoxin
_____	**40.** poisoning	_____	**45.**	decontamination

A. an exposure to a non-pharmacological toxic substance
B. entry of a substance into the body via a break in the skin
C. bacterial exotoxin that produces GI symptoms and diseases such as food poisoning
D. entry of a substance into the body via the respiratory tract
E. entry of a substance into the body via the GI tract
F. any chemical that causes adverse effects on an organism exposed to it
G. dosage range between effective and toxic dosages
H. need to progressively increase dosage to achieve same effect
I. potentially lethal syndrome found when alcohol withdrawn from chronic abusers
J. process of minimizing toxicity by reducing amount of toxin absorbed into the body

Chapter 35

Hematology

Review of Chapter Objectives

After reading this chapter, you should be able to:

1. Identify the anatomy and physiology of the hematopoietic system. (see Chapter 12)

The components of the hematopoietic system include the blood, bone marrow, liver, spleen, and kidneys. The process of hematopoiesis forms the cellular components of blood. In the fetus, this first takes place outside the bone marrow in the liver, spleen, lymph nodes, and thymus. By the fourth month of gestation, the bone marrow begins to produce blood cells. After birth and across the span of life, bone marrow continues to fulfill this critical function barring the development of some pathological process.

In hematopoiesis, the stem cell reproduces to maintain a constant population of cells. Some stem cells further differentiate into myeloid multipotent stem cells that, in turn, differentiate into unipotent progenitors, which ultimately mature into the formed elements of blood: red blood cells (RBCs), white blood cells (WBCs), and platelets. Pluripotent stem cells may also differentiate into common lymphoid stem cells, ultimately becoming lymphocytes. Erythropoietin, the hormone responsible for red blood cell production, is produced by the kidneys and, to a lesser extent, the liver. The liver also removes toxins from the blood and produces many of the clotting factors and proteins in plasma. The spleen plays an important role in the immune system with its cells that scavenge abnormal blood cells and bacteria.

2. Discuss the following: (see Chapter 12)

Plasma
Plasma is a thick, pale yellow fluid consisting predominately of water, electrolytes, and proteins. It also contains some fats, carbohydrates, and chemical messengers. Plasma is the medium that carries the formed elements of the blood cells.

Red blood cells (erythrocytes)
Erythropoiesis—the process of RBC production—is triggered by the secretion of erythropoietin. The secretion occurs whenever the kidney's renal cells sense hypoxia. Erythropoietin, in turn, causes the bone marrow to produce more red blood cells, which increases the oxygen-carrying capacity of the blood.Red blood cells have a life span of about 4 months, although hemorrhage, hemolysis (RBC destruction), or sequestration by the liver or spleen may significantly reduce this time. The spleen and liver contain macrophages (a specialized type of scavenger white blood cell) that can remove damaged or abnormal cells from circulation.

Hemoglobin
Hemoglobin is an iron compound found in the red blood cells. It has a great affinity for oxygen and helps transport oxygen from the pulmonary capillaries to the tissues. One gram of hemoglobin can carry 1.34 milliliters of oxygen.

Hematocrit

Hematocrit is the packed cell volume of red blood cells per unit of blood. This measurement is obtained by spinning a blood sample in a centrifuge to separate the cellular elements from the plasma. Red cells—the heaviest component of the blood (due to the hemoglobin's iron)—settles to the bottom of the tube. The white blood cells form the next layer, while plasma floats on top. The height of the RBCs is divided by the total height of the tube's contents (cellular components + plasma) and is reported as a percentage. The normal range is from 40–52 percent, although women tend to have slightly lower levels than men.

White blood cells

White blood cells originate in the bone marrow from undifferentiated stem cells. The process by which the stem cells differentiate into the various immature forms of white blood cells—known as -blasts—is known as leukopoiesis. The three main -blasts include granulocytes, monocytes, and lymphocytes. While leukocytes provide protection from foreign invasion, each type of white blood cell has its own unique function. Healthy people have between 5 000–9 000 white blood cells per milliliter of blood. The presence of illness, however, can cause that number to rise to more than 16,000.

Granulocytic white blood cells include three types—eosinophils, neutrophils, and basophils. Basophils act as storage sites for the body's histamine. When stimulated, the basophils degranulate and release the histamine, typically in an allergic reaction. Eosinophils can inactivate the chemical mediators of an acute allergic reaction, thus modulating the anaphylactic response. The main purpose of neutrophils is to fight infection.

Monocytes, the second main grouping of white blood cells, serve as "trash collectors." They move throughout the body engulfing both foreign invaders and dead neutrophils. Some monocytes remain in circulation, while others migrate to other sites to further mature into macrophages. Monocytes and macrophages also secrete growth factors to stimulate the formation of red blood cells and granulocytes. Some macrophages become fixed within tissues of the liver, spleen, lungs, and lymphatic system, becoming part of the reticuloendothelial system. Here they have the capability of stimulating lymphocyte production in an immune response.

Lymphocytes, the third main grouping of white blood cells, circulate in the blood. They are also found in the lymph fluid and nodes, bone marrow, spleen, liver, lungs, skin, and intestine. These highly specialized cells contain surface receptor sites specific to a single antigen and initiate an immune response in order to rid the body of infectious agents.

Platelets, clotting, and fibrinolysis

Platelets, or thrombocytes, function to form a plug at an initial bleeding site and to secrete several factors important to clotting. Normally, platelets number between 150 000–450 000 per milliliter. They are derived from megakaryocytes that come from an undifferentiated stem cell in the bone marrow. They can survive from 7–10 days, after which they are removed from circulation by the spleen.

Damage to cells or to the *tunica intima* (innermost lining of the blood vessels) triggers clotting, or the "coagulation cascade." Cascading can be activated by either an intrinsic pathway (trauma to blood cells from turbulence) or an extrinsic pathway (damage to vessels).

Following the intrinsic pathway, platelets release substances that lead to the formation of prothrombin activator. In the presence of calcium, the prothrombin converts to thrombin, which in turn converts fibrinogen to stable fibrin. The fibrin traps blood cells and more platelets to form a clot. Following the extrinsic pathway, smooth muscle fibers in the *tunica media* (middle lining of the blood vessels) contract. The resulting vasoconstriction reduces the size of the injury, which reduces blood flow through the area. This action limits blood loss and allows platelet aggregation (formation of a platelet plug) and the subsequent conversion of the prothrombin activator.

Clotting factors or proteins are primarily produced in the liver and circulate in an inactive state. Prothrombin and fibrinogen are the best known of these factors. Damaged cells send out a chemical message that activates a specific clotting factor. This activates each protein in a sequence geared toward stable clot formation.

An enzyme on the surface of the platelet membrane makes it sticky. This stickiness allows platelet aggregation to occur.

Fibrinolysis, the process through which plasmin dismantles a blood clot, does not signal the end of the coagulation cascade. Once a fibrin clot is formed, it releases a chemical called plasminogen, which is subsequently converted to plasmin. Plasmin begins dismantling or lysing a clot, which may take hours or days. This allows the scarring process to take place.

Hemostasis

Hemostasis involves three mechanisms to prevent or control blood loss: (1) vascular spasms that reduce the size of a vascular tear, (2) platelet plugs (an aggregate of platelets that adheres to collagen), and (3) the formation of stable fibrin clots (coagulation).

3. Identify the following: (see Chapter 13)

Inflammatory process

The inflammatory process is a nonspecific defense mechanism that wards off damage caused by some microorganism or trauma. The process helps localize damage, while simultaneously destroying the source and facilitating repair. The process may be triggered by various agents—infectious, chemical, or immunologic—or by trauma. Following local tissue injury, chemical messengers are released. These chemicals attract white blood cells, increase capillary permeability, and cause vasodilatation, which in turn produces the redness, swelling, warmth, and pain associated with inflammation.

Systemic inflammation is another type of inflammatory process. It occurs as a result of bacterial infection. Fever, which commonly accompanies systemic inflammation, is thought to occur in response to the chemical mediators released by macrophages seeking to rid the body of an infectious agent. These same mediators act on the brain, triggering sympathetic nervous system stimulation and causing heat conservation, vasoconstriction, and fever.

Cellular and humoral immunity

Lymphocytes, the primary cells of the immune system, include two types—T cells and B cells. T cells, which mature in the thymus, are responsible for handling mediated or cellular immunity. In humoral immunity, B cells produce antibodies to combat infection. Cellular immunity is responsible for antigen-triggered release of effector cells. This type of immunity causes the following: (1) delayed hypersensitivity reactions, (2) transplant rejection, and (3) defense against intracellular organisms. Humoral immunity occurs when an antigen triggers the development and release of specific antibodies necessary for the body's defense.

Alterations in immunologic response

A variety of factors—drugs, diseases, genetic conditions, and infection—can trigger alterations in the body's immunologic response. Genetics and viral infection, for example, can cause the immune system to develop antibodies against the body's own tissues, which leads to a variety of localized or systemic diseases. Immunosuppressive drugs, like those used to prevent transplant rejection, and cancer chemotherapy agents (as well as cancer itself) can also cause alterations, the most significant of which is a reduce ability to fight infections. Alterations in immunity may also be acquired through infection with the human immunodeficiency virus (HIV), which has an affinity for T lymphocytes, rendering the body at great risk of opportunistic infections.

Regardless of the cause, alterations in immunologic response and the resultant risk of infection make it imperative for the EMS provider to protect the patient from disease-causing agents. You must practice good hand washing techniques, correct IV procedures, and proper wound care.

4. Identify blood groups.   pp. 725-726

The presence of certain antigens (proteins) on the surface of a donor's red blood cells allows the patient's body to recognize it as "self" or "not self." Following a transfusion, antibodies in the patient's own blood attack any foreign antigens that may be present in the transfused blood, causing a reaction. The presence or absence of such antigens and antibodies provides us with the blood typing system used today—a system designed to prevent reactions to transfusions.

To see how this system works, consider these cases. Someone with A antigen on his or her red blood cells would have anti-B antibodies. This person is said to have type A blood. Conversely, someone with B antigens would have anti-A antibodies, resulting in type B blood. Other people have both A and B antigens, but neither anti-A or anti-B antibodies. Their blood type is AB. With regard to transfusions, these individuals are known as universal recipients because they lack any antibodies to attack foreign blood cells. Yet other people have neither A nor B antigens, but have both anti-A and anti-B antibodies. Their blood type is O. Individuals with type O blood are called universal donors because their blood has no antigens to trigger a reaction.

In addition to the presence of A and B antigens, blood typing must take into account another factor—the Rh antigen found on red blood cells. People with the Rh factor are said to be Rh positive; people without it are said to be Rh negative. When identifying an individual on the basis of blood type, all of these elements are taken into account. For example, one person may be O positive, while another might be AB negative.

5. List erythrocyte disorders. pp. 733-735

Erythrocyte disorders include anemia, sickle cell disease, and polycythemia. Of the three, anemia is the most common disorder. It is typically classified as a hematocrit (red blood cell count) of less than 37 percent in women and 40 percent in men. The reduction may be due to blood loss, the destruction of red blood cells (hemolytic anemia), or diseases that limit the production of red blood cells. Anemia is not a disease, but the sign of an underlying problem.

Sickle cell anemia is an inherited disorder of red blood cell production, so named because the red blood cells become sickle-shaped when oxygen levels are low. The cells are less flexible and increase the viscosity of the blood, which in turn leads to vasooclussive crisis and multiple organ damage; The C-shaped cells survive for only a short time, typically 10–20 days.
Polycythemia is an abnormally high hematocrit due to excess production of red blood cells. It is rare and most frequently occurs in persons over 50 years of age. The increased hematocrit predisposes the patient to thrombosis and platelet dysfunction.

6. List leukocyte disorders. pp. 735-737

Disorders or problems of the white blood cells (leukocytes) have a significant impact on the body's defense system. These problems include leukopenia (too few white blood cells) or leukocytosis (too many white blood cells). A variation of leukopenia is neutropenia in which there are too few neutrophils; this is potentially dangerous, as the absolute count for neutrophils is an excellent indicator of the immune system's status. Improper white cell formation may also cause disorders such as leukemia (cancer of the hematopoietic cells) or lymphoma (cancer of the lymphatic system).

7. List platelet and clotting disorders pp. 737-739

The common platelet disorders include thrombocytosis, thrombocytopenia, hemophilia, and von Willebrand's disease. Thrombocytosis is an increase in the production and number of platelets secondary to other disorders and usually leaves the patient asymptomatic.

Thrombocytopenia is an abnormal decrease in the number of platelets. It is due to decreased platelet production, sequestration of platelets in the spleen, destruction of platelets, or any combination of the three. *Acute idiopathic thrombocytopenia purpura (ITP)* results from destruction of platelets by the immune system. It is most commonly seen in children following a viral infection or in adult women with autoimmune disease.

Hemophilia is a blood disorder in which one of the proteins necessary for blood clotting is missing or defective. When a person with hemophilia is injured, the bleeding will take longer to stop because the body cannot form stable fibrin clots. Prolonged hemorrhage may result, even from what might otherwise be a minor wound.

Von Willebrand's disease is a condition in which the vWF component of factor VIII is deficient. This factor is necessary for normal platelet adhesion—an essential part of the clotting process. The disease is not associated with the deep muscle or joint bleeding of hemophilia, nor is it usually as serious, although nosebleeds, excessive menstruation, and gastrointestinal bleeds can occur.

8. Describe how acquired factor deficiencies may occur.   **pp. 737-739**

People who lack clotting factors can have bleeding disorders, which can occur as a result of genetics or medications. Some medications such as aspirin, dipyridamole (Persantine) and ticlopidine (Ticlid) decrease the stickiness of platelets by altering the surface enzyme that allows platelet aggregation. Others such as heparin and warfarin (Coumadin) cause changes within the clotting cascade to prevent clot formation. Heparin, working together with antithrombin III (a naturally occurring thrombin inactivator), inactivates thrombin to prevent formation of the fibrin clot. Coumadin blocks the activity of vitamin K, which is necessary to generate the activated forms of clotting factors II, VII, IX, and X, thus effectively interrupting the clotting cascade.

9. Identify the components of physical assessment as they relate to the hematology system. pp. 727-732

Many times hematological disorders are discovered and diagnosed when the patient seeks assistance for another medical condition, as the signs and symptoms associated with hematological problems may be quite varied. Patients with infection, white blood cell abnormalities (immunocompromised and prone to infection), or transfusion reactions may present with febrile symptoms. Acute hemodynamic compromise can be found in patients with anemia secondary to acute blood loss, coagulation disorders, or autoimmune disease. Confirmation of hematological disorders is usually dependent on laboratory analysis, but a complete history will go a long way toward developing an accurate diagnosis.

Additional specific considerations include mental status, dizziness, vertigo, or syncope, all of which may be indicative of anemia. Visual problems should alert you to the possibility of autoimmune disorders or sickle cell disease.

Skin color may be another indicator of hematological problems. Jaundice may indicate liver disease or hemolysis of red blood cells, while polycythemia is often associated with a florid (reddish) appearance, as pallor is with anemia. Observe for petechiae or purpura and bruising. Itching is commonly associated with hematological problems because of an excess of bilirubin resulting from liver disease or a breakdown of hemoglobin. Many patients report itching over a bruise. Look for evidence of prolonged bleeding, such as multiple bandages over a relatively minor wound.
Palpate the lymph nodes of the neck, clavicle, axilla, and groin. Enlarged lymph nodes are commonly seen in conjunction with hematopoietic disorders.

Gastrointestinal effects may be quite varied. Patients with clotting disorders may report epistaxis, bleeding gums, or melena. Many patients with clotting disorders report atraumatic bleeding of the gums. Ulcerations of the gums and oral mucosa as well as thrush (viral infection of the mouth) are often seen with immunocompromised patients. Abdominal pain is often seen in patients with hematological disorders. You may also be able to discern hepatic or splenic enlargement on your abdominal exam.

You should always ask about joint pain and examine the major joints closely in any patient who you suspect may have hematological problems. Minor trauma can cause significant hemarthrosis in patients with clotting disorders such as hemophilia. Many patients with autoimmune disorders frequently complain of arthralgia (joint pain) in all of their major joints.

You may see a variety of cardiorespiratory presentations that are linked to hematological disorders. Signs of hypoxia, such as tachypnea, tachycardia, and even chest pain, may be indicative of anemia. Occasionally, patients with bleeding disorders may develop hemoptysis. As always, you should be alert to signs and symptoms of shock and be prepared to initiate prompt therapy.

Genitourinary signs and symptoms associated with hematological problems may include hematuria, bleeding into the scrotal sac, excessive menstrual bleeding, and infection. Sickle cell disease is the most common cause for priapism seen in the emergency setting. Recognize that a detailed physical exam of the genitourinary system is not appropriate in the prehospital setting.

10. Describe the pathology and clinical manifestations and prognosis associated with:

Anemia   pp. 733-734
The most common disease associated with red blood cells is defined as a hematocrit of less than 37 percent in women and less than 40 percent in men. The majority of patients remain asymptomatic

until their hematocrit drops below 30 percent. Anemia is either due to a reduction in the total number of RBCs or quality of hemoglobin. It may also be due to acute or chronic blood loss. Anemia is a sign of an underlying disease process that is either destroying RBCs and hemoglobin or decreasing their production. Anemias may be hereditary or acquired.

The signs and symptoms associated with anemia are related to the associated hypoxia that results from the decrease in RBCs or hemoglobin. Depending on the rapidity of onset, signs and symptoms may be subtle or dramatic, determined to some degree by the patient's age and underlying state of health. Signs and symptoms may include fatigue, dizziness, headache, pallor, and tachycardia, or dyspnea with exertion. If the anemia develops rapidly it may overwhelm the body's compensatory mechanisms, in which case you may observe postural or frank hypotension, tachycardia, peripheral vasoconstriction, and decreased mental status.

Anemia may be self-limited or can be a lifelong illness requiring transfusions on a recurring and periodic basis. Confirmation of the illness and determination of its cause will be predictive of its prognosis.

Leukemia   pp. 736-737

Cancers of the hematopoietic cells occur when the precursors of white blood cells in the bone marrow begin to replicate abnormally. Initially, the proliferation of WBCs is confined to the bone marrow but then spreads to the peripheral circulation. Leukemia is classified by the type of cell involved and may be either acute or chronic. Examples include acute or chronic lymphocytic leukemia, acute or chronic myelogenous leukemia, or hairy cell leukemia. Although leukemias may occur across the life span, some are more commonly associated with specific age groups. For instance, acute lymphocytic leukemia (ALL) is seen predominately in children and young adults, while chronic lymphocytic leukemia (CLL) is most common in the sixth and seventh decades of life.

The signs and symptoms of leukemia are variable, although anemia and thrombocytopenia (decreased number of platelets) are common. These patients often appear acutely ill, complain of fatigue, and are febrile due to secondary infection. Lymph nodes will be enlarged. The history often includes weight loss and anorexia, as well as a feeling of abdominal fullness or pain that occurs as a result of liver and spleen enlargement.

The management of leukemia is a marvel of modern medicine as treatments such as chemotherapy, radiation therapy, and bone marrow transplantation have resulted in cures of specific types. Where ALL was once a virtual death sentence, now more than 50 percent of the pediatric patients live a normal life with the disease cured or in remission.

Lymphomas   p. 737

Lymphomas are cancers of the lymphatic system. Malignant lymphoma is classified by the cell type involved, which indicates the stem cell from which the malignancy arises. The cancer may be either Hodgkin's or non-Hodgkin's lymphoma. In 2003 there were 6 400 people diagnosed with non-Hodgkin's lymphoma in Canada and 2 800 deaths attributed to the disease.

The most common presenting sign of non-Hodgkin's lymphoma is painless swelling of the lymph nodes, while those with Hodgkin's lymphoma typically have no related symptoms. Some patients report fever, night sweats, anorexia, weight loss, and pruritis.

The long-term survival rate is much better with Hodgkin's lymphoma. Many people with this disease who were treated with radiation, chemotherapy, or both are considered cured.

Polycythemia   p. 735

Polycythemia is an abnormally high hematocrit due to excess production of red blood cells. A relatively rare disorder, it typically occurs in people over the age of 50. It can also develop secondary to dehydration. The increased red blood cell load increases the patient's risk of thrombosis, which causes most polycythemia-related deaths.

The signs and symptoms of polycythemia vary. The primary finding is a hematocrit of 50 percent or greater, which is usually accompanied by an increased number of white blood cells and platelets. The large number of RBCs may cause platelet dysfunction resulting in bleeding abnormalities such as epistaxis, spontaneous bruising, and gastrointestinal bleeding. Other complaints may include headache, dizziness, blurred vision, and itching. Severe cases can result in congestive heart failure.

Disseminated intravascular coagulopathy   p. 739

Disseminated intravascular coagulopathy (DIC), also called consumption coagulopathy, is a disorder of coagulation caused by the systemic activation of the coagulation cascade. Normally, inhibitory mechanisms localize coagulation to the affected area through a combination of rapid blood flow and absorption of the fibrin clot. In DIC, circulating thrombin cleaves to fibrinogen, forming fibrin clots throughout the circulation. This condition results in widespread thrombosis and, occasionally, end-organ ischemia.

Bleeding, the most frequent sign of DIC, occurs due to the reduced fibrinogen level, consumption of coagulation factors, and thrombocytopenia. It most commonly results from sepsis, hypotension, obstetrical complications, severe tissue injury, brain injury, cancer, and major hemolytic transfusion reactions. The patient may exhibit a purpuric rash, often over the chest and abdomen. The disease is quite grave and has a poor prognosis.

Hemophilia   pp. 738-739

Hemophilia is a disorder in which one of the proteins necessary for blood clotting is missing or defective. A deficiency of factor VIII is called hemophilia A, which is the most common inherited disorder of hemostasis. The severity of the disease is related to the amount of available circulating factor VIII, and patients are classified as mild, moderate, or severe on that basis. A deficiency of factor IX is known as hemophilia B or Christmas disease, which is more rare but also more severe than hemophilia A.

Hemophilia is a sex-linked inherited bleeding disorder. The gene with the defective encoding is carried on the X chromosome; this means that if the mother is a carrier, her son will inherit this disorder. Conversely, female offspring who inherit the defective gene from their mother will be carriers, but will not exhibit the clotting defect. In order for a female to exhibit the defect, she must inherit the defect from both parents, that is, a mother who is a carrier and a father who has hemophilia. Hemophilia A affects 1 in 10 000 males.

The signs and symptoms of hemophilia include prolonged bleeding, numerous bruises, deep muscle bleeding characterized as pain or a "pulled muscle," and bleeding in the joints known as hemarthrosis.

Sickle cell disease   pp. 734-735

This disease is an inherited disorder of RBC production that causes hemoglobin to be produced in a "C" or sickle shape during low oxygen states. These patients also have a hemolytic anemia as a result of destruction of abnormal red blood cells. The average life span of sickled cells is about 1/6 that of a normal red cell—approximately 10–20 days versus 120 days. Additionally, the sickled shape increases the blood's viscosity, leading to sludging and obstruction of capillaries and small vessels. Blockage of blood flow to various tissues and organs is common usually following periods of stress. The process, called a vasoocclusive crisis, is characteristic of the disease and over time leads to organ damage, particularly in the cardiovascular, renal, and neurologic systems.

Sickle cell disease primarily affects African Americans, although other ethnic groups may also be affected, such as Puerto Ricans and people of Spanish, French, Italian, Greek, or Turkish ancestry. If both parents carry the sickle cell gene, the chances are 1 in 4 that their child will have normal hemoglobin.

Patients will develop three types of problems. Vasoocclusive crisis causes severe abdominal and joint pain, priapism, and renal or cerebrovascular infarcts. Hematological crises present with a drop in hemoglobin, sequestration of RBCs in the spleen, and problems with bone marrow function. Infectious crises mark the third type of problem as the patients are functionally immunosuppressed and the loss of splenic function makes them vulnerable to infection. Infections become increasingly common and often are the cause of death.

Multiple myeloma   p. 739-740

Multiple myeloma is a cancerous disorder of plasma cells, the type of B cell responsible for producing immunoglobulins (antibodies). Rarely seen in patients under the age of 40, approximately 14,000 new cases are diagnosed each year.

Usually, multiple myeloma begins with a change or mutation in a plasma cell in the bone marrow. These cancerous cells crowd out the normal healthy cells and lead to a reduction in blood cell production. The patient then becomes anemic and prone to infection. The first sign is often a pain in the back or ribs as the diseased marrow weakens the bones and as a result, pathological fractures may occur. The resulting anemia leads to fatigue, and reduced platelet production places the patient at risk of bleeding. Calcium levels rise as a result of the bone destruction, and this often leads to renal failure.

11. Given several preprogrammed patients with hematological problems, provide the appropriate assessment, management, and transport. pp. 724-740

Throughout your classroom, clinical, and field training, you will encounter a variety of real and simulated patients with hematological problems. Use the information provided in this chapter of your text, as well as the application of this information as demonstrated by your instructors, preceptors, and mentors to enhance your ability to assess, manage, and transport these patients.

CONTENT SELF-EVALUATION

Multiple Choice

1. The surface protein on a blood cell that allows blood to be typed is known as a(n):
   - A. antibody.
   - B. antigen.
   - C. thrombocyte.
   - D. granulocyte.
   - E. monocyte.

2. The rarest blood type in Canada is:
   - A. A.
   - B. AB.
   - C. B.
   - D. O.
   - E. none of the above

3. The blood type known as a universal donor is:
   - A. A.
   - B. AB.
   - C. B.
   - D. O.
   - E. none of the above

4. The process of red blood cell destruction is known as:
   - A. sequestration.
   - B. fibrinolysis.
   - C. hemolysis.
   - D. hematopoiesis.
   - E. phagocytosis.

5. Tiny red dots found on the skin that may be indicative of hematological disorders are called:
   - A. purpura.
   - B. jaundice.
   - C. ecchymosis.
   - D. petechiae.
   - E. bruises.

6. An excess of bilirubin, either from liver disease or the breakdown of hemoglobin, can cause:
   - A. gingivitis.
   - B. generalized sepsis.
   - C. arthralgia.
   - D. priapism.
   - E. pruritis.

7. Often, one of the earliest indications of hematological problems is:
   - A. gingivitis.
   - B. generalized sepsis.
   - C. arthralgia.
   - D. priapism.
   - E. pruritis.

8. Which disease may result in slower blood clotting?
   - A. AIDS
   - B. cholecystitis
   - C. cirrhosis
   - D. pancreatitis
   - E. malaria

9. The condition in which patients with hemophilia develop swollen, discolored, and painful joints with minimal trauma is:

- **A.** leukotaxis.
- **B.** dysthralgia.
- **C.** ecchymotic arthralgia.
- **D.** hemarthrosis.
- **E.** arthralgia.

10. A deficiency of _____ is linked to anemia.

- **A.** calcium
- **B.** copper
- **C.** iron
- **D.** potassium
- **E.** magnesium

11. A hematocrit of 50 percent or greater is the principal finding in:

- **A.** anemia.
- **B.** leukopenia.
- **C.** polycythemia.
- **D.** thrombocytopenia.
- **E.** non-Hodgkin's lymphoma.

12. Painless swelling of lymph nodes is the most common presenting sign of:

- **A.** anemia.
- **B.** leukopenia.
- **C.** polycythemia.
- **D.** thrombocytopenia.
- **E.** non-Hodgkin's lymphoma.

13. An abnormal decrease in the number of platelets, which can be induced by many drugs, is:

- **A.** anemia.
- **B.** leukopenia.
- **C.** polycythemia.
- **D.** thrombocytopenia.
- **E.** non-Hodgkin's lymphoma.

14. Patients with hemophilia A are deficient in blood clotting factor:

- **A.** VII.
- **B.** VIII.
- **C.** IX.
- **D.** X.
- **E.** XII.

15. The disease referred to as consumption coagulation is often caused by any of the following EXCEPT:

- **A.** hemolytic transfusion reactions.
- **B.** hypertension.
- **C.** obstetrical complications.
- **D.** sepsis.
- **E.** hypotension.

True/False

16. Approximate 45% of the Canadian population has type B blood type.

- **A.** True
- **B.** False

17. Patients that are anemic often present with polycthemia.

- **A.** True
- **B.** False

18. Liver disease can slow blood clotting, most evident in a prolonged prothrombin (PT) time.

- **A.** True
- **B.** False

19. Thrush in adults is commonly associated with AIDS.

- **A.** True
- **B.** False

20. Aplastic anemia is a vitamin B12 deficiency which is necessary for correct red blood cell division during its development.
   A.   True
   B.   False

21. Common signs and symptoms of polycythemia include epistaxis, spontaneous bruising and GI bleeding.
   A.   True
   B.   False

22. A reduction in the number of neutrophils (neutropenia) predisposes the patient to bacterial and fungal infections.
   A.   True
   B.   False

33. Hemophilia A is also known as the Christmas disease..
   A.   True
   B.   False

24. A deficiency of factor VII is called hemophilia.
   A.   True
   B.   False

25. Von Willebrand's disease is an inherited disease where a component of factor VIII is deficient.
   A.   True
   B.   False

Matching

Write the letter of the term in the space provided next to the appropriate description.

A.	polycythemia	F.	neutropenia
B.	antigen	G.	sickle cell anemia
C.	leukemia	H.	thrombocytosis
D.	leukopenia	I.	von Willebrand's disease
E.	anemia	J.	disseminated intravascular coagulation

26. an inherited disorder of the red blood cells

27. excessive red blood cells

28. an abnormal increase in the number of platelets

29. a reduction in the number of neutrophils

30. condition in which the vWF component of factor VIII is deficient

31. protein on the surface of donor's red blood cells that the patient's body recognizes as "not self"

32. a disorder of coagulation caused by systemic activation of the coagulation cascade

33. too few white blood cells

34. an inadequate number of red blood cells

35. a cancer of the hematopoietic cells

Chapter 36

Environmental Emergencies

Review of Chapter Objectives

After reading this chapter, you should be able to:

1. Define "environmental emergency."   **p. 743**

An environmental emergency is a medical condition caused by or exacerbated by environmental factors such as weather, terrain, atmospheric pressure, or other local factors.

2. Identify risk factors most predisposing to environmental emergencies.   **p. 743**

General risk factors that place an individual at greater risk for an environmental emergency include age (very young and very old), poor general health, fatigue, predisposing medical conditions, and certain prescription or over-the-counter medications. Among drowning and near-drowning cases, alcohol use by an adult victim or the supervising adult is common.

3. Identify environmental factors that may cause illness or exacerbate a pre-existing illness or complicate treatment or transport decisions.   **p. 743**

Environments with certain characteristics are more likely to have emergencies: For instance, deserts may have tremendous variation in temperature between the hottest part of the day and overnight. Other such factors include current season, local weather patterns, atmospheric (high altitude) or hydrostatic (underwater) pressure, and the type of terrain. Rough or isolated terrain may significantly increase time for EMS response and for transport to the appropriate treating facility.

4. Define "homeostasis" and relate the concept to environmental influences.   **pp. 743-744**

Homeostasis is the body's ability to maintain a steady and normal internal environment despite changing external conditions. In this chapter, external conditions that are explored in the context of environmental emergency are (1) extremes in temperature, (2) drowning (fresh-water or saltwater), (3) atmospheric (high altitude) or hydrostatic (underwater diving) pressure, and (4) nuclear radiation.

5. Identify normal, critically high, and critically low body temperatures.   **pp. 745-746, 777**

In the core of the body, temperature usually varies within 1° of 37°C. Heat exhaustion occurs at core temperatures above 37.8°C, and heatstroke can occur at 40.6°C and higher. In contrast, mild hypothermia is associated with core temperatures of roughly 32–35°C. Severe hypothermia develops when core temperature drops below 32°C.

6. Describe several methods of temperature monitoring.   **p. 746**

Core body temperature can be monitored with a tympanic or rectal thermometer. Peripheral body temperature, which is usually a little bit lower, can be measured with use of an oral thermometer or a thermometer placed under the armpit (an axillary temperature). Approximate peripheral temperature or change in peripheral temperature can often be discerned by touch.

7. Describe human thermal regulation, including system components, substances used, and wastes generated.   pp. 744-747, 753

The human body does not generate "cold," it generates heat, and this process is called thermogenesis. There are three types of thermogenesis: The most basic and vital type is thermoregulatory thermogenesis, in which the nervous system and endocrine system work together to control the rate of cellular metabolism, which directly changes the rate of internal heat production. In work-induced thermogenesis, heat is produced through the work of skeletal muscles during exercise. In a cool or cold environment, muscles will produce some additional heat through shivering. The last type of heat generation is diet-induced thermogenesis, and it reflects the heat generated by cells as they process food and nutrients and eventually metabolize the breakdown products.

The body's thermal regulation is achieved through coordination of the nervous and endocrine systems. This is intuitively logical because these two systems are the control systems for all major body functions. Cells in the hypothalamus, a structure at the base of the brain, have the ability to act as a thermostat. As nerve cells, they sense the temperature of the core blood passing by them and they can receive messages from temperature sensors located in other parts of the body. Additional sensor cells for core temperature are located in the spinal cord, abdomen, and around the great veins in the chest. Peripheral sensors are in the skin and subcutaneous tissue.

On a cool day, peripheral temperature may drop. When the hypothalamic cells get the message, the cells act as endocrine cells, producing and secreting a hormone into the blood that acts to increase work-induced thermogenesis. Heat is produced through shivering. Also piloerection, or "goose bumps," the standing of small hairs, results in decreased air flow over the skin surface. If the environment is so cold that both peripheral and core temperature drop, the hypothalamic cells secrete hormones that increase heat production through all three means: thermoregulatory, work-induced, and diet-induced thermogenesis. (In the last, body cells burn fats and thus produce more heat.) In addition, core temperature, which is critical for survival, is maintained in part by reducing blood flow (and thus, heat) to the most peripheral tissues, the skin and subcutaneous tissues. In contrast, when the thermostat cells sense peripheral temperature is too high (as when you exercise vigorously), they stop releasing the hormone that stimulates thermogenesis. Not only is heat production slowed, but mechanisms to dissipate heat into the external environment are also activated. These include dilation of blood vessels in the skin and subcutaneous tissue (why people flush in the heat) and sweating.

This method of control, in which the production of a substance (in this case, heat) is turned off by the presence of that substance, is called negative feedback. Heat feeds back on the thermostat cells to turn off production of more heat. Think about the thermostat and furnace in a house. They work in a very similar fashion.

Thermogenesis consumes nutrient fuel for cells—fats, proteins, and carbohydrates—and it results in waste products such as carbon dioxide and water (from cellular respiration and fat breakdown) and urea (from protein breakdown). Extensive skeletal muscle use may also result in lactic acid accumulation. Heat dissipation through sweating consumes water, urea, and salts that are lost onto the skin surface.

8. List the common forms of heat and cold disorders.   pp. 747-760

The common heat disorders are variants of hyperthermia, elevated core body temperature: In terms of increasing severity, these conditions are heat (muscle) cramps, heat exhaustion, and heatstroke. Cold disorders are frostbite, trench foot, and hypothermia.

9. List the common predisposing factors and preventive measures associated with heat and cold disorders.   pp. 748-749, 754

Important predisposing factors for hyperthermia include age, general health, and medications. Both the very young and the very old have less responsive heat regulating systems and can tolerate less variation in their core body temperature. Persons who have diabetes with autonomic neuropathy are at higher risk for hyperthermia because damage to the autonomic nervous system may interfere with proper messaging to the CNS about temperature and may interfere with the heat-dissipating processes of vasodilation and sweating. Several groups of medications can affect body temperature. Diuretics predispose to dehydration, which impairs ability to sweat. Beta blockers interfere with vasodilation, impair ability to increase heart rate in response to volume loss, and may interfere with temperature messages to the CNS. Psychotropics and antihistamines interfere with thermoregulation within the CNS. Additional factors include acclimatization to local conditions, length and intensity of heat exposure, and environmental factors such as humidity and wind. Preventive measures for heat disorders include three major elements. First, maintenance of adequate fluid intake is vital, and remember that thirst alone is an inadequate indicator for dehydration. Second, you should allow yourself time for acclimatization to the hot environment, which results in more perspiration with lower salt concentration, thus conserving body-fluid volume. Last, it is important to limit exposure to hot environments.

Important predisposing factors for hypothermia are the same: age, general health, and medications. Both the very young and the very old have less responsive heat generating systems to combat cold exposure and cannot tolerate cold environments. The elderly may become hypothermic in environments that are only somewhat cool to others. Persons with inadequately treated hypothyroidism have suppressed metabolisms, which prevents proper responsiveness to cold. In addition, malnutrition, hypoglycemia, Parkinson's disease, fatigue, and other medical conditions can interfere with the body's ability to combat cold exposure. Drugs that interfere with heat-generating mechanisms include narcotics, alcohol, phenothiazines, barbiturates, antiseizure medications, antihistamines and other allergy medications, antipsychotics, sedatives, antidepressants, and various analgesics such as aspirin, acetaminophen, and NSAIDs. Additional factors include prolonged or intense exposure, which directly affects both morbidity and mortality, and coexisting weather conditions (such as high humidity, brisk winds, or accompanying rain, all of which magnify the effect of cold). Preventive measures can decrease the morbidity of cold-related injury, and these include dressing warmly, being rested, which maximizes the ability of the heat-generating mechanisms to replenish energy reserves, appropriate eating at proper intervals to support metabolism, and limitation of exposure to cold environments.

10. Define heat illness, hypothermia, frostbite, near-drowning, decompression illness, and altitude illness.   pp. 747, 753, 759, 761, 766, 771

• *Heat illness* is increased core body temperature (CBT) due to inadequate thermolysis (heat dissipation).
• *Hypothermia* is a state of low body temperature, particularly low core body temperature.
• *Frostbite* is environmentally induced freezing of body tissues causing destruction of cells.
• *Near-drowning* is an incident of potentially fatal submersion in liquid which did not result in death or in which death occurred more than 24 hours after submersion.
• *Decompression illness* is the development of nitrogen bubbles within body tissues due to a rapid reduction of air pressure when a diver returns to the surface; this is commonly called "the bends."
• *High altitude illness* is caused by a decrease in ambient pressure causing a low-oxygen environment and resultant hypoxia.

11. Describe the pathophysiology, signs and symptoms, and predisposing factors, preventive actions, and treatment for heat cramps, heat exhaustion, heatstroke, and fever. pp. 749-753

Heat cramps are caused by overexertion and dehydration in a hot environment. They occur when the temperature- and exercise-induced sweating (which consumes water and electrolytes including sodium) depletes the body of so much water and electrolytes that the actively exercising skeletal muscle fibers cramp. Signs and symptoms include cramping in fingers, arms, legs, or abdominal muscles. Patients are generally mentally alert with a feeling of weakness, but they may be dizzy or faint. Vital signs are stable, although temperature may be normal or slightly elevated. Skin is likely to be moist and warm. Note that heat cramps may be painful but they are NOT considered to be an actual heat illness. Treatment for heat cramps is usually easily accomplished. First, remove the patient from the hot environment to a cooler one such as a shady area or an air-conditioned ambulance. For severe cramps, you can administer an oral saline solution (approximately 4 tsp salt to one litre water) or a sports electrolyte drink. Do NOT use salt tablets, which are not absorbed readily and can irritate the stomach causing ulceration or hypernatremia. If the patient cannot take liquids readily, an IV of normal saline may be needed. Palliative care may include muscle massage or moist towels over patient's head and the cramping muscles.

Heat exhaustion, which is considered a mild heat illness, is an acute reaction to heat exposure, and it is the most common heat-related illness seen by EMS providers. The loss of water and electrolytes (notably sodium) from working in a hot environment, combined with general vasodilation as a heat-dissipating mechanism, leads to a decreased circulating blood volume, venous pooling, and reduced cardiac output. The presenting symptoms are due to dehydration and sodium loss secondary to sweating. Because the symptoms are not unique to heat exhaustion, diagnosis requires presentation in the appropriate environmental setting. Remember that untreated heat exhaustion can progress to heatstroke. The signs and symptoms of heat exhaustion include increased body temperature (over 37.8°C), cool clammy skin with heavy perspiration, rapid, shallow breathing, and a weak pulse. Signs of active thermolysis may include diarrhea and muscle cramps. The patient will feel weak and, in some cases, may lose consciousness. There also may be CNS symptoms such as headache, anxiety, paresthesia, and impaired judgment or even psychosis. The general predisposing factors and preventive measures for all heat-related disorders are discussed with objective 9. Treatment includes removal of the patient from the hot environment and placement in a supine position. For severe cramps, you can administer an oral saline solution (approximately 4 tsp salt per one litre of water) or a sports electrolyte drink. Do NOT use salt tablets, as discussed above. If the patient cannot take liquids readily, an IV of normal saline may be needed. Remove some clothing and fan the patient to increase heat dissipation. Be careful not to cool the patient to the point of chilling him or her. Stop fanning if shivering develops, and consider covering the patient lightly. If shock is suspected, treat accordingly. If symptoms do not resolve, consider the possibility of increased core body temperature and evolution of heatstroke.

Heatstroke is a true environmental emergency, one in which the body's hypothalamic temperature regulation is lost and there is uncompensated hyperthermia resulting in cell death and damage to the brain, liver, and kidneys. Generally, heatstroke is characterized by body temperature above 40.6°C, CNS disturbances, and (usually) cessation of perspiration. It is thought that sweating stops either because of destruction of sweat glands or because of sensory overload resulting in their temporary dysfunction. Patients may present with signs and symptoms including cessation of sweating, hot skin that is either moist or dry (depending on whether sweat has dried), very high core temperatures, deep respirations that become shallow and rapid respirations that may later slow, a rapid, full pulse that may slow later, hypotension with low or absent diastolic reading, confusion or disorientation or unconsciousness, and possible seizures. Field management centers on immediate cooling of the patient's body and replacement of fluids. First, remove the patient from the environment; if this is not done, other measures will be only minimally useful. Initiate rapid active body cooling to a target temperature of 39°C. This can be accomplished en route to the hospital. Remove the patient's clothing and cover with sheets soaked in tepid water. If necessary, either fanning or misting may be used. Be sure you avoid overcooling because this can trigger reflex hypothermia. Tepid water avoids the risk of producing reflex peripheral vasoconstriction and shivering that can be produced by exposure to cold water. In addition, use high-flow oxygen and assist respirations if they are shallow. Use pulse oximetry if available. Administer fluid therapy orally (if possible) or IV. In many cases, orally will suffice. Remember in this setting that electrolyte replacement is not nearly as necessary as water/volume replacement. If IVs are needed, start one or two and make the initial infusion with the line(s) wide open. Be sure to monitor the ECG because dysrhythmias can develop at any time. Avoid vasopressors and anticholinergic drugs because they may inhibit sweating and can contribute to development of a hyperthermic state in high-humidity, high-temperature environments. Lastly, monitor body temperature for trends toward target temperature or for other shift.

Fever (or pyrexia) is defined simply as elevation of body temperature above the normal for the individual. The body develops fever when pathogens cause infection, in turn stimulating productions of pyrogens, substances produced either by the pathogen or by cells involved in an inflammatory or immune response to the pathogen. Pyrogens produce fever by resetting the hypothalamic thermostat to a high level. The increase in temperature is largely due to increased metabolic activity. When production of pyrogen stops (or pathogen attack stops), the thermostat resets to normal and fever ends. Although fever typically presents in a setting of infectious disease, it may be difficult to distinguish from heatstroke, particularly if there is no history available and CNS signs are apparent. If you are unsure of diagnosis, treat for heatstroke. Treatment for fever should be undertaken when the patient is uncomfortable or when a child has a history of febrile seizures. Remove extra layers of clothing or bedclothes to allow body cooling. Consider use of an antipyretic agent such as acetaminophen or ibuprofen. Acetaminophen is available in rectal suppository form if vomiting is a concern. Note that sponge baths and cool-water immersion should not be used because they can cause a rapid drop in temperature with reflex shivering and increase in body temperature.

12. Describe the contribution of dehydration to the development of heat disorders.   p. 752

Dehydration often accompanies heat disorders because it inhibits vasodilation and heat dissipation (thermolysis). Dehydration leads to orthostatic hypotension and the following symptoms: nausea, vomiting, abdominal distress, vision disturbances, decreased urine output, poor skin turgor, and signs of hypovolemic shock. These may present along with the signs and symptoms of heatstroke. When assessment suggests dehydration, rehydration is critical. IV fluids may be needed, especially when the patient has altered mental status or is nauseated. An adult with moderate to severe dehydration may require 2–3 litres of IV fluids or more.

13. Describe the differences between classical and exertional heatstroke.   p. 751

Heatstroke is often divided into two types: classic and exertional. In classic heatstroke, the patient probably has chronic disorders, and increased core body temperature is due to deficient thermoregulatory function. Predisposing conditions include age, diabetes, and other medical conditions. In classic heatstroke, hot, red, dry skin is common. In contrast, exertional heatstroke often occurs in persons in good general health, and the increased core body temperature is due to overwhelming heat stress. Contextually, there is excessive ambient temperature, excessive exertion, prolonged exposure, and poor acclimatization. In exertional heatstroke, skin may well be moist from prior sweat. If heatstroke is tied to exertion, you may find severe metabolic acidosis caused by lactic acid accumulation. Hyperkalemia may also develop due to release of potassium from injured muscle cells, renal failure, or metabolic acidosis.

14. Identify the fundamental thermoregulatory difference between fever and heatstroke.   p. 752

The fundamental difference is that the trigger for temperature disruption is endogenous (internal) in fever and exogenous (external) in heatstroke. In fever, the hypothalamic thermostat is actually reset to a high level by pyrogens, substances associated with infection and the body's responses to it. The thermostat resets to the normal level when pyrogens disappear from the body. In heatstroke, exposure to high ambient temperatures depletes the body of the materials necessary for compensation (such as water and electrolytes for perspiration) and then causes the hypothalamic thermoregulatory processes to be lost. The ensuing uncompensated hyperthermia, with very high core body temperatures, begins the process of organ damage (if untreated) with potential for death.

15. Discuss the role of fluid therapy in the treatment of heat disorders. p. 752

Objective 12 discusses the role of dehydration in heat disorders. Because dehydration plays an increasingly significant role in heat cramps, heat exhaustion, and heatstroke, rehydration becomes increasingly pivotal to treatment success. Remember in milder forms of heat disorders, such as heat cramps, that the patient's perception of thirst is a poor indication of the degree of dehydration present. Fluid, whether it is administered orally or IV, is important in restoring the body's thermolytic abilities. In heat exhaustion and heatstroke, replacement of fluid (often by IV due to patient nausea, inability to swallow, or inability to take in fluids orally fast enough to be successful) is critical. Remember that an adult with moderate to severe dehydration can require 2–3 liters or more of replacement fluid.

16. Describe the pathophysiology, predisposing factors, signs, symptoms, and management of the following:

a.   hypothermia   pp. 753-759

Hypothermia is defined as a state of low core body temperature, which can be due to inadequate heat generation, excessive cold stress, or a combination of both. Hypothermia can be discussed in several contexts. In both forms signs and symptoms of hypothermia are present. Onset of symptoms can be acute (falling through ice into a lake), subacute (hikers trapped on a mountain during a winter snowstorm), or chronic (homeless individuals living outdoors during the winter). In many cases of acute and subacute hypothermia, the individual may not have any underlying predisposing factors for hypothermia: The pathophysiology of hypothermia rests on exposure to unsurvivable cold (as in the example of falling in the lake) or extended exposure to very cold conditions (the hiking example). In both settings, the body's ability for thermogenesis is simply overwhelmed. In other cases, an individual with impaired capacity for compensation is exposed to normal or cool conditions and develops hypothermia when a healthy individual would not or develops hypothermia before a healthy person would do so. Medical conditions that predispose to hypothermia include inadequately treated hypothyroidism, which depresses the body's metabolic rate, brain tumors or head trauma, which may impair hypothalamic function, as well as myocardial infarction, diabetes, hypoglycemia, drugs, poor nutrition, sepsis, or very young or old age.

Signs and symptoms of hypothermia are given in Table 36-2 (text page 756). Your assessment of an individual with mild hypothermia will likely reveal lethargy, shivering, lack of coordination, pale, cold, dry skin, and an early rise in blood pressure, heart rate, and respiratory rates. In severe hypothermia, you may find no shivering, loss of voluntary muscle control, hypotension, and an unpredictable pulse and respiration. On the ECG, you may find dysrhythmias. The most common presenting dysrhythmia is atrial fibrillation. With progressive cooling of the body core, a variety of dysrhythmias may appear, with eventual bradycardia or asystole. Note: The severely hypothermic patient requires assessment of pulse and respirations for at least 30 seconds every 1–2 minutes. Management includes: (1) removal of wet garments; (2) protection against further heat loss and wind chill (calling for passive external warming with blankets, moisture barriers, etc.); (3) maintenance of patient in horizontal position; (4) avoidance of rough handling, which can trigger dysrhythmias; (5) monitoring of core temperature; and (6) monitoring of cardiac rhythm. Persons with mild hypothermia may be rewarmed with active external techniques such as warmed blankets or heat packs. In contrast, active rewarming of the severely hypothermic patient is best carried out in the hospital because of the possibility of complications such as ventricular fibrillation. If transport to the hospital will require more than 15 minutes, you may need to begin active rewarming in the field.

b.   superficial and deep frostbite   pp. 759-760

Frostbite is an environmentally induced freezing of body tissues. As tissues freeze due to the excessive cold, ice crystals form within cells and water is drawn from cells into the extracellular space. As the ice crystals expand, cells are destroyed. Damage to blood vessels from ice-crystal formation causes loss of vascular integrity, which results in further tissue swelling and loss of distal blood flow. Peripheral tissues are more exposed to cold and thus more likely to be involved in frostbite. Thus, frostbite is largely seen in the extremities and in areas of the head and face. Predisposing factors are the same as those for hypothermia, and they are discussed with objective 10. The role of predisposing factors is often straightforward in terms of pathophysiology. A patient with diabetes, for instance, may have impaired peripheral circulation, and this relatively low flow of warm blood may make the extremities more vulnerable to frostbite. Two types of frostbite are defined based on the extent of tissue freezing: superficial and deep frostbite. Superficial frostbite (also called frostnip) involves some freezing of epidermal tissue, resulting in initial redness followed by blanching and diminished sensation. Deep frostbite involves both the epidermal and subcutaneous layers; there is a white, hardened appearance. Sensation is lost. Subfreezing temperatures are necessary for frostbite (otherwise, cellular water wouldn't freeze) but are not necessary for hypothermia. You will find that many patients with frostbite also do have hypothermia. You will also find that there is tremendous variation in presentation of frostbite. Some patients will feel little pain at the outset, whereas other will complain of bitter pain. Physical exam is a better indicator of the extent of frostbite. In superficial frostbite, there will be some degree of compliance felt beneath the frozen layer upon palpation; in deep frostbite, the frozen part will be hard and noncompliant. Treatment involves the following steps. First, do not thaw the affected area if there is any possibility of refreezing and do not massage the frozen area or rub with snow. Both may result in more extensive damage. Do administer analgesia prior to thawing, and do transport to the hospital for rewarming by immersion. Do cover the thawed part with loosely applied, dry, sterile dressings and elevate and immobilize the thawed part. Do not puncture or drain blisters, and do not rewarm frozen feet if they are required for walking out of a hazardous situation.

c. near-drowning pp. 761-764

Near-drowning is defined as submersion that is survived for at least 24 hours. The pathophysiology parallels that of drowning. Following submersion, a conscious person will have complete apnea for up to three minutes as an involuntary reflex as he struggles to keep his head above water, and during this period blood is shunted to the heart and brain. During apnea, $PaCO_2$ will rise to greater than 50 mmHg while PaO_2 falls to less than 50 mmHg. The hypoxic stimulus eventually overrides the sedative effects of the hypercarbia, resulting in CNS stimulation. While conscious, the panicky victim typically swallows a lot of water into the stomach, stimulating severe laryngospasm and bronchospasm. Especially in near-drowning victims, this effect prevents significant influx of water into the lungs (and is thus termed a dry drowning or near-drowning). Another effect of laryngospasm is worsening hypoxia, which causes a deepening coma. Morbidity or delayed mortality in near-drowning is primarily due to asphyxia from airway obstruction secondary to water in the airways (if a wet event) or laryngospasm and bronchospasm (if a dry near-drowning). Water in the lungs of a near-drowning survivor may cause lower-airway disease. A number of factors affect survival, and these include the cleanliness of the water, the duration of submersion, and the age and general health of the victim. Children have a longer survival time and a greater probability of successful resuscitation. Most significant is water temperature. In general, the colder the water, the greater the chance for survival. Usually, you expect brain death after 4–6 minutes without oxygen. However, some patients in cold water, may be resuscitated after 30 minutes or more in cardiac arrest. A possible physiologic factor in this phenomenon is the mammalian diving reflex. When a person dives into cold water, the submersion of the face inhibits breathing, drops heart rate, and causes vasoconstriction in tissues relatively resistant to asphyxia even as blood flow to the heart and brain continue. The colder the water, the greater the shunting of blood to brain and heart. This is the origin of the saying "the cold water drowning victim is not dead until he is warm and dead."

Field treatment for near-drownings in either saltwater or fresh water is similar: The first goal is to correct the profound hypoxia. Treatment includes the following steps: Remove the patient from the water. If possible, initiate ventilation while the victim is still in the water. Note that both steps require a trained, equipped rescue swimmer. Suspect head and neck injury if there was a fall or a dive involved; rapidly place victim on long backboard and use C-spine precautions. Then, protect from heat loss by removing wet clothing, laying the patient on a warm surface, and covering the body to the extent possible. The remaining steps are familiar to all resuscitations: Examine for airway patency, breathing, and pulse. If needed, begin CPR and defibrillation. Manage the airway as needed with suctioning and airway adjuncts. Administer 100% oxygen. Use respiratory rewarming, if available and if transport time will exceed 15 minutes. Establish an IV of lactated Ringer's or normal saline for venous access and run at 75 mL/hr. Follow ACLS protocols if the patient is normothermic. If hypothermic, the patient should be treated for hypothermia as discussed in the text. Note: Resuscitation is NOT indicated if immersion is known to have been extremely prolonged (unless hypothermia IS present) or if there is evidence of decomposition. All near-drowning victims should be admitted for observation for possible late complications including adult respiratory distress syndrome (ARDS).

d. decompression illness pp. 766, 767-769

Decompression illness, or the bends, is due to nitrogen bubbles coming out of solution in the blood and tissues, causing increased pressure on various body structures and occluding circulation in small blood vessels. This occurs in joints, tendons, the spinal cord, skin, brain, and inner ear. The trigger is a rapid ascent after exposure to a depth of 12 metres or more for a time sufficient to allow body tissues to become saturated with nitrogen. Predisposing factors for the individual include older age, obesity, fatigue, alcohol consumption before or after dive, and a history of medical problems. General factors are cold water diving, diving in rough water, strenuous diving conditions, history of previous decompression incident, overstaying time at a given dive depth, diving at 24 metres or more, too rapid an ascent, heavy exercise before or after dive, flying after diving (within 24 hours), or driving to high altitude after dive. Signs and symptoms include joint and abdominal pain, fatigue, paresthesia, and CNS disturbances. If the nitrogen bubbles occlude blood flow such that areas of local ischemia develop, tissue damage may occur.

Patients with decompression illness usually seek treatment within 12 hours of ascent, but some may not seek help until 24 hours afterward. Early oxygen therapy may reduce symptoms substantially, and divers who are given high-concentration oxygen have a significantly better treatment outcome. Prehospital management includes a number of steps. First, assess ABCs and administer CPR, if needed. Administer oxygen at 100% concentration with a nonrebreather mask. Intubate if the patient is unconscious. Keep the patient in a supine position and protect him or her from excessive heat or cold, wetness, or noxious fumes. If the patient is conscious and alert, give nonalcoholic liquids such as fruit juice or oral balanced salt solutions. Evaluate and stabilize the patient at the nearest emergency department prior to transfer to a recompression chamber for definitive therapy. Begin IV fluid replacement with electrolyte solutions if the patient is unconscious or seriously injured, otherwise, use lactated Ringer's solution. DO NOT use 5% dextrose in water. If there is evidence of CNS involvement, give dexamethasone, heparin, or diazepam as instructed by medical direction. If air evacuation is used, cabin pressure must be maintained at sea level to avoid worsening of the illness. Be sure to send the diving equipment for examination, if possible.

e.   diving emergency   pp. 764-771

The underlying physiology of diving emergencies is based on dissolution of gases in water, specifically, oxygen, carbon dioxide, and other gases dissolved in a diver's blood and body tissues. Pressure increases during descent, causing more gas to dissolve. During ascent, decreasing pressure allows gases to come out of solution, and they are eliminated gradually through respiration. If ascent is too rapid, however, dissolved gases, primarily nitrogen, come out of solution and expand in volume quickly, forming bubbles in the blood, brain, spinal cord, inner ear, muscles, and joints. Scuba diving injuries are due to barotrauma (changes in pressure), pulmonary over-pressure, arterial gas embolism, decompression illness, cold, panic, or a combination. Accidents generally occur at one of four phases of the dive: on the surface, during descent, at the bottom, or during ascent. Risk factors at the surface include presence of lines or kelp in which a diver can become entangled, cold water, which might induce shivering or even blackout, and boats or other large objects in the area. Barotrauma during descent is a factor in emergencies occurring during that period. If the diver cannot equilibrate the pressure between the nasopharynx and middle ear, he or she can experience severe pain, ringing in the ears, dizziness, and hearing loss, any of which can cause disorientation or panic, leading to an emergency. A similar problem of disequilibration can occur in the sinuses, producing frontal headache or pain below the eyes. Emergencies at the bottom often involve nitrogen narcosis, a state of stupor commonly called "rapture of the deep." Other emergencies occur when a diver begins to run out of oxygen and panics. Injury during ascent can involve barotrauma or decompression illness. The most serious form of barotrauma is pulmonary over-pressure, a condition in which expansion of air within the alveoli is greater than the tissue can handle and rupture of alveoli occur. If this occurs, the lung sustains structural damage and air entering the circulatory system can cause an arterial gas embolism. Pneumomediastinum (air in the mediastinum) and pneumothorax can also occur.

In a diving emergency, gather all evidence of air embolism and decompression illness together. Specific questions center on the timing and nature of the phases of the dive, as well as the diver's experience and state of equipment. Signs and symptoms of pulmonary over-pressure include substernal chest pain, respiratory distress, and diminished breath sounds. Treatment is the same as for pneumothorax of any other origin (see Chapter 27, "Pulmonology"). The signs and symptoms of arterial gas embolism (AGE) begin within 2–10 minutes of ascent with a rapid, dramatic onset of sharp tearing pain and other symptoms related to the specific organ system affected by lack of blood flow. The most common presentation resembles that of a stroke, with confusion, vertigo, visual disturbances, and loss of consciousness. Presentation may include hemiplegia as well as cardiopulmonary collapse. The key to diagnosis is the history of the dive. Treatment after assessment of ABCs includes use of 100% oxygen via nonrebreather mask, placement of patient in supine position, frequent monitoring of vitals, IV fluids at keep-vein-open rate, and use of a corticosteroid if ordered by medical direction. Transport to a recompression chamber as rapidly as possible under conditions that keep air pressure at that of sea level. Pneumomediastinum produces substernal chest pain, irregular pulse, abnormal heart sounds, reduced blood pressure and narrow pulse pressure, and change in voice. Cyanosis may or may not be present. Field management includes use of high-concentration oxygen via nonrebreather mask, IV with lactated Ringer's or normal saline per medical direction, and transport to an emergency department. Nitrogen narcosis causes the same concerns regarding mental and physical function as present with any other type of intoxication, with the addition of a person's functioning underwater during a dive. Altered level of consciousness and impaired judgment are key in assessment. Treatment involves return to shallow depth as this produces self-resolution.

Less frequent diving problems include oxygen toxicity due to prolonged exposure to high partial pressures of oxygen, hyperventilation, and hypercapnia due to inadequate clearance of carbon dioxide through the breathing equipment. Oxygen toxicity can lead to lung damage or even seizures. Hyperventilation due to excitement or panic may lead to muscle cramps or even decreased level of consciousness. Hypercapnia may also lead to unconsciousness. Finally, poorly prepared air tanks may be contaminated with other gases, which can increase the risk of hypoxia, narcosis, and accidental injury.

f.   altitude illness   pp.

In contrast to diving emergencies, high altitude illnesses are due to decreased ambient pressure creating a low-oxygen environment. As barometric pressure decreases at higher altitudes, lower oxygen availability can both trigger related disorders and aggravate existing medical

conditions such as angina, congestive heart failure, COPD, and hypertension. Even in very healthy individuals, rapid ascent to high altitudes without time for acclimatization can cause illness. It is difficult to predict who will be affected by altitude illness: The predictor is hypoxic ventilatory response. There are two medications that may act to prevent altitude illness: acetazolamide and nifedipine. High altitude illness begins to be manifest at approximately 8,000 ft (2,400 m) above sea level. Aspen, Colorado is located at 2,438 m, and it has 26% less oxygen per volume of air than at sea level. The range considered high altitude is 4,900–11,500 ft. Here, the hypoxic environment causes decreased exercise tolerance, although without major disruption of normal oxygen transport in the blood. The range for very high altitude is 11,500–18,000 ft, and this causes extreme hypoxia during exercise or sleep. Extreme altitude (greater than 18,000 ft) will cause severe illness in virtually everyone. Some signs and symptoms of altitude illness include malaise, anorexia, headache, sleep disturbance, and respiratory distress that worsens with exertion. Specific disorders include acute mountain sickness, high altitude pulmonary edema, and high altitude cerebral edema.

Acute mountain sickness (AMS) usually manifests in an unacclimatized person who ascends rapidly to an altitude of 2,000 m (6,600 ft) or higher. Signs and symptoms include lightheadedness, breathlessness, weakness, headache, and nausea and vomiting. More serious signs can develop, especially if the person continues to ascend: weakness to the point of requiring assistance to dress and eat, severe vomiting, decreased urine output, shortness of breath, and altered level of consciousness. Mild AMS is self-limiting and often improves in 1–2 days if no further ascent occurs. Treatment for AMS consists of halting ascent or possibly lowering altitude, use of acetazolamide and anti-nauseants as needed. Supplemental oxygen will relieve symptoms but is typically used only in severe cases. Definitive treatment for all high altitude illnesses is descent.

High altitude pulmonary edema (HAPE) results from increased pulmonary pressure and hypertension caused by changed blood flow in higher altitude. Children are most susceptible, and men are more susceptible than women. Initial symptoms include dry cough, mild shortness of breath on exertion, and slight crackles in the lungs. Symptoms of progression include severe dyspnea and cyanosis, coughing productive of frothy sputum, and weakness that may progress to coma and death. In its early stages, HAPE is completely reversed by descent and use of oxygen. If immediate descent isn't possible, oxygen can completely reverse HAPE but requires 36–72 hours to do so. Such a supply is rarely available to mountain climbers. An alternative is a portable hyperbaric bag, the use of which simulates a descent of roughly 5,000 ft. Acetazolamide may decrease symptoms. Other medications such as morphine, nifedipine, and furosemide may be useful but carry risk for complications such as hypotension and dehydration.

The exact cause of high altitude cerebral edema (HACE) is unknown. It usually presents as deteriorating neurological status in a patient with AMS or HAPE. The increased fluid in the brain tissue causes increased intracranial pressure. Symptoms include altered mental status, ataxia, decreased level of consciousness, and coma. If descent isn't possible, oxygen and steroids and a hyperbaric bag may help. If coma develops, it may persist for days after descent to sea level, but it usually resolves, although it may leave residual disability.

17. Identify differences between mild, severe, chronic, and acute hypothermia. p. 754

As discussed with objective 17a, mild hypothermia is defined by a core temperature greater than 32°C in the presence of signs/symptoms of hypothermia, Acute hypothermia involves sudden exposure to a cold environment as can happen when someone falls through the ice on a frozen lake. Chronic hypothermia may occur in predisposed persons in ambient temperatures inadequately cold to produce hypothermia in a healthy, appropriately dressed individual. In North America., look for it among homeless persons who have endured frequent and prolonged cold stress outdoors.

18. Discuss the impact of severe hypothermia on standard BCLS and ACLS algorithms and transport considerations. pp. 755-759

Severe hypothermia (core temperature less than 30°C) mandates a switch from passive rewarming and some degree of active external rewarming to active internal rewarming, which may include use of warm IV fluids, warm, humid oxygen, peritoneal lavage, extracorporeal rewarming, and esophageal rewarming tubes. If pulse or breathing is absent, severe hypothermia mandates continuance of CPR but withholding of IV fluids and limitation of electrical conversion to three times maximum. Drug metabolism in the severely hypothermic patient is significantly decreased, and levels may accumulate that will become toxic when the patient is rewarmed. In addition.

19. Differentiate between fresh-water and saltwater immersion as they relate to near-drowning. pp. 762-763

There are differences between fresh-water and saltwater near-drowning because of the difference in the salt content of the water. You should know, however, that although the pathophysiology is different, there is no difference in the end result or in field management. In fresh-water settings, a massive amount of hypotonic water diffuses across the alveolar/capillary interface, resulting in hemodilution, an expansion in blood plasma volume with relative reduction in erythrocyte concentration. Hemodilution produces a thickening of the alveolar walls with inflammatory cells, hemorrhagic pneumonitis, and destruction of surfactant. Surfactant is the lipid substance secreted by lung cells that regulates surface tension on the fluid lining the alveoli, helping to keep them open. Loss of surfactant leads to fluid buildup in the small airways with atelectasis. Because some blood flowing through the lungs is now not oxygenated, hypoxemia results. Saltwater settings are different because the ambient water is hypertonic to that in the body. Thus, water is drawn from the bloodstream into the alveoli, producing pulmonary edema and profound shunting. Hypoxemia again results. In addition, saltwater near-drownings feature respiratory and metabolic acidosis due to retention of carbon dioxide and the development of anaerobic metabolism.

20. Discuss the incidence of "wet" versus "dry" drownings and the differences in their management. p. 761-762

While conscious, the panicky victim typically swallows a lot of water into the stomach, stimulating severe laryngospasm and bronchospasm. Especially in near-drowning victims, this effect prevents significant influx of water into the lungs (and is thus termed a dry drowning or near-drowning). Another effect of laryngospasm is worsening hypoxia, which causes a deepening coma. Morbidity or delayed mortality in near-drowning is primarily due to asphyxia from airway obstruction secondary to water in the airways (if a wet event) or laryngospasm and bronchospasm (if a dry near-drowning). Water in the lungs of a near-drowning survivor may cause lower-airway disease. Dry drownings occur in about 10 percent of drowning victims, which means wet drownings are by far more common.

21. Discuss the complications and protective role of hypothermia in the context of near-drowning. pp. 761, 763-764

In general, the colder the water, the greater the patient's chance for survival. Usually, you expect brain death after 4–6 minutes without oxygen. However, some patients in cold water may be resuscitated after 30 minutes or more in cardiac arrest. A possible physiologic factor in this phenomenon is the mammalian diving reflex. When a person dives into cold water, the submersion of the face inhibits breathing, drops heart rate, and causes vasoconstriction in tissues relatively resistant to asphyxia even as blood flow to the heart and brain continues. The colder the water, the greater the shunting of blood to brain and heart. This is the origin of the saying "the cold water drowning victim is not dead until he is warm and dead."

22. Define self-contained underwater breathing apparatus (scuba). p. 764

Scuba is the commonly known abbreviation for self-contained underwater breathing apparatus, a portable system that contains compressed air that is delivered to a diver so he or she can breathe underwater.

23. Describe the laws of gases and relate them to diving emergencies and altitude illness. pp. 764-765

Three laws pertaining to the behavior of gases under different physical conditions relate to environmental emergencies.

• *Boyle's law* states that a volume of gas is inversely proportional to its pressure when temperature remains constant. As you increase pressure (as happens during a dive), gas is compressed into increasingly smaller volumes. One liter of air at the surface fills 500 mL at 9.9 metres of water depth, and the same one liter fills only 250 mL at 19.8 metres. As a diver ascends, pressure decreases toward that at the surface and the gas present in tissues and in the blood expands to occupy ever greater volumes. The reason controlled ascent is so important is that the sudden dissolution of gas into bubble form associated with rapid assent causes occlusion of small blood vessels by bubbles, the disorder known as decompression illness. With increasing altitudes, the problem is the reverse. The gas molecules in air expand to occupy an increasingly larger volume, and thus a lungful of air contains ever less gas (including oxygen) at higher altitudes, and hypoxemia and tissue hypoxia can result.

• *Dalton's law* states that the total pressure of a mixture of gases (such as air) is equal to the sum of the partial pressures of each individual gas. Air is roughly 78% nitrogen, 21% oxygen, and 1% carbon dioxide and other trace gases. As altitude changes (upward or downward), those proportions remain the same. The fraction of oxygen in air does not change.

• *Henry's law* states that the amount of a gas dissolved in a given volume of fluid is proportional to the pressure of the gas above it. This law is most relevant to diving. As a person descends to greater depths, oxygen is increasingly used up in cellular metabolism, whereas nitrogen, which is inert, does not change in quantity. Instead, it dissolves into body water. As the person ascends, those gases (particularly nitrogen, because it is present in the greatest amount) come out of the blood and tissues and form bubbles. The correct rate of ascent allows the gas to form bubbles at a rate for which the body can compensate.

24. Differentiate between the various diving emergencies.   pp. 764-771

Briefly, one disorder, nitrogen narcosis, is unrelated to change in pressure (barotrauma). Instead, it reflects the sedative and intoxicating effect of nitrogen on the CNS. Disorders related to barotrauma include decompression illness during rapid ascent, in which nitrogen bubbles forming in blood and other body fluids cause severe pain and the possibility of areas of ischemia secondary to occlusion of small blood vessels by bubbles. Lung overinflation associated with rapid ascent can cause pulmonary over-pressure accidents, in which air expansion can rupture alveoli, resulting in hemorrhage and reduced oxygen and carbon dioxide transport, as well as complications due to air leakage.

25. Identify the various conditions that may result from pulmonary over-pressure accidents.   pp. 776-777, 769

Lung overinflation associated with rapid ascent can cause pulmonary over-pressure accidents, in which air expansion can rupture alveoli, resulting in hemorrhage and reduced oxygen and carbon dioxide transport, as well as air leakage into the mediastinum, a condition termed pneumomediastinum. Another condition associated with pulmonary over-pressure is arterial gas embolism (AGE), in which a large bubble of free air can enter the circulation, travel through the left side of the heart, and eventually lodge at some point in the systemic circulation, setting up the possibility of cardiac, pulmonary, or cerebral compromise.

26. Describe the function of the Divers Alert Network (DAN) and how its members may aid in the management of diving-related illnesses.   pp. 771

The Divers Alert Network (DAN) serves as a non-profit consultant for diving-related health concerns, and it can be contacted through Duke University Medical Center in North Carolina. There are both emergency (919-684-8111) and non-emergency (919-684-2948) telephone numbers.

27. Describe the specific function and benefit of hyperbaric oxygen therapy for the management of diving accidents.   p. 768

Decompression illness may require recompression, which can be accomplished by placing the patient in a hyperbaric oxygen chamber (a chamber in which pressure of oxygen is maintained at greater-than-atmospheric levels). In this setting, nitrogen redissolves, relieving the illness. Controlled decompression then allows the nitrogen to come out of solution and be eliminated without forming bubbles. Arterial gas embolism also requires prompt treatment in a recompression chamber so the air embolism can dissolve, relieving the ischemia associated with its occlusion of a blood vessel. These are the only diving-related conditions for which hyperbaric oxygen is standard. In some cases, it may also be required for patients with pulmonary over-pressure.

28. Define acute mountain sickness (AMS), high altitude pulmonary edema (HAPE), and high altitude cerebral edema (HACE).   pp. 773-775

• *Acute mountain sickness (AMS)* represents sudden-onset hypoxia in a person unacclimatized to the current altitude. Signs and symptoms are generally mild and the illness often resolves spontaneously within 1–2 days of living at the higher altitude. AMS usually develops after a rapid ascent to an altitude of 2,000 m or higher.

• *High altitude pulmonary edema (HAPE)* is a more serious condition caused by increased pulmonary pressure and hypertension due to altitude-induced changes in blood flow. Either immediate descent or 36–72 hours of supplemental oxygen usually relieves the condition.

• *High altitude cerebral edema (HACE)* reflects increased intracranial pressure due to increased fluid in the brain. The pathophysiologic mechanism is unclear. Even with proper treatment, residual disability may result if coma developed before definitive treatment (descent, oxygen, steroids) could improve the patient's condition.

29. Discuss the symptomatic variations presented in progressive altitude illnesses. pp. 773-775

The symptoms associated with AMS are so mild that the patient may never request treatment, and they resemble those associated with severe overexertion (in both cases because root cause is insufficient oxygen and stressed body systems). In HAPE, symptoms of similar severity (cough, shortness of breath on exertion) progress to those of a clearly serious illness: dyspnea, possibly with cyanosis, and coughing productive of frothy sputum. Weakness can progress to coma. The presentation of HACE may follow presentation of AMS or HAPE. The presentation of HACE itself reflects the progressive neurologic deterioration associated with increased intracranial pressure: altered mental status and decreasing level of consciousness, ataxia, and coma.

30. Discuss the pharmacology appropriate for the treatment of altitude illnesses. P.773

If AMS requires medication, treatment usually consists of acetazolamide and anti-nauseants such as prochlorperazine. Supplemental oxygen will relieve symptoms but is usually reserved for severe cases. HAPE in its early stages can be treated with rapid descent and supplemental oxygen. If descent is not an option, oxygen in combination with a portable hyperbaric bag is useful; pharmacological adjuncts include acetazolamide, morphine, nifedipine, and furosemide. Acetazolamide carries the least risk for complications. HACE is treated with descent, oxygen with a hyperbaric bag, and steroids to reduce intracranial swelling.

31. Given several preprogrammed simulated environmental emergency patients, provide the appropriate assessment, management, and transportation. pp. 743-799

Attention to the ABCs is always important, and this doesn't change with environmental emergencies. The need to move the patient from the harmful environment to one conducive to recovery is special, although not unique (as with inhalation toxicological emergencies). Among the heat disorders, heatstroke is the most serious, and rapid transport is always required.

Hypothermia always requires transport to a hospital setting. The urgency in rewarming varies with the degree of hypothermia, as do some potential complications on rewarming such as cardiac dysrhythmias. Superficial and deep frostbite differ in the depth of tissue affected by freezing; care while en route to the hospital is similar. Early recognition is important to the EMS provider, but prevention is the most important of all steps.

Near-drownings require immediate care and rapid transport to the hospital. Although more than 90% of near-drowning patients survive without sequelae, ARDS can occur as a potentially deadly late complication. Emergencies related to air pressure (diving and altitude) can vary in severity and setting, but immediate care and removal to an appropriate environment as soon as possible are key to treatment. Again, these emergencies are better prevented than treated. Knowing what resources are available in the area is important to treating any of these types of emergencies.

CONTENT SELF-EVALUATION

Multiple Choice

_____ 1. General risk factors that predispose a person to developing an environmental illness include all of the following EXCEPT:
  A. predisposing medical conditions such as diabetes.
  B. fatigue.
  C. high levels of fluid intake.
  D. use of certain over-the-counter or prescription medications.
  E. age: either very young or old persons.

2. Which process is NOT one that results in body heat loss into the environment?

    A.   evaporation   **D.**   radiation
    B.   convection   **E.**   diffusion
    C.   respiration

3. Which group of medications does NOT predispose a person to hyperthermia?

    A.   psychotropics   **D.**   beta blockers
    B.   antiepileptics   **E.**   antihistamines
    C.   diuretics

4. Medical conditions that may predispose to hypothermia include all of the following EXCEPT:

    A.   hypothyroidism.   **D.**   thin body build.
    B.   malnutrition.   **E.**   hypoglycemia.
    C.   Parkinson's disease.

5. Which is NOT appropriate as a rewarming measure for mild to moderate hypothermia?

    A.   warmed blankets   **D.**   heat packs
    B.   warmed IV fluids   **E.**   heat lamp
    C.   peritoneal lavage

6. Management guidelines for frostbite include all of the following negatives EXCEPT:

    A.   Do not thaw affected area if possibility of refreezing exists.
    B.   Do not massage the frozen area or rub with snow.
    C.   Do not puncture or drain any blisters.
    D.   Do not warm frozen feet if patient will need to walk out of hostile environment.
    E.   Do not give analgesia prior to thawing.

7. Resuscitation of a drowning victim is not indicated when:

    A.   respirations have ceased.
    B.   cardiac asystole exists.
    C.   the patient has been pulled from freezing water and is very cold himself.
    D.   immersion is known to have been extremely long.
    E.   head or neck injury due to trauma is evident.

8. Which gas law is most applicable to decompression illness?

    A.   Boyle's law   **D.**   Ohm's law
    B.   Dalton's law   **E.**   Venturi's law
    C.   Henry's law

9. Which of the following might be administered IV to a near-drowning patient?

    A.   plasmanate   **D.** D_5W
    B.   dextran   **E.**   hetastarch
    C.   lactated Ringer's

10. One of the most severe complications of near-downing is:

    A.   "the squeeze."   **D.**   barotrauma.
    B.   ARDS.   **E.**   pneumomediastinum.
    C.   DAN.

11. The condition whose chief signs and symptoms include altered levels of consciousness and impaired judgment is:

    A.   AGE.   **D.**   pneumomediastinum.
    B.   "the squeeze."   **E.**   nitrogen narcosis.
    C.   "the bends."

12. The condition whose signs and symptoms include substernal chest pain, irregular pulse, abnormal heart sounds, reduced blood pressure and narrow pulse pressure, and a change in voice is:
    A. AGE.
    B. "the squeeze."
    C. "the bends."
    D. pneumomediastinum.
    E. nitrogen narcosis.

13. The condition whose signs and symptoms include altered mental status, ataxia, decreased level of consciousness, and coma is:
    A. AGE.
    B. DAN.
    C. HACE.
    D. HAPE.
    E. AMS.

14. The unit of local tissue energy deposition in cases of radiation exposure is the:
    A. Geiger.
    B. RAD.
    C. QF.
    D. gamma.
    E. radioisotope.

15. A naked person can be exposed to an external environment ranging anywhere from ___ C to 62 C.
    A. 8
    B. 3.
    C. 5
    D. 15.
    E. 0

16. Which part of the brain is responsible to temperature control?
    A. cerebellum
    B. optic chiasma
    C. hypothalamus
    D. corpus callosum
    E. thalamus

17. At what temperature does the body suffer from heat exhaustion? :
    A. 37.8 C
    B. 38.6 C
    C. 40.6 C
    D.. below 32 C
    E. above 40.6 C

18. Mild hypothermia is associate with which of the following temperature ranges?
    A. 30.2-34.6 C
    B. 31.4-35.8 C
    C. 32.4-34.8 C
    D. 32.2-35.8 C
    E. 33.3-36.5 C

19. Measures to prevent heat disorders include all but which of the following.
    A. limit exposure
    B. preventative planning
    C. apply sunscreen
    D. maintaining adequate fluid intake
    E. allow time to acclimatize

20. Which of the following is NOT an Individual factor contributing to the development of decompression illness?
    A. fatigue
    B. sex
    C. obesity
    D. age
    E. history of medical problems

True/False

_____ 21. Homeostasis is the body's ability to maintain a steady, normal internal environment in the face of changing external conditions.
  A. True
  B. False

_____ 22. Thirst is an adequate indicator of dehydration.
  A. True
  B. False

_____ 23. Dehydration is often intimately associated with heat disorders because it inhibits peripheral vasodilation and limits sweating.
  A. True
  B. False

_____ 24. In situations where it is unclear whether the diagnosis is fever or heatstroke, always treat for both conditions.
  A. True
  B. False

_____ 25. Rewarming is not the mirror image of the cooling process.
  A. True
  B. False

_____ 26. The physiology of fresh-water and saltwater drownings differs, and these differences contribute to differences in prognosis and field management.
  A. True
  B. False

_____ 27. In Canada, approximately 10 000 persons die annually due to drowning.
  A. True
  B. False

_____ 28. Boyles law states that the volume of a gas in inversely proportional to its pressure if the temperature is kept constant.
  A. True
  B. False

_____ 29. In a patient suffering from High altitude cerebral edema, there is decreased fluid in the brain tissue causing an increase in intracranial pressure (ICP).
  A. True
  B. False

_____ 30. In the treatment of environmental emergencies, it is paramount that we remove the environmental influence causing the problem.
  A. True
  B. False

Matching

Write the letter of the clinical characteristics in the space provided next to the appropriate disorder.

_____	31.	heat exhaustion	_____ 36.	pulmonary over-pressure
_____	32.	deep frostbite	_____ 37.	nitrogen narcosis
_____	33.	high altitude cerebral edema	_____ 38.	mild hypothermia
_____	34.	severe hypothermia	_____ 39.	decompression illness
_____	35.	acute mountain sickness (early phase)	_____ 40.	high altitude pulmonary edema

A. moderately decreased core temperature, shivering, lethargy, early rise in heart and respiratory rates

B. dry cough and dyspnea progressing to cough productive of frothy sputum and severe dyspnea

C. severe pain and CNS disturbances that develop during a rapid ascent from a dive to depth below 12 metres

D. environmentally induced freezing of skin and subcutaneous tissues with hardness on palpation, no sensation

E. altered mental status and decreasing level of consciousness, ataxia

F. substernal chest pain that develops during ascent, often from shallow depths, associated with respiratory distress and diminished breath sounds

G. lightheadedness, shortness of breath, nausea after rapid ascent to altitude of 3160 metres or more

H. stuporous state that develops during deep dives rather than during descent or ascent

I. somewhat increased core temperature, rapid, shallow respirations, weak pulses

J. severely decreased core temperature, no shivering, hypotension, dysrhythmias, undetectable pulse and respirations

Chapter 37

Infectious Disease

Review of Chapter Objectives

After reading this chapter, you should be able to:

1. **Describe the specific anatomy and physiology pertinent to infectious and communicable diseases.   pp.782-787; also see Chapter 13**

The body's first line of defense against many infectious agents is the skin. Additionally, components of the respiratory system also assist in this endeavor by creating turbulent airflow, while nasal hairs trap pathogens and mucus in the lower airways also traps and kills pathogens. Cilia in the airways move the mucus to the mouth and nose for expulsion. Other bacteria are removed from the body via feces and urine. However, there are three body systems that specifically protect against disease; these are the immune system, the complement system, and the lymphatic system.

The immune system fights disease by protecting the body from foreign invaders in a mechanism initiated by the inflammatory response and involving white blood cells. There are two types of immune system response: cell-mediated immunity that employs T lymphocytes and humoral immunity that depends on the B lymphocytes to form antibodies. The complement system recognizes surface proteins, providing alternative pathways to combat infection. The lymphatic system is a secondary circulatory system that collects overflow fluid from tissue spaces and filters it before returning it to the circulatory system. The spleen is an essential organ of the lymphatic system whose white pulp generates antibodies and produces B and T lymphocytes, while the red pulp removes unwanted particulate matter, such as old or damaged red blood cells.

2. **Define specific terminology identified with infectious/communicable diseases. pp. 782-830**

Infectious diseases are illnesses caused by infestations of biological organisms, such as bacteria, viruses, fungi, protozoans, or helminths. Microorganisms that normally reside in our bodies without causing disease are referred to as normal flora and protect us from pathogens (disease-causing organisms). Opportunistic pathogens are ordinarily non-harmful bacteria that cause disease only under unusual circumstances, such as a weakened immune system.

3. **Discuss public health principles relevant to infectious/communicable diseases. pp. 782-783**

The task of public health epidemiologists is to study how infectious diseases affect populations, as well as to predict and describe how disease moves from individuals to populations and determine what the impact of the disease is on the population. Paramedics must evaluate the host (patient), what they believe to be the infectious agent, and the environment. Based on that assessment, they may opt to use more aggressive personal protective equipment. They must also consider the patient, those in the patient's environment, and the environment where the patient is being transported all to be at risk for infection.

4. Identify public health agencies involved in the prevention and management of disease outbreaks.   p. 783

Local agencies including hospitals, fire departments, and EMS agencies cooperate with provincial and local health departments to monitor and report the incidence and prevalence of disease. Additionally, Health Canada has a Population and Public Health Branch (PPHB) that is responsible for policies, programs, and research relating to disease surveillances, prevention, and control, health promotion and community action.

5. List and describe the steps of an infectious process.   p. 790

The elements of disease transmission include the interactions of host, infectious agent, and environment. Infectious agents invade hosts by either direct or indirect transmission, and may be bloodborne, airborne, or transmitted by fecal-oral route. Factors that affect the likelihood that an exposed individual will become infected and then actually develop disease include correct mode of entry, virulence (strength), number of organisms transmitted, and host resistance.

6. Discuss the risks associated with infection.   pp. 782, 787-790

Infection is the presence of an agent within the host, without necessarily causing disease. Not all exposures result in transmission of microorganisms, nor are all infectious agents communicable. Risk of infection is considered theoretical if transmission is acknowledged to be possible but has not actually been reported. It is considered measurable if factors in the infectious agent's transmission and associated risks have been identified from reported data. Generally, the risk of disease transmission increases if a patient has open wounds, increased secretions, active coughing, or any ongoing invasive treatment where exposure to an infectious body fluid is likely.

7. List and describe the stages of infectious diseases. pp. 787-790

Exposure to an infectious agent may result in contamination or penetration. Penetration implies that infection has occurred, but infection should never be equated with disease. Once infected, the host goes through a latent period when he cannot transmit an infectious agent to someone else. This is followed by the communicable period when the host may exhibit signs of clinical disease and can transmit the infectious agent to another host. The time between exposure and the appearance of symptoms is known as the incubation period, which may range from a few days to months or years.

Most viruses and bacteria have antigens that stimulate the body to produce antibodies. The presence of these antibodies in the blood indicates exposure to the particular disease that they fight. This process is known as seroconversion. The window phase refers to the time between exposure and seroconversion. The disease period is the duration from the onset of signs and symptoms of disease until the resolution of symptoms or death.

8. List and describe infectious agents, including bacteria, viruses, fungi, protozoans, and ☐elminthes (worms).   Pp. 783-787

• *Bacteria:* microscopic single-celled organisms (1–20 micrometers in length) that can be differentiated by their reaction to a chemical staining process; classified by type as spheres (cocci), rods, spirals.
• *Viruses:* disease-causing organisms that are much smaller than bacteria and are only visible with an electron microscope; obligate intracellular parasites, they can grow and reproduce only within a host cell.
• *Fungi:* plant-like microorganisms, most of which are not pathogenic.
• *Protozoans:* single-celled parasitic organisms with flexible membranes and ability to move; rarely a cause of disease in humans, but commonly considered opportunistic pathogens in those patients with compromised immune function.
• *Helminths (worms):* parasitic organisms that live in or on another organism and are common causes of disease where sanitation is poor; various forms include pinworms, hookworms, trichinella.

9. **Describe characteristics of the immune system, including the categories of white blood cells, the reticuloendothelial system (RES), and the complement system. (see Chapters 13 and 31)**

The immune system is the body's mechanism for defending against foreign invaders. The various cells involved in the immune response are sometimes collectively referred to as the reticuloendothelial system (RES) because their locations are so widely scattered throughout the body. Reticulo means network and endothelial refers to certain cells that line blood vessels, the heart, and various body cavities. Key to the immune system's response is the ability to differentiate "self" from "nonself." Once an invader is recognized as "nonself," a series of actions is initiated to eradicate the foreign material; this process is known as the inflammatory response. This response involves selected leukocytes (white blood cells) that attack the infectious agent in a process called phagocytosis. Neutrophils act first and then 12–24 hours later are followed by macrophages. The macrophages release chemotactic factors, which trigger additional immune system responses.

The complement system provides an alternative pathway to deal with foreign invaders more quickly than is accomplished through cell-mediated or humoral immunity. This system of at least 20 proteins works with antibody formation and the inflammatory reaction to combat infection by starting a cascade of biochemical events triggered by tissue injury.

10. **Describe the processes of the immune system defenses, including humoral and cell-mediated immunity. (see Chapters 13 and 31)**

There are two types of immune system response: cell-mediated immunity, which generates various forms of T lymphocytes that react against specific antigens, and humoral-mediated immunity, which results from antibodies (immunoglobulins) formed from mature B lymphocytes in the lymph nodes and bone marrow. Humoral immunity is responsible for the immune system properties of memory and specificity. Other classes of white blood cells, monocytes, eosinophils, basophils, and natural killer (NK) cells, also participate in the general immune response. There are five classes of human antibodies: IgG—major class of immunoglobulin in the immune response; it crosses the placental barrier and thus plays an important role in producing immunity prior to birth; IgM—formed early in most immune responses; IgA—primary immunoglobulin in exocrine secretions; IgD—acts as an antigen receptor and is present on the surface of B lymphocytes; IgE—attaches itself to mast cells in the respiratory and intestinal tracts, playing a critical role in allergic reactions.

11. **In specific diseases, identify and discuss the issues of personal isolation. p. 800**

Understanding the mechanism for disease transmission, as well as the relationship between infectious agent, host, and environment, will allow the EMS provider to make appropriate decisions regarding personal protection against disease. To supplement the body's natural defenses against disease, paramedics must protect themselves against infectious exposures. Prevention is the most effective approach to infectious disease. All body fluids are possibly infectious, and universal precautions should be followed at all times.

12. **Describe and discuss the rationale for the various types of personal protection equipment. pp. 790-795**

Personal protective equipment provides an additional barrier to exposure, thus minimizing the risk of infection from bloodborne and airborne organisms. Isolating all body substances and avoiding contact with them further reduces risk of exposure. Using disposable items for patient care also decreases risk, as does exercising caution around "sharps." Thorough and vigorous hand washing also goes a long way to reduce inadvertent contamination. Dispose of biohazard wastes as proscribed by local laws and regulations. Decontaminate and disinfect infected equipment according to local SOPs and protocols.

13. **Discuss what constitutes a significant exposure to an infectious agent. p. 795**

All exposures to blood, blood products or any potentially infectious material should be immediately reported to the designated infectious disease control officer (IDCO), according to local protocol. The nature of the exposure is assessed based on route (percutaneous, mucosal, or cutaneous), dose, and nature of the infectious agent. For instance, in the case of HIV, the highest risk exposure involves percutaneous exposure with a large volume of blood, a high antibody titer against a retrovirus in the source patient, deep percutaneous injury, or actual intramuscular injection.

14. Describe the assessment of a patient suspected of, or identified as having, an infectious/communicable disease. pp. 795-797

When assessing any patient, you should maintain a high index of suspicion that an infectious agent may be involved. Evaluate every environment for its suitability to transmit infectious agents and always maintain appropriate BSI.

Be alert to clues about the potential for infectious disease based on the patient's past medical history and medication use, as well as his or her chief complaint and the history of present illness. Look for general indicators of infection, such as unusual skin signs or rashes, fever, weakness, profuse sweating, malaise, or dehydration. Follow the standard format for assessing medical patients.

15. Discuss the proper disposal of contaminated supplies such as sharps, gauze, sponges, and tourniquets.   pp. 790-795

Any patient care supplies (gauze, sponges, and tourniquets) that have been contaminated by blood or body fluids should be disposed of as biohazard waste in leak-proof biohazard bags and in accordance with local protocol. Dispose of all contaminated sharps in properly labeled puncture-resistant containers.

16. Discuss disinfection of patient care equipment and areas where patient care occurred. p. 794

Decontaminate infected equipment according to local protocols in the appropriate designated area. The decontamination process begins with the removal of surface dirt and debris using soap and water, then disinfect as appropriate, and finally sterilize if required. There are four levels of decontamination:

• *low-level disinfection*—appropriate for routine cleaning and removing visible body fluids
• *intermediate-level disinfection*—appropriate for cleaning equipment that has been in contact with intact skin
• *high-level disinfection*—required for all reusable devices that have come in contact with mucous membranes
• *sterilization*—required for all contaminated invasive instruments

17. Discuss the seroconversion rate after direct significant HIV exposure.   p. 798

HIV is detected through the presence of antibodies specific to HIV. When a person develops antibodies after exposure to a disease, his previously negative test will be positive indicating that seroconversion has taken place. The estimated probability of a health care worker becoming infected by a work-related exposure to virus-containing blood is 0.2 to 0.44%.

18. Discuss the causative agent, body systems affected and potential secondary complications, routes of transmission, susceptibility and resistance, signs and symptoms, patient management and protective measures, and immunization for each of the following:

• **Human immunodeficiency virus (HIV)   pp. 798-780**
—HIV is a retrovirus with affinity for human T lymphocytes with the CD4 marker.
—Transmitted via blood, blood products, and body fluids, HIV enters the body through breaks in the skin, mucous membranes, eyes, or by placental transmission (13–30% transmission rate).
—Destruction of the immune system leads to the development of opportunistic infections and cancers.
—There is no vaccine or cure, although postexposure prophylaxis with triple therapy (two reverse transcriptase inhibitors and one protease inhibitor) may be helpful.
—Practice BSI for all potential blood/body fluid exposures during patient care activities.

• Hepatitis A (HAV)   pp. 801-802

—Hepatitis A virus is transmitted by fecal-oral route. It has an incubation period of 3 to 5 weeks, with greatest probability of transmission in the latter half of that period.

—The disease causes inflammation of the liver (also known as viral or infectious hepatitis) evidenced by general malaise, fever, anorexia, nausea and vomiting, and possibly jaundice, although many infections are asymptomatic.

—Vaccines (Havrix and Vaqta) provide effective active immunization.

—EMS workers should employ universal precautions against bloodborne or fecal-oral transmission.

• Hepatitis B (HBV) pp. 802-803

—Hepatitis B virus is transmitted by direct contact with contaminated blood or body fluids and is very highly infectious. There is a 1.9–40% transmission rate via cutaneous exposure and a rate of 5–35% via needle stick. The HBV incubation period is 8–24 weeks.

—HBV causes inflammation of the liver (also known as serum hepatitis) evidenced by general malaise, fever, anorexia, nausea and vomiting, and possibly jaundice, cirrhosis, and malignancies. Some 60–80% of infections, however, are asymptomatic.

—Vaccines (Recombivax HB, Engerix B) provide effective immunization after completion of series of three IM injections and follow-up antibody screening.

—Employ universal precautions against bloodborne transmission.

• Hepatitis C (HCV) p. 803

—Hepatitis C virus is transmitted by direct contact with contaminated blood or body fluids.

—A majority of patients have chronic hepatitis C, which has the ability to cause active disease years later.

—HCV often causes liver fibrosis, which progresses over the years to cirrhosis.

—Effective vaccines do not yet exist, although there has been some success in treating disease with alpha interferon, often in combination with ribavirin.

—Employ universal precautions against bloodborne transmission.

• Hepatitis D (HDV)   p. 803

—Hepatitis D virus seems only to coexist with hepatitis B.

—HDV virus is transmitted by direct contact with contaminated blood or body fluids.

—HDV causes inflammation of the liver evidenced by general malaise, fever, anorexia, nausea and vomiting, and possibly jaundice, cirrhosis, and malignancies.

—Immunization against HBV confers immunity to HDV.

—Employ universal precautions against bloodborne transmission.

• Hepatitis E   pp. 803-804

—Hepatitis E virus is transmitted, like hepatitis A, by the fecal-oral route; it is more commonly associated with contaminated drinking water.

—Hepatitis E causes inflammation of the liver evidenced by general malaise, fever, anorexia, nausea, and vomiting. It occurs primarily in young adults, with highest rates among pregnant women.

—Employ universal precautions against fecal-oral transmission.

• Tuberculosis (TB) pp. 804-807

—The causative bacteria of the disease is *Mycobacterium tuberculosis.*

—TB is commonly transmitted through airborne droplets but may also be contracted by direct inoculation through mucous membranes and broken skin or by drinking contaminated milk.

—The communicability of TB is variable, with an incubation period of 4 to 12 weeks, although disease usually develops from 6 to 12 months after infection.

—TB primarily affects the respiratory system, including a highly contagious form in the larynx, and may spread to other organ systems causing extrapulmonary TB.

—No vaccine exists, although postexposure prophylaxis is helpful.

—Protect against disease transmission by practicing universal precautions, plus donning an N95 (or HEPA) respirator, as well as employing appropriate respiratory precautions while performing CPR or intubation; masking the patient will also reduce exposure to droplet nuclei.

• **Meningococcal meningitis pp. 811-812**
　　—The causative organism for meningococcal meningitis is *Neisseria meningitidis.*
—The infection asymptomatically colonizes in the upper respiratory tract of healthy individuals and
then is transmitted by respiratory droplets.
—Presentation includes fever, chills, headache, nuchal rigidity with flexion, arthralgia, lethargy,
malaise, altered mental status, vomiting and seizures; characteristic petechiae rash common in
pediatric cases.
—The incubation period from is from 2 to 4 days, but potentially as long as 10 days.
—Meningococcal vaccines are available against some of the serotypes but are not routinely
recommended for routine immunization of health care workers; postexposure drug prophylaxis is
effective.
—Practice universal precautions and using masks on self or patient.

• **Pneumonia　　　pp. 807-808**
—Pneumonia's causative organism may be bacterial, viral, or fungal, although the most common
pathogen is *Streptococcus pneumoniae.*
—It is transmitted by airborne droplet inhalation.
—Acute lung infection is characterized by fever, chills, dyspnea, productive cough, pleuritic chest
pain, and adventitious lung sounds indicative of consolidation.
—An effective vaccine exists for at risk populations: children under 2 years of age, adults over age 65,
and anyone without a spleen. Routine vaccination of EMS personnel is not required.
—Use of respiratory precautions is advised.

• **Tetanus   pp. 823-824**
—*Clostridium tetani* bacillus is the causative organism.
—Tetanus is transmitted by exposure to *C. tetani* spores, which are present in the soil, street dust, and
feces. The condition is often associated with puncture wounds, deep lacerations, or injections.
—Localized symptoms include rigidity of muscles in close proximity to wound. Generalized
symptoms include pain and stiffness of the jaw that may progress to cause muscle spasm and rigidity
of the entire body; respiratory arrest may result.
—The incubation period is variable (usually 3 to 21 days, or 1 to 3 months); shorter periods are linked
to more severe illness.
—Universal precautions should afford sufficient protection, although respiratory protection and
goggles are advised for intubation.
—Vaccinations usually begin in childhood (DTP or diphtheria-tetanus toxoid, pertussis) and every 10
years thereafter; postexposure prophylaxis is often recommended.

• **Rabies　　pp. 821-823**
—The causative organism is the rabies virus, a member of the *Rhabdovirus* family and *Lyssavirus*
genus, which affects the nervous system
—Rabies is transmitted in the saliva of an infected animal by bites, through an opening in the skin, or
by direct contact with a mucous membrane. Once it enters the body, it then travels along motor and
sensory fibers to the spinal ganglia corresponding to the site of invasion and then to the brain, creating
an encephalomyelitis that is almost always fatal.
—Rabies is characterized by a nonspecific prodrome that typically lasts 1 to 4 days (malaise, fever,
chills, sore throat, myalgia, anorexia, nausea, vomiting, and diarrhea); this is followed by the
encephalitic phase that begins with periods of excessive motor activity, followed by confusion,
hallucinations, tetany, and seizures. Focal paralysis appears and if untreated causes death within 2 to 6
days. Attempts to drink water may produce laryngospasm, causing profuse drooling associated with
hydrophobia.
—BSI precautions are appropriate and the use of masks may be prudent.
—Several options for rabies immunization are available and are recommended for animal care
workers. Postexposure prophylaxis should be discussed on a case-by-case basis with a physician.

• **Hantavirus　　　pp. 818-819**
—This family of viruses is carried by rodents such as the deer mouse.
—Transmission is primarily by inhalation of aerosols caused by the stirring up of the dried urine,

saliva, and fecal droppings of these rodents. Contamination of food and autoinoculation after handling objects tainted by rodent droppings may also cause transmission.

—Hantavirus causes hantavirus pulmonary syndrome (HPS) whose signs and symptoms include fatigue, fever, muscle aches, headaches, nausea, vomiting and diarrhea, and—after 4 to 10 days—pulmonary edema occurs. Hemodynamic compromise occurs approximately 5 days after onset.

—There is no vaccine available.

—Wear masks when in dusty, unoccupied buildings for extended periods of time.

• Chickenpox   pp. 810-811
—Chickenpox is caused by the varicella zoster virus (VZV) in the herpesvirus family.

—It is transmitted by airborne droplet inhalation plus direct contact with weeping lesions or contaminated linens.

—Respiratory symptoms include malaise and low-grade fever, followed by a rash that starts on the face and trunk and progresses to the rest of the body including the mucous membranes. The fluid-filled vesicles that form the rash rupture, leaving small ulcers that scab over within a week.

—The incubation period is from 10 to 21 days.

—An effective vaccine exists (Varivax) and is required in some states for admission to elementary school or day care; it is also recommended for susceptible health care workers.

—Employ universal precautions and place masks on patients. Extensive decontamination of the ambulance and any equipment used for patient with chickenpox is strongly recommended.

• Mumps   pp. 814-815
—The mumps virus is a member of the genus *Paramyxovirus*.

—It is transmitted through respiratory droplets and direct contact with saliva of infected patients.

—The infection is characterized by painful enlargement of the salivary glands. It presents as a feverish cold followed by swelling and stiffening of the parotid salivary gland in front of the ear, often bilaterally.

—The incubation period is 12 to 25 days.

—A mumps live-virus vaccine is available and should be administered with measles and rubella (MMR) to all children over 1 year of age.

Medical Emergencies
—Standard BSI precautions are advised; EMS personnel should not work without an established MMR immunity.

• Rubella   p. 815
—The carrier is the rubella virus of the genus *Rubivirus*.

—It is transmitted by inhalation of infective droplets.

—Rubella is generally milder than measles. It is characterized by a low-grade fever and sore throat, and accompanied by a fine, pink rash on the face, trunk, and extremities that lasts about 3 days.

—The incubation period is 12 to 19 days.

—Immunization should be combined with mumps and measles (MMR) and, due to its devastating effects in a developing fetus, every woman should be immunized prior to becoming pregnant.

—Standard BSI precautions are advised; EMS personnel should not work without an established MMR immunity.

• Measles   p. 814
—The carrier is the measles virus of the genus *Morbilli*.

—It is transmitted by droplet inhalation and direct contact.

—Known also as rubeola or hard measles, it is characterized by fever, conjunctivitis, malaise, cough, and nasopharyngeal congestion. Koplik's spots (bluish-white specks with a red halo approximately 1 mm in diameter) appear on the oral mucosa, followed within 24 to 48 hours by a maculopapular rash lasting about 6 days, moving from head to toe.

—The incubation period is 7 to 14 days.

—Immunization is 97–99% percent effective and is usually administered in conjunction with mumps and rubella (MMR).

—Standard BSI precautions are advised, along with vigilant hand washing and masks; EMS personnel should not work without an established MMR immunity.

• Pertussis (whooping cough)   p. 816
—Pertussis is caused by the bacterium *Bordetella pertussis.*
—It is transmitted via respiratory secretions or in an aerosolized form and is highly contagious.
—The disease has a three-phase clinical presentation. The catarrhal phase of 1 to 2 weeks resembles a common cold and fever. In the paroxysmal phase of 1 month or longer, fever subsides and the patient develops a mild cough that quickly becomes severe and violent. Rapid consecutive coughs are accompanied by deep high-pitched inspiration, and coughing produces copious thick mucus and may lead to increased intracranial pressure and, potentially, intracerebral hemorrhage. Finally, in the convalescent phase, the frequency and severity of the coughs decrease, and the patient is no longer contagious.
—The incubation period is 6 to 20 days.
—Mask the patient and observe standard BSI precautions, including postexposure hand washing. Booster doses of DTP (diphtheria-tetanus toxoid, pertussis) should be considered.

• Influenza pp. 813-814
—Influenza is caused by viruses designated types A, B, C.
—It is transmitted by airborne droplet inhalation, direct contact, or autoinoculation.
—The disease is characterized by sudden onset of chills, fever (usually of 3 to 5 days duration), malaise, muscle aches, nasal discharge, and cough that may be severe and of long duration.
—The incubation period is from 1 to 3 days.
—Immunization is available and recommended for the elderly, those who live in institutional settings, military recruits, and health care workers.
—Antiviral agents such as amantadine are available but are only effective against type A.
—Universal BSI precautions and good hand washing are recommended.

• Mononucleosis   p. 817
—The causative organism of mononucleosis is Epstein-Barr virus (EBV).
—It is transmitted by direct oropharyngeal contact with an infected person.
—Clinical presentation includes fatigue, fever, sore throat, oral discharges, and tender, enlarged lymph nodes. Splenomegaly is not uncommon.
—The incubation period is 4 to 6 weeks.
—No vaccine is available.
—Observe universal BSI precautions, and good hand washing practices are recommended.

• Herpes Simplex 1 and 2   pp. 817, 827
—There are two forms of herpes simplex, herpes simplex virus type 1 (HSV-1) and herpes simplex virus type 2 (HSV-2).
—HSV-1 is transmitted in the saliva of carriers.
—HSV-1 affects the oropharynx, face, lips, skin, fingers, and toes, although it can cause meningoencephalitis in newborns and aseptic meningitis in adults. Following an incubation period of 2 to 12 days, fluid-filled vesicles form that soon deteriorate to small ulcers. Lesions may be accompanied by fever, malaise, and dehydration. Lesions usually disappear in 2 to 3 weeks but may recur throughout the patient's life.
—HSV-2 is sexually transmitted, although it may be transmitted during childbirth as the infant moves through the birth canal.
—Presentation of HSV-2 includes vesicular lesions on the genitals, rectum, anus, perineum, or mouth depending on the type of sexual activity. Females may be asymptomatic. Fever and enlarged lymph nodes often accompany initial infection. Lesions last up to several weeks and may recur throughout the patient's lifetime.
—Immunization is not available for either form.
—Universal precautions are absolutely essential, along with good hand washing.

• Syphilis   pp. 826-827

—Syphilis is caused by the spirochete *Treponema pallidum.*

—It is transmitted by direct contact with exudates from other syphilitic lesions of the skin and mucous membranes, semen, blood, saliva, and vaginal discharges.

—The disease has four stages: primary syphilis—painless lesion forms 3 to 6 weeks after exposure; secondary syphilis—bacteremic stage occurs 5 to 6 weeks after lesion heals; maculopapular rash on hands and feet, condyloma latum (painless wart-like lesions on warm, moist skin areas that are very infectious); latent stage—symptoms abate for months to years; tertiary syphilis—wide variety of presentations (cardiovascular, neurologic).

—The incubation period is 3 weeks.

—No immunization is available.

—Universal precautions are absolutely essential along with use of good hand washing practices.

• Gonorrhea   p. 825

—Gonorrhea is caused by a gram-negative bacterium, *Neisseria gonorrhoeae.*

—It is transmitted by direct contact with exudates of mucous membranes, primarily from direct sexual contact.

—Presentation varies: in men, it most commonly causes dysuria and purulent discharge, then epididymitis; in women, there is commonly no pain or discharge unless it develops into pelvic inflammatory disease.

—The incubation period is 10 to 14 days.

—Universal precautions are absolutely essential along with use of good hand washing practices.

• Chlamydia   pp. 827-828

—Chlamydia is caused by a genus of intracellular parasites most like gram-negative bacteria, *Chlamydia trachomatis.*

—It is transmitted by sexual activity and by hand-to-hand transfer of eye secretions; it often coexists with gonorrhea.

—Presentation varies with symptoms in a manner similar to gonorrhea, but less severe: in men, it most commonly causes dysuria and purulent discharge, then epididymitis; women may have no pain or discharge unless it develops into pelvic inflammatory disease.

—The incubation period is 10 to 14 days.

—Universal precautions are absolutely essential along with use of good hand washing practices.

• Scabies   p. 830

—Scabies is caused by infestation of a mite, *Sarcoptes scabiei.*

—The condition is contracted by exposure through close personal contact, from hand holding to sexual contact. Mites remain viable on clothing or bedding for up to 48 hours.

—Upon attaching to a new host, the female burrows into the epidermis to lay eggs within $2 1/2$ minutes. Larvae hatch shortly and are full-grown adults in 10 to 20 days. Primary symptom of the condition is intense itching.

—The incubation period is 2 to 6 weeks after infestation. It remains communicable until all mites and eggs are destroyed.

—No immunization is available.

—Bag and remove all linens immediately. Decontaminate stretcher and patient compartment as for lice. Remove and decontaminate any clothing that may have contacted the patient.

• Lice (Pediculosis) pp. 829-830

—There are three varieties of infestation: *Pediculus humanus var. capitis* (head lice), *Pediculus humanus var. corporis* (body lice), and *Pthirus pubis* (pubic lice or crabs).

—Lice are transmitted by direct contact, which may or may not be associated with sexual activity.

—Eggs hatch within 7 to 10 days.

—Infestation results in parasitic infection of the skin of the scalp, trunk, or pubic area, which is primarily characterized by intense itching. Red macules, papules, and urticaria commonly appear on the shoulders, buttocks, abdomen, or genital areas.

—No immunization is available.

—Spray the ambulance interior close to the cot and the area by the patient's head with an insecticide, preferably one containing permethrin. Wipe and clean all surfaces to remove insecticide residues.

• **Lyme disease   pp. 824-825**
—Lyme disease is caused by the tick-borne spirochete *Borrelia burgdorferi.*
—It is transmitted by the bite of an infected tick.
—A flat, painless red lesion may appear at bite site (and may appear to resemble a bull's eye). This may be accompanied by malaise, headache, and muscle aches; then the spirochete spreads to the skin, nervous system, heart, and joints. Meningitis, cardiac conduction defects, and arthritis are common. Recurrence can appear months to years after initial exposure.
—The incubation period ranges from 3 to 32 days.
—Immunization is available (LYMErix) as a series of three vaccinations.
—Employ universal precautions. Also, when responding in wooded areas, check for ticks, and spray the ambulance compartment with an arthropod-effective insecticide.

• **Gastroenteritis   pp. 819-820**
—Causative organisms for the condition may be viruses, bacteria, and parasites.
—It is highly contagious via the fecal-oral route, including the ingestion of contaminated food or water.
—Prolonged vomiting and diarrhea may cause dehydration and electrolyte disturbances.
—No immunization is available.
—Follow universal precautions and use aggressive hand washing.

19. Discuss other infectious agents known to cause meningitis including streptococcus pneumonia, haemophilus influenza type B, and various varieties of viruses. p. 811

Meningitis is often caused by other infectious agents, particularly *Streptococcus pneumoniae* and *Haemophilus influenzae* type B. *Streptococcus* is the most common cause of adult pneumonia and the leading cause of otitis media in children. Vaccines have proven to be very effective, especially in children. *Haemophilus* was once the leading cause of meningitis in children from 6 months to 3 years of age but the development of a vaccine in the early 1980s has virtually eliminated its incidence. While a variety of viruses have also been known to cause meningitis, in otherwise healthy individuals viral meningitis is a self-limited disease that lasts 7 to 10 days.

20. Identify common pediatric viral diseases. pp. 810-811, 814-815, 817-818

The most common cause of viral illness in children is *respiratory syncytial virus* (RSV), most commonly causing pneumonia and bronchiolitis in infants and young children. Croup and pharyngitis have also been attributed to viruses, such as the parainfluenza virus and rhinovirus. All of these are transmitted by direct inhalation of infected droplets or through exposed mucosal surfaces, as well as autoinoculation from unwashed hands after handling contaminated surfaces.

21. Discuss the characteristics of and organisms associated with febrile and afebrile diseases including bronchiolitis, bronchitis, laryngitis, croup, epiglottitis, and the common cold. pp. 817-819

The common cold (viral rhinitis) is caused by the any of the more than 100 serotypes of rhinovirus. Transmission is caused by direct inhalation of infected droplets or through exposed mucosal surfaces, as well as autoinoculation from unwashed hands after handling contaminated surfaces. The incubation period is from 12 hours to 5 days, with an average of 48 hours. Generally, it is a mild illness characterized by nasal congestion, rhinitis, and cough.

Bronchiolitis, bronchitis, laryngitis, croup, and epiglottitis may have bacterial or viral origins, although epiglottitis is most commonly due to *Haemophilus influenzae, Streptococcus pneumoniae,* or *Staphylococcus aureus,* while croup is usual viral.

All of these are transmitted by direct inhalation of infected droplets or through exposed mucosal surfaces, as well as autoinoculation from unwashed hands after handling contaminated surfaces.

22. Articulate the pathophysiological principles of an infectious process given a case study of a patient with an infectious/communicable disease. pp. 782-830

As already discussed, the interactions between a host, an infectious agent, and the environment are the elements of disease transmission. Recognizing that infectious agents invade hosts through either direct or indirect transmission, you should generally be able to determine which is applicable given the patient presentation. Your role as paramedic is to interrupt disease transmission while providing safe and effective care for your patient, based on your recognition of signs and symptoms and your knowledge of the physiologic priorities for emergency care.

23. Given several preprogrammed infectious disease patients, provide the appropriate body substance isolation procedure, assessment, management, and transport. pp. 782-831

Throughout your training, you will encounter a variety of real and simulated patients with a variety of infectious diseases. Use the information provided in your text as well as the application of this information as demonstrated by your instructors, preceptors, and mentors to enhance your ability to assess, manage, and transport these patients. Remember that prevention is the best approach and, for that reason, you should presume that every patient is potentially infectious and take appropriate precautions to minimize your exposure. Your own personal accountability in the area of infection control is equally important. Do not go to work if you have any signs or symptoms of illness, keep your immunizations up to date, and always practice effective hand washing.

CONTENT SELF-EVALUATION

Multiple Choice

1. Microscopic single-celled organisms that can be differentiated by their reaction to a chemical staining process are called:
   - A. helminths.
   - B. bacteria.
   - C. viruses.
   - D. fungi.
   - E. protozoans.

2. Single-celled parasitic organisms that are a common cause of opportunistic infection are called:
   - A. helminths.
   - B. bacteria.
   - C. viruses.
   - D. fungi.
   - E. protozoans.

3. Visible only by electron microscope, obligate intracellular parasites that resist antibiotic treatment are called:
   - A. helminths.
   - B. bacteria.
   - C. viruses.
   - D. fungi.
   - E. protozoans.

4. All of the following are airborne diseases EXCEPT:
   - A. meningitis.
   - B. tuberculosis.
   - C. measles.
   - D. syphilis.
   - E. influenza.

5. The presence of an infectious agent within the host, without necessarily causing disease, is referred to as:
   - A. infection.
   - B. contamination.
   - C. communicable.
   - D. exposure.
   - E. virulence.

6. All of the following are factors that affect disease transmission EXCEPT:
   A. mode of entry.
   B. virulence.
   C. dose of organism.
   D. host resistance.
   E. type of organism.

7. Surface proteins on viruses and bacteria that stimulate the production of antibodies are called:
   A. pathogens.
   B. prokaryotes.
   C. antigens.
   D. prions.
   E. eukaryotes.

8. The creation of antibodies following an exposure to a disease is called:
   A. incubation.
   B. seroconversion.
   C. latency.
   D. infection.
   E. contamination.

9. At the scene of a motor vehicle accident, all of the following are appropriate infection control measures EXCEPT:
   A. wearing gloves and changing them between patients.
   B. using protective eyewear or face shields to limit splash exposures.
   C. recapping needles to reduce risk of needlestick to others.
   D. decontaminating all reusable equipment.
   E. putting all contaminated dressings in a leak-proof biohazard bag.

10. Risk factors for developing infectious disease include:
    A. immunosuppression.
    B. diabetes.
    C. artificial heart valves.
    D. alcoholism.
    E. all of the above

11. Which of these infectious diseases poses the greatest risk to EMS personnel as a result of work-related exposures?
    A. AIDS
    B. tuberculosis
    C. hepatitis A
    D. hepatitis B
    E. hantavirus

12. The most significant problem associated with HIV is:
    A. opportunistic infection.
    B. hemorrhage.
    C. dementia.
    D. blindness.
    E. splenomegaly.

13. The most common form of hepatitis transmitted by the fecal-oral route is:
    A. hepatitis A.
    B. hepatitis B.
    C. hepatitis C.
    D. hepatitis D.
    E. hepatitis E.

14. Primarily a respiratory disorder, the most common preventable adult infectious disease in the world is:
    A. hepatitis A.
    B. tuberculosis.
    C. HIV.
    D. pneumonia.
    E. influenza.

15. Your 60-year-old patient reports an acute onset of high fever, chills, dyspnea, pleuritic chest pain, and a productive cough. You suspect:
    A. hantavirus.
    B. tuberculosis.
    C. HIV.
    D. pneumonia.
    E. influenza.

16. Your patient has a low-grade fever and malaise and is covered from head to toe with fluid-filled vesicles and small ulcers. You suspect:

A.	measles.	D.	meningitis.
B.	rubella.	E.	scabies.
C.	chickenpox.		

17. Your patient reports an acute onset of high fever, stiff neck, and severe headache. You suspect:

A.	measles.	D.	meningitis.
B.	rubella.	E.	scabies.
C.	chickenpox.		

18. All of the following are viral infections that may be contracted in the EMS setting EXCEPT:

A.	measles.	D.	meningitis.
B.	rubella.	E.	scabies.
C.	chickenpox.		

19. The most important personal precaution against disease transmission is:
- A. effective hand washing.
- B. up-to-date immunizations.
- C. postexposure prophylaxis.
- D. disinfection of equipment.
- E. compliance with infection control policies.

20. Your partner reports a sudden onset of fever, chills, malaise, muscle aches, nasal discharge, and a cough. You suspect:

A.	hantavirus.	D.	pneumonia.
B.	tuberculosis.	E.	influenza.
C.	HIV.		

21. All of the following are causative organisms for food poisoning EXCEPT:

A.	*Escherichia coli.*	D.	*Salmonella.*
B.	*Haemophilus influenzae.*	E.	*Shigella.*
C.	*Campylobacter.*		

22. All of the following are sexually transmitted diseases EXCEPT:

A.	HSV-2.	D.	HPV.
B.	chlamydia.	E.	gonorrhea.
C.	HAV.		

23. Bacteria such as Campylobacter, Salmonella, Shigella or Vibrio cholerae may be implicated in which of the following:
- A. food poisoning
- B. menningitis.
- C. Hepatitis A
- D. syphilis.
- E. gonorrhea.

24. The incubation period for SARS is typically:

A.	5-14 days.	D.	1-3 days.
B.	2-3 weeks.	E.	12 days.
C.	2-7 days.		

25. Signs and symptoms of SARS include all of the following EXCEPT:

A.	difficulty breathing	D.	ARDS.
B.	cough .	E.	myalgia.
C.	temperature <38 C.		

True/False

_____ **26.** All microorganisms that reside in our bodies are pathogenic.
    A. True
    B. False

_____ **27.** Sterilization is the recommended level of decontamination for all equipment used by EMS personnel.
    A. True
    B. False

_____ **28.** The clinical presentation of encephalitis often mimics that of meningitis.
    A. True
    B. False

_____ **29.** Methicillin-resistant staphylococcus aureus and vancomycin-resistant enterococcus are both examples of nosocomial infections .
    A. True
    B. False

_____ **30.** Chancroid is a highly contagious ulcer caused by a gram-positive bacterium.
    A. True
    B. False

_____ **31.** Sexually transmitted diseases include gonorrhea, genital warts, chlamydia and chancroid.
    A. True
    B. False

_____ **32.** Puncture wounds are commonly associated with *C. tetani* infection.
    A. True
    B. False

_____ **33.** Hantavirus is a family of viruses carried by rodents, such as the deer mouse.
    A. True
    B. False

_____ **34.** The clinical presentation of varicella may include Koplik's spots on the oral mucosa.
    A. True
    B. False

_____ **35.** SARS presents as a typical pneumonia.
    A. True
    B. False

Matching

Write the letter of the term in the space provided next to the appropriate description.

A.	impetigo	**F.**	Lyme disease
B.	croup	**G.**	rubella
C.	pertussis	**H.**	Kernig's sign
D.	bacteria	**I.**	varicella
E.	nosocomial	**J.**	chancroid

_____ **36.** chickenpox

_____ **37.** microscopic single-celled organisms

_____ **38.** acquired while in the hospital

_____ **39.** infection of the skin caused by staphylococci or streptococci

_____ **40.** viral illness characterized by inspiratory and expiratory stridor and a seal-bark-like cough

_____ **41.** recurrent inflammatory disorder caused by a tick-borne spirochete

_____ **42.** German measles

_____ **43.** inability to fully extend the knees with hips flexed

_____ **44.** disease characterized by severe, violent coughing

_____ **45.** highly contagious sexually transmitted ulcer

Chapter 38

Psychiatric and Behavioral Disorders

Review of Chapter Objectives

After reading this chapter, you should be able to:

1. **Define behavior and distinguish among normal behavior, abnormal behavior, and the behavioral emergency. pp. 834-835**

Behavior is a person's observable conduct and activity, while a behavioral emergency is a situation in which a patient's behavior becomes so unusual, bizarre, or threatening that it alarms the patient or another person and requires the intervention of EMS and/or mental health personnel. The differentiation between "normal" and "abnormal" behavior is largely subjective and widely variable based on culture, ethnic group, socioeconomic class, environment, and personal interpretation and opinion.

2. **Discuss the prevalence of behavioral and psychiatric disorders. p. 835**

It is estimated that 20 percent of the population has some type of mental health problem and that as many as 1 in 7 will require treatment for an emotional disturbance.

3. **Discuss the pathophysiology of behavioral and psychiatric disorders. pp. 835-836**

The general causes of behavioral and psychiatric disorders are biological (organic), psychosocial, and sociocultural. Biological (organic) causes are related to disease processes or structural changes in the brain. Psychosocial causes are related to the patient's personality, dynamics of unresolved conflict, or crisis management methods. Sociocultural causes are related to the patient's actions and interactions within society. It should be noted that many psychiatric disorders are due to altered brain chemistry.

4. **Discuss the factors that may alter the behavioral or emotional status of an ill or injured individual. pp. 835-836**

Remember that you cannot be sure that a patient is suffering from a purely psychological condition until you have completely ruled out medical conditions, such as hypoglycemia, traumatic injury, and substance abuse. Failure to comply with the prescribed medication regimen may cause exacerbation of a patient's psychiatric condition and lead to the development of a behavioral emergency. Societal events (rape, assault, and acts of violence) may contribute to alterations in someone's emotional status, as can interpersonal events, such as death of a loved one or loss of a relationship.

5. Describe the medical legal considerations for management of emotionally disturbed patients.
   pp. 853-856

The laws of consent specify that any competent person has the right to refuse to consent to treatment. Further, no competent person may be transported against his/her will. Any person who is in imminent danger of harming him-/herself or others is not considered competent to refuse treatment and transport. Most states have laws that allow persons fitting this criterion to be transported against their will to a hospital or approved psychiatric facility for evaluation.

6. Describe the overt behaviors associated with behavioral and psychiatric disorders.
   pp. 840-851

Overt behaviors that may be associated with behavioral emergencies include hand gestures (clenched fists, wringing hands, etc.) or postures (cowering, visible tension, etc.) that you may observe in your patient. The patient may display strange or threatening facial expressions. The patient's speech may reveal disorientation, fixations, unrealistic judgments, or unusual thought processes. Other behaviors you may observe include pacing, picking at one's skin, or appearing to pull things from the air. There are many different kinds of such overt behaviors, and they can differ or overlap depending on the specific disorder.

7. Define the following terms:

• Affect   p. 837
Visible indicators of mood or the impression that someone else may have about one's mood based on one's appearance. For instance, a person with a flat affect gives the appearance of being disinterested and is often lacking facial expression.

• Anger   p. 843
This can be described as feelings of hostility or rage to compensate for an underlying feeling of anxiety.

• Anxiety   pp. 842-843
This is a state of uneasiness, discomfort, apprehension, and restlessness.

• Confusion   p. 837
This is a state of being unclear or unable to make a decision easily.

• Depression   p. 843
This is a profound sadness or feeling of melancholy.

• Fear   p. 837
Fear is a feeling of alarm and discontent in the expectation of danger.

• Mental status   p. 837
This is defined as the state of the patient's cerebral functioning.

• Open-ended question   p. 837
This is the type of question that cannot be answered by "yes" or "no" and requires a longer response from the person being questioned.

• Posture   p. 837
This term refers to the position, attitude, or bearing of the body.

8. Describe verbal techniques useful in managing the emotionally disturbed patient.
   pp. 838-839

The key to dealing with the emotionally disturbed patient is to listen carefully. Place yourself at the patient's level, but keep a safe and proper distance, not invading the patient's personal space. Ask open-ended questions that require your patient to respond in detail. Be comfortable with silence and take whatever time is necessary to get the whole story of the situation. Do not lie to or make fun of the patient. Be nonjudgmental.

9. List the appropriate measures to ensure the safety of the paramedic, the patient, and others. pp. 836-840, 851-853

As with any call, determining scene safety is critical. Many behavioral emergencies, for which you are dispatched, will also warrant mutual response by law enforcement personnel. Gain control of the scene. Remove anyone who agitates the patient or adds confusion to the scene. Examine the environment for signs of violence and potential weapons. Approach every situation cautiously and when feasible observe the patient from a distance first before approaching. Avoid invading the patient's personal space. Watch for signs of aggression. If a patient becomes violent, use of restraint may become necessary; in such cases, carefully follow your service's protocols for such circumstances and be sure to document your actions thoroughly.

10. Describe the circumstances when relatives, bystanders, and others should be removed from the scene. p. 837

It is important to gain control of the scene as quickly as possible. Remove anyone who agitates the patient or adds to the confusion on the scene. Generally, it is a good idea to limit the number of people around the patient. You may even find it necessary to totally clear the room or to move the patient to a quiet area.

11. Describe techniques to systematically gather information from the disturbed patient. pp. 839, 853

Your interpersonal skills are crucial to your success as an EMS professional but never more so than when you are caring for a patient who is having a behavioral emergency. Limit environmental distractions at the scene. Introduce yourself and note how the patient responds to you, altering your approach if the patient becomes agitated. Establish eye contact. Place yourself at the patient's level. Listen carefully. Take your time. Do not physically threaten the patient. Ask open-ended questions. Be truthful with the patient and never play along with hallucinations or delusions. Focus your questioning and assessment on the immediate problem.

12. Identify techniques for physical assessment in a patient with behavioral problems. pp. 837-839

All of the interpersonal skills discussed above that allow you to effectively interview patients will need to be incorporated into your physical assessment activities. Generally, the examination of a behavioral emergency patient is largely conversational. If you need to perform hands-on assessment activities, defer their completion until you have had the opportunity to establish rapport and, even then, do not make any sudden moves that may startle the patient. If a patient is restrained, be sure to monitor him or her frequently and carefully to ensure that the airway is patent and that he or she is not experiencing positional asphyxia.

13. List situations in which you are expected to transport a patient forcibly and against his will. pp. 853-854

Any person who is in imminent danger of harming him-/herself or others is not considered competent to refuse treatment and transport. Patients who are suicidal or homicidal meet this criterion. Most states have laws that allow persons fitting this criterion to be transported against their will for evaluation. The authority to make this decision varies from state to state. Other situations are not so clear-cut and require you to use clinical judgment and follow your service's protocols.

14. Describe restraint methods necessary in managing the emotionally disturbed patient.
pp. 854-856

The primary objective is to restrict the patient's movement to prevent him from harming himself or others. Your own agency's rules will dictate the appropriate technique and method for restraint. The following rules always apply: use minimum necessary force; use appropriate devices; remember that restraint is not punitive; and carefully monitor anyone who is restrained. Before initiating any restraint activities, make sure that you have sufficient help, as this minimizes the potential for injury to the patient or yourself.

15. List the risk factors and behaviors that indicate a patient is at risk for suicide. **p. 850**

All of the following are considered to be risk factors for suicide: previously attempted suicide, depression, age (15 to 24 years of age or over 40), substance abuse, social isolation, major separation trauma, major physical stresses, loss of independence, suicide of a parent. Also significant is having possession of a mechanism for suicide and having a specific plan and/or expressing it.

16. Use the assessment and patient history to differentiate between the various behavioral and psychiatric disorders. **pp. 840-851**

Most psychiatric disorders have two diagnostic elements: symptoms of the disease/disorder and indications that the disease/disorder has impaired major life functions or interfered with the activities of daily living. It is not the role of EMS personnel to diagnose behavioral disorders, as this can be a difficult task even for skilled mental health professionals. The overview of psychiatric disorders is intended to increase your general understanding of behavioral problems.

The most helpful thing you can do is to perform a mental status exam (MSE) as part of your routine assessment. The elements of an MSE include: general appearance, behavioral observations, orientation, memory, sensorium, perceptual processes, mood and affect, intelligence, thought processes, insight, judgment, psychomotor.

17. Given several preprogrammed behavioral emergency patients, provide the appropriate scene size-up, initial assessment, focused assessment, and detailed assessment, then provide the appropriate care and patient transport. **pp. 834-856**

Throughout your training, you will encounter a variety of real and simulated patients with behavioral or psychiatric emergencies. Use the information in the text, as well as the application of this information as demonstrated by your instructors, preceptors, and mentors to enhance your ability to assess, manage, and transport patients with behavioral emergencies. Every emergency call has an element of behavioral emergency in it; your patience and professionalism will help minimize the emotional component for everyone involved.

CONTENT SELF-EVALUATION

Multiple Choice

_____ 1. Organic causes for behavioral emergencies include all of the following EXCEPT:
A.	tumor.	D.	infection.
B.	depression.	E.	hypoglycemia.
C.	substance abuse.		

_____ 2. The term that describes the state of a patient's cerebral functioning is:
A.	affect.	D.	orientation.
B.	mood.	E.	sensorium.
C.	mental status.		

3. The best approach for gaining information from a behavioral emergency patient is to:
   A. ask questions requiring yes or no answers.
   B. talk loudly to establish control.
   C. ask open-ended questions.
   D. physically restrain the patient before questioning.
   E. move quickly to expedite transport and then question.

4. The structured exam designed to quickly evaluate a patient's level of mental functioning is the:
   A. neurologic exam.
   B. mental status exam.
   C. psychiatric evaluation.
   D. Glasgow Coma Score.
   E. stroke assessment scale.

5. The most likely way to provoke violence or aggression in a behavioral emergency patient is to:
   A. listen carefully to his responses.
   B. appear patient and unhurried.
   C. ask open-ended questions.
   D. invade his personal space.
   E. avoid rapid or sudden movements.

6. Panic attack, phobias, and posttraumatic stress syndrome are classified as:
   A. types of schizophrenia.
   B. personality disorders.
   C. variants of depression.
   D. bipolar disorders.
   E. anxiety disorders.

7. The most prevalent form of psychiatric problem is:
   A. schizophrenia.
   B. personality disorder.
   C. depression.
   D. bipolar disorder.
   E. anxiety disorder.

8. Profound sadness, diminished ability to concentrate, and feelings of worthlessness are commonly associated with:
   A. schizophrenia.
   B. personality disorders.
   C. depression.
   D. bipolar disorders.
   E. anxiety disorders.

9. Medications commonly used in the management of schizophrenia are:
   A. antipsychotics.
   B. sedatives.
   C. antihistamines.
   D. antipsychotics and sedatives.
   E. sedatives and antihistamines.

10. Common causes of dementia include all of the following EXCEPT:
   A. Alzheimer's disease.
   B. head trauma.
   C. cardiac seizure.
   D. Parkinson's disease.
   E. AIDS.

11. Hallucinations, delusions, and disorganized thought, speech, and behavior are commonly associated with:
   A. schizophrenia.
   B. personality disorders.
   C. depression.
   D. bipolar disorders.
   E. anxiety disorders.

12. The compelling desire to use a substance, inability to reduce use of a substance, and repeated unsuccessful efforts to quit using that substance are indicators of:
   A. psychological dependence.
   B. physical dependence.
   C. substance tolerance.
   D. factitious disorder.
   E. somatoform disorder.

13. The primary objective in patient restraint is to:
   A. initiate punitive response.
   B. stop dangerous behaviors.
   C. limit patient strength.
   D. reduce legal liability.
   E. encourage patient cooperation.

14. Which of the following can result in a biological psychiatric disorder?
    A.   infections   D.   traumatic events.
    B.   values   E.   abusive parents
    C.   discrimination

15. When conducting an assessment of a patient experiencing a behavioural emergency, what type of questions should be asked?
    A.   threatening.   D.   open-ended
    B.   faster than usual   E.   judgemental
    C.   closed-ended

16. Patients presenting with an acute onset of general clouding of consciousness, inattention and vivid visual hallucinations may be suffering from:
    A.   schizophrenia.   D.   bipolar disorders.
    B.   delirium.   E.   anxiety disorders.
    C.   dementia.

17. Two types of cognitive disorders are:
    A.   schizophrenia and anxiety.   D.   anxiety and depression.
    B.   dementia and delirium.   E.   dementia and Alzheimer's.
    C.   mood and anxiety.

18. Having aphasia, apraxia, or agnosia, may be associated with:
    A.   dementia.   D.   posttraumatic stress syndrome.
    B.   schizophrenia   .   E.   anxiety disorders.
    C.   personality disorder cluster.

19. Common signs of panic attacks include all of the following EXCEPT
    A.   chest pain or discomfort   D.   nausea
    B.   bradycardia   E.   trembling
    C.   diaphoresis

20. Bipolar disorder is also known as:
    A.   obsessive-compulsive   D.   histrionic-depressive
    B.   anti-social   E.   manic-depressive
    C.   paranoid-schizoid

21. A condition characterized by physical symptoms that have no apparent physiological cause and attributable to psychological factors can be classified as which type of disorder?
    A.   factitious disorder   D.   dissociative disorder
    B.   depressive disorder   E.   personality disorder.
    C.   somatoform disorder

22. Treatment of Bipolar disorder includes which of the following pharmacological agents?:
    A.   fluoxetine   D.   lithium
    B.   sertraline   E.   vardenafil HCI
    C.   lorazepam

23. A person who believes he has a defect in his physical appearance is said to have which of the following disorders?
    A.   body dysmorphic disorder   D.   conversion disorder
    B.   hypochondrias   E.   fugue state
    C.   psychogenic amnesia

24. In 1992 the most common method of suicide was:
    A.   poisoning   D.   gunshot.
    B.   strangulation   .   E.   jumping.
    C.   cutting.

25. Treatment of anxiety disorders may include the administration of the which of the following medications?
   A.   lorazepam
   B.   haloperidol
   C.   Ketamine.
   D.   labetalol
   E.   phenobarbital

True/False

26. It is always safe to assume that a patient exhibiting bizarre behavior is suffering from a psychological problem or disease.
   A.   True
   B.   False

27. When a pediatric or geriatric patient is experiencing a behavioral emergency, the paramedic should always consider using chemical restraints.
   A.   True
   B.   False

28. A behavioural emergency is considered abnormal behaviour.
   A.   True
   B.   False

29. Delirium is characterized by a fairly acute onset and is seldom reversible.
   A.   True
   B.   False

30. The symptoms of Schizophrenia may include catatonia or grossly disorganized behaviour.
   A.   True
   B.   False

31. Patients of disorders of impulse control tend to have pleasure gratification after committing an act.
   A.   True
   B.   False

32. Suicidal patients are usually "just looking for attention" and are not really a true emergency.
   A.   True
   B.   False

33. The surest way to make a behavioural emergency patient violent is to invade his "personal space", approximately 1 m around the person.
   A.   True
   B.   False

34. Schizophrenics require ongoing treatment of haloperidol to function normally within society.
   A.   True
   B.   False

35. Dementia may be due to several medical problems including vascular problems.
   A.   True
   B.   False

Matching

Write the letter of the word or phrase in the space provided next to its definition.

A.	delirium	**F.**	catatonia
B.	dementia	**G.**	paranoid
C.	schizophrenia	**H.**	bipolar disorder
D.	delusions	**I.**	personality disorder
E.	hallucinations	**J.**	depersonalization

_____ **36.** Feeling detached from oneself

_____ **37.** Condition characterized by relatively rapid onset of widespread disorganized thought

_____ **38.** Fixed false beliefs

_____ **39.** Condition that results in persistently maladaptive behavior

_____ **40.** Sensory perceptions with no basis in reality

_____ **41.** Condition characterized by one or more manic episodes, with or without subsequent or alternating periods of depression

_____ **42.** Condition characterized by immobility, rigidity, and stupor

_____ **43.** Common disorder involving significant behavioral changes and disorganized thought

_____ **44.** Preoccupation with feelings of persecution

_____ **45.** Condition involving gradual development of memory impairment and cognitive disturbance

Chapter 39

Gynecology

Review of Chapter Objectives

After reading this chapter, you should be able to:

1. Review the anatomic structures and physiology of the female reproductive system. (see Chapter 12)

The most important female reproductive structures are located within the pelvic cavity. Essential to reproduction, these structures include the ovaries, fallopian tubes, uterus, and vagina. The external genitalia have accessory functions, in that they protect body openings and play an important role in sexual functioning.

2. Identify the normal events of the menstrual cycle. (see Chapter 12)

A monthly hormonal cycle prepares the uterus to receive a fertilized egg. The first 2 weeks of the cycle (known as the proliferative phase) are dominated by estrogen causing the uterine lining to thicken. In response to a surge of luteinizing hormone, ovulation takes place and an egg is released from the ovary. The secretory phase is the stage of the menstrual cycle immediately surrounding ovulation. If the egg is not fertilized, the woman's estrogen level drops sharply while the progesterone level dominates. Uterine vascularity increases in anticipation of implantation. If fertilization does not occur, estrogen and progesterone levels fall, triggering vascular changes leaving the endometrium ischemic. The ischemic endometrium is shed during the menstrual phase (menstruation), along with a discharge of blood, mucus, and cellular debris. Menstrual flow usually lasts 3 to 5 days, with an average blood loss of 50 ml.

3. Describe how to assess a patient with a gynecological complaint.   pp. 858-860

The most common gynecological complaints are abdominal pain and vaginal bleeding. Complete your initial assessment in the usual manner and then proceed with a focused history and physical exam. Specific questions will need to be asked that are pertinent to reproductive function and dysfunction. If pertinent, be sure to gather information about her obstetrical history, including pregnancies and deliveries. It is important to document the date of the patient's last menstrual period (LMP). You should also ask what form of birth control, if any, she uses and, if pertinent, whether she uses it regularly. Pay particular attention to the physical exam, which will be limited to assessment of the abdomen and potentially (in the presence of serious bleeding) inspection of the patient's perineum. Gently auscultate and palpate the abdomen. Be sure to note the color, character, and volume of any blood lost. An internal vaginal exam should never be performed in the pre-hospital setting.

4. Explain how to recognize a gynecological emergency.   pp. 858-860

As with any emergency situation, vital signs are useful clues as to your patient's status as well as its severity. Be alert for early signs of shock or a positive tilt test, both of which point to significant blood loss. If possible, estimate blood loss. The use of two sanitary pads per hour is considered significant bleeding.

**5. Describe the general care for any patient experiencing a gynecological emergency.
pp. 860-861**

Management of gynecological emergencies is focused on supportive care. Rely on your initial assessment guidance in your decision making about oxygen therapy, ventilatory support, and vascular access. In the presence of shock, follow your local protocols for fluid resuscitation and use of the PASG. In cases of heavy bleeding, do not pack dressings in the vagina. Continue to monitor the patient's status and bleeding en route to definitive care. Equally important is the psychological support that you give your patient. Protect her modesty and privacy.

6. Describe the pathophysiology, assessment, and management of the following gynecological emergencies.

a.   Pelvic inflammatory disease   pp. 861-862
Pelvic inflammatory disease (PID), the most common cause of nontraumatic abdominal pain in women in the childbearing years, is an infection of the female reproductive tract that is most commonly caused by gonorrhea or chlamydia. Predisposing factors include: multiple sexual partners, prior history of PID, recent gynecological procedure, or an IUD. The patient will look acutely ill and will often present with diffuse lower abdominal pain, and may also have fever, chills, nausea, vomiting, and possibly a foul-smelling vaginal discharge. The patient may also walk with a shuffling gait due to pain. Blood pressure may be normal, and fever may or may not be present. Palpation of the lower abdomen usually elicits moderate to severe pain. The primary management in the field is supportive care and a position of comfort during transport. If the patient appears septic, then administer oxygen and initiate IV therapy.

b.   Ruptured ovarian cyst   p. 862
Cysts are fluid-filled pockets, and, when they develop in the ovary, they can rupture and be a source of abdominal pain. The rupture spills a small amount of blood into the abdomen, irritating the peritoneum and causing abdominal pain and rebound tenderness. Usually the patient complains of moderate to severe unilateral abdominal pain that may radiate to the back; it may be associated with vaginal bleeding. The patient may also report pain during intercourse or a delayed menstrual period. The primary management in the field is supportive care and a position of comfort during transport.

c.   Cystitis p. 862
A bacterial infection of the urinary bladder (cystitis) is a common cause of abdominal pain that may be accompanied by urinary frequency, dysuria, and a low-grade fever. The pain is generally located just above the symphysis pubis unless the infection has spread to the kidneys, in which case there is likely to be flank pain as well. The primary management in the field is supportive care and a position of comfort during transport.

d.   Mittelschmerz   p. 862
Mid-cycle abdominal pain may accompany ovulation. The unilateral lower quadrant pain is usually self-limited and may be accompanied by mid-cycle spotting. Treatment is symptomatic.

e.   Endometritis   p. 862
Endometritis, an infection of the uterine lining, is an occasional complication of miscarriage, childbirth, or gynecologic procedures. Commonly reported signs and symptoms include mild to severe lower abdominal pain, a bloody and foul-smelling discharge, and fever that may mimic PID. The primary management in the field is supportive care and a position of comfort during transport. If the patient appears septic, then administer oxygen and initiate IV therapy.

f.   Endometriosis   pp. 862-863

Endometriosis is a condition in which endometrial tissue is found outside the uterus. Most commonly, it is found in the abdomen and pelvis. Regardless of the site, the tissue responds to the hormones of the menstrual cycle, thus bleeding in a cyclic manner. The condition is most common in women between 30 and 40 and is rare in postmenopausal women. The patient complains of dull, cramping pelvic pain, usually related to menstruation. The primary management in the field is supportive care and a position of comfort during transport.

g.   Ectopic pregnancy   p. 863

Ectopic pregnancy is the implantation of a fetus outside of the uterus, most commonly in the fallopian tubes. Patients usually report severe unilateral abdominal pain that may radiate to the shoulder on the affected side, a late or missed menstrual period, and sometimes vaginal bleeding. As the fetus develops, the tube can rupture, triggering a massive, life-threatening hemorrhage. Absorb the bleeding but do not pack the vagina. Ectopic pregnancy is a surgical emergency, and the primary management in the field is supportive care and a position of comfort during transport, as well as oxygen administration and IV therapy for fluid resuscitation.

h.   Vaginal hemorrhage   p. 863

Nontraumatic vaginal hemorrhage is rarely encountered in the prehospital setting unless it is severe. Do not presume that such bleeding is due to normal menstrual flow. Most commonly, it is due to a spontaneous abortion (miscarriage) and is associated with cramping abdominal pain and the passage of clots and tissue. Other possible causes include cancerous lesions, PID, or the onset of labor. Absorb bleeding but do not pack the vagina. The primary management in the field is supportive care and a position of comfort for the patient, as well as oxygen administration and IV therapy for fluid resuscitation. If the bleeding is due to miscarriage, this will likely be a significant emotional event for your patient, so your kind and considerate care is important.

Traumatic vaginal bleeding may result from sexual assault, blunt-force injuries to the lower abdomen, seat-belt injuries, objects inserted into the vagina, self-attempts at abortion, and lacerations following childbirth. Bleeding in such cases should be managed by direct pressure over a laceration or a cold pack applied to a hematoma. Never pack the vagina. Provide expedited transport to the hospital, with oxygen administration and IV access as necessary.

7. Describe the assessment, care, and emotional support of the sexual assault patient.   pp. 864-866

Sexual assault victims are unique patients with unique needs. The psychological care of these patients is as important, if not more so, than the physical care they may need. Confine your questions to the physical injuries that the patient may have received. Unless your patient is unconscious, do not touch the patient, even to take vital signs, without her permission. Explain what's going to be done before initiating any treatment. Avoid touching the patient other than to take vital signs or to examine other physical injuries. Do not examine the external genitalia of the sexual assault victim unless there is life-threatening hemorrhage. Consider the patient to be a crime scene and protect that scene; handle clothing as little as possible, collect all bloody articles as potential evidence, do not allow the patient to change clothes or bathe and do not clean wounds if possible. Be sure to document the treatment of the sexual assault victim carefully, thoroughly, and objectively.

8. Given several preprogrammed gynecological patients, provide the appropriate assessment, management and transportation.   pp. 858-866

Throughout your classroom, clinical, and field training, you will encounter a variety of real and simulated gynecologic patients. Use the information provided in this chapter of your text, as well as the application of this information as demonstrated by your instructors, preceptors, and mentors to enhance your ability to assess, manage, and transport these patients. Keep in mind that gynecological emergencies are likely to be very stressful situations for your patients, and they will appreciate your gentle, considerate care and professionalism.

CONTENT SELF-EVALUATION

Multiple Choice

_____ 1. Painful discomfort during menstrual periods is known as:
- **A.** menarche.
- **B.** dyspareunia.
- **C.** cystitis.
- **D.** dysmenorrhea.
- **E.** pelvic inflammatory disease.

_____ 2. Which of the following questions is LEAST likely to get an accurate response from a female who is complaining of abdominal pain?
- **A.** Are you currently menstruating?
- **B.** Are you sexually active?
- **C.** Could you be pregnant?
- **D.** Have you ever experienced this pain before when menstruating?
- **E.** Have you experienced dizziness?

_____ 3. The term used to describe the number of deliveries a woman has had is:
- **A.** gravida.
- **B.** gravity.
- **C.** parity.
- **D.** parita.
- **E.** completa.

_____ 4. A palpable abdominal mass found midway between the symphysis pubis and the umbilicus in the lower abdomen of a 25-year-old woman is most likely to be a(n):
- **A.** tumor.
- **B.** intrauterine pregnancy of 5 months gestation.
- **C.** intrauterine pregnancy of 4 months gestation.
- **D.** intrauterine pregnancy of 3 months gestation.
- **E.** ovarian cyst.

_____ 5. Pelvic inflammatory disease is most often caused by:
- **A.** gonorrhea and chlamydia.
- **B.** streptococcus and staphylococcus.
- **C.** gonorrhea and HIV.
- **D.** chlamydia and streptococcus.
- **E.** HIV and staphylococcus.

_____ 6. Mid-cycle abdominal pain associated with ovulation is known as:
- **A.** endometriosis.
- **B.** PID.
- **C.** a miscarriage.
- **D.** cystitis.
- **E.** mittelschmerz.

_____ 7. All of the following signs and symptoms are associated with endometritis EXCEPT:
- **A.** history of gynecologic procedure.
- **B.** severe abdominal pain.
- **C.** fever.
- **D.** bradycardia.
- **E.** bloody, foul-smelling discharge.

_____ 8. All of the following signs and symptoms are associated with a ruptured ovarian cyst EXCEPT:
- **A.** dyspareunia.
- **B.** severe abdominal pain.
- **C.** fever.
- **D.** delayed menstrual period.
- **E.** irregular bleeding.

_____ 9. If a female patient presents with severe unilateral abdominal pain that radiates to the shoulder on one side, a missed menstrual period, and vaginal bleeding, you should suspect:
- **A.** mittelschmerz.
- **B.** ectopic pregnancy.
- **C.** PID.
- **D.** endometriosis.
- **E.** cystitis.

10. A female reports that during intercourse she felt a sudden and sharp tearing sensation. She is now bleeding from the external genitalia, although the bleeding is minimal. Management should include:
   A. asking the woman to hold a dressing over the area and apply direct pressure.
   B. establishing an IV and beginning fluid resuscitation regardless of blood loss.
   C. packing the vagina with sterile dressings.
   D. palpating the interior of the vagina to determine the extent of bleeding.
   E. securing a hot pack over the vaginal opening with tape.

11. The pre-hospital priorities for care of the sexual assault victim include all of the following EXCEPT:
   A. examining for perineal tears.
   B. determining if life-threatening injuries exist.
   C. providing emotional support
   D. preserving evidence.
   E. protecting patient's privacy.

12. The BEST management for a victim of a sexual assault is:
   A. aggressive questioning and internal examination.
   B. discouraging the patient from dressing since this may taint evidence.
   C. examining the genitalia.
   D. psychological and emotional support.
   E. prompt summoning of law enforcement officials.

13. Vaginal bleeding due to a miscarriage is often associated with:
   A. headache.   D. dysmenorrhea.
   B. cramping.   E. dyspareunia.
   C. cystitis

14. Which of the following is NOTa recommended treatment for a patient with non-traumatic vaginal bleeding?
   A. IV access
   B. position for comfort or altered vital signs
   C. application of dressings
   D. pack the vagina
   E. oxygen therapy

15. Significant vaginal bleeding may cause which of the following:
   A. positive tilt-test   D. increased respiratory rate
   B. increased pulse rate   E. all of the above
   C. narrowing pulse pressures

True/False

16. The term used to describe the number of times a woman has been pregnant is parity.
   A. True
   B. False

17. Endometriosis is an infection of the uterine lining.
   A. True
   B. False

18. The most effective means to control vaginal hemorrhage is to apply direct pressure to the perineum.
   A. True
   B. False

_____ **19.** PID is a major risk factor for pelvic adhesions..
    A.   True
    B.   False

_____ **20.** When completing your patient care reports, you should include your opinion as to whether rape occurred.
    A.   True
    B.   False

_____ **21.** In cases of sexual assault, after assessing if physical injuries exist, your should respect the patient's wishes and offer emotional support.
    A.   True
    B.   False

_____ **22.** Straddle injuries are the second most common form of gynecological trauma after sexual assault.
    A.   True
    B.   False

_____ **23.** Sexual assault includes oral-genital sex
    A.   True
    B.   False

_____ **24.** Any patient of reproductive age who still has her uterus should be considered to be pregnant until proven otherwise.
    A.   True
    B.   False

_____ **25.** General management of gynecological emergencies is focused on supportive care.
    A.   True
    B.   False

Matching

Write the letter of the term in the space provided next to the appropriate description.

A.	obstetrics	**F.**	pelvic inflammatory disease
B.	mittelschmerz	**G.**	dysuria
C.	LMP	**H.**	cystisis
D.	dysmenorrhea	**I.**	endometriosis
E.	dyspareunia	**J.**	menorrhagia

_____ **26.** painful menstration

_____ **27.** infection of the urinary bladder

_____ **28.** abdominal pain associated with ovulation

_____ **29.** excessive menstrual flow

_____ **30.** the branch of medicine that deals with the care of women throughout pregnancy

_____ **31.** an acute infection of the reproductive organs that can be caused by bacteria, virus or fungus

_____ **32.** painful urination often associated with cystitis

_____ **33.** painful sexual intercourse

_____ **34.** condition in which endometrial tissues grows outside of the uterus

_____ **35.** last menstrual period

Chapter 40

Obstetrics

Review of Chapter Objectives

After reading this chapter, you should be able to:

1. Describe the anatomic structures and physiology of the reproductive system during pregnancy.   pp. 868-872

The primary "organ of pregnancy" is the placenta, which arises from the site on the uterine wall where the blastocyst (fertilized egg) implants itself. This temporary, blood-rich structure serves as a lifeline for the developing fetus via the umbilical cord. Its functions include the transfer of heat while exchanging oxygen and carbon dioxide, delivering nutrients, and removing waste. The placenta also serves as an endocrine gland throughout the pregnancy, secreting hormones necessary for fetal survival as well as the estrogen and progesterone required to maintain the pregnancy. The placenta is also a protective barrier against harmful substances that might cross the placental barrier to the fetus.

The fetus develops within the amniotic sac, a thin-walled membranous covering containing amniotic fluid that surrounds and protects the fetus during intrauterine life.

2. Identify the normal events of pregnancy. pp. 872-875

Fetal development begins at the moment of conception (fertilization). Normally, the duration of pregnancy is 40 weeks after the date of the mother's last menstrual period or 280 days. This is comparable to 10 lunar months or 9 calendar months. This time period is divided into trimesters, each of 3 calendar months duration.

Implantation of the fertilized egg into the uterine wall occurs during the pre-embryonic stage that lasts approximately 14 days. The embryonic stage begins at day 15 and ends at approximately 8 weeks, by which time all of the body systems have been formed. It is midway through this stage that the fetal heart begins to beat. The period from 8 weeks gestation until delivery is known as the fetal stage. The gender of the infant can usually be determined by 16 weeks, and by the 20th week, fetal heart tones are audible by stethoscope. The mother usually feels fetal movement (quickening) by the 24th week. By the 38th week, the baby is considered to be full term.

3. Describe how to assess an obstetrical patient.   pp. 875-878

The initial assessment for an obstetric patient is the same as for any other patient. Utilization of the SAMPLE history will allow you to obtain specific information about the pregnancy. Ask about gravidity, parity, length of gestation, and EDC (estimated date of confinement or due date). You should also obtain information about past OB/GYN history (e.g., C-section) or complications as well as prenatal care. Determine current medications and any drug allergies as well. It is important to obtain the past medical history because pregnancy may aggravate pre-existing medical problems or trigger new ones such as gestational diabetes. It is possible to estimate the due date by measuring fundal height above the symphysis pubis. Continue the physical exam, which is essentially the same for any patient, while being mindful of the need for modesty and privacy.

4. Identify the stages of labor and the paramedic's role in each stage. pp. 889-890

Labor is the physiologic and mechanical process by which the baby, placenta, and amniotic sac are expelled through the birth canal. The three stages of labor are dilatation, expulsion, and placental. The first stage (dilatation stage) begins with the onset of true labor and ends with the complete dilatation and effacement of the cervix. The second stage (expulsion stage) begins with the complete dilatation of the cervix and ends with the delivery of the baby. The third and final stage of labor (placental stage) begins immediately after the birth of the baby and ends with the delivery of the placenta. The role of the paramedic during labor is to assist in the delivery and to recognize and treat life-threatening problems for the mother or baby.

5. Differentiate between normal and abnormal delivery. pp. 889-901

Normally, most infants present from the birth canal in a headfirst, face-down position (vertex presentation), which allows the infant to be delivered vaginally. Abnormal delivery situations generally preclude vaginal delivery and are likely to require caesarean section, so transport must be expedited. These situations include breech presentation (buttocks present first), prolapsed cord (umbilical cord protrudes from the birth canal), limb presentation (baby's arm or leg protrudes from the birth canal) or occiput posterior presentation (baby's brow is facing forward).

6. Identify and describe complications associated with pregnancy and delivery. pp. 878-889, 901-903

Medical complications of pregnancy include ectopic pregnancy, bleeding problems, supine hypotensive syndrome, gestational diabetes, and hypertensive disorders. Ectopic pregnancy refers to the implantation of the fertilized egg outside of the uterus. Abdominal pain and evidence of intra-abdominal and/or vaginal bleeding usually herald this event. Bleeding is generally differentiated as painful or painless. Vaginal bleeding, accompanied by cramping abdominal pain, prior to the 20th week of gestation is almost always associated with a spontaneous abortion. Painless bleeding is most commonly associated with *placenta previa* where, due to abnormal implantation of the placenta on the uterine wall, labor is accompanied by bleeding. Painful bleeding is the hallmark of *abruptio placenta* or the premature separation of the placenta from the uterine wall. It poses an immediate life threat to mother and child.

Supine hypotensive syndrome occurs most commonly in the third trimester as a result of compression of the inferior vena cava by the gravid uterus. Insulin resistance and decreased glucose tolerance characterize gestational diabetes, occurring in the last 20 weeks of pregnancy. Hypertensive disorders of pregnancy (formerly called toxemia) include preeclampsia or eclampsia and chronic and transient hypertension. Major motor seizures are the hallmark of eclampsia, which is the most serious of the hypertensive disorders, posing a life threat to the mother and child.

Some of complications associated with delivery are discussed in objective 5. Other problems can occur after delivery. One of these is postpartum hemorrhage, which is the loss of 500 cc or more of blood immediately following delivery. A common cause of the condition is lack of uterine muscle tone, and it occurs most frequently in the multigravida, with multiple births, and with the births of large infants. Uterine rupture is another complication of delivery. It can result from blunt abdominal trauma, prolonged uterine contractions, or a surgically scarred uterus. Uterine rupture presents with a patient in excruciating abdominal pain and often in shock. Uterine inversion occurs when the uterus turns inside out after delivery and extends through the cervix. Blood loss from 800 to 1,800 cc occurs, and the patient often experiences profound shock. Pulmonary embolism can also occur after pregnancy as a result of venous thromboembolism. It often presents with sudden dyspnea accompanied by sharp chest pain and a sense of impending doom.

7. Identify predelivery emergencies. pp. 878-889

Recognition of a predelivery emergency is based on information obtained from the focused history and physical exam that relates to the reported abnormality, such as pain, discomfort, or bleeding. While any of the complications listed above has potential to be an emergency, the most likely are *abruptio placenta* and eclampsia, both of which pose potential life threats to mother and child and require prompt and appropriate intervention.

8. State indications of an imminent delivery. p. 889

Increasing frequency and duration of contractions and the sensation of needing to move one's bowels (urge to push) are all signs of impending delivery. However, crowning is the definitive sign that birth is imminent.

9. Identify the contents of an obstetrical kit and explain the use of each item. p. 891

Commercially prepared OB kits are available from a variety of sources and contain the following items for use in the event of a field delivery: toweling or drape material, bulb syringe, two plastic umbilical clamps, and scissors. The toweling is used for draping the patient to minimize contamination of the baby during the birth. A bulb syringe is necessary for suctioning the baby's mouth and nose, while the cord clamps and scissors are used when separating the infant from its mother by clamping and cutting the umbilical cord.

10. Differentiate the management of a patient with predelivery emergencies from a normal delivery.   pp. 878-889

Management of predelivery emergencies requires that the paramedic correctly recognize their presence based on information obtained from the focused history and physical exam and then expedite transport while anticipating the development of shock and maintaining adequate oxygenation, fluid resuscitation as necessary, and, if appropriate, pharmacological intervention. Most of the time, the mother will be transported in the left lateral recumbent position.

11. State the steps in the predelivery preparation of the mother.   pp. 891-892

The first priority is to provide the mother with privacy. Then, time permitting, administer oxygen via a nasal cannula and establish vascular access. Position the mother on her back with knees and hips flexed and buttocks slightly elevated, or the mother may prefer squatting or to be in a semi-Fowler position with knees and hips flexed. Drape the mother's perineum to minimize contamination of the infant during delivery.

12. Establish the relationship between body substance isolation and childbirth. p. 891

Normally, preparation for childbirth in the prehospital setting would entail thoroughly washing hands and forearms before donning a gown, in addition to sterile gloves and goggles. Body substance isolation for childbirth generally includes draping the mother to minimize contamination of the baby during delivery.

13. State the steps to assist in the delivery of a newborn.   pp. 891-894

Key EMS actions during a routine (normal) delivery are primarily supportive, but you should remain vigilant to signs of impending problems. Providing gentle support to the perineum as the delivery progresses decreases the likelihood of an explosive delivery causing vaginal tears and the potential for neonatal head trauma. While supporting the head, gently slide your finger along the head and neck to ensure that the cord is not wrapped around the baby's head and neck. As the head emerges from the vaginal opening, suction the airway (mouth first, then nose) to insure that the airway is clear prior to the neonate taking his first breath. It may be necessary to tear the amniotic sac to release the amniotic fluid and permit the baby to breathe.

Gently guide the baby's head downward to allow delivery of the upper shoulder. Do not pull! Then gently guide the baby's body upward to allow delivery of the lower shoulder. Once the shoulders are delivered, the rest of the body will be quickly delivered. Keep the baby at the level of the mother's hips until the cord has been clamped and cut. Once the body has fully emerged from the birth canal, the baby should again be suctioned until the airway is clear. After clamping the umbilical cord at 10 cm and 15 cm from the baby and cutting in between, carefully dry the baby and wrap in a warming blanket to prevent hypothermia.

14. Describe how to care for the newborn.   pp. 893, 894-896

The essential emergency care of the newborn includes the establishment and maintenance of adequate airway and breathing status and the prevention of heat loss. Support the infant's head and torso, using both hands. Maintain warmth, repeat suctioning of the mouth and nose as needed until the airway is clear, and then assess using the APGAR score. Do not delay resuscitation or transport to perform APGAR scoring.

15. Describe how and when to cut the umbilical cord. pp. 891, 894

Once the baby's body has been delivered, suction the airway until clear while keeping the baby at the level of the mother's hips until the cord has been clamped and cut. Do not "milk" the cord. Supporting the baby's body, place the first umbilical clamp approximately 10 cm from the baby and the second clamp at 15 cm and carefully cut in between.

16. Discuss the steps in the delivery of the placenta.   pp. 893, 894

Following delivery of the baby, the vaginal opening will continue to ooze blood. Do not pull on the umbilical cord! Eventually, the cord will appear to lengthen indicating separation of the placenta from the uterine wall. Once the placenta is expelled through the vaginal opening, it should be placed in a biohazard bag and be transported to the hospital for examination.

17. Describe the management of the mother post-delivery.   p. 894, 901-903

The mother should receive fundal massage to control postpartum bleeding and the perineum should be inspected for tears. Continuously monitor vital signs. If not accomplished prior to delivery, vascular access should be established should fluid resuscitation become necessary.

18. Summarize neonatal resuscitation procedures.   p. 896

If the infant's respirations are below 30 per minute and tactile stimulation does not increase the rate to a normal range (30–60), immediately assist ventilations using a pediatric bag-valve mask with high-flow oxygen. If the heart rate is below 60 and does not increase in response to ventilations, initiate chest compressions. Transport to a facility with neonatal intensive care capabilities.

19. Describe the procedures for handling abnormal deliveries, complications of pregnancy, and maternal complications of labor. pp. 901

Management of abnormal deliveries or complications of pregnancy and labor require that the paramedic correctly recognize the problem and expedite transport while anticipating the development of shock and maintaining adequate oxygenation, fluid resuscitation as necessary and, if appropriate, pharmacological intervention. Most of the time, the mother will be transported in the left lateral recumbent position. When the baby's position (breech presentation, prolapsed cord, or limb presentation) dictates, the mother should be placed on oxygen and then assisted in assuming the knee-chest position. Additionally, in the management of prolapsed cord, two gloved fingers should be placed inside the vagina to prevent the baby's weight from compressing the cord and inhibiting oxygen delivery to the baby.

20. Describe special considerations when meconium is present in amniotic fluid or during delivery.   pp. 878-889, 896-903

The presence of meconium (fetal fecal matter) in the amniotic fluid is indicative of a fetal hypoxic incident. The thicker and darker the color of the meconium staining in the amniotic fluid, the higher the risk of fetal morbidity. Once the head has emerged from the birth canal, suction the mouth and nose thoroughly while still on the perineum. However, if the meconium is thick, visualize the glottis and use an endotracheal tube to suction the hypopharynx and trachea until clear. Failure to suction will cause the meconium to be pushed further down the trachea and into the lungs.

21. Describe special considerations of a premature baby.   pp. 887-889

Premature infants are ill suited for extrauterine life, particularly with regard to their pulmonary function. All of the concerns about caring for a neonate are exaggerated when the neonate is less than 38 weeks gestation. Of greatest concern are airway maintenance, ventilatory support, and oxygen delivery. These critically ill neonates should be taken immediately to a facility with neonatal intensive care capabilities.

22. Given several simulated delivery situations, provide the appropriate assessment, management, and transport for the mother and child.   pp. 868-903

Throughout your training, you will encounter a variety of real and simulated obstetric patients. Use the information provided in this chapter, as well as the application of this information as demonstrated by your instructors, preceptors, and mentors to enhance your ability to assess, manage, and transport these patients. Keep in mind that this is likely to be a stressful situation for your patient, and she will appreciate your kind, considerate care and professionalism.

CONTENT SELF-EVALUATION

Multiple Choice

1. Thickening of the uterine lining in anticipation of implantation of the fertilized egg is stimulated by:
   A.   estrogen.
   B.   progesterone.
   C.   follicle-stimulating hormone.
   D.   luteinizing hormone.
   E.   oxytocin.

2. All of the following are placental functions EXCEPT:
   A.   acting as the "organ of pregnancy."
   B.   production of hormones.
   C.   serving as a protective barrier.
   D.   providing fertilization.
   E.   providing a means of heat transfer.

3. The normal duration of pregnancy is:
   A.   40 weeks.
   B.   280 days.
   C.   10 lunar months.
   D.   9 calendar months.
   E.   all of the above

4. Blood volume increases by what percentage during pregnancy?
   A.   10%
   B.   25%
   C.   30%
   D.   45%
   E.   60%

5. The fetus receives its blood from the placenta by means of the:
   A.   umbilical vein.
   B.   umbilical artery.
   C.   inferior vena cava.
   D.   superior vena cava.
   E.   aorta.

6. Fetal circulation changes to normal circulation with the:
   A.   onset of labor.
   B.   expulsion from the birth canal.
   C.   baby's first breath.
   D.   clamping of the umbilical cord.
   E.   dilation/effacement of the cervix.

7. When performing a focused history on a pregnant patient, which of the following questions would be appropriate?
   A. Are you experiencing any pain or discomfort?
   B. Have you had any vaginal discharge or bleeding?
   C. When is your due date?
   D. Have you ever been pregnant before?
   E. all of the above

8. All of the following are common signs or symptoms of a predelivery emergency EXCEPT:
   A. abdominal pain or trauma.
   B. vaginal bleeding or discharge.
   C. painful deformed extremities.
   D. altered mental status or seizures.
   E. hypertension or hypotension.

9. All of the following are causes of bleeding during pregnancy EXCEPT:
   A. abortion.
   B. ovarian cyst.
   C. ectopic pregnancy.
   D. placenta previa.
   E. abruptio placenta.

10. Treatment of a female patient who is 16 weeks pregnant, is complaining of cramping abdominal pain, and has bright red vaginal bleeding should include all of the following EXCEPT:
    A. packing the vagina to control bleeding.
    B. treating for shock if indicated.
    C. maintaining oxygenation.
    D. providing emotional support.
    E. saving any tissue and clots for evaluation.

11. You suspect the patient in the situation described in question 10 is having a(n):
    A. abortion   .
    B. ovarian cyst.
    C. ectopic pregnancy.
    D. placenta previa.
    E. abruptio placenta.

12. Pelvic inflammatory disease, endometriosis, and tubal ligation are predisposing factors for:
    A. abortion.
    B. ovarian cyst.
    C. ectopic pregnancy.
    D. placenta previa.
    E. abruptio placenta.

13. You find that your patient is 36 weeks pregnant, has an altered mental status, and is reported to have had a major motor seizure, which you suspect is due to:
    A. placenta previa.
    B. eclampsia.
    C. epilepsy.
    D. abruptio placenta.
    E. supine hypotensive syndrome.

14. Care of the patient in question 13 should include all of the following EXCEPT:
    A. administering high-flow oxygen via a nonrebreather mask.
    B. protecting the patient from injury if seizures recur.
    C. minimizing noise and light to prevent seizure activity.
    D. administering magnesium sulfate per protocol.
    E. transporting on right side to protect airway.

15. All of the following are signs and symptoms of an imminent delivery EXCEPT:
    A. the presence of crowning.
    B. contractions occurring every 1–2 minutes.
    C. passage of "bloody show."
    D. sensation of an urge for bowel movement.
    E. rupture of membranes.

16. Your patient has just delivered a healthy baby boy. Following the delivery of the placenta, her vaginal bleeding seems to increase. Which of the following best describes what you should do provide emergency care for this patient?

    A.   Massage the uterus and position your patient on her right side.

    B.   Administer oxygen and firmly massage the uterus.

    C.   Massage the uterus and pack the vagina to control bleeding

    D.   Administer oxygen and pack the vagina with sanitary napkins.

    E.   Provide fluid resuscitation and position patient on her right side.

17. Meconium-stained amniotic fluid should first be managed by:

    A.   immediate transport to the hospital for physician evaluation.

    B.   administration of oxygen to the mother to resolve fetal distress.

    C.   suctioning of the mouth and nose before the infant takes his first breath.

    D.   stimulation of the infant to encourage coughing to clear meconium from airway.

    E.   expediting completion of delivery to decrease fetal distress.

18. Management of a limb presentation should include all of the following EXCEPT:

    A.   administration of high-flow oxygen to the mother.

    B.   immediate transport to the hospital.

    C.   attempting to push the limb back into the vagina.

    D.   positioning the mother with her head down and pelvis elevated.

    E.   providing reassurance to the mother.

19. The administration of an IV fluid bolus to control premature labor is based on increasing intravascular volume and thus causing inhibition of:

    A.   antidiuretic hormone.   **D.**   luteinizing hormone.

    B.   progesterone.   **E.**   follicle-stimulating hormone.

    C.   estrogen.

20. You have just assisted with the delivery of a baby girl. She has shallow, gasping respirations and a heart rate that is less than 100 beats per minute. Which of the following best describes your emergency care for this patient?

    A.   administering "blow by" oxygen and monitoring her pulse for 60 seconds

    B.   assisting ventilations with a BVM and reassessing in 30 seconds

    C.   administering high-flow oxygen with a nonrebreather mask

    D.   assisting ventilations with a BVM and beginning chest compressions

    E.   continuing to monitor and expedite transport

21. Shoulder dystocia is commonly associated with diabetic or obese mothers and:

    A.   prematurity.   **D.**   hormonal deficits.

    B.   hormonal excesses.   **E.**   fetal distress.

    C.   post-term pregnancy.

22. If the uterus protrudes from the vaginal opening following the delivery of the placenta, you should:

    A.   wrap it tightly in dry towels.

    B.   wrap it in dextrose-soaked dressings.

    C.   make no more than 3 attempts to replace it.

    D.   make no more than 1 attempt to replace it.

    E.   cover it with plastic wrap.

23. During the delivery of the baby you observe that the umbilical cord is wrapped tightly around the baby's neck twice. Your best intervention at this time would be to:

    A.   administer morphine sulphate for pain management

    B.   attempt to suction the airway to enable the baby to breathe

    C.   gently guide the baby's head downward to allow delivery of the upper shoulder

    D.   carefully place two umbilical cord clamps approximately 5 cm apart and cut the cord

    E.   massage the uterine fundus to promote blood flow to the baby

24. You have aided in the delivery of a baby boy who appears limp; without response; respirations slow and shallow; heart rate of 88 and body and extremities are blue. Which of the following reflect an accurate APGAR score of this baby?

A.	2		**D.**	5
B.	3		**E.**	6
C.	4			

25. The APGAR score awarded to the patient in question number 25 represents a patient that is:
- **A.** healthy and active.
- **B.** moderately depressed
- **C.** normal
- **D.** severely depressed
- **E.** requiring no immediate intervention

True/False

26. The stage of labor that begins with complete cervical dilatation and ends with the delivery of the fetus is called the dilatation stage.
- **A.** True
- **B.** False

27. Elements of the APGAR assessment include appearance, pulse, grimace, activity and respirations.
- **A.** True
- **B.** False

28. Acrocyanosis in the neonate is always a sign of inadequate oxygenation.
- **A.** True
- **B.** False

29. Normally the umbilical cord contains two arteries and one vein.
- **A.** True
- **B.** False

30. The umbilical vein transports oxygenated blood to the fetus while the umbilical arteries return relatively deoxygenated blood to the placenta.
- **A.** True
- **B.** False

31. Fetal heart tones (FHTs) can be detected by stethoscope as early as 12 weeks.
- **A.** True
- **B.** False

32. Diabetics are at an increased risk of developing preeclampsia and hypertension.
- **A.** True
- **B.** False

33. Pregnant women are at increased risk of developing gallstones as a result of hormonal influences that delay emptying of the gallbladder.
- **A.** True
- **B.** False

34. Approximately 75% of ectopic pregnancies are implanted in the fallopian tube..
- **A.** True
- **B.** False

_____ **35.** Vaginal examinations should be completed on all patients with suspected placenta previa..
  A. True
  B. False

Matching

Write the letter of the definition in the space provided next to the term it describes.

_____	**36.**	amniotic sac	_____	**41.**	effacement
_____	**37.**	ovulation	_____	**42.**	Braxton-Hicks contractions
_____	**38.**	fetus	_____	**43.**	parity
_____	**39.**	placenta	_____	**44.**	tocolysis
_____	**40.**	umbilical cord	_____	**45.**	puerperium

A. Unborn infant from the third month of pregnancy to birth
B. Fetal lifeline, a placental extension through which the child is nourished
C. Organ of pregnancy for the exchange of oxygen and waste products
D. Transparent membrane forming the sac which holds the fetus
E. Release of an egg from the ovary
F. The time period surrounding the birth of the fetus
G. Thinning and shortening of the cervix during labor
H. Number of pregnancies carried to term
I. Process of stopping labor
J. Painless, irregular uterine contractions

Essentials of Paramedic Care

Division 5

Special Considerations

Chapter 41

Neonatology

Review of Chapter Objectives

With each chapter of the Workbook, we identify the objectives and the important elements of the text content. You should review these items and refer to the pages listed if any points are not clear.

After reading this chapter, you should be able to:

1. Define newborn and neonate.   **p. 907**

A newborn is a baby in the first few hours of its life, also called a *newly born infant.* A neonate is a baby less than one month old.

2. Identify important antepartum factors that can affect childbirth.   **p. 908**

Antepartum factors are those that occur before the onset of labor. Examples of important antepartum factors that can adversely affect childbirth include multiple gestation, inadequate prenatal care, a mother who is younger than 16 years of age or older than 35, a history of perinatal morbidity or mortality, post-term gestation, drugs or medications, and a mother with a history of toxemia, hypertension, or diabetes.

3. Identify important intrapartum factors that can determine high-risk newborn patients.   **p. 908**

Intrapartum factors are those that occur during childbirth. Examples of intrapartum factors that can help determine high-risk newborn patients include a mother with premature labor, meconium-stained amniotic fluid, rupture of membranes more than 24 hours prior to delivery, use of narcotics within four hours of delivery, an abnormal presentation, prolonged labor or precipitous delivery, and a prolapsed cord or bleeding.

4. Identify the factors that lead to premature birth and low-birth-weight newborns.   **pp. 924, 926, 929-930**

A premature or low-birth-weight newborn is an infant born prior to 37 weeks of gestation or with a birth weight ranging from 0.6 to 2.2 kg. Factors that lead to premature birth or low-birth-weight newborns include, among others, maternal narcotic use or trauma. For a full list of factors, see Chapter 40, "Obstetrics."

5. Distinguish between primary and secondary apnea.   **p. 909**

When an infant is born, it may experience hypoxia. This is usually relieved by the initial gasps for air. If this asphyxia continues, respiratory movement may cease altogether. The infant may then enter a period of apnea known as *primary apnea.* In most cases, simple stimulation and exposure to oxygen will reverse bradycardia and assist in the development of pulmonary perfusion. With ongoing asphyxia, the infant will enter a period known as *secondary apnea.* Always assume that apnea in the newborn is secondary apnea and rapidly treat it with ventilatory assistance.

6. Discuss pulmonary perfusion and asphyxia.   **p. 909**

With the first breaths, the lungs rapidly fill with air, which displaces the remaining fetal fluid. The pulmonary arterioles and capillaries open, decreasing pulmonary vascular resistance. The blood is now diverted from the ductus arteriosus to the pulmonary circulation. However, if hypoxia or severe acidosis occurs, the pulmonary vascular bed may constrict and the ductus may reopen. This will retrigger fetal circulation with its attendant shunting, ongoing hypoxia, and ultimately asphyxia (if the situation is not managed quickly and correctly).

7. Identify the primary signs utilized for evaluating a newborn during resuscitation.   **p. 918**

The newborn should be assessed immediately after birth. The primary signs used for evaluating a newborn during resuscitation include respiratory rate, heart rate, and skin color. The newborn's respiratory rate should average 40–60 breaths per minute. The normal heart rate is between 150 and 180 beats per minute at birth, slowing to 130–140 beats per minute thereafter. A pulse less than 100 beats per minute indicates distress and requires emergency intervention. Some cyanosis of the extremities is common immediately after birth. However, if the newborn is cyanotic in the central part of the body or if peripheral cyanosis persists, the newborn must be treated with 100% oxygen.

8. Identify the appropriate use of the APGAR scale. pp. 911-912

The APGAR scale—designed for use at 1 and 5 minutes after birth—helps distinguish between newborns who need only routine care and those who need greater assistance. The system also predicts long-term survival. A severely distressed newborn (one with an APGAR score of less than 4) requires immediate resuscitation.

9. Calculate the APGAR score given various newborn situations.   **(see Chapter 40)**

To calculate the APGAR score, a value of 0, 1, or 2 is given for each of the following categories: pulse rate (heart rate), grimace (irritability), activity (muscle tone), and respiratory rate.

10. Formulate an appropriate treatment plan for providing initial care to a newborn.   **p.**

Treatment of the newborn begins by preparing the environment and assembling the equipment needed for delivery and immediate care of the newborn. The initial care of the newborn follows the same priorities as for all patients. Complete the initial assessment first. Correct any problems detected in the initial assessment before proceeding to the next step. The majority of term newborns require no resuscitation beyond suctioning of the airway, mild stimulation, and maintenance of body temperature by drying and warming with blankets.

11. Describe the indications, equipment needed, application, and evaluation of the following management techniques for the newborn in distress:

     a.   **Blow-by oxygen p. 921**
     Blow-by oxygen—the process of blowing oxygen across a newborn's face—is applied if central cyanosis is present or if the adequacy of ventilations is uncertain. If possible, the oxygen should be warmed and humidified.

     b.   **Ventilatory assistance   p.921**
     Positive-pressure ventilation should be applied to a newborn if any of the following conditions exist: heart rate less than 100 beats per minute, apnea, or persistence of central cyanosis after administration of supplemental oxygen. A bag-valve-mask unit is the device of choice. A self-inflating bag of appropriate size should be used (450 mL is optimal). If prolonged ventilation is required, it may be necessary to disable the pop-off valve.

c. Endotracheal intubation pp. 916, 918, 919

This technique involves placement of an endotracheal (ET) tube into the trachea of a newborn, usually for suctioning meconium. Endotracheal intubation requires appropriately sized tubes without cuffs and a laryngoscope. After suctioning, a fresh tube should be inserted for mechanical ventilation. (See Procedure 41-2 for more details.) Endotracheal intubation should be carried out in the following situations: The bag-valve mask does not work, tracheal suctioning is needed, prolonged ventilation will be required, a diaphragmatic hernia is suspected, or an inadequate respiratory effort is found.

d. Orogastric tube p. 922

An orogastric, or nasogastric, tube is used to relieve significant gastric distention, most often caused by a leak around an uncuffed endotracheal tube. The tube should be inserted through the nose or mouth, then through the esophagus into the stomach. An endotracheal tube should be in place to avoid misplacing the gastric tube into the trachea. Make sure the newborn is well oxygenated and that the tube is correctly measured (from the tip of the newborn's nose, around the ear, to the xiphoid process). Lubricate the end of the tube before inserting and then check placement by injecting 10 cc of air into the tube and auscultating a bubbling sound (or sound of rushing air) over the epigastrium.

e. Chest compressions pp. 922-923

Chest compressions should be applied to newborns with heart rates of less than 60 beats per minute. Begin chest compressions by encircling the newborn's chest, placing both thumbs on the lower one-third of the sternum. Compress the sternum 1.5 to 2.0 cm at a rate of 120 times per minute. Maintain a ratio of three compressions to one ventilation. Reassess the newborn after 20 cycles of compressions (1-minute intervals). Discontinue compressions if the spontaneous heart rate exceeds 60 beats per minute.

f. Vascular access pp. 923-924

Vascular access—a method for administering fluids and drugs—should be considered if ventilation and oxygenation fail to correct cardiopulmonary arrests or in cases of persistent bradycardia, hypovolemia, respiratory depression secondary to narcotics, and metabolic acidosis. Vascular access can most readily be managed by using the umbilical vein. The umbilical cord contains three vessels—two arteries and one vein, with the vein being the largest of the three. Equipment for venous access includes a scalpel blade, a 5 French umbilical catheter, a three-way stopcock, umbilical tape, and saline. Be sure to save enough of the umbilical stump (cut to 1 cm above the abdomen) in case neonatal personnel have to place additional lines. Also, if the catheter is inserted too far, it may become wedged against the liver, and it will not function.

12. Discuss the routes of medication administration for the newborn. pp. 923-924

Medications for the newborn may be administered by peripheral vein cannulation, intraosseous cannulation, umbilical vein cannulation, and endotracheal tube.

13. Discuss the signs of hypovolemia in a newborn. P. 931

Hypovolemia is the leading cause of shock in the newborn. It may result from dehydration, hemorrhage, or third-spacing of fluids, with dehydration being by far the most common cause. Signs of hypovolemia include pale color, cool skin, diminished peripheral pulses, delayed capillary refill (despite a normal ambient temperature), mental status changes, and diminished urination (oliguria).

14. Discuss the initial steps in resuscitation of a newborn. pp. 915-924

Resuscitation of the newborn follows an inverted pyramid. In chronological order, initial steps include drying, warming, positioning, suctioning, and tactical stimulation; administration of supplemental oxygen; bag-valve ventilation; and chest compressions. If these steps fail, advanced measures include intubation and administration of medications.

15. Discuss the effects of maternal narcotic usage on the newborn.   pp. 924, 926

Maternal narcotic use has been shown to produce low-birth-weight infants. Such infants may demonstrate withdrawal symptoms—tremors, startles, and decreased alertness. They also face a serious risk of respiratory depression at birth.

16. Determine the appropriate treatment for the newborn with narcotic depression.   p. 924

Naloxone, which is extremely safe even at high doses, is the treatment of choice for respiratory depression secondary to maternal narcotic use *within four hours of delivery*. Ventilatory support must be provided prior to administration of naloxone. Due to the long duration of the narcotic, which may exceed the duration of the naloxone, repeat administration will be needed. Keep in mind, however, that the naloxone may induce a withdrawal reaction in an infant born to a *narcotic-addicted* mother. Medical direction may advise that naloxone NOT be administered if the mother is drug addicted, recommending prolonged ventilatory support instead.

17. Discuss appropriate transport guidelines for a newborn.   p. 926

Paramedics are frequently called upon to transport a high-risk newborn from a facility where stabilization has occurred to a neonatal intensive care unit. During transport you will help maintain the newborn's body temperature, control oxygen administration, and maintain ventilatory support. Often, a transport isolette with its own heat, light, and oxygen source is available. If a self-contained isolette is not available for transport, you might wrap the newborn in several blankets, keep the infant's head covered, and place hot-water bottles containing water heated to no more than 40°C near, but not touching, the newborn. DO NOT use chemical packs to keep the newborn warm.

18. Determine appropriate receiving facilities for low and high-risk newborns. p. 926

Low-risk newborns need to be taken to a hospital with an obstetrical unit, whereas high-risk newborns are often taken directly or transferred to a facility with a neonatal intensive care unit (NICU).

19. Describe the epidemiology, including the incidence, morbidity/mortality, risk factors and prevention strategies, pathophysiology, assessment findings, and management for the following neonatal problems:

a.   Meconium aspiration   pp. 912, 916, 926-927
Meconium-stained amniotic fluid occurs in approximately 10–15 percent of deliveries, mostly in post-term or small-for-gestational-age newborns. Meconium aspiration accounts for a significant proportion of neonatal deaths. Fetal distress and hypoxia can cause meconium to be passed into the amniotic fluid. Either *in utero* or more often with the first breath, thick meconium is aspirated into the lungs, resulting in small airway obstruction and aspiration pneumonia. The infant may have respiratory distress within the first hours, or even the first minutes, of life as evidenced by tachypnea, retraction, grunting, and cyanosis in severely affected newborns. The partial obstruction of some airways may lead to a pneumothorax.

An infant born through thin meconium may not require treatment, but depressed infants born through thick, particulate (pea-soup) meconium-stained fluid should be intubated immediately, prior to the first ventilation. Before stimulating such infants to breathe, apply suction with a meconium aspirator attached to an endotracheal tube. Connect to suction at 100 cc/H$_2$O or less to remove meconium from the airway. Withdraw the ET tube as suction is applied. It may be necessary to repeat this procedure to clear the airway. The patient should then be taken to a facility that can manage a high-risk neonate.

b.   Apnea p. 928
This condition is a common finding in the pre-term infant or infants weighing under 1 500 grams, infants exposed to drugs, or infants born after prolonged or difficult labor and delivery. Typically, the infant fails to breathe spontaneously after stimulation, or the infant experiences respiratory pauses of greater than 20 seconds. Apnea can be due to hypoxia, hypothermia, narcotic or central nervous system depressants, weakness of the respiratory muscles, septicemia, metabolic disorders, or central nervous system disorders.

Management begins with tactile stimulation, followed by bag-valve-mask ventilation, with the pop-off valve disabled. If the infant does not breathe on its own, or if the heart rate is below 60 with adequate ventilation and chest compressions, perform tracheal intubation with direct visualization. Gain circulatory access, and monitor the heart rate continuously. If the apnea is due to a narcotic administered within the past four hours, consider naloxone. Remember, however, that the use of a narcotic antagonist is generally contraindicated if the mother is a drug abuser. Throughout the treatment, keep the infant warm to prevent hypothermia.

c.   Diaphragmatic hernia   pp. 928-929

This is a rare condition seen in approximately 1 out of every 2 200 live births. The defect is caused by the failure of the pleurperitoneal canal to close completely. The survival rate for newborns who require mechanical ventilation in the first 18 to 24 hours is approximately 50 percent, and it approaches 100 percent if there is no distress in the first 24 hours of life.

Protrusion of abdominal viscera through the hernia into the thoracic cavity occurs in varying degrees. Assessment findings may include little to severe distress present from birth, dyspnea and cyanosis unresponsive to ventilations, small, flat (scaphoid) abdomen, bowel sounds in the chest, and heart sounds displaced to the right. If you suspect a diaphragmatic hernia, position the infant with its head and thorax higher than the abdomen and feet. This will help to displace the abdominal organs downward. Place a nasogastric or orogastric tube and apply low, intermittent suctioning. DO NOT use bag-valve-mask ventilation, which can worsen the condition by causing gastric distension. If necessary, cautiously administer positive-pressure ventilation through an endotracheal tube. A diaphragmatic hernia usually requires surgical repair, which should be explained to the parents along with the need for quick transport.

d.   Bradycardia   p. 929

Bradycardia is most commonly caused by hypoxia in newborns. However, the bradycardia may also be due to several other factors, including increased intracranial pressure, hypothyroidism, or acidosis. In cases of hypoxia, the infant experiences minimal risk if the hypoxia is corrected quickly. In providing treatment, follow the procedures in the inverted pyramid. Resist the inclination to treat the bradycardia with pharmacological measures alone. Keep the newborn warm and transport to the nearest facility.

e.   Prematurity   pp. 929-930

A premature newborn is an infant born prior to 37 weeks of gestation or with weight ranging from 0.6 to 2.2 kg. Mortality decreases weekly with gestation beyond the onset of fetal viability. Premature newborns are at greater risk of respiratory suppression, head or brain injury caused by hypoxemia, changes in blood pressure, intraventricular hemorrhage, and fluctuations in serum osmolarity. They are also more susceptible to hypothermia than full-term newborns. The degree of immaturity determines the physical characteristics of a premature newborn. Premature newborns often appear to have a larger head relative to body size. They may have large trunks and short extremities, transparent skin, and few wrinkles.

Prematurity should not be a factor in short-term treatment. Resuscitation should be attempted if there is any sign of life, and the measures of resuscitation should be the same as those for newborns of normal weight and maturity. Maintain a patent airway and avoid potential aspiration of gastric contents.

f.   Respiratory distress or cyanosis   p. 930

Prematurity is the single most common factor causing respiratory distress and cyanosis in the newborn. The problem occurs most frequently in infants less than 1 200 grams and 30 weeks of gestation. Premature infants have an immature central respiratory control center and are easily affected by environmental or metabolic changes. There are many factors contributing to respiratory distress, including lung or heart disease, central nervous system disorders, meconium aspiration, metabolic problems, obstruction of the nasal passages, shock and sepsis, and diaphragmatic hernia. Expect the following assessment findings: tachypnea, paradoxical breathing, intercostal retractions, nasal flaring, and expiratory grunt.

In providing treatment, follow the inverted pyramid, paying particular attention to airway and ventilation. Suction as needed and provide a high concentration of oxygen. If prolonged ventilation will be required, consider placing an ET tube. Perform chest compressions, if indicated. Consider dextrose ($D_{25}W$) if the newborn is hypoglycemic. Maintain body temperature and transport to the most appropriate facility.

g. Seizures pp. 931-932

Neonatal seizures differ from seizures in a child or an adult, because generalized tonic-clonic convulsions rarely occur in the first month of life. Types of seizures in the neonate include:

- *Subtle seizures*—consist of chewing motions and excessive salivation, blinking, sucking, swimming movements of the arms, pedaling movements of the legs, apnea, and color changes.
- *Tonic seizures*—characterized by rigid posturing of the extremities and trunk; sometimes associated with fixed deviation of the eyes.
- *Focal clonic seizures*—consist of rhythmic twitching of muscle groups in the extremities and face.
- *Multi focal seizures*—exhibit signs similar to focal clonic seizures except multiple muscle groups are involved and clonic activity randomly migrates.
- *Myoclonic seizures*—characterized by brief focal or generalized jerks of the extremities or parts of the body that tend to involve distal muscle groups.

The causes of neonatal seizures include sepsis, fever, hypoglycemia, hypoxic ischemic encephalopathy, metabolic disturbances, meningitis, development abnormalities, or drug withdrawal. Assessment findings of seizures include decreased level of consciousness and seizure activity as already described. Treatment focuses on airway management, oxygen saturation, and administration of an anti-convulsant. You might administer a benzodiazepine (usually lorazepam) for status epilepticus or dextrose ($D_{25}W$) for hypoglycemia.

h. Fever p. 932

Neonates do not develop fever as easily as older children. Therefore, any fever in a neonate requires extensive evaluation because it is more likely to be caused by a life-threatening condition such as pneumonia, sepsis, or meningitis. In fact, fever may be the only sign of meningitis in a neonate. Because of their immature development, they do not exhibit the classic symptoms such as a stiff neck. Assessment findings of a fever include changes in mental status (irritability or somnolence), decreased feeding, skin warm to the touch, and rashes or petechia. Term infants may form beads of sweat on their brow, but not on the rest of their body. Premature infants, on the other hand, will have no visible sweat at all.

Treatment of the neonate with a fever will, for the most part, be limited to ensuring a patent airway and adequate ventilation. Do not use cold packs, as they may drop the temperature too quickly and cause seizures. If the newborn becomes bradycardic, provide chest compressions.

i. Hypothermia pp. 932-933

Hypothermia presents a common and life-threatening condition for newborns. The increased surface-to-volume relationship in newborns makes them extremely sensitive to environmental temperatures, especially right after delivery when they are wet. In treating hypothermia—a body temperature below 35°C —try to control the loss of heat through evaporation, conduction, convection, and radiation. Also remember that hypothermia can be an indicator of sepsis in the newborn. Regardless of the cause, the increase in the metabolic demands can produce a variety of related conditions including metabolic acidosis, pulmonary hypertension, and hypoxemia.

In assessing hypothermic newborns, remember that they do not shiver. Instead, expect the following findings: pale color, skin cool to the touch (especially in the extremities), acrocyanosis, respiratory distress, possible apnea, bradycardia, central cyanosis, initial irritability, and lethargy in later stages. Management focuses on ensuring adequate ventilations and oxygenation. Chest compressions may be necessary with bradycardia.

j. Hypoglycemia pp. 933-934

Newborns are the only age group that can develop severe hypoglycemia and not have diabetes mellitus. Hypoglycemia is more common in premature or small-for-gestational-age infants, the smaller twin, and newborns of diabetic mothers, as these infants have decreased glucose utilization. Hypoglycemia may be due to a number of factors, including inadequate glucose intake or increased glucose utilization, stress (which can cause blood sugar to fall to a critical level), respiratory illnesses, hypothermia, toxemia, CNS hemorrhage, asphyxia, meningitis, and sepsis. Infants receiving glucose infusions can develop hypoglycemia if the infusion is suddenly stopped.

Infants with hypoglycemia may be asymptomatic, or they may exhibit symptoms such as apnea, color changes, respiratory distress, lethargy, seizures, acidosis, and poor myocardial contractility. Assessment findings may include twitching or seizures, limpness, lethargy, eye-rolling, high-pitched cry, apnea, irregular respirations, and possible cyanosis. Treatment begins with management of airway and ventilations. Administer chest compressions, if needed. With medical direction, administer dextrose ($D_{25}W$). Remember—persistent hypoglycemia is a serious condition and can have catastrophic effects on the brain.

k.   Vomiting   p. 934

Vomiting in a neonate may result from a variety of causes and rarely presents as an isolated symptom. Vomiting—the forceful ejection of stomach contents—rarely occurs during the first weeks of life and may be confused with regurgitation or "spitting up." Causes of vomiting include a tracheoesophageal fistula, an upper gastrointestinal obstruction, increased intracranial pressure, or an infection. Vomiting containing dark blood signals a life-threatening illness. Keep in mind, however, that vomiting of mucus—which may occasionally be streaked with blood—in the first few hours after birth is not uncommon.

Assessment findings may include distended stomach, signs of infection, increased ICP, or drug withdrawal. Because vomitus can be aspirated, management considerations focus on ensuring a patent airway to prevent aspiration. If you detect respiratory difficulty, suction or clear the vomitus from the airway and oxygenate as needed. Fluid administration may be necessary to prevent dehydration. Remember that, as with older patients, vagal stimulation may cause bradycardia in the neonate.

l.   Diarrhea   pp. 934-935

Diarrhea can cause severe dehydration and electrolyte imbalances in the neonate. Normally five to six stools per day can be expected, especially in breast-fed infants. Causes of diarrhea in a neonate include bacterial or viral infection, gastroenteritis, lactose intolerance, phototherapy, neonatal abstinence syndrome (NAS), thyrotoxicosis, and cystic fibrosis. In managing an infant with diarrhea, remember BSI precautions. Management consists of maintenance of airway and ventilations, adequate oxygenation, and chest compressions, if indicated. With medical direction, fluid therapy might be administered to prevent or treat dehydration.

m.   Common birth injuries   pp. 935-936

A birth injury occurs in an estimated 2 to 7 of every 1,000 live births in Canada. About 3 of every 100 000 infants die of birth trauma. Risk factors for birth injury include prematurity, postmaturity, cephalopelvic disproportion, prolonged labor, breech presentation, explosive delivery, and a diabetic mother.

Birth injuries can take various forms. Cranial injuries may include molding of the head and overriding of the parietal bones, erythema, abrasions, ecchymosis, subcutaneous fat necrosis, subconjunctival and retinal hemorrhage, subperiosteal hemorrhage, and fracture of the skull. Often the infant will develop a large scalp hematoma, called a *caput succedaneum,* during the birth process, but this condition will usually resolve over a week's time. Other birth injuries include peripheral nerve injury, injury to the liver, rupture of the spleen, adrenal hemorrhage, fractures of the clavicle or extremities, and hypoxia-ischemia.

Assessment findings may include diffuse (sometimes ecchymotic) edematous swelling of soft tissues around the scalp, paralysis below the level of the spinal cord injury, paralysis of the upper arm with or without paralysis of the forearm, diaphragmatic paralysis, movement on only one side of the face when crying, inability to move the arm freely on the side of the fractured clavicle, lack of spontaneous movement of the affected extremity, hypoxia, and shock. Management of a newborn who has suffered a birth injury is specific to injury but always centers on protection of the airway, provision of adequate ventilation, and chest compressions, if necessary.

n. Cardiac arrest   p. 936

The incidence of neonatal cardiac arrest is related primarily to hypoxia. The condition can be caused by primary or secondary apnea, bradycardia, persistent fetal circulation, or pulmonary hypertension. Unless appropriate interventions are initiated immediately, the outcome is poor.

Risk factors for cardiac arrest in newborns include bradycardia, intrauterine asphyxia, prematurity, drugs administered to or taken by the mother, congenital neuromuscular diseases, congenital malformations, and intrapartum hypoxemia. Assessment findings may include peripheral cyanosis, inadequate respiratory effort, and ineffective or absent heart rate. In managing the neonatal cardiac arrest, follow the inverted pyramid for resuscitation and administer drugs or fluids according to medical direction.

o. Post-arrest management p. 936

Post-arrest management involves maintenance of the infant's body temperature, prompt transport to the appropriate facility, and delicate handling of the parents or caregivers.

20. Given several neonatal emergencies, provide the appropriate procedures for assessment, management, and transport.   pp. 907-936

During your classroom, clinical, and field training, you will assess and develop a management plan for the real and simulated patients you attend. Use the information presented in this chapter, the information on neonatal emergencies in the field provided by your instructors, and the guidance given by your clinical and field preceptors to develop the skills needed to assess, manage, and transport the newborn and neonate patient. Continue to refine these skills once your training ends and you begin your career as a paramedic.

CONTENT SELF-EVALUATION

Multiple Choice

1. Examples of antepartum factors indicating possible complications in newborns would include multiple gestation and:
    A. premature labor.   D. prolapsed cord.
    B. inadequate prenatal care.   E. prolonged labor.
    C. abnormal presentation.

2. Examples of intrapartum factors indicating possible complications in newborns would include the use of narcotics within four hours of delivery and:
    A. meconium-stained amniotic fluid.   D. toxemia or diabetes.
    B. post-term gestation.   E. a mother over 35 years old.
    C. a mother under 16 years old.

3. When the fetus is in the uterus, the respiratory system is:
    A. working at a very rapid speed.   D. essentially functional.
    B. working at a very slow speed.   E. flushed with meconium.
    C. essentially nonfunctional.

4. Factors that stimulate the baby's first breath include:
    A. mild acidosis.
    B. hypoxia.
    C. hypothermia.
    D. initiation of stretch reflexes in the lungs.
    E. all of the above

5. Persistent fetal circulation is a condition in which the:
   A. ductus arteriosus remains closed.   D. both A and C
   B. ductus arteriosus reopens.   E. both B and C
   C. pulmonary vascular bed dilates.

6. Most of the fetal development that could lead to congenital problems occurs during the:
   A. first trimester.   D. onset of labor.
   B. second trimester.   E. intrapartum period.
   C. third trimester.

7. A congenital hernia of the umbilicus found in the neonate is called a(n):
   A. choanal atresia.   D. meningomyelocele.
   B. Pierre Robin Syndrome.   E. omphalocele.
   C. spina bifida.

8. A congenital condition characterized by a small jaw combined with a cleft palate, downward displacement of the tongue, and an absent gag reflex is called a(n):
   A. cleft lip.   D. Pierre Robin Syndrome.
   B. omphalocele.   E. choanal atresia.
   C. cleft palate.

9. The G in APGAR stands for:
   A. gravida.   D. gray tone.
   B. gestation.   E. none of the above
   C. grimace.

10. A dark green material found in the intestine of the full-term newborn is called:
    A. bile.   D. vomitus.
    B. meconium.   E. hyperbilirubinemia.
    C. mucus.

11. Loss of heat by the newborn can occur through:
    A. evaporation.   D. radiation.
    B. convection.   E. all of the above
    C. conduction.

12. Prior to cutting the umbilical cord, it should not be "milked" as this can cause:
    A. polycythemia.   D. hemophilia.
    B. anemia.   E. both A and C
    C. hyperbilirubinemia.

13. An increase in the level of bilirubin in the blood can cause:
    A. jaundice.   D. flushing.
    B. pallor.   E. anemia.
    C. cyanosis.

14. EMS units should contain all of the following equipment in their neonatal resuscitation kit EXCEPT a(n):
    A. meconium aspirator.
    B. laryngoscope with size 3 and 4 blades.
    C. device to secure the endotracheal tube.
    D. umbilical catheter and 10 mL syringe.
    E. DeLee suction trap.

15. Following the inverted pyramid of neonatal resuscitation, which would be done first?
    A. intubation   D. drying and warming
    B. bag-valve-mask ventilations E. administration of medications
    C. chest compressions

16. The danger of deep suctioning a newborn is that it can cause a(n):
- **A.** vagal response.
- **B.** increased heart rate.
- **C.** decreased respiratory rate.
- **D.** allergic reaction.
- **E.** tachypnea.

17. Normal newborn respirations are approximately _____ times a minute.
- **A.** 10–30
- **B.** 20–50
- **C.** 30–60
- **D.** 40–70
- **E.** 60–90

18. Which of the following represents hemodynamic changes in the newborn at birth?
- **A.** lungs expand allowing fetal lung fluid to enter, allowing an increase in the amount of blood flow through the lungs
- **B.** lungs expand as they are filled with air, promoting fetal lung fluid to leave the alveoli, while arterioles open increasing the amount of blood flow through the lungs
- **C.** lungs expand as they are filled with air, promoting fetal lung fluid to leave the bronchioles increasing the amount of blood flow through the lungs
- **D.** lungs constrict absorbing fetal lung fluid while decreasing the amount of blood shunted through the foramen ovale
- **E.** arterioles dilate and blood flow increases while decreasing pulmonary blood flow

19. Which of the following is the most common birth defect involving the nose and is due to the presence of a bony or membranous septum between the nasal cavity and the pharynx?
- **A.** cleft palate
- **B.** Pierre Robin syndrome
- **C.** choanal atresia
- **D.** cleft lip
- **E.** omphalocele.

20. The best treatment for the defect described in question 19 would be:
- **A.** vigorous suctioning
- **B.** mechanical ventilations.
- **C.** a nasal airway
- **D.** chest compressions
- **E.** an oral airway

21. One should expect a normal newborn heart rate to be _____ beats per minute:
- **A.** 120-140
- **B.** 130-160
- **C.** 150-180
- **D.** less than 100
- **E.** 160-190

22. While performing chest compressions on a neonate, the depth of the compression should be:
- **A.** 1.0-2.5 cm
- **B.** 0.5-2.5 cm
- **C.** 2.5-3.0 cm
- **D.** 1.5-2.0 cm
- **E.** none of the above

23. The compression to ventilation ratio of a neonatal resuscitation is:
- **A.** 3 :1
- **B.** 2 :1
- **C.** 1:1
- **D.** 4 :1
- **E.** 5 :1

24. When ventilating a newborn, the proper positioning of a mask should:
- **A.** cover the nose and mouth.
- **B.** cover the eyes, nose and mouth
- **C.** cover the nose only
- **D.** cover the mouth only
- **E.** cover the nose and eyes

25. Initial pressures required to ventilate a newborn may be as high as:
- **A.** 40 cm/H2O.
- **B.** 50 cm/H2O.
- **C.** 60 cm/H2O.
- **D.** 70 cm/H2O
- **E.** none of the above

True/False

_____ **26.** Always assume that apnea in the newborn is secondary apnea and rapidly treat it with ventilatory assistance.
     A. True
     B. False

_____ **27.** Some infants are born with a defect in their spinal cord. In some cases, the spinal cord and associated structures may be exposed. This abnormality is called diaphragmatic hernia.
     A. True
     B. False

_____ **28.** The APGAR score should be assigned at 1 and 10 minutes after the infant's birth.
     A. True
     B. False

_____ **29.** Immediately after birth, the newborn's core temperature can drop 1 C or more from its birth temperature.
     A. True
     B. False

_____ **30.** The most important indicator of neonatal distress is the fetal respiratory rate.
     A. True
     B. False

_____ **31.** In distressed newborns, monitor the heart rate with external electronic monitors.
     A. True
     B. False

_____ **32.** Suctioning of a newborn should last no longer than 10 seconds.
     A. True
     B. False

_____ **33.** Insertion of an endotracheal tube is recommended when prolonged ventilation of a newborn will be required.
     A. True
     B. False

_____ **34.** During hemodynamic changes in the newborn at birth, blood flow through the ductus arteriosus flows through the lungs leading to the eventual closure of the ductus.
     A. True
     B. False

_____ **35.** A newborn has a relatively fixed stroke volume.
     A. True
     B. False

Matching

Write the letter of the term in the space provided next to the appropriate description.

A.	neonate	**F.**	meningomyelocele
B.	meconium	**G.**	acrocyanosis
C.	extrauterine	**H.**	intrapartum
D.	cleft lip	**I.**	thyrotoxicosis
E.	polycythemia	**J.**	ductus arteriosis

_____ **36.** channel between the main pulmonary artery and the aorta of the fetus

_____ **37.** an infant from time of birth to one month of age

_____ **38.** herniation of the spinal cord and membranes through a defect in the spinal column

_____ **39.** outside the uterus

_____ **40.** an excess of red blood cells

_____ **41.** occurring during childbirth

_____ **42.** cyanosis of the extremities

_____ **43.** condition characterized by tachycardia, and rapid metabolism

_____ **44.** congenital vertical fissure in the upper lip

_____ **45.** dark green material found in the intestine of a full-term newborn

Chapter 42

Pediatrics

Review of Chapter Objectives

After reading this chapter, you should be able to:

1. Discuss the paramedic's role in the reduction of infant and childhood morbidity and mortality from acute illness and injury.   pp. 939-940

When considering the reduction of pediatric morbidity and mortality, your role as a paramedic centers around two key concepts. First, you must realize that pediatric injuries have become a major health concern. Second, you should remember that children are at a higher risk of injury than adults and that they are more likely to be adversely affected by the injuries that they suffer.

In addition to pediatric injuries, paramedics are often responsible for treating the ill child. There are many aspects of disease and disease processes that are unique to children. It is important that the paramedic be familiar with these, as early intervention is often the key to reduced morbidity and mortality.

2. Identify methods/mechanisms that prevent injuries to infants and children. pp. 939-940

As a paramedic, you can help reduce the rate of injury by taking advantage of opportunities to share "teaching points" in your daily life, both personally and professionally. Take part in, or offer to organize, school or community programs in injury prevention or health care. Engage student interest in the EMS profession by volunteering to speak at "career days," emphasizing those aspects of your job that relate to young people. Use nonurgent ambulance calls as a chance to educate family members or caregivers on the importance of "child-proofing" a home or neighborhood. Work with appropriate agencies in initiating or conducting safety inspections, block watches, and more.

3. Identify the common family responses to acute illness and injury of an infant or child. pp. 941-942

As you might expect, the reaction of parents or caregivers to a pediatric emergency will vary. Initial responses by parents or caregivers might include shock, grief, denial, anger, guilt, fear, or complete loss of control. Their behavior may change during the course of the emergency.

4. Describe techniques for successful interaction with families of acutely ill or injured infants and children.   pp. 941-942

Communication is the key to successful interaction with families of acutely ill or injured pediatric patients. Preferably only one paramedic will speak with adults at the scene. This will avoid any chance of conflicting information and allow a second paramedic to focus on the child. If parents or caregivers sense your confidence and professionalism, they will regain control and trust your suggestions for care. As with the child, most parents and caregivers feel overwhelmed by fear.

If conditions permit, you should allow one of the parents or caregivers to remain with the child at all times. Some family members may be extremely emotional in emergency situations. The child will react more positively to a family member who appears calm and reassuring. If a parent or caregiver is "out of control," have another person take him or her away from the immediate area to settle down. Maintain a reasonable level of suspicion if a child shows a pattern of injuries, some old and some new. In such cases, the parent or caregiver may try to cover up what may be an abusive situation. They may also try to block examination and treatment.

5. Identify key anatomical, physiological, growth, and developmental characteristics of infants and children and their implications. **pp. 942-945**

Children are broken into age groups because they differ in terms of anatomical, physiological, growth, and developmental characteristics. The following are some of the differences:

Newborns (first hours after birth). The term "newborn" refers to a baby in the first hours of extrauterine life. These patients are assessed using the APGAR scoring system, which was described in Chapters 40 and 41. Resuscitation of the newborn generally follows the inverted pyramid and the guidelines established in the Neonatal Advanced Life Support (NALS) curriculum.

Neonates (ages birth to 1 month). The neonate typically loses up to 10 percent of its birth weight as it adjusts to extrauterine life. This lost weight, however, is ordinarily recovered within 10 days. Gestational age affects early growth. Children born at term (40 weeks) should follow accepted developmental guidelines. Infants born prematurely will not be as developed, either neurologically or physically, as their term counterparts.

The neonatal stage of development centers on reflexes. The neonate's personality also begins to form. Obviously, the history must be obtained from the parents or caregivers. However, it is also important to observe the child. Common illnesses in this age group include jaundice, vomiting, and respiratory distress. The approach to this age group should include several factors. First, the child should always be kept warm. Observe skin color, tone, and respiratory activity. The absence of tears when crying may indicate dehydration. The lungs should be auscultated early during this exam, while the infant is quiet.

Infants (ages 1 to 5 months). Infants should have doubled their birth weight by 5 to 6 months of age and can follow the movement of others with their eyes. Muscle control develops in a cephalo-caudal ("head-to-tail") progression, with control spreading from the trunk toward the extremities. Although the infant's personality continues to form, it still centers strongly on the parents or caregivers. Concentrate on keeping these patients warm and comfortable, allowing them to remain the parent's or caregiver's lap, if possible. A pacifier or bottle can be used to help keep the baby quiet during the examination.

Infants (ages 6 to 12 months). Patients in this age group are active and enjoy exploring the world with their mouths. In this stage of development, the risk of foreign body airway obstruction (FBAO) becomes a serious concern. Infants 6 months and older have more fully formed personalities and express themselves more readily than younger babies. They have a considerable anxiety toward strangers. They don't like lying on their backs, and they tend to cling to their mother, though the father "will do." Common illnesses and accidents include febrile seizures, vomiting, diarrhea, dehydration, bronchiolitis, car accidents, croup, child abuse, poisonings, falls, airway obstructions, and meningitis. These children should be examined while sitting in the lap of the parent or caregiver. The exam should progress in a toe-to-head order, since starting at the face may upset the child. If time and conditions permit, allow the child to become familiar with you before beginning the examination.

Toddlers (ages 1 to 3 years). Great strides in gross motor development occur during this stage. Children tend to run underneath or stand on almost anything. As they grow older, toddlers become braver and more curious or stubborn. They begin to stray away from the parents or caregivers more frequently. Yet these remain the only people who can comfort them quickly, and most children will cling to a parent or caregiver if frightened. At ages 1 to 3, language development begins. Although the majority of the history comes from interaction with the parent or caregiver, it is possible to ask the toddler simple questions.

Accidents of all types are the leading cause of injury deaths in pediatric patients ages 1 to 15. Common accidents in this age group include motor vehicle collisions, homicides, burn injuries, drownings, and pedestrian accidents. Common illnesses and injuries in the toddler age group include vomiting, diarrhea, febrile seizures, poisonings, falls, child abuse, croup, and meningitis. Keep in mind that FBAO is still a high risk for toddlers.

Be cautious when treating toddlers. Approach toddlers slowly and try to gain their confidence. Conduct the exam in a toe-to-head order. The child may be difficult to examine and may resist being touched. Be sure to tell the child if something will hurt. If at all possible, avoid procedures on the dominant arm/hand, which the child will try to pull away.

Preschoolers (ages 3 to 5 years). Children in this age group show a tremendous increase in fine and gross motor development. Language skills increase greatly. However, if frightened, these children often refuse to speak. They usually have vivid imaginations and may see monsters as part of their world. Preschoolers may have tempers and will express them. During this stage of development, children fear mutilation and may feel threatened by treatment. Avoid frightening or misleading comments. When evaluating a child in this age group, question the child first, keeping in mind that imagination may interfere with the facts. The child often has a distorted sense of time, and thus you must rely on the parents or caregivers to fill in the gaps. Common illnesses and accidents in this age group include croup, asthma, poisonings, auto accidents, burns, child abuse, ingestion of foreign bodies, drownings, epiglottitis, febrile seizures, and meningitis.

Start the examination with the chest and evaluate the head last. Do not lie or try to trick the patient. Avoid baby talk. If time and situation permit, give the preschooler health care choices.

School-age children (ages 6 to 12 years). School-age children are active and carefree. Growth spurts sometimes lead to clumsiness. The personality continues to develop, and these children are proud and protective of their parents and caregivers. Common illnesses and injuries for this age group include drownings, auto accidents, bicycle accidents, falls, fractures, sports injuries, child abuse, and burns.

When examining school-age children, give them responsibility for providing the history. However, remember that children may be reluctant to provide information if they sustained an injury while doing something forbidden. The parents or caregivers can fill in the pertinent details. During assessment, respect the modesty of school-age children. Also, remember to be honest and tell the child what is wrong.

Adolescents (ages 13 to 18). Adolescence covers the period from the end of childhood to the start of adulthood (age 18). It begins with puberty, roughly at age 13 for males and 11 for females. Puberty is highly child specific and can begin at various ages. Adolescents vary significantly in their development. Those over age 15 are physically nearer to adults in terms of their vital signs but emotionally may still be children. Regardless of physical maturity, remember that teenagers as a group are "body conscious." The slightest possibility of a lasting scar may be a tremendous issue to the adolescent patient. Common illnesses and injuries in this age group include mononucleosis, asthma, auto collisions, sports injuries, drug and alcohol problems, suicide gestures, and sexual abuse. Remember that pregnancy is also possible in female adolescents.

In examining an adolescent patient, it may be wise to conduct the interview away from the parents or caregivers. If you must perform a detailed physical exam, respect the teenager's sense of privacy. If the patient exhibits modesty or bodily shame, have a paramedic of the same sex as the teenager conduct the exam. Although patients in this age group are not legally adults, keep in mind that most of them see themselves as grown up and will take offense at the use of the word "child."

6. **Outline differences in adult and childhood anatomy, physiology, and "normal" age-group-related vital signs.   pp. 945-949, 953**

Anatomical or physiological differences in infants and children as compared with adults include:
• A proportionally larger tongue
• Smaller airway structures
• Abundant secretions
• Deciduous (baby) teeth

- Flatter nose and face
- Head heavier relative to body and less-developed neck structures and muscles
- Fontanelle and open sutures (soft spots) palpable on top of a young infant's head
- Thinner, softer brain tissue
- Head larger in proportion to the body
- Shorter, narrower, more elastic (flexible) trachea
- Shorter neck
- Abdominal breathers with a faster respiratory rate
- In the case of newborns, breathe primarily through the nose (obligate nose breathers)
- Larger body surface relative to their body mass
- Softer bones
- More exposed spleen and liver
- More easily dehydrated
- Less blood and in greater danger of developing severe shock or bleeding to death from a relatively minor wound
- Immature temperature control mechanism (unstable in babies)

Age-related differences in vital signs include:

- Pulse rates (average) by age group:
    —Newborn: 100–180
    —Infant 0–5 months: 100–160
    —Infant 6–12 months: 100–160
    —Toddler 1–3 years: 80–110
    —Preschooler 3–5 years: 80–110
    —School-age child 6–10 years: 65–110
    —Early adolescent 11–14 years: 60–90

- Respiratory rates (average) by age group:
    —Newborn: 30–60
    —Infant 0–5 months: 30–60
    —Infant 6–12 months: 30–60
    —Preschooler 3–5 years: 22–34
    —School-age child 6–10 years: 18–30
    —Early adolescent 11–14 years: 12–26

- Blood pressure (average/mmHg at rest) by age group:

	Systolic Approx. 90 plus 2 3 age	Diastolic Approx. 2/3 systolic
—Preschooler 3–5 years:	average 98 (78–116)	average 65
—School-age child 6–10 years:	average 105 (80–122)	average 69
—Early adolescent 11–14 years:	average 114 (88–140)	average 76

7. Describe techniques for successful assessment and treatment of infants and children. pp. 957-959

Many of the components of the initial patient assessment can be done during a visual examination of the scene ("assessment from the doorway"). Whenever possible, involve the parent or caregiver in efforts to calm or comfort the child. Depending on the situation, you may decide to allow the parent or caregiver to remain with the child during treatment and transport. The developmental stage of the patient and the coping skills of the parents or guardians will be key factors in making this decision.

When interacting with parents or other responsible adults, pay attention to the way in which parents or caregivers interact with the child. Are the interactions appropriate to the emergency? Are family members concerned? Are they angry? Are they overly emotional or entirely indifferent? From the time of dispatch, you will continually acquire information relative to the patient's condition. As with all patients, personal safety must be your first priority. In treating pediatric patients, follow the same guidelines in approaching the scene as you would with any other patient. Observe for potentially hazardous situations, and make sure you take appropriate BSI precautions. Remember that infants and young children are at especially high risk of an infectious process.

8. Discuss the appropriate equipment used to obtain pediatric vital signs.   pp. 957-959

Remember that poorly taken vital signs are of less value than no vital signs at all. Therefore, you must have the correct equipment to obtain pediatric vital signs. Items include appropriate-sized BP cuffs, a pediatric stethoscope, and so on. Modern noninvasive monitoring devices all have their application to emergency care. These devices may include pulse oximeter, automated blood pressure devices, self-registering thermometers, and ECGs. However, these devices may frighten a child. Before applying any monitoring device, explain what you are going to do and then demonstrate the device.

9. Determine appropriate airway adjuncts, ventilation devices, and endotracheal intubation equipment; their proper use; and complications of use for infants and children. pp. 961-964

As a general rule, use airway adjuncts in pediatric patients only if prolonged artificial ventilations are required. There are two reasons for this. First, infants and children often improve quickly through the administration of 100% oxygen. Second, airway adjuncts may create greater complications in children than in adults.

Keeping this in mind, be sure to have available the appropriate-sized airway adjuncts for each pediatric age group. Basic equipment includes oral and nasal airways, a pediatric BVM, smaller sized suction catheters, smaller sized masks for the BVM, age-appropriate nasogastric tubes, and a pediatric laryngoscope, blades, and ET tubes. It is also a good idea to carry a Braslow® tape, which, after measuring the child's height, displays the appropriate sizes of tubes.

The biggest complication of airway management for the pediatric patient is the possibility of overinflation, which allows air to gather in the stomach. Gastric distention can cause pressure on the diaphragm, making full expansion of the lungs difficult. For specific techniques in airway management in the pediatric patient, review the steps and scans in the textbook, especially those dealing with advanced airway and ventilatory management.

10. List the indications and methods of gastric decompression for infants and children. pp. 969-970, 971

If gastric distention is present in a pediatric patient, you may consider placing a nasogastric tube (NG tube). In infants and children, gastric distention may result from overly aggressive artificial ventilations or from air swallowing. Placement of an NG tube will allow you to decompress the stomach and the proximal bowel of air. An NG tube can also be used to empty the stomach of blood or other substances. Indications for use of nasogastric intubation include an inability to achieve adequate tidal volumes during ventilation due to gastric distention and the presence of gastric distention in an unresponsive patient.

As with nasopharyngeal airways, an NG tube is contraindicated in pediatric patients who have sustained head or facial trauma. Because the NG tube might migrate into the cranial sinuses, consider the use of an orogastric tube instead. Other contraindications include possible soft-tissue damage in the nose and inducement of vomiting.

In determining the correct length of NG tube, measure the tube from the top of the nose, over the ear, to the tip of the xiphoid process. To insert an NG tube, you should:

• Oxygenate and continue to ventilate, if possible.
• Measure the NG tube from the tip of the nose, over the ear, to the tip of the xiphoid process.
• Lubricate the end of the tube. Then pass it gently downward along the nasal floor to the stomach.
• Auscultate over the epigastrium to confirm correct placement. Listen for bubbling while injecting 10–20 cc of air into the tube.
• Use suction to aspirate stomach contents.
• Secure the tube in place.

11. Define pediatric respiratory distress, failure, and arrest.   pp. 977-978

The severity of respiratory compromise can be quickly classified into the following categories:

Respiratory distress. The mildest form of respiratory impairment is classified as respiratory distress. The most noticeable finding is the increased work of breathing. The signs and symptoms of respiratory distress include a normal mental status deteriorating to irritability or anxiety, tachypnea, retractions, nasal flaring (in infants), good muscle tone, head bobbing, grunting, and cyanosis that improves with supplemental oxygen. If not corrected immediately, respiratory distress will lead to respiratory failure.

Respiratory failure. Respiratory failure occurs when the respiratory system is not able to meet the demands of the body for oxygen intake and for carbon dioxide removal. It is characterized by inadequate ventilation and oxygenation. During respiratory failure, the carbon dioxide level begins to rise as the body is not able to remove it. This ultimately leads to respiratory acidosis. The signs and symptoms of respiratory failure include irritability or anxiety deteriorating to lethargy, marked tachypnea later deteriorating to bradypnea, marked retractions later deteriorating to agonal respirations, poor muscle tone, marked tachycardia later deteriorating to bradycardia, and central cyanosis. Respiratory failure is a very ominous sign. If immediate intervention is not provided, the child will deteriorate to full respiratory arrest.

Respiratory arrest. The end result of respiratory impairment, if untreated, is respiratory arrest. The cessation of breathing typically follows a period of bradypnea and agonal respirations. The signs and symptoms of respiratory arrest include unresponsiveness deteriorating to coma, bradypnea deteriorating to apnea, absent chest wall movement, bradycardia deteriorating to asystole, and profound cyanosis. Respiratory arrest will quickly deteriorate to full cardiopulmonary arrest if appropriate interventions are not made. The child's chances of survival markedly decrease when cardiopulmonary arrest occurs.

12. Differentiate between upper airway obstruction and lower airway disease.   pp. 979-986

Obstruction of the upper airway can be caused by many factors and may be partial or complete. Obstruction can result from inflamed or swollen tissues, which may be caused by infection or by aspirating a foreign body. Two medical conditions that can lead to upper airway obstruction in pediatric patients include croup and epiglottitis. Appropriate care depends on prompt and immediate identification of the disorder and its severity.

Suspect lower airway distress when the following conditions exist: an absence of stridor, presence of wheezing during exhalation, and increased work of breathing. Common causes of lower airway disease include respiratory diseases such as asthma, bronchiolitis, and pneumonia. Although infrequent, you may also encounter cases of foreign body lower airway aspiration, especially in toddlers and preschoolers.

13. Describe the general approach to the treatment of children with respiratory distress, failure, or arrest from upper airway obstruction or lower airway disease.   pp. 977-979

The general approach to the child with respiratory distress or failure from an upper or lower airway problem is to assess the child in the least stressful way possible and to administer oxygen. If the child has a complete upper airway obstruction, the appropriate FBAO maneuvers will need to be quickly done. If the child is in respiratory arrest, begin BVM resuscitation and consider the need for ET tube insertion. An NG tube may be useful to minimize gastric distention. If the child is in respiratory failure, assisted ventilations should also be considered.

In cases of upper airway obstruction, keep this precaution in mind: Because it is difficult to distinguish between croup from epiglottitis in the prehospital setting, never examine the oropharynx. If epiglottitis is present, examination of the oropharynx may result in laryngospasm and complete airway obstruction. In fact, if the patient is maintaining his or her airway, *do not put anything into the child's mouth,* including a thermometer. In the case of foreign body aspiration, do not attempt to look into the child's mouth if the obstruction is partial. Instead make the child comfortable and administer humidified oxygen. If the obstruction is complete, clear the airway with accepted basic life support techniques. However, DO NOT perform blind finger sweeps, as this can push a foreign body deeper into the airway.

When treating lower airway diseases, the primary goal is to support ventilations through the use of supplemental, humidified oxygen and appropriate pharmacological therapy such as bronchodilator medications (asthma and bronchiolitis). If prolonged ventilation will be required, perform endotracheal intubation.

14. Discuss the common causes and relative severity of hypoperfusion in infants and children. pp. 986-987

The second major cause of pediatric cardiopulmonary arrest—after respiratory impairment—is shock. Shock can most simply be defined as inadequate perfusion of the tissues with oxygen and other essential nutrients and inadequate removal of metabolic waste products.

When compared with the incidence of shock in adults, shock is an unusual occurrence in children because their blood vessels constrict so efficiently. However, when the blood pressure does drop, it drops so far and so fast that the child may quickly develop cardiopulmonary arrest. A number of factors place infants and young children at risk for shock. Newborns and neonates will develop shock as a result of a loss of body heat. Other causes include dehydration (from vomiting and/or diarrhea), infection (particularly septicemia), trauma, and blood loss. Less common causes of shock in infants and children include allergic reactions, poisoning, and cardiac events.

As in adults, the severity of shock in a pediatric patient is classified as compensated shock, decompensated shock, and irreversible shock. It can also be categorized as *cardiogenic* or *noncardiogenic*. Cardiogenic shock results from an inability of the heart to maintain an adequate cardiac output to the circulatory tissues. Cardiogenic shock in a pediatric patient is ominous and often fatal. Noncardiogenic shock—types of shock that result from causes other than inadequate cardiac output—is more frequently encountered in pediatric patients, because they have a much lower incidence of cardiac problems that adults. Causes of noncardiogenic shock may include hemorrhage, abdominal trauma, systemic bacterial infection, spinal cord injury, and others.

15. Identify the major classifications of pediatric cardiac rhythms. pp. 991-994

Dysrhythmias in children are uncommon. When dysrhythmias occur, bradydysrhythmias are the most common. Supraventricular tachydysrhythmias are very uncommon. Dysrhythmias can cause pump failure, ultimately leading to cardiogenic shock. Children have a very limited capacity to increase stroke volume. The primary mechanism through which they increase cardiac output is through changes in the heart rate. The treatment of dysrhythmias is specific for the dysrhythmia in question.

16. Discuss the primary etiologies of cardiopulmonary arrest in infants and children. pp. 977-978, 986

The primary causes of cardiopulmonary arrest in infants and children include untreated respiratory failure, immaturity of the cardiac conductive system, bradycardia, hypoxia, vagal stimulation (rare), drug overdose, drowning, multiple system trauma, electrocution, pericardial tamponade, tension pneumothorax, acidosis, hypothermia, hypoglycemia, and FBAO.

17. Discuss age-appropriate sites, equipment, techniques, and complications of vascular access for infants and children. pp. 970, 972-973

Intravenous techniques for children are basically the same as for adults. (See Chapter 7, "Medication Administration.") However, additional veins may be accessed in an infant. These include veins of the neck and scalp, as well as of the arms, hands, and feet. The external jugular vein, however, should only be used in life-threatening situations.

The use of intraosseous (IO) infusion has become popular in the pediatric patient. This is especially true when large volumes of fluid must be administered, as occurs in hypovolemic shock, and when other means of venous access are unavailable. The indications for IO include the existence of shock or cardiac arrest, an unresponsive patient, or an unsuccessful attempt at a peripheral IV insertion. The contraindications for IO infusion include the presence of a fracture in the bone chosen for infusion and a fracture of the pelvis or extremity fracture in the bone proximal to the chosen site. In performing IO perfusion, you can use a standard 16- or 18-gauge needle (either hypodermic or spinal). However, an intraosseous needle is preferred and significantly better. Basic steps are as follows: Prep the anterior surface of the leg below the knee with antiseptic solution (povidone iodine), and insert the needle in twisting fashion 1–3 centimeters below the tuberosity. Insertion should be slightly inferior in direction (to avoid the growth plate) and perpendicular to the skin. Signs of correct placement of the needle into the marrow cavity include a lack of resistance as the needle passes through the bony cortex, the ability of the needle to stand upright without support, the ability to aspirate bone marrow into a syringe, or free flow of the infusion without infiltration into the subcutaneous tissues.

18. Describe the primary etiologies of altered level of consciousness in infants and children. pp. 976-1003, 1008, 1009

The primary causes of an altered level of consciousness in infants and children include infection (fever), traumatic brain injury, respiratory failure (hypoxia), hypoperfusion, and dysrhythmias. Although metabolic causes such as seizures and hypoglycemia are fairly uncommon, they can and do produce altered levels of consciousness in children. Shunt failures may also present as altered mental status.

19. Identify common lethal mechanisms of injury in infants and children. pp. 1003-1005

The most common pediatric mechanisms of injury (MOI) include falls, motor vehicle crashes, car vs. pedestrian collisions, drownings and near drownings, penetrating injuries, burns, and physical abuse.

20. Discuss anatomical features of children that predispose or protect them from certain injuries. pp. 1009-1011

Head. Small children have larger heads in proportion to the rest of their bodies. For this reason, when they fall or are thrown through the air, they often land head first, predisposing them to serious head injury. The larger relative mass of the head and lack of neck muscle strength also provide increased momentum in acceleration-deceleration injuries and a greater stress on the cervical spine. Because the skull is softer and more compliant in infants and young children than in adults, brain injuries occur more readily.
Chest and abdomen. Infants and young children lack the rigid rib cages of adults. Therefore, they suffer fewer rib fractures and more intrathoracic injuries. Remember that chest injuries are the second most common cause of pediatric trauma death. Because of the compliance of the chest wall, severe intrathoracic injury can be present without signs of external injury. Likewise, their relatively underdeveloped abdominal musculature affords minimal protection to the viscera, particularly the spleen.
Extremities. Because children have more flexible bones than adults, they tend to have incomplete fractures such as bend fractures, buckle fractures, and greenstick fractures. Therefore, you should treat "sprains" and "strains" as fractures and immobilize accordingly. In younger children, the bone growth plates have not yet closed. Some growth plate fractures can lead to permanent disability if not managed correctly.
Body surface area. There are three distinguishing features of the pediatric patient's skin and BSA. First, the skin of an infant or child is thinner than that of an adult. Second, infants and children generally have less subcutaneous fat. Finally, they have a larger body-surface-area-to-weight ratio. As a result of these features, children risk greater injury from extremes in temperature or thermal exposure. They lose fluids and heat more quickly than adults and have a greater likelihood of dehydration and hypothermia. They also burn more easily and deeper than adults, which explains why burns are one of the leading causes of death among pediatric trauma patients.

21. Describe aspects of infant and child airway management that are affected by potential cervical spine injury. pp. 975, 1006

An infant's open airway is in the neutral or extended position but not in the hyperextended position. This needs to be kept in mind when positioning the infant who may have sustained a neck injury where there can be little to no movement of the neck for fear of worsening the potential neck injury. Children under the age of 6 usually have large heads in proportion to the rest of their bodies. Therefore, it is often necessary to pad behind the shoulders when a cervical collar is applied as a part of the spinal immobilization. Keep infants, toddlers, and preschoolers with the cervical spine in a neutral in-line position by placing padding from the shoulders to the hips.

Always make sure that you use appropriate-sized pediatric immobilization equipment. These supplies may include rigid cervical collars, towel or blanket rolls, foam head blocks, commercial pediatric immobilization devices, vest-type or short wooden backboards, and long boards with the appropriate padding.

22. Identify infant and child trauma patients who require spinal immobilization.
pp. 1006-1007

Children are not small adults. Although spinal injuries are not as common as in adults, they do occur, especially because of a child's disproportionately larger and heavier head. Any time an infant or child sustains a significant head injury, assume that a neck injury may be present. Children can suffer a spinal cord injury with no noticeable damage to the vertebral column as seen on cervical spine X-rays. Thus, negative cervical spine X-rays do not necessary assure that a spinal cord injury does not exist. As a result, children should remain immobilized until a spinal cord injury has been ruled out by hospital personnel.

Remember that many children, especially those under age 5, will protest or fight restraints. Try to minimize the emotional stress by having a parent or caregiver stand near or touch the child.

23. Discuss fluid management and shock treatment for infant and child trauma patients.
pp. 987-990, 1007

Fluid management and shock treatment for pediatric trauma patients should include administration of supplemental oxygen and establishment of intravenous access. However, DO NOT delay transport to gain venous access. Management of the airway and breathing takes priority over management of circulation, as circulatory compromise is less common in children than in adults.

When obtaining vascular access, remember the following:

• If possible, insert a large-bore catheter into a peripheral vein.
• Intraosseous access in children less than 6 years of age is an alternative when a peripheral IV cannot be obtained.
• Once venous access is obtained, administer an initial fluid bolus of 20 mL/kg of lactated Ringer's or normal saline.
• Reassess the patient's vital signs and re-bolus with another 80–100 mL/kg if there is no improvement.
• If improvement does not occur after the second bolus, there is likely to be a significant blood loss that may require surgical intervention. Rapid transport is essential.

24. Determine when pain management and sedation are appropriate for infants and children.
p. 1008

Many pediatric injuries are painful and analgesics are indicated. These include burns, long bone fractures, dislocations, and others. Unless there is a contraindication, pediatric patients should receive analgesics. Commonly used analgesics include meperidine, morphine, and fentanyl. It is best to avoid using synthetic analgesics, as their effects on children are unpredictable. Also, certain pediatric emergencies may benefit from sedation. These include such problems as penetrating eye injuries, prolonged rescue from entrapment in machinery, cardioversion, and other painful procedures. Always consult medical direction if you feel pediatric analgesia or sedation may be required.

25. Define child abuse, child neglect, and sudden infant death syndrome (SIDS). pp. 1012-1016, 1011

Child abuse is the intentional effort by a parent or caregiver to harm a child physically, psychologically, or sexually. Abuse can also take the form of **child neglect** (either physical or emotional), in which the physical, mental, and/or emotional well being of the child is ignored.

Sudden infant death syndrome (SIDS) is defined as the sudden death of an infant during the first year of life from an illness of unknown etiology, with peak incidence occurring at 2–4 months.

26. Discuss the parent/caregiver responses to the death of an infant or child. p. 1012

The responses of the parent or caregiver to the death of a child include the normal grief reactions. Initially, there may be shock, disbelief, and denial. Other times, the parents or caregivers may express anger, rage, hostility, blame, or guilt. Often, there is a feeling or inadequacy as well as helplessness, confusion, and fear. The grief process is likely to last for years, as in the case of a SIDS death.

27. Define children with special health care needs and technology-assisted children. pp. 1016-1020

In recent years medical technology has lowered infant mortality rates and allowed a greater number of children with special needs to live at home. Some of these infants and children include:

• Premature babies
• Infants and children with lung disease, heart disease, or neurological disorders
• Infants and children with chronic diseases, such as cystic fibrosis, asthma, childhood cancers, cerebral palsy, and others
• Infants and children with altered functions from birth (e.g., spina bifida, congenital birth defects, and cerebral palsy)

On some calls, you may be asked to treat technology-assisted children who depend, in varying degrees, upon special equipment. Commonly found devices include tracheostomy tubes, apnea monitors, home artificial ventilators, central intravenous lines, gastric feeding tubes, gastrostomy tubes, and shunts. (For more on these devices, see Chapter 46, "Acute Interventions for the Chronic-Care Patient.")

28. Discuss basic cardiac life support (CPR) guidelines for infants and children. p. 960

The CPR guidelines for infants and children are available at he Brady website at: www.bradybooks.com . This site will provide the most up-to-date information on these standards.

29. Integrate advanced life support skills with basic cardiac life support for infants and children. pp. 965-975

This is a skills objective that should be practiced in the classroom lab setting. You should work through simulated "mega-codes" that involve both BLS and ALS responders administering all the appropriate treatments as specified in their regional protocols and the American Heart Association's PALS algorithms.

30. Discuss the indications, dosage, route of administration, and special considerations for medication administration in infants and children. pp. 973-975

When administering medications to any patient of any age, the paramedic needs to know the indications, contraindications, correct dose, correct route of administration, and any expected side effects of the medication. Specifically, when administering the medications to infants and children, be very careful and accurate with the dose. Most medication doses are weight specific, so it will be necessary to have a rough idea of the weight of the patient or to use some other tool such as the Braslow tape.

The objectives of medication therapy in pediatric patients include:
• Correction of hypoxemia
• Increased perfusion pressure during chest compressions
• Stimulation of spontaneous or more forceful cardiac contractions
• Acceleration of the heart rate
• Correction of metabolic acidosis
• Management of pain (see objective 25)
• Treatment of seizures (see objective 33)

In administering medications to pediatric patients, consult with medical direction.

31. Discuss appropriate transport guidelines for low- and high-risk infants and children. pp. 975-976

In managing a pediatric patient, never delay transport to perform a procedure that can be done en route to the hospital. After deciding upon necessary interventions—first BLS, then ALS—determine the appropriate receiving facility. In reaching your decision, consider three factors: time of transport, specialized facilities, and specialized personnel. If you live in an area with specialized prehospital crews such as Critical Care Crews and Neonatal Nurses, their availability should weigh in your decision. Consider whether the patient would benefit by transfer to one of these crews. (For more on transport guides for low- and high-risk infants, see Chapter 41, "Neonatology.")

32. Describe the epidemiology, including the incidence, morbidity/mortality risk factors, prevention strategies, pathophysiology, assessment, and treatment of infants and children with:

a.   Respiratory distress/failure   pp. 977-978
Respiratory emergencies constitute the most common reason EMS is called to care for a pediatric patient. Respiratory illnesses can cause respiratory compromise due to their effect on the alveolar/capillary interface. Some illnesses are quite minor, causing only minor symptoms, while others can be rapidly fatal. Your approach to the child with a respiratory emergency will depend upon the severity of respiratory compromise. If the child is alert and talking, then you can take a more relaxed approach. However, if the child is ill-appearing and exhibiting marked respiratory difficulty, then you have to immediately intervene to prevent respiratory arrest and possible cardiopulmonary arrest.

Pediatric patients with late respiratory failure or respiratory arrest require aggressive treatment. This includes:

• Establishment of an airway
• Administration of high-flow supplemental oxygen
• Mechanical ventilation with a bag-valve-mask device attached to a reservoir delivering 100% oxygen
• Endotracheal intubation if mechanical ventilation does not rapidly improve the patient's condition
• Consideration of gastric decompression with an orogastric or nasogastric tube if abdominal distension is impeding ventilation
• Consideration of needle decompression of the chest if a tension pneumothorax is suspected
• Consideration of cricothyrotomy if complete obstruction is present and the airway cannot be obtained by any other method
• Obtain venous access, and transport to a facility equipped to handle critically ill children

b.   Hypoperfusion   pp. 986-990
As noted, shock is the second major cause of pediatric cardiopulmonary arrest. For an overview of the causes and degrees of severity of hypoperfusion in infants and children, see objective 15.

The definitive care of shock takes place in the emergency department of a hospital. Because shock is a life-threatening condition in pediatric patients, it is important to recognize early signs and symptoms—or even the possibility of shock in a situation where the signs and symptoms may not have yet developed. In a situation in which you suspect a possibility of shock, provide oxygen to boost tissue perfusion and transport as quickly as possible. Also, keep the patient in a supine position and take steps to protect the child from hypothermia and agitation that might worsen the condition. In some cases (compensated shock), fluid therapy as ordered by medical direction can buy time until the patient arrives an appropriate treatment center. (See objective 24 for more on fluid therapy and shock management.)

c. Cardiac dysrhythmias   pp. 991-994
Dysrhythmias in children are uncommon. When dysrhythmias occur, bradydysrhythmias are the most common. Supraventricular tachydysrhythmias are very uncommon. Dysrhythmias can cause pump failure, ultimately leading to cardiogenic shock. Children have a very limited capacity to increase stroke volume. The primary mechanism through which they increase cardiac output is through changes in the heart rate. The treatment of dysrhythmias is specific for the dysrhythmia in question.

d. Neurological emergencies   pp. 994, 996-997
Neurological emergencies in childhood are fairly uncommon. However, seizures can and do occur. In fact, they are a frequent reason for summoning EMS. In addition to seizures, meningitis tends to show up more often in children than in adults. Although your chances of encountering either of these two diseases are small, both are life threatening and should be promptly identified and treated.

Seizures. The etiology for seizures is often unknown. However, several risk factors have been identified. They include fever, hypoxia, infections, idiopathic epilepsy (epilepsy of unknown origin), electrolyte disturbances, head trauma, hypoglycemia, toxic ingestions or exposure, tumor, or CNS malformations. Management of pediatric seizure is essentially the same as for the seizing adult. Place patients on the floor or on the bed. Be sure to lay them on their side, away from furniture. Do not restrain patients, but take steps to protect them from injury. Maintain the airway, but do not force anything, such as a bite stick, between the teeth. Administer supplemental oxygen. Then take and record all vital signs. If the patient is febrile, remove excess layers of clothing, while avoiding extreme cooling. If status epilepticus is present, institute the following steps:

• Start an IV of normal saline or lactated Ringer's and perform a glucometer evaluation.
• Administer diazepam as follows:
—*Children 1 month to 5 years:* 0.2–0.5 mg slow IV push every 2–5 minutes up to a maximum of 2.5 milligrams.
—*Children 5 years and older:* 1 mg slow IV push every 2–5 minutes to a maximum of 5 milligrams.

• Contact medical direction for additional dosing. Diazepam can be administered rectally if an IV cannot be established.

• If the seizure appears to be due to a fever and a long transport time is anticipated, medical direction may request the administration of acetaminophen to lower the fever. Acetaminophen is supplied as an elixir or as suppositories. The dose should be 15 mg/kg body weight.

Meningitis. Meningitis is an infection of the meninges, the lining of the brain and spinal cord. Meningitis can result from both a virus and a bacteria. These infections can be rapidly fatal if they are not promptly recognized and treated appropriately. Prehospital care of the pediatric patient with meningitis is supportive. Rapidly complete the initial assessment and transport the child to the emergency department. If shock is present, treat the child with IV fluids (20 mL/kg) and oxygen.

e. Trauma   pp. 1003-1011
Trauma is the number one cause of death in infants and children. Most pediatric injuries result from blunt trauma. Children have thinner body walls that allow forces to be more readily transmitted to body contents, increasing the possibility of injury to internal tissues and organs. If

you serve in an urban area, you can expect to see a higher incidence of penetrating trauma, mostly intentional and mostly from gunfire or knife wounds. There is also a significant incidence of penetrating trauma outside the cities (mostly unintentional) from hunting accidents and agricultural accidents.

Although pediatric patients can be injured in the same way as adults, children tend to more susceptible to certain types of injuries than grownups. Falls, for example, are the single most common cause of injury in children. Other mechanisms of injury include motor vehicle collisions, car vs. pedestrian collisions, drownings and near drownings, penetrating injuries, burns, and physical abuse.

The treatment of trauma is injury specific. It involves management of the ABCS, management of the injury (e.g., spinal immobilization, splinting of fractures, control of bleeding), and treatment for possible shock.

f. Abuse and neglect   pp. 1012-1016

Child abuse is the second leading cause of death in infants less than 6 months of age. In 1998, there were 135 573 child maltreatment investigations in Canada. There are several characteristics common among abused children. Often the child is seen as "special" and different from others. Premature infants and twins stand a higher risk of abuse than other children. Many abused children are less than 5 years of age. Physically and mentally handicapped children as well as those with special needs are at greater risk. So are uncommunicative children. Boys are more often abused than girls. A child who is not what the parents wanted (e.g., the "wrong" gender) is at increased risk of abuse, too.

Signs of abuse or neglect can be startling. As a guide, the following findings should trigger a high index of suspicion:
• Any obvious or suspected fractures in a child under 2 years of age
• Injuries in various stages of healing, especially burns and bruises
• More injuries than usually seen in children of the same age or size
• Injuries scattered on many areas of the body
• Bruises or burns in patterns that suggest intentional infliction
• Increased intracranial pressure in an infant
• Suspected intra-abdominal trauma in a young child
• Any injury that does not fit with the description of the cause given
Information in the medical history may also raise the index of suspicion. Examples include:
• A history that does not match the nature or severity of the injury
• Vague parental accounts or accounts that change during the interview
• Accusations that the child injured himself or herself intentionally
• Delay in seeking help
• Child dressed inappropriately for the situation
• Revealing comment by bystanders, especially siblings

Suspect child neglect if you spot any of the following conditions:
• Extreme malnutrition
• Multiple insect bites
• Long-standing skin infections
• Extreme lack of cleanliness
• Verbal or social skills far below those you would expect for a child of similar age and background
• Lack of appropriate medical care

In cases of child abuse or neglect, the goals of management include appropriate treatment of injuries, protection of the child from further abuse, and notification of proper authorities.

g. Special health care needs, including technology-assisted children   pp. 1016-1020

For most of human history, infants and children with devastating congenital conditions or diseases died or remained confined to a hospital. In recent decades, however, medical technology has lowered infant mortality rates and allowed a greater number of children with special needs to live at home. For examples of children with special needs and some of the technological devices used to assist them, see objective 28.

In treating pediatric patients with special needs, remember that they require the same assessment as other patients. (Recall that in the initial assessment, "disability" refers to a patient's neurological status—not to the child's special need.) Keep in mind that the child's special need is often an ongoing process, which may make the parent or caregiver an excellent source of information. In most cases, you should concentrate on the acute problem—the reason for the call. In managing patients with special needs, try to keep several thoughts in mind.

• Avoid using the term "disability" (in reference to the child's special need). Instead, think of the patient's many abilities.
• Never assume that the patient cannot understand what you are saying.
• Involve the parents, caregivers, or the patient, if appropriate, in treatment. They manage the illness or congenital condition on a daily basis.
• Treat the patient with a special need with the same respect as any other patient.

h.   SIDS   pp. 1011-1012

The incidence of SIDS in Canada is approximately 1 deaths per 1 000 births. It is the leading cause of death between 2 weeks and 1 year of age, with peak incidence occurring at 2–4 months. SIDS occurs most frequently in the fall and winter months. It tends to be more common in males than in females. It is more prevalent in premature and low birth-weight infants, in infants of young mothers, and in infants whose mothers did not receive prenatal care. Infants of mothers who used cocaine, methadone, or heroin during pregnancy are at greater risk. Occasionally, a mild upper respiratory infection will be reported prior to the death. SIDS is not caused by external suffocation from blankets or pillows. Neither is it related to allergies to cow's milk or regurgitation and aspiration of stomach contents. It is not thought to be hereditary.

Current theories vary about the etiology of SIDS. Some authorities feel it may result from an immature respiratory center in the brain that leads the child to simply stop breathing. Others think there may be an airway obstruction in the posterior pharynx as a result of pharyngeal relaxation during sleep, a hypermobile mandible, or an enlarged tongue. Studies strongly link SIDS to a prone sleeping position. Soft bedding, waterbed mattresses, smoking in the home, and/or an overheated environment are other potential associations. A small percentage of SIDS may be abuse related.

Unless the infant is obviously dead, undertake active and aggressive care of the infant to assure the family or caregivers that everything possible is being done. A first responder or other personnel should be assigned to assist the parents or caregivers and to explain the procedure. At all points, use the baby's name.

33. Given several pre-programmed simulated pediatric patients, provide the appropriate assessment, treatment, and transport.   pp. 939-1020

During your classroom, clinical, and field training, you will be presented with real and simulated pediatric patients and assess and treat them. Use the information provided in this chapter and the information and skills you gain from your instructors and clinical and field preceptors to develop your skill on caring for these patients. Continue to refine newly learned skills once your training ends and you begin your paramedic career.

CONTENT SELF-EVALUATION

Multiple Choice

1. The leading cause of death in pediatric patients in Canada is:
   - A. AIDS.
   - B. asthma.
   - C. trauma.
   - D. neglect.
   - E. cardiac arrest.

2. Factors that account for high rates of pediatric injury include all of the following EXCEPT:
   - A. weather.
   - B. geography.
   - C. dangers in the home.
   - D. HMOs.
   - E. motor vehicle accidents.

3. A specific course through continuing education aimed at improving the assessment and treatment of pediatric patients who suffer from life-threatening illnesses and injuries is called:
   - A. EMSC.
   - B. PBTLS.
   - C. PALS.
   - D. APLS.
   - E. TRIPP.

4. The most common response of children to illness or injury is:
   - A. denial.
   - B. fear.
   - C. excitement.
   - D. indifference.
   - E. grief.

5. Treatment of a pediatric patient begins with:
   - A. obtaining vital signs.
   - B. placement of an ET tube.
   - C. administration of oxygen.
   - D. focused head-to-toe exam.
   - E. communications and psychological support.

6. While caring for the pediatric patient, whenever possible, the paramedic should:
   - A. avoid discussing painful procedures.
   - B. administer high-flow oxygen.
   - C. allow a parent or caregiver to stay with the child.
   - D. use correct medical and anatomical terms.
   - E. stand in an authoritative posture.

7. The term neonate describes a baby that is:
   - A. newly born.
   - B. 10 days or less in age.
   - C. up to 1 month in age.
   - D. 1 to 5 months in age.
   - E. 6 months or more in age.

8. The age group for which foreign body airway obstruction (FBAO) becomes a concern is:
   - A. infants ages 1–5 months.
   - B. infants ages 6–12 months.
   - C. toddlers.
   - D. preschoolers.
   - E. school-age children.

9. An infant's airway differs from that of an adult in all of the following ways EXCEPT that it:
   - A. is narrower at all levels.
   - B. has a softer and more flexible trachea.
   - C. is less likely to be blocked by secretions.
   - D. has a greater likelihood of soft-tissue injury.
   - E. is more prone to obstruction by the tongue.

10. In comparing pediatric heart and respiratory rates with those of an adult, infants and young children have:
   A.   about the same heart and respiratory rates as an adult.
   B.   slower heart rates and slower respiratory rates.
   C.   slower heart rates and faster respiratory rates.
   D.   faster heart rates and slower respiratory rates.
   E.   faster heart rates and faster respiratory rates.

11. Unlike an adult, the trachea of a child can collapse if the neck and head are hyperextended because:
   A.   the trachea is softer and more flexible.
   B.   a child's tongue takes up more space proportionately.
   C.   the cricoid rings are firmer.
   D.   a child's larynx is higher.
   E.   the airway is wider at all levels.

12. The two abdominal organs that are most likely to suffer traumatic injury in a pediatric patient are the:
   A.   kidney and gallbladder.   D.   colon and appendix.
   B.   liver and spleen.   E.   bladder and pancreas.
   C.   stomach and small intestine.

13. A child's larger body-surface-area-to-weight ratio causes a pediatric patient to be:
   A.   resilient to temperature changes. D.   prone to excess subcutaneous fat.
   B.   prone to hypothermia.   E.   less likely to lose fluids quickly.
   C.   difficult to assess.

14. Although infants and children have a circulating blood volume proportionately larger than adults, their absolute blood volume is:
   A.   about the same.   D.   rate dependent.
   B.   smaller.   E.   variable.
   C.   even larger.

15. In an infant or small child, tachypnea, an abnormally rapid rate of breathing, may indicate:
   A.   fear.   D.   exposure to cold.
   B.   pain.   E.   all of the above
   C.   inadequate oxygenation.

16. A respiratory rate of 18–30 breaths per minute would be considered normal for a(n):
   A.   newborn.   D.   preschooler.
   B.   6-month old infant.   E.   school-age child.
   C.   toddler.

17. Which of the following approaches is the correct method for conducting the physical examination of an infant or a very young child?
   A.   toe-to-head   D.   chest-to-head
   B.   head-to-chest   E.   both A and B
   C.   head-to-toe

18. To obtain the blood pressure of a pediatric patient, the cuff should be _____ the width of the patient's arm.
   A.   one-fourth   D.   two-thirds
   B.   one-third   E.   three-fourths
   C.   one-half

19. Medication administration in the pediatric patient is modified to the patient's:
   A.   age.   E.   level of distress.
   B.   height.   D.   level of consciousness.
   C.   weight.

20. The hallmark of pediatric management is:
- **A.** frequent pulse checks.
- **B.** prompt transport.
- **C.** administration of fluids.
- **D.** adequate oxygenation.
- **E.** diagnosis of medical conditions.

21. As a rule, an oropharyngeal airway should only be used on pediatric patients who:
- **A.** have sustained head or facial trauma.
- **B.** are known to suffer from seizures.
- **C.** show signs of cardiac arrest.
- **D.** exhibit a vagal response.
- **E.** lack a gag reflex.

22. The only indication for cricothyrotomy in the pediatric patient is:
- **A.** a foreign body airway obstruction.
- **B.** desire to suction the airway.
- **C.** failure to obtain an airway by any other method.
- **D.** desire to ventilate by a BVM.
- **E.** both A and C

23. Indications for performing an endotracheal intubation in a pediatric patient include all of the following EXCEPT the:
- **A.** need to gain access for suctioning.
- **B.** necessity of providing a route for drug administration.
- **C.** need for prolonged artificial ventilations.
- **D.** failure to provide adequate ventilations with a BVM.
- **E.** all of the above

24. The optimal positioning of the head for pediatric intubation in the absence of a spinal injury is:
- **A.** neutral.
- **B.** hyperextended.
- **C.** sniffing.
- **D.** head-tilt.
- **E.** spine.

25. If gastric distention is present in a pediatric patient, a paramedic might consider placing a(n):
- **A.** oropharyngeal airway.
- **B.** nasopharyngeal airway.
- **C.** needle cricothyrotomy.
- **D.** nasogastric tube.
- **E.** endotracheal tube.

26. The indications for use of intraosseous infusion include all of the following EXCEPT:
- **A.** a patient less than 7 years old.
- **B.** existence of shock or cardiac arrest.
- **C.** presence of a facture in the pelvis.
- **D.** an unresponsive patient.
- **E.** failure to place a peripheral IV.

27. All of the following are symptoms of epiglottitis EXCEPT:
- **A.** a rapid onset.
- **B.** occasional stridor.
- **C.** a barking cough
- **D.** drooling.
- **E.** a fever of approximately 38.8-40 C.

28. In treating a patient with epiglottitis, a paramedic should:
- **A.** take blood pressure regularly.
- **B.** attempt to visualize the oropharynx.
- **C.** take the child's temperature orally.
- **D.** place the child in a supine position.
- **E.** none of the above

29. Common causes of lower airway distress include all of the following EXCEPT:
- **A.** pneumonia.
- **B.** asthma.
- **C.** croup.
- **D.** bronchiolitis.
- **E.** status asthmaticus.

30. When a child experiences a severe asthma attack without wheezing, this is:
- **A.** an ominous sign.
- **B.** because of a lack of expectorant.
- **C.** a sign of improvement.
- **D.** because of an inability to cough.
- **E.** common, and should not alarm the paramedic.

31. All of the following are signs and symptoms of shock in a child EXCEPT:
- **A.** pale, cool, clammy skin.
- **B.** impaired mental status.
- **C.** absence of tears when crying.
- **D.** increased urination.
- **E.** a rapid respiratory rate.

32. When dysrhythmias do occur in children, the most common form is a(n):
- **A.** bradydysrhythmia.
- **B.** supraventricular tachydysrhythmia.
- **C.** ventricular tachydysrhythmia.
- **D.** asystole.
- **E.** ventricular fibrillation.

33. A pediatric patient is seen by a paramedic for a seizure. Assessment and history reveal that the child has a fever of 38.4 C, was very sleepy and irritable before the seizure, and has had no similar episodes. The child complained of a stiff neck and headache earlier in the day. You suspect that the episode may have been caused by:
- **A.** febrile convulsions.
- **B.** meningitis.
- **C.** hypoglycemia.
- **D.** hypoxia.
- **E.** hyperglycemia.

34. Whenever a glucometer reading reveals a blood sugar of less than 4.0 mmol/L, a paramedic might suspect:
- **A.** hypoxia.
- **B.** hyperglycemia.
- **C.** hypoglycemia.
- **D.** ketoacidosis.
- **E.** dehydration.

35. The single most common cause of trauma-related injuries in children is:
- **A.** motor-vehicle collisions.
- **B.** burns.
- **C.** falls.
- **D.** physical abuse.
- **E.** drownings.

36. Appropriate-sized pediatric immobilization equipment includes all of the following EXCEPT:
- **A.** towel or blanket roll.
- **B.** vest-type device (KED).
- **C.** sandbag.
- **D.** straps and cravats.
- **E.** padding.

37. All of the following are true statements about SIDS EXCEPT that it:
- **A.** occurs most frequently in the fall and winter.
- **B.** is not caused by external suffocation by blankets.
- **C.** tends to be more common in females than in males.
- **D.** is not thought to be hereditary.
- **E.** is possibly linked to a prone sleeping position.

38. Child abuse can take the form of:
- **A.** psychological abuse.
- **B.** physical abuse.
- **C.** sexual abuse.
- **D.** neglect.
- **E.** all of the above

39. In cases of suspected child abuse, management goals include all of the following EXCEPT:
    A. protection of the child from further injury.
    B. notification of proper authorities.
    C. appropriate treatment of injuries.
    D. cross-examination of the parents or caregivers.
    E. documentation of all findings and statements.

40. A surgical connection that runs from the brain to the abdomen in a pediatric patient is called a(n):
    A. central IV.   D. inner cannula.
    B. tracheostomy.   E. epigastric tube.
    C. shunt.

True/False

41. The pediatric assessment triangle focuses on airway, breathing, and circulation.
    A. True
    B. False

42. Poorly taken vital signs are of less value than no vital signs at all.
    A. True
    B. False

43. In obtaining vascular access in a pediatric patient, the external jugular vein should only be used in life-threatening situations.
    A. True
    B. False

44. You are more likely to use electrical therapy on pediatric patients than adult patients.
    A. True
    B. False

45. Cardiogenic shock is more frequently encountered in pre-hospital pediatric care than noncardiogenic shock.
    A. True
    B. False

46. At ages 1-3, language development begins and children can understand better than they can speak.
    A. True
    B. False

47. Cardiopulmonary arrest in children is usually not a sudden event
    A. True
    B. False

48. Back blows are the definitive treatment for children older than one year of age who have a complete airway obstruction.
    A. True
    B. False

49. The child in decompensated shock is critically ill, and death will ensue rapidly without aggressive intervention..
    A. True
    B. False

_____ 50. Pediatrics who are post-ictal on arrival of paramedics should be assessed and left at scene if all vitals are stable.
  A.   True
  B.   False

Matching

Write the letter of the term in the space provided next to the appropriate description.

A.	asthma	F.	growth plate
B.	hypoglycemia	G.	bacterial tracheitis
C.	croup	H.	epiglottitis
D.	buckle fractures	I.	cardiogenic shock
E.	bronchiolitis	J.	<7 years old

_____ 51. abnormally low concentration of glucose in the blood

_____ 52. the epiphyseal plate

_____ 53. condition marked by recurrent attacks of dyspnea due to spasmodic constriction of the bronchi

_____ 54. viral infection of the medium-sized airways, occurring most frequently during the first year of life

_____ 55. bacterial infection of the epiglottis

_____ 56. fractures characterized by a raised or bulging projection at the fracture site

_____ 57. intraosseous infusion can be initiated

_____ 58. the inability of the heart to meet the metabolic needs of the body resulting in poor tissue perfusion

_____ 59. infection most likely to appear after episodes of croup

_____ 60. laryngotracheobronchitis

Chapter 43

Geriatric Emergencies

Review of Chapter Objectives

After reading this chapter, you should be able to:

1. **Discuss the demographics demonstrating the increasing size of the elderly population in Canada.   pp. 1023-1025**

Between 1971 and 1996, the number of elderly people has grown one and one-half times in Canada. By 1996, persons aged 65+ made up 12 per cent of the population.. In 2031, when the post–World War II baby boomers enter their 80s, more than 7.8 million people will be age 65 or older.

2. **Assess the various living environments of the elderly patients.   p. 1024**

The elderly live in both independent and dependent living environments. Many continue to live alone or with their partner until well into their 80s or 90s. The "oldest" old are the most likely to live alone, and, in fact, nearly half of those age 85 and older live by themselves. The great majority of these people—an estimated 78 percent—are women. This is because married men tend to die before their wives, and widowed men tend to remarry more often than widowed women. Elderly persons living alone represent one of the most impoverished and vulnerable parts of society.

3. **Discuss society's view of aging and the social, financial, and ethical issues facing the elderly. pp. 1024**

After years of working and/or raising a family, an elderly person must not only find new roles to fulfill but, in many cases, must overcome the societal label of "old person." A lot of elderly people disprove ageism—and all the stereotypes it engenders—by living happy, productive, and active lives. Others, however, feel a sense of social isolation or uselessness. Physical and financial difficulties reinforce these feelings and help create an emotional context in which illnesses can occur. Successful medical treatment of elderly patients involves an understanding of the broader social content in which they live.

As a group, most elderly people worry about income, aggravated by fixed retirement payments or loss of benefits when a partner dies. Tight finances and limited mobility may prevent an independent elderly person from maintaining adequate nutrition and safety. As a result, elderly patients may be at increased risk of accidental hypothermia, carbon monoxide poisoning, or fires. They may also reduce their medications, or "half dose," to save money. In the course of caring for elderly patients, ethical concerns frequently arise. You may be confronted with multiple decision makers, particularly in dependent living environments. You may also have a question about the patient's competency to give informed consent or refusal of treatment. Finally, you may be faced with advanced directives, such as "living wills" and Do Not Resuscitate (DNR) orders.

In treating the elderly, remember that the best intervention is prevention. The goal of any health care service, including EMS, should be to help keep people from becoming sick or injured in the first place. As a paramedic, you can reduce morbidity among the elderly by taking part in community education programs and by cooperating with agencies or organizations that support the elderly. The specific resources may differ from community, to community, but some possibilities include senior centers, Meals on Wheels, religious organizations with programs for the elderly, governmental agencies, or national and state associations such as the Alzheimer's Association, or the Association for Senior Citizens.

Many EMS agencies have developed a means for referring elderly patients to appropriate follow-up services. Consider preparing a checklist with descriptions of services in your area as well as the names of contact people and their phone numbers. The checklists can be given to elderly patients as needed.

4. Discuss common emotional and psychological reactions to aging, including causes and manifestations. pp. 1023-1029

When behavioral or psychological problems develop later in life, they are often dismissed as normal age-related changes. This attitude denies an elderly person the opportunity to correct a treatable condition and/or overlooks an underlying physical disorder. Studies have shown that the elderly retain their basic personalities and their adaptive cognitive abilities. Intellectual decline and regressive behavior are not normal age-related changes and could in fact have a physiological cause, such as head trauma.

It is important to keep in mind the emotionally stressful situations facing many elderly people such as isolation, loneliness, loss of independence, loss of strength, fear of the future, and more. The elderly are at risk for alcoholism as well as facing a higher incidence of secondary depression as a result of neuroleptic medications such as Haldol or Thorazine.

The emotional well-being of the elderly impacts upon their overall physical health. Therefore, it is important that you note evidence of altered behavior in any elderly patient that you assess and examine. Also, keep in mind that many emotional conditions, such as depression, are normal reactions to stressful situations and can be resolved with appropriate counseling and treatment. Finally, remember that medical disorders in the elderly often present as functional impairment and should be treated as an early warning of a possibly undetected medical problem.

5. Apply the pathophysiology of multi-system failure to the assessment and management of medical conditions of the elderly patient. p. 1026

The body becomes less efficient with age, increasing the likelihood of malfunction. The body of an elderly patient is susceptible to all the disorders of young people, but its maintenance, defense, and repair processes are weaker. As a result, the elderly often suffer from more than one illness or disease at a time. On average, six medical disorders may coexist in an elderly person and perhaps even more in the old-old. Furthermore, disease in one organ system may result in the deterioration of other systems, compounding existing acute and/or chronic conditions.

Because of concomitant diseases (comorbidity) in the elderly, complaints may not be specific to any one disorder. Common complaints of the elderly include fatigue and weakness, dizziness/vertigo/syncope, falls, headaches, insomnia, dysphagia, loss of appetite, inability to void, and/or constipation/diarrhea.

Elderly patients often accept medical problems as a part of aging and fail to monitor changes in their condition. In some cases, such as a silent myocardial infarction, pain may be diminished or absent. In others, a complaint may seem trivial, such as constipation.
Although many medical problems in the young and middle-aged populations present with a standard set of signs and symptoms, the changes involved in aging lead to different presentations. In pneumonia, for example, some classic symptoms such as fever, chest pain, and a cough may be diminished or absent.

6. Compare the pharmacokinetics of an elderly patient to that of a young patient, including drug distribution, metabolism, and excretion. pp. 1026-1027

In general, a person's sensitivity to drugs increases with age. When compared with younger patients, the elderly experience more adverse drug reactions, more drug-drug interactions, and more drug-disease interactions. Because of age-related pharmacokinetic changes such as a loss of body fluids and atrophy of organs, drugs concentrate more readily in the plasma and tissues of elderly patients. As a result, drug dosages often must be adjusted to prevent toxicity. Additionally, due to differences in the GI tract, medications are metabolized and excreted at a slower rate in the elderly patient.

7. Discuss the impact of polypharmacy, dosing errors, increased drug sensitivity, and medication non-compliance on assessment and management of the elderly patient. pp. 1026-1027

If medications are not correctly monitored, polypharmacy can cause a number of problems among the elderly. In taking a medical history of an elderly patient, remember to ask questions to determine if the patient is taking a prescribed medication as directed. Noncompliance with drug therapy, usually underadherence, is common among the elderly. Up to 40 percent do not take medications as prescribed. Of these individuals, 35 percent experience some type of medical problem.

Factors that can decrease compliance in the elderly include limited income, memory loss (due to decreased or diseased neural activity), limited mobility, sensory impairment (cannot hear/read/understand directions), multiple or complicated drug therapies, fear of toxicity, child-proof containers (especially difficult for arthritic patients), and lengthy drug therapy plans.

8. Discuss the use and effects of commonly prescribed drugs for the elderly patient. pp. 1026-1027, 1064-1066

Functional changes in the kidneys, liver, and gastrointestinal system slow the absorption and elimination of many medications in the elderly. In addition, the various compensatory mechanisms that help buffer against medication side effects are less effective in the elderly than in younger patients.

Approximately 30 percent of all hospital admissions are related to drug-induced illness. About 50 percent of all drug-related deaths occur in people over the age of 60. Accidental overdoses may occur more frequently in the aged due to confusion, vision impairment, self-selection of medications, forgetfulness, and concurrent drug use. Intentional drug overdose also occurs in attempts at self-destruction. Another complicating factor is the abuse of alcohol among the elderly.

9. Discuss the problem of mobility in the elderly, and develop strategies to prevent falls. pp. 1027-1028

Regular exercise and a good diet are two of the most effective prevention measures for ensuring mobility among the elderly. Some elderly may suffer from a severe medical problem, such as crippling arthritis. They may fear for their personal safety, either from accidental injury or intentional injury, such as robbery. Certain medications also may increase their lethargy. Whatever the cause, a lack of mobility can have detrimental physical and emotional effects. Some of these include poor nutrition, difficulty with elimination, poor skin integrity, a greater predisposition for falls, loss of independence and/or confidence, depression from "feeling old," and isolation.

Falls present an especially serious problem for the elderly. Fall-related injuries represent the leading cause of accidental death among the elderly and the seventh highest cause of death overall. As a result, the paramedic should consider strategies for making a home safe for the elderly and point these out to the elderly patient or family of the elderly patient, whichever may be appropriate. Examples of hazards that can easily be corrected include torn or slippery rugs, chairs without armrests, chairs with low backs, chairs with wheels, obstructing furniture, slippery bathtubs, dim lighting, high cabinet shelves, missing handrails on stairways, and high steps on stairways.

10. Discuss age-related changes in sensations in the elderly, and describe the implications of these changes for communication and patient assessment. pp. 1028, 1031-1033

Most elderly patients suffer from some form of age-related sensory changes. Normal physiological changes may include impaired vision or blindness, impaired or loss of hearing, an altered sense of taste or smell, and/or a lower sensitivity to pain or touch. Any of these conditions can affect your ability to communicate with the patient. In general, be prepared to spend more time obtaining histories from elderly patients.

11. Discuss the problems with continence and elimination in the elderly patient, and develop communication strategies to provide psychological support.   pp. 1028-1029

The elderly often find it embarrassing to talk about problems with continence and elimination. They may feel stigmatized, isolated, and/or helpless. When confronted with these problems, DO NOT make a big deal out of them. Respect the patient's dignity, and assure the person that, in many cases, the problem is treatable.

Remember, too, that problems with continence and elimination are not necessarily caused by aging. They may be the result of drug therapy or medical conditions such as diabetes. As a result, in assessing a patient with incontinence or constipation, inquire about their medications and any chronic medical disorders. Also keep in mind the variety of other conditions that can result from problems with continence or elimination. In the case of incontinence, for example, a patient may experience rashes, skin infections, skin breakdown (ulcers), urinary tract infections, sepsis, and falls or fractures (caused by a frequent need to eliminate). In elderly people with cerebrovascular disease or impaired baroreceptor reflexes, efforts to force a bowel movement can lead to a transient ischemic attack (TIA) or syncope.

12. Discuss factors that may complicate the assessment of the elderly patient.   pp.1026, 1030-1034

In assessing an elderly patient, keep in mind the variety of causes of functional impairment. If identified early, an environmental or disease-related condition can often be reversed. Your success depends upon a thorough understanding of age-related changes and the implications of these changes for patient assessment and management. You will need to recall at all times the complications that can arise from comorbidity (having more than one disease at a time) and polypharmacy (concurrent use of a number of drugs).

Communications challenges may also complicate the assessment. Patients may be blind, have speech difficulties, or have some kind of hearing loss that can make assessment more difficult. They also often have a lower sensitivity to pain or touch.

In general, assessment of the elderly patient follows the same basic approach used with any other patient. However, you should keep in mind these points:

• Set a context for illness, taking into account the patient's living situation, level of activity, network of social support, level of dependence, medication history (both prescriptive and nonprescriptive), and sleep patterns.

• Pay close attention to an elderly person's nutrition, noting conditions that may complicate or discourage eating.

• Keep in mind that elderly patients may minimize or fail to report important symptoms. Therefore, try to distinguish the patient's chief complaint from the patient's primary problem.

• Because of presence of multiple chronic diseases, treat the patient on a "threat-to-life" basis.

• Recall at all times that alterations in the temperature-regulating mechanism can result in a lack of fever, or a minimal fever, even in the presence of a severe infection.

• When confronted with a confused patient, try to determine whether the patient's mental status represents a significant change from normal for them. DO NOT assume that a confused, disoriented patient is "just senile," thus failing to assess for a serious underlying problem.

• Remember that some patients are often easily fatigued and cannot tolerate a long physical examination. Also, because of problems with temperature regulation, the patient may be wearing several layers of clothing.

• Be aware that the elderly patient may minimize or deny symptoms because of a fear of institutionalization or a loss of self-sufficiency.

• Try to distinguish signs of chronic disease from acute problems. For example:

—Peripheral pulses may be difficult to evaluate because of peripheral vascular disease and arthritis.

—The elderly may have nonpathological crackles (rales) upon lung auscultation.

—The elderly often exhibit an increase in mouth breathing and a loss of skin elasticity, which may be confused with dehydration.

—Dependent edema may be caused by inactivity, not congestive heart failure.

13. Discuss the principles that should be employed when assessing and communicating with the elderly. pp. 1028, 1030-1034

To improve your skill at assessing and communicating with the elderly, keep in mind these principles.

• Always introduce yourself.
• Speak slowly, distinctly, and respectfully.
• Speak to the patient first, rather than to family members, caregivers, or bystanders.
• Speak face to face, at eye level with eye contact.
• Locate the patient's hearing aid or eyeglasses, if needed.
• DO NOT shout at the patient. This will not help if the patient is deaf, and it may distort sounds for the patient who has some level of hearing.
• Write notes, if necessary.
• Allow the patient to put on the stethoscope, while you speak into it like a microphone.
• Turn on the room lights.
• If a patient has forgotten to put in dentures, politely ask the person to do so.
• Display verbal and nonverbal signs of concern and empathy.
• Remain polite at all times.
• Preserve the person's dignity.
• Always explain what you are doing and why.
• Use your power of observation to recognize anxiety—tempo of speech, eye contact, tone of voice—during the telling of the history.

14. Compare the assessment of a young patient with that of an elderly patient. pp. 1030-1031, 1035-1041

The assessment of the older person differs from that of a younger person in a number of ways. The elderly often have complicated medical histories that entail numerous chronic conditions. They also usually take multiple medications (both prescribed and nonprescribed), which in turn may produce a variety of physical and/or psychological side effects. As stated in previous objectives, remain sensitive to the special fears of an elderly patient, particularly the fear of increased dependency, and unique stresses of that age group, such as loss of long-term partners or friends. Allow for the extra time necessitated by communication challenges. DO NOT rush the elderly patient through an assessment unless it is absolutely necessary because of a life-threatening condition.

15. Discuss common complaints of elderly patients. pp. 1026, 1041-1046

Common complaints of elderly patients include fatigue and weakness, dizziness, vertigo or syncope, falls, headaches, insomnia, dysphagia, loss of appetite, inability to void, and constipation or diarrhea. Many of these complaints in and of themselves would not be too serious. However, given the context of complicated medical histories of the elderly, each of these complaints are important and should be followed up and taken very seriously.

16. Discuss the normal and abnormal changes of age in relation to the:

a. Pulmonary system pp. 1035-1037
The effects of aging on the respiratory system begin as early as age 30. Without regular exercise and/or training, the lungs start to lose their ability to defend themselves and to carry out their prime function of ventilation. Age-related changes in the respiratory system include decreased chest wall compliance, loss of lung elasticity, increased air trapping due to collapse of the smaller airways, and reduced strength and endurance of the respiratory muscles. In addition, there is a decrease in an effective cough reflex and the activity of the cilia. The decline of these two defense mechanisms leave the lungs more susceptible to recurring infection. Other factors that may affect pulmonary function in the elderly are kyphosis (exaggeration of the normal posterior curvature of the spine), chronic exposure to pollutants, and long-term cigarette smoking.

b.   Cardiovascular system   pp. 1037-1038

A number of variables unrelated to aging influence cardiovascular functions—diet, smoking and alcohol use, education, socioeconomic status, and even personality traits. Of particular importance is the level of physical activity.

This said, the cardiovascular system still experiences, in varying degrees, age-related deterioration. Changes include a loss of elasticity and hardening of the arteries, an increase in the size and bulk of the left ventricle (hypertrophy), development of fibrosis (formation of fiber-like connective/scar tissue), and changes in the rate, rhythm, and overall efficiency of the heart.

c.   Nervous system p. 1038

Unlike cells in other organ systems, cells in the central nervous system cannot reproduce. The brain can lose as much as 45 percent of its cells in certain areas of the cortex. Overall, there is an average 10 percent reduction in brain weight from age 20 to age 90. Keep in mind, however, that reductions in brain weight and ventricular size are not well correlated with intelligence, and elderly people may still be capable of highly creative and productive thought. In addition to shrinkage of brain tissue, the elderly may experience some memory loss, clinical depression, altered mental status, and impaired balance. Keep in mind that these changes vary greatly and may not be seen in all elderly patients, even at the close of very long lives.

d.   Endocrine system   pp. 1038, 1039

The elderly experience a variety of age-related hormonal changes. Women, for example, experience menopause, the result of reductions in estrogen production. Men also experience a decline in levels of testosterone. In addition, the elderly commonly experience a decline in insulin sensitivity and/or an increase in insulin resistance. Finally, thyroid disorders, especially hypothyroidism and thyroid nodules, increase with age as well.

e.   Gastrointestinal system p. 1039

Age affects the gastrointestinal system in various ways. The volume of saliva may decrease by as much as 33 percent, leading to complaints of dry mouth, nutritional deficiencies, and a predisposition to choking. Gastric secretions may decrease to as little as 20 percent of the quantity present in younger people. Esophageal and intestinal motility also decrease, making swallowing more difficult and delaying digestive processes. The production of hydrochloric acid also declines, further disrupting digestion and, in some adults, contributing to nutritional anemia. Gums atrophy and the number of taste buds decrease, reducing even further the desire to eat.

Other conditions may also develop. Hiatal hernias are not age-related per se, but can have serious consequences for the elderly. The hernias may incarcerate, strangulate, or, in the most severe cases, result in massive GI hemorrhage. A diminished liver function, which is associated with aging, can delay or impede detoxification. It also can reduce the production of clotting proteins, which in turn leads to bleeding abnormalities.

f.   Thermoregulatory system   p. 1039

As people age, the thermoregulatory system becomes altered or impaired. Aging seems to reduce the effectiveness of sweating in cooling the body. Older people tend to sweat at higher core temperatures and have less sweat output per gland than younger people. As people age, they also experience deterioration of the autonomic nervous system, including a decrease in shivering and lower resting peripheral blood flow. In addition, the elderly may have a diminished perception of the cold. Drugs and disease can further alter an elderly patient's response to temperature extremes, resulting in hyperthermia or accidental hypothermia.

g.   Integumentary system   pp. 1040, 1057

As people age, the skin loses collagen, a connective tissue that gives elasticity and support to the skin. Without this support, the skin is subject to a great number of injuries from bumping or tearing. In addition, the skin thins as people age. Because cells reproduce more slowly, older patients often suffer more severe skin injuries than younger patients and healing takes a longer time. As a rule, the elderly are at a higher risk of secondary infections, skin tumors, drug-induced eruptions, and fungal or viral infections. Decades of exposure to the sun also makes the elderly vulnerable to melanoma and other sun-related carcinomas.

h. Musculoskeletal system   pp. 1040, 1058

An aging person may lose as much as 2–3 inches of height from narrowing of the intervertebral disks and osteoporosis (softening of bone tissue due to the loss of essential minerals). This is especially evident in the vertebral bodies, thus causing a change in posture. The posture of the aged individual often reveals an increase in the curvature of the thoracic spine (kyphosis) and slight flexion of the knee and hip joints. The demineralization of bone makes the elderly patient much more susceptible to hip and other fractures.

In addition to skeletal changes, a decrease in skeletal muscle weight commonly occurs with age—especially with sedentary individuals. To compensate, elderly women develop a narrow, short gait, while older men develop a wide gait. These changes make the elderly more susceptible to falls.

17. Describe the incidence, morbidity/mortality, risk factors, prevention strategies, pathophysiology, assessment, need for intervention and transport, and management of the elderly medical patient with:

a.   Pneumonia, chronic obstructive disease, and pulmonary embolism   pp. 1042-1045

Pneumonia. Pneumonia is an infection of the lung usually caused by a bacterium or virus. Aspiration pneumonia is also common in the elderly due to difficulty in swallowing.

Pneumonia is the fourth leading cause of death in people age 65 and older. Its incidence increases with age at a rate of 10 percent for each decade beyond age 20. It is found in 60 percent of autopsies performed on the elderly. Reasons for the high incidence of pneumonia among the elderly include decreased immune response, reduced pulmonary function, increased colonization of the pharynx by gram-negative bacteria, abnormal or ineffective cough reflex, and decreased effectiveness of mucociliary cells of the upper respiratory system. The elderly who are at the greatest risk for contracting pneumonia are frail adults and those with multiple chronic diseases or compromised immunity.

Common signs and symptoms of pneumonia include increasing dyspnea, congestion, fever, chills, tachypnea, sputum production, and altered mental status. Occasionally, abdominal pain may be the only symptom.

Prevention strategies include prophylactic treatment with antibiotics. Efforts should also be taken to reduce exposure to infectious patients and to promote patient mobility. Once a person has contracted the disease, treatment includes management of all life threats, maintenance of adequate oxygenation, and transport to the hospital for diagnosis and further management.

Chronic obstructive pulmonary disease (COPD). COPD is really a collection of diseases characterized by chronic airflow obstruction with reversible and/or irreversible components. Although each COPD has its own distinct features, elderly patients commonly have two or more types at the same time. COPD usually refers to some combination of emphysema, chronic bronchitis, and, to a lesser degree, asthma. Pneumonia, as well as other respiratory disorders, can further complicate chronic obstructive pulmonary disease in the elderly.

In the Canada, COPD is among the leading causes of death. Its prevalence has been increasing over the past 20 years due to factors such as genetic predisposition, exposure to environmental pollutants, existence of a childhood respiratory disease, and cigarette smoking (a contributing factor in up to 80 percent of all COPD cases).

The physiology of COPD varies but may include inflammation of the air passages with increased mucus production or actual destruction of the alveoli. Usual signs and symptoms include a cough, increased sputum production, dyspnea, accessory muscle use, pursed-lip breathing, tripod positioning, exercise intolerance, wheezing, pleuritic chest pain, and tachypnea.

The most effective prevention involves elimination of tobacco products and reduced exposure to cigarette smoke. Once the disease is present, appropriate self-care measures include exercise, avoidance of infections, appropriate use of medications, avoidance of unnecessary stress, and, when necessary, calling EMS. When confronted with an elderly patient with COPD, treatment is essentially the same as for all age groups: supplemental oxygen and possibly drug therapy, usually for reducing dyspnea.

Pulmonary embolism (PE). Pulmonary embolism should always be considered as a possible cause of respiratory distress in the elderly. Although statistics for the elderly are unavailable, in Canada nearly 11 percent of PE deaths take place in the first hour, and another 38 percent in the second hour.

Blood clots are the most frequent cause of a PE. However, the condition may also be caused by fat, air, bone marrow, tumor cells, or foreign bodies. Risk factors for developing pulmonary embolism include deep venous thrombosis; prolonged immobility (common among the elderly); malignancy (tumors); paralysis; fractures of the pelvis, hip, or leg; obesity; trauma to the leg vessels; major surgery; presence of a venous catheter; use of estrogen (in women); and atrial fibrillation.

Definitive diagnosis of a pulmonary embolism takes place in a hospital setting. However, the condition should be suspected in a patient with the acute onset of dyspnea. Often, it is accompanied by pleuritic chest pain and right heart failure. If the PE is massive, you can expect severe dyspnea, cardiac dysrhythmias, and ultimately cardiovascular collapse.

The goals of field treatment are to manage and minimize complications of the condition. General treatment considerations include delivery of high-flow oxygen via mask, maintaining oxygen levels above an SaO$_2$ of 90 percent. Establishment of an IV for possible administration of medications, upon advice from medical direction, is appropriate. However, vigorous fluid therapy should be avoided, if possible. Rapid transport is essential. Position the patient in an upright position and avoid lifting the patient by the legs or knees, which may dislodge thrombi in the lower extremities. During transport, monitor changes in skin color, pulse oximetry, and breathing rate and rhythm.

b.   Myocardial infarction, heart failure, dysrhythmias, aneurysm, and hypertension pp. 1045-1049

The leading cause of death in the elderly is cardiovascular disease. Assessment and treatment of cardiovascular disease in the elderly patient is often complicated by non-age-related factors and disease processes in other organ systems. Commonly found cardiovascular disorders in the elderly include the following. (Additional disorders, including syncope, can be found in the text.)

Myocardial infarction (MI). Myocardial infarction involves actual death of muscle tissue due to partial or complete occlusion of one or more of the coronary arteries. The greatest number of patients hospitalized for acute MI are older than age 65. The elderly patient with MI is less likely to present with classic symptoms, such as chest pain, than a younger counterpart. Atypical presentations that may be seen in the elderly include the absence of pain, exercise intolerance, confusion/dizziness, syncope, dyspnea (common in patients over age 85), neck or dental pain, epigastric pain, and fatigue/weakness.

The mortality rate associated with myocardial infarction doubles after age 70. Elderly patients are more likely to suffer silent myocardial infarction. They also tend to have larger myocardial infarctions. The majority of the deaths that occur in the first few hours after a myocardial infarction are due to dysrhythmias such as ventricular fibrillation.
Field management is the same as that listed for angina, except that the nitro often does not work and morphine may be necessary if the patient's BP tolerates it. It may also be necessary to manage dysrhythmias and hypotension with medications. These patients need to be quickly evaluated and transported to a facility that can administer clot busters or provide emergency cardiac catheterization and angioplasty, if necessary.

Heart failure. Heart failure takes place when the cardiac output cannot meet the body's metabolic demands. The incidence rises exponentially after age 60 and is the most common diagnosis in hospitalized patients over the age of 65. The causes of heart failure fall in one of four categories— impairment to flow, inadequate cardiac filling, volume overload, and myocardial failure. Factors that place the elderly at risk for heart failure include prolonged myocardial contractions, noncompliance with drug therapy, anemia, ischemia, thermoregulatory disorders, hypoxia, infection, and use of nonsteroidal anti-inflammatory drugs.

Signs and symptoms of heart failure vary. In most patients, regardless of age, some form of edema exists. Assessment findings for the elderly may include musculoskeletal injury, fatigue (left failure), two-pillow orthopnea, dyspnea on exertion, dry hacking cough progressing to a productive cough, dependent edema (right failure), nocturia, anorexia, hepatomegaly (enlarged liver), and ascites.

Nonpharmacologic management of heart failure includes modifications in diet, exercise, and reduction in weight, if necessary. Pharmacologic management may include treatment with diuretics, vasodilators, antihypertensive agents, or inotropic agents. Check to see if the patient is already on any of these medications and if the patient is compliant with scheduled doses.

Dysrhythmias. Many cardiac dysrhythmias develop with age, but atrial fibrillation is the most common dysrhythmia encountered. Dysrhythmias occur primarily as a result of the degeneration of the patient's conductive system. Anything that decreases myocardial blood flow can produce a dysrhythmia. They may also be caused by electrolyte abnormalities.

To complicate matters further, the elderly do not tolerate extremes in heart rate as well as a younger person would. In addition, dysrhythmias can lead to falls due to cerebral hypoperfusion. They can also result in congestive heart failure (CHF) or a transient ischemic attack (TIA). Treatment considerations depend upon the type of dysrhythmia. Patients may already have a pacemaker in place. In such cases, keep in mind that pacemakers have a low but significant rate of complications such as a failed battery, fibrosis around the catheter site, lead fracture, or electrode dislodgment. In a number of situations, drug therapy is indicated. Whenever you discover a dysrhythmia, remember that an abnormal or disordered heart rhythm may be the only clinical finding in an elderly patient suffering acute myocardial infarction.

Aneurysms. An aneurysm, or rupture of the vessel, often results from aortic dissection—a degeneration of the wall of the aorta, either in the thoracic or abdominal cavity. Approximately 80 percent of thoracic aneurysms are due to atherosclerosis combined with hypertension. The remaining cases occur secondary to other factors, including Marfan's syndrome or blunt trauma to the chest. Patients with dissections will often present with tearing chest pain radiating through to the back or, if a rupture/aneurysm occurs, cardiac arrest.

The distal portion of the aorta is the most common site for an abdominal aneurysm. Approximately one in 250 people over age 50 dies from a ruptured abdominal aneurysm. Patients may present with tearing abdominal pain or unexplained low back pain. Pulses in the legs are diminished or absent and the lower extremities feel cold to the touch. There may be sensory abnormalities such as numbness, tingling, or pain in the legs. The patient may fall when attempting to stand.

Treatment of the aneurysm depends upon the size, location, and severity of the condition. In the case of thoracic aortic dissection, continuous IV infusion and/or administration of drug therapy to lower the arterial pressure and to diminish the velocity of left ventricle contraction may be indicated. Rapid transport is essential, especially for the older patient who most commonly requires care and observation in an intensive care unit.

Hypertension. Because hypertension is not widely seen in less developed nations, experts believe that the condition is not a normal age-related change. Today more than 50 percent of Canadians over age 65 have clinically diagnosed hypertension—defined as blood pressure greater than 140/90 mmHg. Prolonged elevated blood pressure will eventually damage the heart, brain, or kidneys. As a result of hypertension, elderly patients are at a greater risk for heart failure, stroke, blindness, renal failure, coronary heart disease, and peripheral vascular disease. In men with blood pressure greater than 160/95 mmHg, the risk of mortality nearly doubles.

Hypertension increases with atherosclerosis, which is more common in the elderly than other age groups. Other contributing factors include obesity and diabetes. The condition is often a "silent" disease because it produces no clinically obvious signs or symptoms. It may be associated with nonspecific complaints such as headache, tinnitus, epistaxis (nosebleed), slow tremors, and nausea or vomiting.

Hypertension can be prevented or controlled through diet, exercise, cessation of smoking, and compliance with medications. Management of the condition depends upon its severity and the existence of other conditions. For example, hypertension is often treated with beta-blockers—medications that are contraindicated in patients with chronic obstructive lung disease, asthma, or heart block greater than first degree. Diuretics, another common drug used for treating hypertension, should be prescribed with care for patients on digitalis. Keep in mind that centrally acting agents are more likely to produce negative side effects in the elderly. Unlike younger patients, the elderly may experience depression, forgetfulness, sleep problems, or vivid dreams and/or hallucinations.

c. Cerebral vascular disease, delirium, dementia, Alzheimer's disease, and Parkinson's disease pp. 1049-1054

Cerebral vascular disease (CVA). Cerebral vascular disease (stroke/brain attack) is the forth leading cause of death in Canada. Annually, about 40 0000-50 000 people suffer strokes in Canada. Incidence of stroke and the likelihood of dying from a stroke increases with age. Occlusive stroke is statistically more common in the elderly and relatively uncommon in younger individuals. Older patients are at higher risk of stroke because of atherosclerosis, hypertension, immobility, limb paralysis, congestive heart failure, and atrial fibrillation. Transient ischemic attacks (TIAs) are also more common in older patients, more than one-third of whom will develop a major, permanent stroke.

Strokes fall into one of two categories. Brain ischemia—injury to brain tissue caused by an inadequate supply of oxygen and nutrients—accounts for about 80 percent of all strokes. Brain hemorrhage, the second major category, may be either subarachnoid hemorrhage or intracerebral hemorrhage. Because of the various kinds of strokes, signs and symptoms can present in many ways—altered mental status, coma, paralysis, slurred speech, a change in mood, and seizures. Stroke should be highly suspected in any elderly patient with a sudden change in mental status. Keep two things in mind when treating stroke. One, complete the Glasgow Coma Scale for later comparison at the ED. Second, transport the patient as rapidly as possible. In the case of stroke, "time is brain tissue." By far the most preferred treatment is prevention. Preventive strategies include control of hypertension, treatment of cardiac disorders, treatment of blood disorders, cessation of smoking, cessation of recreational drugs, moderate use of alcohol, regular exercise, and good eating habits.

Delirium, dementia and Alzheimer's disease. Approximately 12 percent of all Canadians over the age of 65 have some degree of dementia or delirium. Dementia is chronic global mental impairment, often progressive or irreversible. The best-known form of dementia is Alzheimer's disease, a condition that affects thousands of Canadians. Delirium is a global mental impairment of sudden onset and self-limited duration.

Possible causes of delirium include subdural hematoma, tumors and other mass lesions, drug-induced changes or alcohol intoxication, CNS infections, electrolyte abnormalities, cardiac failure, fever, metabolic disorders (including hypoglycemia), chronic endocrine abnormalities (including hypothyroidism and hyperthyroidism), and post-concussion syndrome. Common signs and symptoms include acute onset of anxiety, an inability to focus, disordered thinking, irritability, inappropriate behavior, fearfulness, excessive energy, or psychotic behavior such as hallucinations or paranoia. Aphasic or speaking errors and/or prominent slurring may be present.

Dementia is more prevalent in the elderly than delirium. Over 50 percent of all nursing home patients have dementia. The mental deterioration is often called "organic brain syndrome," "senile dementia," or "senility." Causes of dementia include small strokes, atherosclerosis, age-related neurological changes, neurological diseases, certain hereditary diseases, and Alzheimer's disease. Signs and symptoms include progressive disorientation, shortened attention span, aphasia or nonsense talking, and hallucinations.

Alzheimer's disease, a particular type of dementia, is a chronic degenerative disorder that attacks the brain and results in impaired memory, thinking, and behavior. It goes through stages, each with different signs and symptoms, the culmination of which is death.

Parkinson's disease. Parkinson's disease is a degenerative disorder involving changes in muscle response, including tremors, loss of facial expressions, and gait disturbances. It usually appears in people over the age of 50 and peaks at age 70. The disease affects 100 000 Canadians each year. The causes include viral encephalitis, atherosclerosis of cerebral vessels, reaction to certain drugs or toxins (antipsychotics or carbon monoxide), metabolic disorders (anoxia), tumors, head trauma, and degenerative disorders (Shy-Drager syndrome).

There is no known cure for Parkinson's disease. In calls involving a Parkinson's patient, observe for conditions that may have involved the EMS system, such as a fall or the inability to move. Manage treatable conditions and transport as needed.

d.   Diabetes and thyroid diseases   pp. 1054-1055

Diabetes. An estimated 20 percent of older adults have diabetes mellitus, primarily Type II diabetes. Almost 40 percent have some type of glucose intolerance. Reasons the elderly develop this disorder include poor diet, decreased physical activity, loss of lean body mass, impaired insulin production, and resistance by body cells to the actions of insulin. The condition may present, in the early stages, with such vague constitutional symptoms as fatigue or weakness. Allowed to progress, diabetes can result in neuropathy and visual impairment.

Elderly patients on insulin risk hypoglycemia, especially if they accidentally take too much insulin or do not eat enough food following injection. The lack of good nutrition can be particularly troublesome to elderly diabetic patients. They often find it difficult to prepare meals, fail to enjoy food because of diminished taste, have trouble chewing food, or are unable to purchase adequate and/or enough food because of limited income.

Many diabetics use self-monitoring devices to monitor their glucose levels. Self-treatment involves diet, exercise, and the use of sulfonylurea agents and/or insulin. In EMS calls involving diabetic or hypoglycemic elderly patients, follow care steps similar to those taken with younger patients. However, remember that diabetes places the elderly at increased risk of other complications, including atherosclerosis, delayed healing, retinopathy (disorders of the retina), altered renal function, and severe peripheral vascular disease, leading to foot ulcers and even amputations. In the case of hypoglycemia, DO NOT rule out alcohol as a complicating factor.

Thyroid diseases. With normal aging, the thyroid gland undergoes moderate atrophy and changes in hormone production. An estimated 2 to 5 percent of the people over 65 experience hypothyroidism, a condition resulting from inadequate levels of thyroid hormones. It affects women in greater numbers than men, and the prevalence rises with age.

Less than 33 percent of the elderly present with typical signs and symptoms of hypothyroidism. When they do, their complaints are often attributed to aging. Common nonspecific complaints in the elderly include mental confusion, anorexia, falls, incontinence, decreased mobility, and muscle or joint pain. Treatment involves thyroid hormone replacement. Hyperthyroidism is less common among the elderly but may result from medication errors such as an overdose of thyroid hormone replacement. The typical symptom of heat intolerance is often present. Otherwise, hyperthyroidism presents atypically in the elderly with nonspecific features or complaints such as atrial fibrillation, failure to thrive (weight loss and apathy combined), abdominal distress, diarrhea, exhaustion, and depression.

Diagnosis and treatment of thyroid disorders does not take place in the field. Elderly patients with known thyroid problems should be encouraged to go to the hospital for medical evaluation.

e.   Gastrointestinal problems, GI hemorrhage, and bowel obstruction pp. 1055-1057

Gastrointestinal problems. Gastrointestinal emergencies are common among the elderly. The most frequent emergency is GI bleeding. However, older people will also describe a variety of other gastrointestinal complaints—nausea, poor appetite, diarrhea, and constipation, to name a few. Remember that like other presenting complaints in the elderly, these conditions may be symptomatic of a more serious disease.

Prompt management of a GI emergency is essential for old and young alike. However, keep in mind that older patients are more intolerant of hypotension and anoxia than younger patients. The elderly also face a significant risk of hemorrhage and shock. Treatment of GI emergencies in the elderly includes airway management, support of breathing and circulation, high-flow oxygen therapy, IV fluid replacement with a crystalloid solution, PASG placement (if indicated), and, above all else, rapid transport.

GI hemorrhage. Gastrointestinal hemorrhage falls into two general categories: upper GI bleed and lower GI bleed. Upper GI bleeds include peptic ulcer disease, gastritis, esophageal varices, and Mallory-Weiss tears. Lower GI bleeds include diverticulosis, tumors, ischemic colitis, and arterio-venous malformations.

Signs of significant gastrointestinal blood loss include the presence of "coffee ground" emesis, black tar-like stools (melena), obvious blood in the emesis or stool, orthostatic hypotension, pulse greater than 100 (unless on beta blockers), and confusion. GI bleeding in the elderly is a true emergency and requires prompt transport to an appropriate medical facility.

Bowel obstruction. Bowel obstructions in the elderly typically involve the small bowel and may be caused by tumors, prior abdominal surgery, use of certain medications, and occasionally the presence of vertebral compression fractures. The patient will typically complain of diffuse abdominal pain, bloating, nausea, and vomiting. The abdomen may feel distended when palpated. Bowel sounds may be hypoactive or absent. If the obstruction has been present for a prolonged period, the patient may have fever, weakness, various electrolyte imbalances, and shock.

An even more serious condition arises with mesenteric infarct, which occurs when a portion of the bowel does not receive enough blood to survive. Certain age-related changes—atrial fibrillation or atherosclerosis—predispose the elderly to a clot lodging in one of the mesenteric arteries serving the bowel. In addition, age-related changes in the bowel itself can promote swelling that effectively cuts off blood flow. Primary signs and symptoms include pain out of proportion to the physical exam, bloody diarrhea, some tachycardia, and abdominal distention. A mesenteric infarct, or dead bowel, attracts interstitial and intravascular fluids, thus removing them from use and increasing the likelihood of shock. Necrotic products are released to the peritoneal cavity, leading to massive infection. The prognosis is poor, due, in part, to decreased physiologic reserves on the part of older patients.

f.   Skin diseases and pressure ulcers   pp. 1057-1058

Skin diseases. Age-related changes in the immune system make the elderly more prone to certain chronic skin diseases and infections. Elderly patients commonly complain about pruritus or itching. This condition can be caused by dermatitis or environmental conditions. Keep in mind that generalized itching can also be a sign of systemic diseases, particularly liver or renal disorders.

Slower healing and compromised tissue perfusion in the elderly make them more susceptible to bacterial infection of wounds, appearing as cellutitis, impetigo, and, in the case of immunocompromised adults, staphylococcal scalded skin. The elderly also experience a higher incidence of fungal infections and suffer higher rates of herpes zoster (shingles), which peaks between ages 50 and 70.

In treating skin disorders, remember that many conditions may be drug induced. For example, antihistamines and corticosteroids are two to three times more likely to provoke adverse reactions in the elderly than in younger adults. In most cases, encourage the patient to seek a medical evaluation to rule out drug complications or an underlying disease.

Pressure ulcers. Most pressure ulcers (bedsores) occur in people over age 70. Pressure ulcers typically develop from the waist down, usually over bony prominences, in bedridden patients. They most commonly result from tissue hypoxia and affect the skin, subcutaneous tissues, and muscle. Factors that can increase the risk of this condition include external compression of tissues, altered sensory perception, maceration (caused by excessive moisture), decreased activity or mobility, poor nutrition, and friction or shear.

To reduce the development of pressure ulcers or to alleviate their condition, assist the patient in changing position frequently, especially during extended transport. Use a pull sheet to move the patient, reducing the likelihood of tearing. Reduce the possibility of shearing by padding areas of skin prone to movement. Unless a life-threatening condition exists, take time to clean and dry areas of excessive moisture. Clean ulcers with normal saline solution and cover with hydrocolloid or hydrogel dressings, if available. With severe ulcers, pack with loosely woven gauze moistened with normal saline.

g.   Osteoarthritis and osteoporosis   p. 1058

Osteoarthritis. Osteoarthritis is the leading cause of disability among people age 65 and older. Contributing factors to this disease include age-related wear and tear, loss of muscle mass, obesity, primary disorders of the joint (such as inflammatory arthritis), trauma, and congenital abnormalities (such as hip dysplasia).

Osteoarthritis initially presents as joint pain. As the disease progresses, pain may be accompanied by diminished mobility, joint deformity, and crepitus (grating sensations), and ultimately tenderness during passive motion or upon palpation. Prevention strategies include stretching exercises and activities that strengthen stress-absorbing tendons. Immobilization, even for short periods, can accelerate the condition. Surgery—i.e., total joint replacement—is the last resort.

Osteoporosis. Osteoporosis affects an estimated 1.4 million Canadians and is largely responsible for fractures of the hip, wrist, and vertebral bones following a fall or other injury. Risk factors include:

• *Age.* Bone mass usually starts to decline after the third decade of life, and decreased bone density generally becomes a treatment consideration at about age 50.

• *Gender.* Women are more than twice as likely as men to develop the disease, especially if they experience early menopause (before age 45) and do not take estrogen replacement therapy.

• *Race.* Whites and Asians are more likely to develop osteoporosis than African Americans and Latinos, who have higher bone mass at skeletal peak.

• *Body weight.* Increased skeletal weight is thought to promote bone density, putting thin people at greater risk of developing the disease than obese people. However, weight-bearing exercise can have the same effect.

• *Family history.* Genetic factors—i.e., peak mass attainment—may affect the occurrence of the disease.

• *Miscellaneous.* Late menarche, nulliparity, and use of caffeine, alcohol, and cigarettes are all thought to be important determinants of bone mass.

Unless a bone density test has been conducted, people are usually asymptotic until a fracture occurs. Management includes prevention of fractures through exercise and drug therapy, such as administration of calcium, vitamin D, estrogen, and other medications or minerals.

h.   Hypothermia and hyperthermia   pp. 1061-1062

Hypothermia. Thermoregulatory emergencies represent some of the most common EMS calls involving the elderly. As a group, the elderly are vulnerable to low temperatures, suffering many winter deaths annually, primarily from hypothermia and "winter risks" such as pneumonia and influenza. Factors that predispose the elderly to hypothermia include accidental exposure to cold, CNS disorders, head trauma, stroke, endocrine disorders (particularly hypoglycemia and diabetes), drugs that interfere with heat production, malnutrition or starvation, chronic illness, forced inactivity as a result of a medical condition, low or fixed income (which discourages use of home heating), inflammatory dermatitis, and A-V shunts.

Hypothermic patients may exhibit slow speech, cold skin, confusion, and sleepiness. In early stages, vitals may reveal hypertension and an increased heart rate. As hypothermia progresses, however, blood pressure drops and the heart rate slows, sometimes to a barely detectable level. Keep in mind that the elderly patient with hypothermia often does not shiver. Check the abdomen and back to see if the skin is cool to the touch or, if your unit has a low-temperature thermometer, check the patient's core temperature.

Treatment is focused on rewarming the patient and rapid transport. Once the elderly develop hypothermia, they become progressively impaired, with their condition worsening other chronic medical problems. Remain alert for complications, most commonly cardiac arrest or ventricular fibrillation.

Hyperthermia. Age-related changes in the sweat glands and increased incidence of heart disease place the elderly at risk of heat stress. They may develop heat cramps, heat exhaustion, or heat stroke. Risk factors for severe hyperthermia include altered sensory output, inadequate liquid intake, decreased functioning of the thermoregulatory center, commonly prescribed medications that inhibit sweating (such as antihistamines and tricyclic antidepressants), low or fixed incomes (which may result in a lack of fans or air conditioning), alcoholism, concomitant medical disorders, and use of diuretics (which increase fluid loss).

Early heatstroke may present with nonspecific signs and symptoms such as nausea, light-headedness, dizziness, headache, and high fever. Prevention strategies include adequate fluid intake, reduced activity, shelter in an air conditioned environment, and use of light clothing. If hyperthermia develops, however, rapid treatment and transport are necessary.

i. **Toxicological problems, including drug toxicity, substance abuse, alcohol abuse, and drug abuse   pp. 1062-1066**

Toxicological problems. Aging alters pharmacokinetics and pharmacodynamics in the elderly. Functional changes in the kidneys, liver, and GI system slow the absorption and elimination of many medications. In addition, the various compensatory mechanisms that help buffer against medication side effects are less effective in the elderly than in younger patients.

Approximately 30 percent of all hospital admissions are related to drug-induced illnesses. About 50 percent of all drug-related deaths occur in people over age 60. Accidental overdoses may occur more frequently in the aged due to confusion, vision impairment, self-selection of medications, forgetfulness, and concurrent drug use. Intentional drug overdose also occurs in attempts at self-destruction. Another complicating factor is the abuse of alcohol in the elderly.

In assessing the elderly patient, always take these steps:

• Obtain a full list of medications currently taken by the patient.
• Elicit any medications that are newly prescribed.
• Obtain a good past medical history, including prior renal or hepatic depression.
• Know your medications, their routes of elimination, and their potential side effects.
• If possible, always take all medications to the hospital along with the patient.

Some of the drugs or substances that have been identified as commonly causing toxicity in the elderly include:
• *Lidocaine.* Lidocaine is recommended for the treatment of ventricular dysrhythmias in the acute setting, especially in acute myocardial infarction and in dysrhythmias that arise from cardiac surgery or catheterization. Patients with liver or kidney problems will have problems metabolizing this drug. Lidocaine toxicity is characterized by vision disturbances, GI effects, tinnitus, trembling, breathing difficulties, dizziness or syncope, seizures, and bradycardiac dysrhythmias. Since the cardiac antidysrhythmics in general can cause a decrease in cardiac function and output, observe for shortness of breath, lightheadedness, loss of consciousness, fatigue, chest discomfort, and palpitations.
• *Beta-blockers.* Beta-blockers are widely used to treat hypertension, angina pectoris, and cardiac dysrhythmias. Elderly patients, however, are susceptible to CNS side effects such as depression, lethargy, and sleep disorders. Because geriatric patients often have pre-existing cardiovascular problems that can cause decreased cardiac function and output, beta-blockers will limit the heart's ability to respond to postural changes, causing orthostatic hypotension. Beta-blockers also limit the heart's ability to increase contractile force and cardiac output whenever a sympathetic response is necessary in situations such as exercise or hypovolemia. This can be detrimental to the trauma patient who is hemorrhaging and cannot mount the sympathetic response necessary to maintain perfusion of vital organs.

Treatment of beta-blocker overdoses includes general supportive measures, the removal of gastric contents, support of the ABCs, fluids, and administration of nonadrenergic inotropic agents such as glucagons for hypotension. Excessive bradycardia can be countered with atropine.
• *Antihypertensives/diuretics.* These medications act on the kidneys to increase urine flow and the excretion of water and sodium. They are used primarily in the treatment of hypertension and congestive heart failure. Of these drugs, furosemide is the most widely used diuretic in the elderly. The elimination half-life of furosemide is markedly prolonged in the patient with acute pulmonary edema and renal and hepatic failure. As a result, the geriatric patient is at risk for a drug buildup. Excessive urination caused by the drug may put the elderly at risk for postural hypotension, circulatory collapse, potassium depletion, and renal function impairment. To reduce this risk, a smaller dose is often prescribed and the patient usually takes a daily potassium supplement.
• *Angiotensin-converting enzyme (ACE) inhibitors.* ACE inhibitors are used for the management of hypertension and congestive heart failure. Geriatric patients generally respond well to treatment with ACE inhibitors. However, these drugs can cause chronic hypotension in patients with severe

heart failure who are also taking high-dose loop diuretics. ACE inhibitors can also cause plasma volume reduction and hypotension with prolonged vomiting and diarrhea in the elderly patient. Some hemodialysis patients can experience anaphylactic reactions if treated with ACE inhibitors. Other side effects of ACE inhibitors include dizziness or lightheadedness upon standing, presence of a rash, muscle cramps, swelling of the hands, face, or eyes, cough, headache, stomach upset, and fatigue.

• *Digitalis (digoxin, lanoxin).* Digoxin is the most widely used cardiac glycoside for the management of congestive heart failure, atrial fibrillation, atrial flutter, paroxysmal atrial tachycardia, and cardiogenic shock. The drug is unique in that it has a positive inotropic effect and a negative chronotropic effect. Because digoxin has a low margin of safety and a narrow therapeutic index, the amount of drug required to produce a desired effect is very close to the toxic range. Digoxin toxicity in the elderly can result from accidental or intentional ingestion. In the renally impaired elderly patient, any change in kidney function usually warrants an alteration in the dosing of digoxin. Diuretics, which are often given to patients with congestive heart failure, cause the loss of large amounts of potassium in the urine. If potassium is not adequately replenished in the patient taking digoxin, toxicity will develop.

Signs and symptoms of digoxin toxicity include visual disturbances, fatigue, weakness, nausea, loss of appetite, abdominal discomfort, dizziness, abnormal dreams, headache, and vomiting. Low potassium (hypokalemia) is also common with chronic digoxin toxicity due to concurrent diuretic therapy. Dysrhythmias commonly associated with digoxin toxicity include sinoatrial (SA) exit block, SA arrest, second- or third-degree AV block, atrial fibrillation with a slow ventricular response, accelerated AV junctional rhythms, patterns of premature ventricular contractions, ventricular tachycardia, and atrial tachycardia with AV block.

The management of digoxin toxicity includes gastric lavage with activated charcoal, correction of confirmed hypokalemia with K+ supplements, treatment of bradycardias with atropine or pacing, and the treatment of rapid ventricular rhythms with lidocaine. Digoxin-specific FAB fragment antibodies (Digibind), an antidote for digoxin toxicity, is used in the treatment of potentially life-threatening situations.

• *Antipsychotics/antidepressants.* Psychotropic medications comprise a variety of agents that affect mood, behavior, and other aspects of mental function. The elderly often experience a high incidence of psychiatric disorders and may take any number of medications, including antidepressants, anti-anxiety agents, sedative-hypnotic agents, and antipsychotics.

Antidepressant use in the elderly may result in side effects such as sedation, lethargy, and muscle weakness. Some antidepressants tend to produce anticholinergic effects, including dry mouth, constipation, urinary retention, and confusion. Newly prescribed tricyclic antidepressants can also cause orthostatic hypotension, which can be compounded if the geriatric patient is taking diuretics or other antihypertensive medications. Side effects such as sedation and confusion may also impair the patient's cognitive abilities and possibly endanger the elderly patient who lives alone.

Antipsychotic medications produce a number of minor side effects such as sedation and anticholinergic effects. Extrapyramidal side effects can also occur, including restlessness and involuntary muscle movements, particularly in the face, jaw, and extremities.

Field treatment for overdose of antipsychotics and antidepressants is aimed primarily at the ABCs, with special emphasis on airway management.

• *Medications for Parkinson's disease.* Drug treatment for Parkinson's disease is aimed at restoring the balance of neurotransmitters in the basal ganglia. Toxicity of Parkinson's drugs commonly presents as dyskinesia (the inability to execute voluntary movements) and psychological disturbances such as visual hallucinations and nightmares. When these medications are first taken, orthostatic hypotension may also occur. The goal of field management is aimed at decreasing the patient's anxiety and providing a supportive environment. Remember that patients with gross involuntary motor movements are at risk for aspiration and choking.

• *Anti-seizure medications.* Seizure disorders are not uncommon in the elderly, and the selection of anti-seizure medication depends upon the type of seizure present in the patient. The most common side effect of anti-seizure medications is sedation. Other side effects include GI distress, headache, dizziness, lack of coordination, and dermatological reactions (rashes). Recommended treatment involves airway management and supportive therapy.

• *Analgesics and anti-inflammatory agents.* Treatment of pain and inflammation for chronic conditions such as rheumatoid arthritis and osteoarthritis includes narcotics and non-narcotic analgesics and corticosteroids. Adverse side effects of these drugs include sedation, mood changes, nausea, vomiting, and constipation. Orthostatic hypotension and respiratory depression may also occur. Over long periods of time, patients may develop drug tolerance and physical dependence on narcotic agents. In the case of corticosteroids, side effects may include hypertension, peptic ulcer, aggravation of diabetes mellitus, glaucoma, increased risk of infection, and suppression of normally produced corticosteroids.

Substance abuse, drug abuse, alcohol abuse. In general, the factors that contribute to substance abuse among the elderly are different than those of younger people. They include age-related changes, loss of employment, loss of spouse or partner, malnutrition, loneliness, moving from a long-loved home, and multiple prescriptions.

The elderly who become physically and/or psychologically dependent upon drugs or alcohol are more likely to hide their dependence and less likely to seek help than other age groups. Common signs and symptoms of drug abuse include memory changes, drowsiness, decreased vision/hearing, orthostatic hypotension, poor dexterity, mood changes, falling, restlessness, and weight loss. Pertinent findings for alcohol abuse include mood swings, denial and hostility (when questioned about alcohol), confusion, history of falls, anorexia, insomnia, visible anxiety, and nausea.

Treatment follows many of the same steps as for any other patient with a pattern of substance abuse. DO NOT judge the patient. Manage the ABCs and evaluate the need for fluid therapy or medications to accommodate withdrawal. Transport the patient to the hospital for further evaluation and referral.

j.   Psychological disorders, including depression and suicide   pp. 1066-1068

Psychological disorders. When behavioral or psychological problems develop later in life, they are often dismissed as normal age-related changes. This attitude denies an elderly person the opportunity to correct a treatable condition and may overlook an underlying physical disorder. It is important to keep in mind the emotionally stressful situations facing many elderly people— isolation, loneliness, loss of self-dependence, loss of strength, and fear of the future. The elderly also face a higher incidence of secondary depression as a result of neuroleptic medications such as Haldol and Thorazine. Some of the common classifications of psychological disorders related to age include organic brain syndrome, affective disorders, neurotic disorders, and paranoid disorders.

Depression and suicide. Up to 15 percent of the non-institutionalized elderly experience depression. Within institutions, that figures rises to about 30 percent. In general, depressed patients should receive supportive care, with caregivers delicately raising questions about suicidal thoughts

In cases of seriously depressed patients, elicit behavior patterns from family, friends, or caregivers. Warning signs may include curtailing activities and self-care, breaking from medical or exercise regimens, grieving a personal loss, expressing feelings of uselessness, putting affairs in order, and stock-piling medications. Be particularly alert to suicide among the acutely ill, especially those in a home-care setting.
Your first priorities in the management of a suicidal elderly patient are to protect yourself and then to protect the patient from self-harm. Conduct a brief interview with the patient, if possible, to determine the need for further action. DO NOT leave the suicidal patient alone. Administer medications with caution, keeping in mind polypharmacy and drug interactions in the elderly. (Consult with medical direction.) *All suicidal elderly patients should be transported to the hospital.*

18. **Describe the incidence, morbidity/mortality, risk factors, prevention strategies, pathophysiology, assessment, need for intervention and transport, and management of the elderly trauma patient with:**

a.   Orthopedic injuries   pp. 1071-1072

The elderly suffer the greatest mortality and greatest incidence of disability from falls. Approximately 33 percent of the falls in the elderly result in at least one fractured bone. The most common fall-related fracture is a fracture of the hip or pelvis. Falls also result in a variety of stress fractures in the elderly, including fractures of the proximal humerus, distal radius, proximal tibia, and thoracic and lumbar bodies. In treating orthopedic injuries, remember to ask questions aimed at detecting an underlying medical condition.

b.   Burns   pp. 1072-1073

People age 60 and older are more likely to suffer death from burns than any other age group except neonates and infants. Factors that help explain the high mortality rate among the elderly include age-related changes that slow reaction time, pre-existing diseases that increase the risk of medical complications, age-related skin changes (thinning) that increase the severity of burns, immunological and metabolic changes that increase the risk of infection, and reductions in physiologic function and the reduced reserves of several organ systems that make the elderly more vulnerable to systemic stress.

Management of the elderly burn patient follows the same general procedures as other patients. However, remember that the elderly are at increased risk of shock. Administration of fluids is important to prevent renal tubular damage. Assess hydration in the initial hours after the burn injury by blood pressure, pulse, and urine output. Keep in mind that complications in the elderly may manifest themselves in the days and weeks following the incident. For serious burns to heal, the body may use up to 20,000 calories a day. Elderly patients, with altered metabolisms and complications such as diabetes, may not be able to meet this demand, increasing the chances for infection and systemic failure. Part of your job may be to prepare the family for such a delayed response.

c.   Head injuries   p. 1073

As people age, the brain decreases in size and weight. The skull, however, remains constant in size, allowing the brain more room to move, thus increasing the likelihood of brain injury. Because of this, the signs and symptoms of brain injury may develop more slowly in the elderly patient, sometimes over days or weeks. In fact, the patient may often have forgotten the offending incident.

The cervical spine is also more susceptible to injury due to osteoporosis and spondylosis—a degeneration of the vertebral body. In addition, arthritic changes can gradually compress the nerve rootlets or spinal cord. Thus, injury to the spine in the elderly makes them much more susceptible to spinal cord injury. Therefore, it is important to provide older patients with suspected spinal-cord injury, especially those involved in motor vehicle collisions, with immediate manual cervical stabilization at the time of initial assessment.

19. Given several pre-programmed simulated geriatric patients with various complaints, provide the appropriate assessment, management, and transport.   pp. 1023-1073

During your classroom, clinical, and field training, you will assess real and simulated geriatric patients and develop a management plan for them. Use the information presented in this text chapter, the information on assessment of geriatric patients in the field presented by your instructors, and the guidance given by your clinical and field preceptors to develop good patient assessment skills. Continue to refine these skills once your training ends and you begin your career as a paramedic.

CONTENT SELF-EVALUATION

Multiple Choice

1. All of the following are responsible for the growing number of elderly people in the Canada—and the projected increase in the number of elderly patients treated by EMS services—EXCEPT a(n):
   A. increase in the mean survival rate of older persons.
   B. increase in the birth rate.
   C. absence of major wars.
   D. improved health care.
   E. higher standard of living.

2. The scientific study of the effects of aging and of age-related diseases on humans is known as:
   A. geriatrics.
   B. ageism.
   C. gerontology.
   D. eldercare.
   E. gerontotherapeutics.

3. The existence of multiple diseases in the elderly is known as:
   A. functional impairment.
   B. dysphagia.
   C. comorbidity.
   D. polypharmacy.
   E. senility.

4. Common complaints in the elderly include:
   A. falls, weakness, syncope.
   B. fractures, drowning, diabetes.
   C. GSW, croup, nausea.
   D. MVC, meningitis, poisoning.
   E. fever, epiglottitis, febrile seizures.

5. Drugs concentrate more readily in the plasma and tissues of elderly patients because of:
   A. diminished neurologic function.
   B. increased body fluid.
   C. atrophy of organs.
   D. more efficient compensatory mechanisms.
   E. increased renal function.

6. Factors that can decrease medication compliance in the elderly include all of the following EXCEPT:
   A. limited mobility.
   B. fear of toxicity.
   C. child-proof containers.
   D. multiple-compartment pill boxes.
   E. sensory impairment.

7. Factors that can increase medication compliance in the elderly include:
   A. compliance counseling.
   B. a belief that an illness is serious.
   C. clear, simple directions.
   D. blister-pack packaging.
   E. all of the above

8. Which of the following is the leading cause of accidental deaths among the elderly?
   A. drownings
   B. fall-related injuries
   C. motor vehicle collisions
   D. gunshot wounds
   E. poisonings

9. Intrinsic factors that can cause an elderly person to fall include all of the following EXCEPT:
   A. dizziness.
   B. slippery floors.
   C. decreased mental status.
   D. impaired vision.
   E. CNS problems.

10. Extrinsic factors that can cause an elderly person to fall include:

    A.   an altered gait.
    B.   a sense of weakness.
    C.   a lack of hand rails.
    D.   use of certain medications.
    E.   a history of repeated falls.

11. The inability to retain urine or feces because of loss of sphincter control or because of cerebral or spinal lesions is called:

    A.   diarrhea.
    B.   involuntary elimination.
    C.   diuresis.
    D.   incontinence.
    E.   uremia.

12. Possible causes of elimination problems in the elderly include:

    A.   diverticular disease.
    B.   constipation.
    C.   colorectal cancer.
    D.   use of opioids.
    E.   all of the above

13. One of the most common reasons that elderly patients underestimate the severity of a primary medical problem is that they have a(n):

    A.   shrinkage of structures in the ear.
    B.   clouding and thickening of lenses in the eyes.
    C.   lowered sensitivity to pain.
    D.   deterioration of the teeth and gums.
    E.   altered sense of taste.

14. All of the following factors play a part in forming a general assessment of the elderly patient EXCEPT:

    A.   average cost of rent.
    B.   medication history.
    C.   living situations.
    D.   sleep patterns.
    E.   level of nutrition.

15. Conditions that may discourage eating among the elderly include:

    A.   breathing or respiratory problems.
    B.   nausea or vomiting.
    C.   poor dental care.
    D.   alcohol or drug abuse.
    E.   all of the above

16. Which of the following is a byproduct of malnutrition?

    A.   electrolyte abnormalities
    B.   dehydration
    C.   vitamin deficiencies
    D.   hypoglycemia
    E.   all of the above

17. A medical condition in which eye pressure increases and ultimately diminishes sight is known as:

    A.   Meniere's disease.
    B.   tinnitus.
    C.   cataracts.
    D.   glaucoma.
    E.   retinitis.

18. A disease of the inner ear characterized by vertigo, nerve deafness, and a roar or buzzing in the ear is called:

    A.   Meniere's disease.
    B.   tinnitus.
    C.   cataracts.
    D.   glaucoma.
    E.   cerumen.

19. To improve communication with an elderly patient, you should try to:

    A.   display verbal and nonverbal signs of concern.
    B.   dim the room lights.
    C.   avoid looking directly into the patient's eyes.
    D.   first talk to family members, then the patient.
    E.   remain as quiet as possible.

20. Both senility and organic brain syndrome may manifest themselves as:

    A.   distractibility.   **D.**   restlessness.

    B.   excitability.   **E.**   all of the above

    C.   hostility.

21. Changes in mental status in the elderly patient may be due to which of the following?

    A.   traumatic head injury   **D.**   infection

    B.   dementia   **E.**   all of the above

    C.   decreased sugar level

22. To help reduce an elderly patient's fears, you should:

    A.   downplay the patient's fears.

    B.   ignore nonverbal messages.

    C.   discourage the expression of feelings.

    D.   confirm what the patient has said.

    E.   instruct the patient to calm down.

23. Compared to younger people, the skin of elderly people:

    A.   is thicker and oilier.   **D.**   is less subject to fungal infections.

    B.   heals more quickly.   **E.**   perspires less.

    C.   tears less easily.

24. Age-related changes to the respiratory system include all of the following EXCEPT:

    A.   increased chest wall compliance.   **D.**   increased air trapping.

    B.   diminished breathing capacity.   **E.**   reduced gag reflex.

    C.   reduced strength and endurance.

25. The decrease of an effective cough reflex and the activity of the _____ make the elderly more prone to respiratory infection.

    A.   gag reflex   **D.**   bronchioles

    B.   alveoli   **E.**   vagal response

    C.   cilia

26. An exaggeration of the normal posterior curvature of the spine is called:

    A.   scoliosis.   **D.**   hypertrophy.

    B.   kyphosis.   **E.**   spondylosis.

    C.   fibrosis.

27. An increase in the size and bulk of the left ventricle wall in some elderly patients is an example of:

    A.   kyphosis.   **D.**   fibrosis.

    B.   anoxia hypoxemia.   **E.**   Marfan's syndrome.

    C.   hypertrophy.

28. In managing elderly patients with complaints related to the cardiovascular system, take all of the following steps EXCEPT:

    A.   inquire about age-related dosages.

    B.   provide high-concentration supplemental oxygen.

    C.   walk the patient slowly to the rig.

    D.   remain empathetic to the patient's fears.

    E.   start an IV for medication administration.

29. All of the following are age-related changes to the nervous system EXCEPT:

    A.   decreased reaction time.   **D.**   shrinkage of brain tissue.

    B.   increased brain weight.   **E.**   recent memory loss.

    C.   impaired balance.

30. Age-related changes in the gastrointestinal system include all of the following EXCEPT:

    A.   impaired swallowing.   **D.**   a predisposition to choking.

    B.   diminished digestive functions.   **E.**   increased gastric secretions.

    C.   decreased liver efficiency.

31. A protrusion of the stomach upward into the mediastinal cavity through the diaphragm is known as:
  A.   a hiatal hernia.
  B.   Marfan's syndrome.
  C.   a diaphragmatic hernia.
  D.   an inguinal hernia.
  E.   an epigastric hernia.

32. Reasons that the elderly develop pneumonia more frequently than younger people include all of the following EXCEPT a(n):
  A.   decreased immune response.
  B.   increased pulmonary function.
  C.   abnormal or ineffective cough reflex.
  D.   decreased activity of mucociliary cells.
  E.   decreased colonization of the pharynx by gram-negative bacteria.

33. The usual signs and symptoms of COPD include:
  A.   cough and wheezing.
  B.   dyspnea and tachypnea.
  C.   exercise intolerance.
  D.   pleuritic chest pain.
  E.   all of the above

34. The most effective prevention of COPD involves:
  A.   elimination of smoking.
  B.   lowering blood sugar.
  C.   reducing physical activity.
  D.   lowering blood pressure.
  E.   use of supplemental oxygen.

35. Your elderly patient is complaining of acute onset of sharp chest pain and shortness of breath. The patient was recently released from the hospital for a leg fracture. What is the most likely suspected disorder?
  A.   pneumonia
  B.   pulmonary embolism
  C.   heart attack
  D.   COPD
  E.   pulmonary edema

36. Although all of the following can contribute to a pulmonary embolism, the condition is most frequently caused by:
  A.   fat.
  B.   bone marrow.
  C.   blood clots.
  D.   tumor cells.
  E.   air.

37. The leading cause of death in the elderly is:
  A.   pneumonia.
  B.   stroke.
  C.   cardiovascular disease.
  D.   Alzheimer's disease.
  E.   COPD.

38. All of the following are atypical presentations of a myocardial infarction in the elderly EXCEPT:
  A.   syncope.
  B.   tearing chest pain.
  C.   dyspnea.
  D.   neck or dental pain.
  E.   exercise intolerance.

39. Assessment findings specific to the elderly such as anorexia, nocturia, dependent edema, and hepatomegaly may be found in a patient with:
  A.   a pulmonary embolism.
  B.   heart failure.
  C.   hypertension.
  D.   an aneurysm.
  E.   syncope.

40. An abnormal dilation of a blood vessel, usually an artery, due to a congenital defect or weakness in the wall of the vessel is called:
  A.   an aneurysm.
  B.   an infarct.
  C.   thrombosis.
  D.   an embolism.
  E.   a hernia.

41. A series of symptoms resulting from decreased blood flow to the brain that are caused by a sudden decrease in cardiac output from a heart block are known as:
  - A. autonomic dysfunction.
  - B. Stokes-Adams syndrome.
  - C. sick sinus syndrome.
  - D. dying heart muscle.
  - E. Marfan's syndrome.

42. Injury to or death of brain tissue resulting from interruption of cerebral blood flow and oxygenation is called a(n):
  - A. subarachnoid hemorrhage.
  - B. autonomic dysfunction.
  - C. TIA.
  - D. stroke.
  - E. intracerebral hemorrhage.

43. Common causes of seizures in the elderly include all of the following EXCEPT:
  - A. head trauma.
  - B. alcohol withdrawal.
  - C. spinal injury.
  - D. stroke.
  - E. hypoglycemia.

44. A progressive, degenerative disease that attacks the brain and results in impaired memory, thinking, and behavior is called:
  - A. dementia.
  - B. Parkinson's disease.
  - C. delirium.
  - D. Alzheimer's disease.
  - E. aphasia.

45. A chronic, degenerative nervous disease characterized by tremors, muscular weakness and rigidity, and loss of postural reflexes is called:
  - A. Parkinson's disease.
  - B. Shy-Drager syndrome.
  - C. Alzheimer's disease.
  - D. sick sinus syndrome.
  - E. grand mal seizure.

46. All of the following are forms of upper GI bleed EXCEPT:
  - A. peptic ulcer disease.
  - B. ischemic colitis.
  - C. esophageal varices.
  - D. gastritis.
  - E. peptic ulcer disease.

47. An example of a lower GI bleed is:
  - A. a Mallory-Weiss tear.
  - B. diverticulosis.
  - C. peptic ulcer disease.
  - D. a bowel obstruction.
  - E. a mesenteric infarct.

48. An inflammation of the colon due to impaired or decreased blood supply is called:
  - A. diverticulosis.
  - B. ischemic colitis.
  - C. arterio-venous malformation.
  - D. colostomy.
  - E. gastritis.

49. The acute skin eruption caused by a reactivation of latent varicella virus that peaks between ages 50 and 70 is known as:
  - A. shingles.
  - B. pruritus.
  - C. maceration.
  - D. herpes zoster.
  - E. both A and D

50. Risk factors for osteoporosis include all of the following EXCEPT:
  - A. African or Latino ancestry.
  - B. low body weight.
  - C. early menopause
  - D. family history of fractures.
  - E. use of caffeine, alcohol, and cigarettes.

True/False

_____ **51.** When compared to younger patients, the elderly experience fewer adverse drug reactions.
     A. True
     B. False

_____ **52.** A lack of mobility can have detrimental physical and emotional effects on the elderly.
     A. True
     B. False

_____ **53.** In elderly people with cerebrovascular disease or impaired baroreceptor reflexes, efforts to force a bowel movement can lead to a transient ischemic attack.
     A. True
     B. False

_____ **54.** The elderly are more prone to environmental thermal problems due to changes in the sweat glands.
     A. True
     B. False

_____ **55.** When assessing an elderly person, if they are confused or disoriented, you can conclude that the patient is senile.
     A. True
     B. False

_____ **56.** The abnormal dilation of veins in the lower esophagus common in patients with cirrhosis of the liver is called esophageal varices.
     A. True
     B. False

_____ **57.** The elderly have a greater risk of trauma-related complications due a decrease in blood volume.
     A. True
     B. False

_____ **58.** In treating respiratory disorders in the elderly patient, do not fluid overload.
     A. True
     B. False

_____ **59.** The elderly are less susceptible to subdural hematomas than younger people.
     A. True
     B. False

_____ **60.** An elderly patient in an institutional setting is up to 50 times more likely to contract pneumonia that an elderly patient receiving home care.
     A. True
     B. False

Matching

Write the letter of the term in the space provided next to the appropriate description.

A.	epistaxis	**F.**	dysphoria
B.	varicosities	**G.**	urosepsis
C.	sick sinus syndrome	**H.**	nocturia
D.	vertigo	**I.**	polycythemia
E.	mesenteric infarct	**J.**	delirium

_____ **61.** acute alteration in mental functioning that is often reversible

_____ **62.** septicemia originating from the urinary tract

_____ **63.** medical term for a nose bleed

_____ **64.** excessive urination, usually at night

_____ **65.** death of tissue in the peritoneal fold that encircles the small intestine

_____ **66.** exaggerated feeling of depression or unrest

_____ **67.** excess of red blood cells

_____ **68.** abnormal dilation of a vein

_____ **69.** group of disorders characterized by dysfunction of the SA node

_____ **70.** sensation of faintness or dizziness causing loss of balance

Chapter 44

Abuse and Assault

Review of Chapter Objectives

After reading this chapter, you should be able to:

1. Discuss the incidence of abuse and assault.   **p. 1075**

Because of underreporting, it is difficult to provide accurate statistics on the incidence of abuse and assault in Canada today. That makes the available figures even more overwhelming in their seriousness. To grasp the magnitude of the problem, consider these facts:

• Fifty-one percent of all Canadian women have experienced at least one incident of sexual abuse.
• Twenty-five percent of all female postsecondary students in 1993 had been physically and/oe sexually assaulted by a male date or boyfriend
• Elder abuse occurs at an incidence of between 700 000 and 1.1 million annually.

2. Describe the categories of abuse. pp. 1075-1085

Partner abuse
Partner abuse results when a man or woman subjects a domestic partner to some form of physical or psychological violence. The victim may be a husband or wife, someone who shares a residence, or simply a boyfriend or girlfriend.

Elder abuse
There are basically two types of elder abuse—domestic and institutional. *Domestic elder abuse* takes place when an elder is being cared for in a home-based setting, usually by relatives. *Institutional elder abuse* occurs when an elder is being cared for by a person with a legal or contractual responsibility to provide care, such as paid caregivers, nursing home staff, or other professionals. Both types of abuse can be either acts of commission (acts of physical, sexual, or emotional violence) or acts of omission (neglect).

Child abuse
Child abuse may range from physical or emotional impairment to neglect of a child's most basic needs. It can occur from infancy to age 18 and can be inflicted by any number of caregivers—parents, foster parents, step-parents, babysitters, siblings, step-siblings, or other relatives or friends charged with a child's care.

Sexual abuse/assault
Sexual abuse, which is a form of physical abuse, can occur in almost any setting with a male or female of any age. It involves forced sexual contact and includes date rape and such contact within marriage. Although the legal definitions of sexual assault vary from state to state, courts generally interpret it as unwanted sexual contact, whether it be genital, oral, rectal, or manual. *Rape* is usually defined as penile penetration of the genitalia or rectum (however slight) without the consent of the victim. Both forms of sexual violence are prosecuted as crimes, with rape constituting a felony offense.

3. Discuss examples of spouse, elder, child, and sexual abuse. pp. 1075-1085

Examples of spouse/partner abuse
Partner abuse can fall into several categories. The most obvious form is physical abuse, which involves the application of force in ways too many to list. In addition to direct injury, physical abuse may exacerbate existing medical conditions, such as hypertension, diabetes, or asthma. Verbal abuse, which consists of words chosen to control or harm a person, may leave no physical mark. However, it damages a person's self-esteem and can lead to depression, substance abuse, or other self-destructive behavior. As noted in objective 2, partner abuse can also take the form of sexual abuse—unwanted, forced sexual contact between two people.

Examples of elder abuse
Elder abuse can also be physical, verbal, or sexual. In some cases, signs of elder abuse are subtle, such as theft of the victim's belongings or loss of freedom. Other signs, such as wounds, untreated decubitus ulcers, or poor hygiene, are more obvious. (For other examples of elder abuse, see Chapter 43.)

Examples of child abuse
As pointed out in Chapters 41 and 42, abused children suffer every imaginable mistreatment. They can be shaken, thrown, burned or scalded, and battered with almost any kind of object. They can be denied food, clean clothing, medical care, or even access to a toilet. The damage done to a child can last a lifetime and perpetuate a cycle of violence for generations to come.

Examples of sexual abuse/assault
Sexual abuse/assault typically involves a male assailant and a female victim, but not always. Forced sexual contact can range from exposure to fondling to rape to sexual torture. It may involve one assailant or multiple assailants. It can be an isolated act or an ongoing occurrence. Sexual abuse/assault can result in injuries, infections, sexually transmitted diseases, and unwanted pregnancies. The psychological damage is deep and long-lasting. Shame, anger, and a lack of trust may persist for years—or even a lifetime.

4. Describe the characteristics associated with the profile of a typical spouse, elder, or child abuser and the typical assailant of sexual abuse. pp. 1077, 1079, 1080-1081

Profile of spouse/partner abusers
Partner abuse occurs in all demographic groups. However, abuse is more common in lower socio-economic levels in which wage earners have trouble paying bills, holding down jobs, or keeping pace with technological changes. Typically the abuser does not like being out of control but at the same time feels powerless to change. A spouse or partner abuser usually exhibits an overly aggressive personality—an outgrowth of low self-esteem. They often feel insecure and jealous, flying into sudden and unpredictable rages. Use of alcohol or drugs increases the likelihood that the abuser will lose control and many not even remember his or her actions.

In the aftermath of an abusive incident, the abuser often feels a sense of remorse and shame. The person may seek to relieve his or her guilt by promising to change or even seeking help. For a time, the abuser may appear charming or loving, convincing an abused spouse or partner to think the pattern has finally been broken. All too often, however, the cycle of violence repeats itself in just a few days, weeks, or months.

Profile of elder abusers
Like partner abuse, elder abuse cuts across all demographic groups. As a result, it is difficult to profile the people who are most likely to abuse elders. However, there are several characteristics found in abusers of the elderly. Often, the perpetrators exhibit alcoholic behavior, drug addiction, or some mental impairment. The abuser may also be dependent upon the income or assistance of the elder—a situation that can cause resentment, anger, and, in some cases, violence. According to one study, in cases of domestic elder abuse, the most typical abusers are adult children who are overstressed by care of the elder and/or who were abused themselves.

Profile of child abusers

As with other types of abusers, you cannot relate child abuse to social class, income, or education. However, most abusers share one common trait: They were physically or emotionally abused as children. They often would prefer to use other forms of discipline, but under stress they regress to the earliest and most familiar patterns. Once they have resorted to physical discipline, the punishments become more severe and more frequent.

In cases of reported physical abuse, perpetrators tend to be men. However, the statistics for men and women even out when neglect is taken into account. Although potential child abusers can include a wide variety of caregivers, one or both parents are the most likely abusers. Frequent behavioral traits include use or abuse of alcohol and/or drugs, immaturity, self-absorption, and an inability to emotionally identify with the child.

Typical assailants of sexual abuse

Once again, sexual assailants can come from almost any background. However, the violent victimizers of children are substantially more likely than the victimizers of adults to have been physically or sexually abused as children. Many assailants, particularly adolescents and abusive adults, think domination is part of any relationship. Such thinking can lead to date rape or marital rape. In a significant number of all cases, the assailants are under the influence of alcohol or drugs.

5. Identify the profile of the "at-risk" spouse, elder, and child. pp. 1077, 1079, 1081, 1084-1085

At-risk spouses/partners

The primary risk factor for abuse is a family history of violence toward a spouse or partner. According to studies, pregnancy also appears to play a role, with 45 percent of abused women suffering some form of abuse during pregnancy. Substance abuse and emotional disorders play a role as well.

At-risk elders

A number of factors place the elderly at risk of abuse. Some of these include increased dependency on others (as a result of longer life spans), decreased productivity in later years, physical and mental impairments (especially among the "old old"), limited resources for long-term care of the elderly, strained family resources, and stress on middle-aged caregivers responsible for two generations—children and parents.

In general, elder abuse occurs most frequently among people who are dependent upon others for their care, especially among those elders who are mentally or physically challenged. Elders in poor health are more likely to be abused than elders in good health. This situation results, in part, from their inability to report the abuse. Yet another risk factor is family history, or a cycle of violence among family members. Finally, the potential for elder abuse increases proportionally with the personal problems of the caregivers. Abusers of the elderly tend to have more difficulties, either financial or emotional, than non-abusers.

At-risk children

As indicated in Chapter 42, abused children share several characteristics. Often, the child is seen as "special" and different from others. Premature infants and twins stand a higher risk of abuse than other children. Many abused children are less than 5 years of age. Physically and mentally challenged children as well as those with special needs are at greater risk. So are uncommunicative (e.g., autistic) children. Boys are more often abused than girls. A child who is not what the parents wanted (e.g., the "wrong" gender) is at increased risk of abuse, too.

6. Discuss the assessment and management of the abused patient. pp. 1077-1078, 1079-1081, 1084-1086

Your primary responsibility on a call involving an abusive situation is safety—both your own and that of the patient. You should never enter a scene if your safety is compromised, and you should leave the scene as soon as you feel unsafe.

You can expect the victims of abuse to feel threatened as a result of the violence they have suffered. One of your main duties is to provide a safe environment for an already traumatized patient. Sometimes you can provide safety merely by your official presence. Other times, you may have to move the patient to the ambulance so you can relocate to a different environment. In still other situations, you may have to summon additional personnel, such as law enforcement.

Specific assessment and management considerations will depend upon the type of abuse encountered. In cases of partner abuse, use direct questions, if possible, to convey an awareness that the person's partner may have contributed to the injury. In cases of suspected child abuse, examine the patient for identifiable patterns of physical mistreatment or neglect and record your objective observations. In cases of sexual abuse, use open-ended questions to reestablish a sense of control. If possible, allow a same-sex crew member to maintain contact with the victim.

Regardless of the situation, keep in mind that the patient has been harmed by another human being, in many cases a person that he or she knows intimately. Try to transport the patient to the hospital. If you cannot do so, either because of patient refusal or intervention by the suspected abuser, be sure to report your suspicions to the appropriate authorities or agencies.

7. Discuss the legal aspects associated with abuse situations.   pp. 1078, 1084, 1086-1087

Abuse and assault constitute crimes. Although their nature and the extent of the crime often depends upon local laws, you have a responsibility to report suspected cases. Because the assailants may be detained only a short time, you also have an obligation to find out about the victim and witness protection programs available in your area.

Study the local laws and protocols regarding cases of abuse and assault. All provinces or territories require EMS personnel to report even a suspicion of abuse or assault. Regardless of where you live, take time to learn the rules and regulations that affect your practice, both for your sake and for the sake of your patient.

8. Identify community resources that are able to assist victims of abuse and assault. pp. 1078, 1086

Specialized resources include both private and provincially or federally funded programs. Make a point of learning about hospital units for the victims of sexual assault, public and private shelters for battered persons, and local agencies responsible for youth and their families.

9. Discuss the documentation necessary when caring for abused and assaulted patients. pp. 1078, 1084, 1086

It is important that you carefully and objectively document all your findings. Your actions can affect the outcome of a case or prosecution of a crime. If the patient tells you something about the abuser or assailant, mark it with quotation marks on the patient care report. In the case of rape, patients should not urinate, defecate, douche, bathe, eat, drink, or smoke. Some jurisdictions have specific rules for evidence protection, such as using paper bags to collect evidence or placing bags over the patient's hands to preserve trace evidence. Remember that any evidence you collect must remain in your custody until you can give it directly to a law enforcement official to preserve the *chain of evidence.* Regardless of the emotions evoked by the call, when documenting the incident, you must be completely factual and nonjudgmental.

CONTENT SELF-EVALUATION

Multiple Choice

_____   1.   The most widespread and best known form of abuse involves the abuse of:

    A.   women by men.   **D.**   elders by their children.

    B.   children by their mothers.   **E.**   same-sex partners.

    C.   children by their fathers.

2. Many victims of abuse hesitate or fail to report the problem because of a:
   - A. fear of reprisal.
   - B. lack of knowledge.
   - C. fear of humiliation.
   - D. lack of financial resources.
   - E. all of the above

3. By far the most common characteristic of abusers—whether they be partner abusers, child abusers, or elder abusers—is a:
   - A. history of substance abuse.
   - B. lack of employment.
   - C. family history of violence.
   - D. lack of education.
   - E. mental impairment.

4. In assessing the battered patient, all of the following are appropriate actions EXCEPT:
   - A. direct questioning.
   - B. asking the victim why she or he doesn't leave.
   - C. rehearsing the quickest way to leave the home.
   - D. nonjudgmental questioning.
   - E. reminding the patient that assault is a crime.

5. All of the following are causes of elder abuse EXCEPT:
   - A. stress on middle-aged caregivers.
   - B. decreased life expectancies.
   - C. physical and mental impairments.
   - D. limited resources for long-term care.
   - E. decreased productivity in later years.

6. Which of the following are two main types of elder abuse?
   - A. neglect and domestic
   - B. emotional and financial
   - C. domestic and institutional
   - D. mental and institutional
   - E. financial and domestic

7. The perpetrators of domestic elder abuse tend to be:
   - A. paid caregivers.
   - B. siblings.
   - C. adult children.
   - D. spouses.
   - E. friends or neighbors.

8. In cases of child abuse, the most likely abusers are:
   - A. babysitters.
   - B. siblings.
   - C. strangers
   - D. one or both parents.
   - E. friends charged with the child's care..

9. All of the following are characteristics of abused children EXCEPT:
   - A. sudden behavioral changes.
   - B. neediness.
   - C. absence of nearly all emotions.
   - D. unusual wariness.
   - E. concern over a parent's absence.

10. One of the signs of intentional scalding of a child is:
   - A. staphylococcal scalded skin.
   - B. hematological disorders.
   - C. multiple splatter marks.
   - D. multiple bruises.
   - E. absence of splash burns.

11. Children rarely exhibit accidental fractures to the:
   - A. head.
   - B. ribs.
   - C. legs.
   - D. arms.
   - E. hands or feet.

12. Which type of injury claims the largest number of lives among abused children?
   - A. malnutrition
   - B. head injuries
   - C. burns
   - D. chest injury
   - E. abdominal injuries

13. When talking to a rape victim, you can help the patient regain a sense of self-control by asking _____ questions.

A.	open-ended	**D.**	non-personal
B.	closed-ended	**E.**	leading
C.	indirect		

14. Sexual Assault Nurse Examiners are specially trained health care workers who can:
- **A.** help with the pre-hospital care report.
- **B.** protect the patient against the assailant.
- **C.** provide information on the protection of evidence.
- **D.** protect EMS crews against legal suits.
- **E.** none of the above

15. All provinces and territories require health care workers to report suspected cases of:

A.	child abuse.	**D.**	spousal abuse.
B.	rape.	**E.**	partner abuse.
C.	elder abuse.		

True/False

16. Partner abuse is defined as physical or emotional violence from a man or woman toward a coworker.
- **A.** True
- **B.** False

17. Forty-five percent of pregnant women suffer some form of battery during pregnancy.
- **A.** True
- **B.** False

18. The group most likely to be victims of sexual assault or rape are adolescent females under age 18.
- **A.** True
- **B.** False

19. The victims of rape most commonly describe their assailant as a stranger.
- **A.** True
- **B.** False

20. In managing a rape case, honor the patient's request to bathe or shower.
- **A.** True
- **B.** False

21. Close to eighty percent of all women who experienced sexual assault have survived more than one violent incident.
- **A.** True
- **B.** False

22. One reason for not reporting abuse is fear of humiliation.
- **A.** True
- **B.** False

23. Direct questioning usually works best in assessing the battered patient.
- **A.** True
- **B.** False

24. Child abuse does not include neglecting the child's basic needs.
- **A.** True
- **B.** False

25. Common conditions mistaken for abuse may include chicken pox, or hematological disorders that cause easy bruising.
    A.   True
    B.   False

Matching

Write the letter of the term in the space provided next to the appropriate description.

A.	partner abuse	**F.**	domestic elder abuse
B.	rape	**G.**	7.5%
C.	sexual assault	**H.**	excessively passive behaviour
D.	fear of reprisal	**I.**	substance abuse
E.	child abuse	**J.**	instituitional elder abuse

26. physical or emotional violence or neglect when an elder is being cared for in a home-based setting

27. a reason for not reporting abuse

28. penile penetration of the genitalia or rectum without the consent of the victim

29. physical or emotional violence or neglect toward a person from infancy to 18 years of age

30. percentage of perpetrators of domestic elder abuse who are friends or neighbours

31. physical or emotional violence from a man or woman toward a domestic partner

32. physical or emotional violence or neglect when an elder is being cared for by a person paid to provide care

33. characteristics of abused children under the age of six

34. unwanted oral, genital, rectal, or manual sexual contact

35. the result of the numbing effect of excessive effects alcohol and/or drugs

Chapter 45

The Challenged Patient

Review of Chapter Objectives

After reading this chapter, you should be able to:

1. Describe the various etiologies and types of hearing impairments.   pp. 1090-1091

There are basically two types of deafness—*conductive deafness* and *sensorineural deafness.* Conductive deafness results from any condition that prevents sound waves from being transmitted from the external ear to the middle or inner ear. The condition may be temporary or permanent. If caught early, many forms of conductive deafness may be treated and cured. Sensorineural deafness, on the other hand, is often incurable. The condition arises from the inability of nerve impulses to reach the auditory center of the brain because of nerve damage either to the inner ear or to the brain. In the case of infants and children, sensorineural deafness often results from congenital defects or birth injuries.

2. Recognize the patient with a hearing impairment. p. 1091

It is very important to detect deafness early in your assessment. A partially deaf person may ask questions repeatedly, misunderstand answers to questions, or respond inappropriately. Such reactions can easily be mistaken for head injury, leading to misdirected treatment.

    The most obvious sign of deafness is a hearing aid. Unfortunately, hearing aids do not work for all types of deafness. Also, many people do not wear hearing aids, even when they have been prescribed. In addition, deaf people may have poor diction, due to partial hearing loss or hearing loss later in life. They might use their hands to gesture or use sign language. Deaf people may ask you to speak louder or they may speak excessively loud themselves. Finally, deaf people will commonly face you so that they can read your lips.

3. Anticipate accommodations that may be needed in order to properly manage the patient with a hearing impairment. pp. 1091-1092

When managing a patient with a hearing impairment, you can do several things to ease communications.
• Begin by identifying yourself and making sure the patient knows that you are speaking to him or her.
• Address deaf patients face to face, giving them the opportunity to read your lips and interpret your expression.
• Speak slowly in a normal voice. Never yell or use exaggerated gestures, which often distort your facial and body language.
• Keep in mind that nearly 80 percent of hearing loss is related to high-pitched sounds. As a result, you might use a low-pitched voice to speak directly into the patient's ear.
• Make sure background noise is reduced as much as possible.
• If necessary, find or adjust a hearing aid.
• Be innovative. Put the stethoscope on the patient and try speaking into it. Don't forget the most simple and effective means of communication—a pen and paper.
• If necessary and if time allows, draw pictures to illustrate procedures.

• If the patient knows sign language, usually American Sign Language (ASL), utilize an interpreter, documenting the name of the person who did the interpreting and the information received.

4. **Describe the various etiologies and types, recognize patients with, and anticipate accommodations that may be needed in order to properly manage each of the following conditions:**

   a.   **visual impairments   pp. 1092-1093**

   When caring for the patient with a visual impairment, it is important to note if the impairment is a permanent disability or if it is a new symptom caused by the illness or injury for which you were called. Visual impairments have a number of etiologies—injury, disease, congenital conditions, infection (such as cytomegalovirus [CMV]), and degeneration of the retina, optic nerve, or nerve pathways.

   Depending on the degree of impairment and a person's adjustment to the loss of vision, you may or may not recognize the condition right away. In cases of obvious blindness, identify yourself as you approach the patient so that the person knows you are there. Also describe everything you are doing. Take into account any special tools that assist a visually impaired person with daily living, most notably guide dogs and/or canes. Depending upon local protocols, arrange to transport the guide dog to the hospital with the patient. If the patient is ambulatory, have the person take your arm for guidance rather than taking the patient's arm.

   b.   **speech impairments   pp. 1093-1094**

   When performing an assessment, you may come across a patient who is awake, alert, and oriented but cannot communicate with you due to a speech impairment. Possible miscommunication can hinder both the treatment administered and the information provided to the receiving facility. You may encounter four types of speech impairments. They include:

   • **Language disorders.** A language disorder is an impaired ability to understand the spoken or written word. In children, language disorders result from a number of causes such as congenital learning disorders, cerebral palsy, hearing impairments, or inadequate language stimulation during the first year of life (delayed speaking ability). In adults, language disorders may result from a variety of illnesses or injuries—stroke, aneurysm, head injury, brain tumor, hearing loss, or some kind of emotional trauma. The loss of ability to communicate in speech, writing, or signs is known as aphasia. Aphasia can manifest itself in the following ways.

   Sensory aphasia—a person can no longer understand the spoken word. Patients with sensory aphasia will not respond to your questions because they cannot understand what you are saying. *Motor aphasia*—a person can no longer use the symbols of speech. Patients with motor aphasia, also known as expressive aphasia, will understand what you say but cannot clearly articulate a response.

   Global aphasia—occurs when a person has both sensory and motor aphasia. These patients can neither understand nor respond to your questions. A brain tumor in the Broca's region can cause this condition.

   • **Articulation disorders.** Articulation disorders, also known as dysarthria, affect the way a person's speech is heard by others. These disorders occur when sounds are produced or put together incorrectly or in a way that makes it difficult to understand the spoken word. Articulation disorders may start at an early age, when the child learns to say words incorrectly or when a hearing impairment is involved. This type of disturbance can occur in both children and adults when neural damage causes a disturbance in the nerve pathways leading from the brain to the larynx, mouth, or lips.

   • **Voice production disorders.** When a patient has a voice production disorder, the quality of the person's voice is affected. This can be caused by trauma due to overuse of the vocal cords or infection. Cancer of the larynx can also cause a speech failure by impeding air from passing through the vocal cords. A patient with a production disorder will exhibit hoarseness, harshness, an inappropriate pitch, or abnormal nasal resonance.

   • **Fluency disorders.** Fluency disorders present as stuttering. Although the cause of stuttering is not fully understood, the condition is found more often in men than in women. When speaking with patients who stutter, do not interrupt or finish their answers out of frustration and do not correct the way they speak.

When speaking to a patient with a speech impairment, never assume that the person lacks intelligence. Do not rush the patient or predict an answer. Try to form questions that require short, direct answers. When asking questions, look directly at the patient. If you cannot understand what the person has said, politely ask him or her to repeat it. Never pretend to understand when you don't. You might miss valuable information related to the call. If all else fails, give the patient the opportunity to write responses to your questions.

c.   obesity pp. 1094-1095

Over 40 percent of the Canadian population are considered obese, while many more are heavier than their ideal body weight. Obesity occurs for a number of reasons. In many cases, diet, exercise, and life styles result in a caloric intake that exceeds daily energy needs. Genetic factors also predispose a person toward obesity. In rare cases, an obese patient may have a low basal metabolic rate, which causes the body to burn calories at a slower rate. In such cases, the condition may have been produced by an illness, such as hyperthyroidism.

Managing an obese patient presents a number of challenges. Beside the obvious difficulty of lifting and moving these patients, excess weight can exacerbate the complaint for which you were called. Obesity can also lead to a number of serious medical conditions, including hypertension, heart disease, stroke, diabetes, and joint and muscle problems. In conducting a history, you will need to question patients carefully to make sure they are not mistakenly attributing signs and symptoms to their weight.

When doing your patient assessment, you may need to accommodate for the patient's weight. It may be necessary to auscultate lung sounds anteriorly on a patient who is too obese to lean forward. If the patient's adipose tissue presents an obstruction, you may need to place ECG monitoring electrodes on the arms and thighs instead of on the chest. Also be sure to have plenty of assistance for lifting and keep in mind that many of the litters and stretchers are not rated for extremely large patients. Finally, alert the emergency department of the need for extra lifting assistance and special stretchers upon arrival.

d.   paraplegia/quadriplegia p. 1096

During your career, you may respond to a call and find that your patient is paralyzed from a previous traumatic or medical event. You will have to treat the chief complaint while taking into account the accommodations that must be made when treating a patient who cannot move some or all of his or her extremities.

A paralyzed patient may be paraplegic or quadriplegic. A paraplegic patient has been paralyzed from the waist down, while a quadriplegic patient has paralysis of all four extremities. In addition, spinal cord injuries in the area of C3 to C5 and above may also paralyze the patient's respiratory muscles and compromise the ability to breathe.

In managing a paraplegic or quadriplegic patient, be prepared for a number of common devices. These include a home ventilator, tracheostomy, halo traction, or colostomy. Be sure to make accommodations for these—and any other assisting devices—when you transport the patient. (For more on acute interventions for physically disabled and other chronic care patients, see Chapter 46.)

e.   mental illness and mental/emotional impairments p. 1096

Mental and emotional illnesses or impairments present a special challenge to the EMS provider. The disorders may range from the psychoses caused by complex biochemical brain diseases, such as bipolar disorder (manic depression), to the personality disorders related to personality development, to a traumatic experience. Emotional impairments can include such conditions as hysteria, compulsive behavior, or anxiety.

f.   developmentally disabled   pp. 1096-1098

People with developmental disabilities are those individuals with impaired or insufficient development of the brain who are unable to learn at the usual rate. Developmental disabilities can occur for a variety of reasons. They can be genetic, such as Down syndrome, or they can be the product of a brain injury caused by some hypoxic or traumatic event. Such injuries can take place before birth, during birth, or anytime thereafter.

Except for patients with Down syndrome, it may be difficult to recognize someone with a developmental disability unless the person lives in a group home or other special residential setting. Remember that a person with a developmental disability can recognize body language, tone, and disrespect just like anyone else. Treat him or her as you would any other patient, listening to his/her answers, particularly if you suspect physical or emotional abuse.

If a patient has a severe cognitive disability, you may need to rely on others to obtain the chief complaint and history. Also, many children or young people with learning disabilities have been taught to be wary of strangers who may seek to touch them. You have to establish a basis of trust with the patient, perhaps by making it clear that you are a member of the medical community or by asking for the support of a person the patient does trust. Also, some people with developmental disabilities have been judged "stupid" or "bad" for behavior that results in an accident and they may try to cover up the events that led up to a call.

At all times, keep in mind that a person with a developmental disability may not understand what is happening. The ambulance, special equipment, and even your uniform may confuse or scare them. In cases of severe disabilities, it will be important to keep the primary caregivers with you at all times, even in the back of the ambulance.

g. Down syndrome pp. 1097-1098

Down syndrome results from an extra chromosome, usually on chromosome 21 or 22. Although the cause is unknown, the chromosomal abnormality increases with the age of the mother, especially after age 40. It also occurs at a higher rate in parents with a chromosomal abnormality, such as the translocation of chromosome 21 to chromosome 14.

Typically Down syndrome presents with easily recognized physical features. They include eyes sloped up at the outer corners, folds of skin on either side of the nose that cover the inner corner of the eye, small face and features, large and protruding tongue, flattening on the back of the head, and short and broad hands.

In addition to mild to moderate developmental disability, Down syndrome patients may have other physical ailments, such as heart defects, intestinal defects, and chronic lung problems. Down syndrome people are also at high risk of developing cataracts, blindness, and Alzheimer's disease at an early age.

When assessing the Down syndrome patient, consider the level of his or her developmental delay and follow the general guidelines mentioned in objective 4f. Transport to the hospital should be uneventful, especially if the caregiver comes along.

h. emotional impairment and i. emotional/mental impairment p. 1096

5. **Describe, identify possible presenting signs, and anticipate accommodations for the following diseases/illnesses:**

a. arthritis p. 1099

The three most common types of arthritis include:
- *Juvenile rheumatoid arthritis (JRA)*—a connective tissue disorder that strikes before age 16
- *Rheumatoid arthritis*—an autoimmune disorder
- *Osteoarthritis*—a degenerative joint disease, the most common arthritis seen in elderly people

All forms cause painful swelling and irritation of the joints, making everyday tasks sometimes impossible. Treatment of arthritis includes aspirin, nonsteroidal anti-inflammatory drugs (NSAIDS), and/or corticosteroids. It is important for you to recognize the side effects of these medications in case you have been called upon to treat a medication side effect rather than the disease. NSAIDS can cause stomach upset and vomiting, with or without bloody emesis. Corticosteroids, such as prednisone, can cause hyperglycemia, bloody emesis, and decreased immunity. You should also take note of all the patient's medications so that you do not administer a medication that can interact with the ones already taken by the patient.

When transporting arthritis patients, keep in mind their high level of discomfort. Use pillows to elevate affected extremities. The most comfortable position might not be the best position to start an IV, but try to make the patient as comfortable as possible.

b. cancer pp. 1099-1100

Cancer is caused by the abnormal growth of cells in normal tissue. The primary site of origin of the cancer determines the type of cancer the patient has. It may be difficult for you to recognize a cancer patient because the disease often has few obvious signs and symptoms. Rather, the treatments for the disease take on telltale signs, such as anorexia leading to weight loss or alopecia (hair loss). Tattoos may be left on the skin by radiation oncologists to mark positioning of radiation therapy equipment. In addition, physical changes, such as loss of a breast (mastectomy), may be obvious.

Management of the cancer patient can present a special challenge. Many patients undergoing chemotherapy treatments become neutropenic—a condition in which chemotherapy creates a dangerously low neutrophil (white blood cell) count. If patients have recently received chemotherapy, assume that they are neutropenic and take every precaution to protect them from infection. Keep a mask on the patient both during transport and during transfer at the emergency department.

In treating cancer patients, also keep in mind that their veins may have become scarred and difficult to access due to frequent IV starts, blood draws, and caustic chemotherapy transfusions. Cancer patients may also have an implanted infusion port, found just below the skin, with the catheter inserted into the subclavian vein or brachial artery. You need special training to access these ports and should not attempt to access them unless you have such training and the approval of medical direction.

Cancer patients may also have a peripheral access device such as a Groshong catheter or Hickman catheter. In this situation, it may simply be a matter of flushing the line and then hooking up your IV fluids to this external catheter. Whatever you decide to do, involve the patient, who has already lost a lot of control over his or her treatment, in the decision-making process.

c.   cerebral palsy   pp. 1100-1101

Cerebral palsy (CP) is a group of disorders caused by damage to the cerebrum in utero or by trauma during birth. Prenatal exposure of the mother to German measles can cause cerebral palsy, as well as any condition leading to fetal hypoxia. Premature birth or brain damage from a difficult delivery can also lead to cerebral palsy. Other causes include encephalitis, meningitis, or head injury during a fall or abuse of an infant.

There are three main types of cerebral palsy—spastic paralysis, athetosis, and ataxia. In treating patients with cerebral palsy, keep this fact in mind: Many people with atheotoid and diplegic CP are highly intelligent. Do not assume that a person with cerebral palsy cannot communicate with you.

When transporting cerebral palsy patients, make accommodations to prevent further injury. If they experience severe contractions, the patients may not rest comfortably on a stretcher. Use pillows and extra blankets to pad extremities that are not in proper alignment. Have suction available if a patient drools. If a patient has difficulty communicating, make sure that the caregiver helps in your assessment. Be alert for cerebral palsy patients who sign. If you do not know how to sign, find somebody who does and alert the emergency department.

d.   cystic fibrosis   pp. 1101-1102

Cystic fibrosis (CF) is an inherited disorder involving the exocrine glands primarily in the lungs and digestive system. Thick mucus forms in the lungs, causing bronchial obstruction and atelectasis in the small ducts of the alveoli. In addition, the thick mucus causes blockages in the small ducts of the pancreas, leading to decrease in the pancreatic enzymes needed to absorb nutrients.

Obtaining a complete medical history is important to the recognition of a CF patient. A unique characteristic of CF is the high concentration of chloride in the sweat, leading to the use of a diagnostic test known as the "sweat test." A CF patient may also complain of frequent lung infections, clay-colored stools, or clubbing of the fingers or toes.

Because of the high probability of respiratory distress in a CF patient, some form of oxygen therapy may be necessary. You may need to have a family member or caregiver hold blow-by oxygen (rather than use a mask) if this is all the patient will tolerate. Suctioning may be necessary to help the patient clear the thick secretions. If the patient is taking antibiotics to prevent infection and using inhalers or Mucomyst to thin secretions, bring these medications to the hospital. Above all else, keep in mind that these patients have been chronically ill for their entire lives. The last thing they or their loved ones want is another trip to the hospital.

Because of a poor prognosis, most of the CF patients that you see will be children or adolescents. A child with cystic fibrosis is still a child. So remember everything that you have learned about the treatment of pediatric patients and apply it to the developmental stage of the CF patient that you are treating.

e.   multiple sclerosis   p. 1102

Multiple sclerosis (MS) is a disorder of the central nervous system that usually strikes between the ages of 20 and 40, affecting women more than men. The exact cause of MS is unknown, but it is considered to be an autoimmune disorder. Characteristically, repeated inflammation of the myelin sheath surrounding the nerves leads to scar tissue, which in turn blocks nerve impulses to the affected area.

The onset of MS is slow. It starts as a change in the strength of a muscle and a numbness or tingling in the affected muscle. Patients may develop problems with gait, slurred speech, and clumsiness. They may experience double vision due to weakness of the eye muscles or eye pain due to neuritis of the optic nerve. As symptoms progress, they become more permanent, leading the MS patient to become increasingly weak and more vulnerable to lung or urinary infections.

Transporting of the MS patient to the hospital may require supportive care, such as oxygen therapy. Make sure the patient is comfortable and help position the patient as needed. Bring any assistive devices, such as a wheelchair or cane, so that the patient can maintain as much independence as possible.

f.   muscular dystrophy   p. 1102

Muscular dystrophy (MD) is a group of hereditary disorders characterized by progressive weakness and wasting of muscle mass. It is a genetic disorder, leading to gradual degeneration of muscle fibers. The most common form of MD is Duchenne muscular dystrophy, which typically affects boys between the ages of 3 and 6. It leads to progressive muscle weakness in the legs and pelvis and to paralysis by age 12. Ultimately, the disease affects the respiratory muscles and heart, causing death. The other various MD disorders are classified by the age of the patient at onset of symptoms and by the muscles affected.

Since MD is a hereditary disease, you should obtain a complete family history. You should also note the particular muscle groups that the patient cannot move. Again, since MD patients are primarily children, choose age-appropriate language. Respiratory support may be needed, especially in later stages of the disease.

g.   myasthenia gravis   p. 1104

Myasthenia gravis is an autoimmune disease characterized by chronic weakness of voluntary muscles and progressive fatigue. The condition results from a problem with the neurotransmitters, which causes a blocking of nerve signals to the muscles. It occurs most frequently in women between ages 20 and 50.

A patient with myasthenia gravis may complain of a complete lack of energy, especially in the evening. The disease commonly involves muscles in the face. You may note eyelid drooping or difficulty chewing or swallowing. The patient may also complain of double vision.
In severe cases of myasthenia gravis, a patient may experience paralysis of the respiratory muscles, leading to respiratory arrest. These patients may need assisted ventilations en route to the emergency facility.

h.   poliomyelitis   pp. 1102-1103

Poliomyelitis is a communicable disease affecting the gray matter in the brain and spinal cord. Although it is highly contagious, immunization has made outbreaks of polio extremely rare in developed nations. However, it is important to be aware of the disease, since many people born before development of the polio vaccine in the 1950s were affected by the disease.

Although most patients recover from polio, they are left with permanent paralysis of the affected muscles. You may recognize a polio victim by the use of assistive devices for ambulation or by the reduced size of the affected limb due to muscle atrophy. Some patients may have experienced paralysis of the respiratory muscles, requiring assisted ventilations. Patients on long-term ventilators will typically have tracheotomies.

Along with polio, you should know about a related disorder called post-polio syndrome. Post-polio syndrome affects those patients who suffered severely from polio more than 30 years ago. Patients with this condition quickly tire, especially after exercise, and develop an intolerance for cold in their extremities.

Many patients with polio or post-polio syndrome may insist on walking to the ambulance but should not be encouraged to do so. Because they may not have required hospitalization for polio since childhood, you will have to alleviate their anxiety, keeping in mind their fears of a renewed loss of independence.

i. spina bifida pp. 1103-1104
Spina bifida is a congenital abnormality that falls under the category of a neural tube defect. It presents when there is a defect in the closure of the backbone and the spinal canal. In spina bifida occulta, the patient exhibits few outward signs of the deformity. In spina bifida cystica, the failure of the closure allows the spinal cord and covering membranes to protrude from the back, causing an obvious deformity.

Symptoms depend upon which part of the spinal cord is protruding through the back. The patient may have paralysis of both lower extremities and lack of bowel or bladder control. A large percentage of the children with this disease also have hydrocephalus, requiring a surgical shunt to help drain excess fluid from the brain.

When treating spina bifida patients, keep several things in mind. Recent research has shown that between 18 and 73 percent of children and adolescents with spina bifida have latex allergies. For safety, assume that all patients with spina bifida have this problem. In transporting spina bifida patients, be sure to bring along any devices that aid them. If you are called to treat an infant, safe transport to the hospital should be done in a car seat, unless contraindicated.

j. patients with a previous head injury p. 1103
Patients with a previous head injury may not be easily recognized until they begin to speak. They may display similar symptoms to those of stroke, but without the hemiparesis (paralysis on one side of the body). Such patients may have aphasia, slurred speech, or loss of vision or hearing, or may develop a learning disability. They may also exhibit short-term memory loss and may not have any recollection of their original injury.

Obtaining a medical history will be extremely important, especially if you are responding to a traumatic event. Note any new symptoms the patient may be having or the recurrence of old ones. If the patient cannot speak, look for obvious physical signs of trauma or for facial expressions of pain. Treatment and transport considerations will depend upon the condition for which you were called.

6. Define, recognize, and anticipate accommodations needed to properly mange patients who:

a. are culturally diverse pp. 1104-1105
Culturally diverse patients may speak a different language or have different traditions or religious beliefs from yours. What may make it difficult for you to treat culturally different patients may not be the differences per se, but your inability to understand them. Do not consider this a reason for refusing treatment. Rather, consider it a learning experience that will prepare you for a similar situation on another run.

As a paramedic, you are ethically required to take care of all patients in the same manner, regardless of their race, religion, gender, ethnic background, or living situation. Remember, the patient who has decision-making abilities has a right to self-determination and can refuse treatment. You should, however, obtain a signed document indicating informed refusal of consent. If your patient does not speak English, communication may be a problem. You may need to rely on a family member to act as an interpreter or on a translator device, such as a telephone language line for non–English speaking people. In such cases, be sure to notify the receiving facility of the need for an interpreter.

b. are terminally ill p.
Caring for a terminally ill patient can be an emotional challenge. Many times, the patient will choose to die at home, but at the last minute the family compromises those wishes by calling EMS. In other cases, the patient may call for an ambulance so that a newly developed condition can be treated or a medication adjusted. (For more on caring for the terminally ill, see Chapter 46.)

c.   have a communicable disease   p. 1105

When treating people with communicable diseases, you should withhold all personal judgment. Although you will need to take BSI precautions just as you would with any patient, keep in mind the heightened sensitivity of a person with a communicable disease. Although most of these patients are familiar with the health care setting, you should still explain that you take these measures with all patients who have a similar disease. Also, you do not need to take additional precautions beyond those required by departmental policy. The patient will generally spot these extra measures and react with feelings of shame, guilt, or anger. (For more on the etiologies and treatment of communicable diseases, see Chapter 37 in Division 4.)

7. Given several challenged patients, provide the appropriate assessment, management, and transportation. pp. 1089-1105

During your classroom, clinical, and field training, you will be presented with real and simulated challenged patients and develop management plans for them. Use the information presented in this text chapter, the information on assessing challenged patients provided by your instructors, and the guidance given by your clinical and field preceptors to develop good skills in caring for the special needs of these patients. Continue to refine newly learned skills once your training ends and you begin your career as a paramedic.

CONTENT SELF-EVALUATION

Multiple Choice

_____ 1. The two main types of deafness are:
    A.   tinnitus and Meniere's disease.   **D.**   clinical and non-clinical.
    B.   conductive and sensorineural.   **E.**   temporary and complete.
    C.   partial and sudden.

_____ 2. An inner ear infection that causes vertigo, nausea, and an unsteady gait is called:
    A.   labyrinthitis.   **D.**   otomycosis.
    B.   otitis media.   **E.**   cerumen.
    C.   presbycusis.

_____ 3. During the patient interview and physical exam, hearing deficits may be mistaken for:
    A.   head injury.   **D.**   effusion syndrome.
    B.   intoxication.   **E.**   drug overdose.
    C.   transducer infection.

_____ 4. When communicating with a deaf patient, consider all of the following strategies EXCEPT:
    A.   speaking slowly in a normal voice.
    B.   using a high-pitched voice to speak directly into the patient's ear.
    C.   reducing background noise.
    D.   using a pen and paper.
    E.   putting a stethoscope on the patient and speaking into it.

_____ 5. The term for removal of the eyeball after trauma, such as a penetrating injury, or certain kinds of illnesses is:
    A.   retinal detachment.   **D.**   orbitotomy.
    B.   enucleation.   **E.**   corneal abrasion.
    C.   optic chiasm.

6. Diabetes can slowly lead to a loss of a vision as a result of:
- A. degeneration of the optic nerve.
- B. disorders in the blood vessels leading to the retina.
- C. degeneration of the eyeball.
- D. cytomegalovirus (CMV).
- E. retinitis.

7. All of the following are types of speech impairments, except:
- A. congenital fluency.
- B. language disorders.
- C. fluency disorders.
- D. articulation disorders.
- E. voice production disorders.

8. A language disorder that can be caused by a stroke or brain injury is known as:
- A. amnesia.
- B. ataxia.
- C. aphagia.
- D. aphasia.
- E. aphonia.

9. Stuttering is an example of a(n):
- A. dyslexic disorder.
- B. fluency disorder.
- C. auditory disorder.
- D. vocal cord disorder.
- E. voice production disorder.

10. If the adipose tissue on an obese patient presents an obstruction, you may need to place ECG monitoring electrodes on the:
- A. chest and back.
- B. hands and feet.
- C. arms and back.
- D. neck and chest.
- E. arms and thighs.

11. Bipolar disorders and biochemical brain diseases are examples of:
- A. emotional and mental impairments.
- B. developmental disabilities.
- C. visual impairments.
- D. articulation disorders.
- E. pathological challenges.

12. People with Down syndrome are risk of developing:
- A. cataracts.
- B. blindness.
- C. early Alzheimer's disease.
- D. heart defects.
- E. all of the above

13. Fetal Alcohol Syndrome (FAS) is sometimes confused with Down syndrome because they both:
- A. produce similar facial characteristics.
- B. are caused by alcohol consumption during pregnancy.
- C. are preventable birth defects.
- D. cause death at an early age
- E. produce hyperactivity.

14. Cancer patients receiving chemotherapy are at high risk for:
- A. syncope.
- B. infection.
- C. altered mental status.
- D. weight gain.
- E. diminished sense of pain.

15. When caring for cerebral palsy patients, you may need to:
- A. treat them as if they have a spinal injury.
- B. change the order of the initial assessment.
- C. use pillows and blankets to pad unaligned extremities.
- D. anticipate brief periods of apnea.
- E. both A and D

16. A group of hereditary disorders characterized by progressive weakness and wasting of muscle tissue is known as:

  A. poliomyelitis.

  B. spina bifida.

  C. multiple sclerosis.

  D. cystic fibrosis.

  E. muscular dystrophy.

17. Most of the cystic fibrosis patients that you see will be:

  A. adults in their 30s and 40s.

  B. elderly patients over age 60.

  C. infants 1 year old and younger.

  D. children and adolescents.

  E. women 20 to 40.

18. A congenital abnormality in which a large percentage of children are born with hydrocephalus is:

  A. Down syndrome.

  B. cerebral palsy.

  C. spina bifida.

  D. fetal alcohol syndrome.

  E. cystic fibrosis.

19. A preventable disorder caused by alcohol consumption during pregnancy is:

  A. JRA.

  B. FAS.

  C. ACE.

  D. TIA.

  E. PE.

20. Research has shown that between 18 and 73 percent of children and adolescents with _____ have a latex allergy.

  A. cerebral palsy

  B. myasthenia gravis

  C. poliomyelitis

  D. spina bifida

  E. Down syndrome

21. A patient with spina bifida may have any of the following conditions EXCEPT:

  A. accumulation of fluid on the brain.

  B. loss of bladder control.

  C. paralysis of the lower extremities.

  D. loss of bowel control.

  E. paralysis on one side of the body.

22. Common complaints from a patient with myasthenia gravis include:

  A. chronic fatigue or lack of energy.

  B. nausea and headache.

  C. shortness of breath and heart palpitations.

  D. dizziness and loss of appetite.

  E. unsteady gait and double vision.

23. Accommodation of a culturally diverse population requires:

  A. patience.

  B. ingenuity.

  C. respect.

  D. use of translators.

  E. all of the above

24. When a patient refuses treatment because of religious reasons, you should:

  A. call the police to intervene.

  B. administer treatment and document your reasons.

  C. ask the person to reconsider his or her religious views.

  D. obtain a signed refusal of treatment and transportation form.

  E. leave the scene.

25. Sensory aphasia is manifested by:

  A. the patient understanding the spoken word.

  B. the patient unable to use the symbols of speech.

  C. the patient no longer understanding the spoken word.

  D. a patient with constant stuttering.

  E. none of the above.

True/False

26. When treating people with communicable diseases, you should take additional precautions beyond those required by departmental policy.
  - **A.** True
  - **B.** False

27. If a homeless person is unable to afford medical bills, it is your job to help the patient get health care regardless of his or her financial situation.
  - **A.** True
  - **B.** False

28. When approaching a patient with a seeing eye dog in a harness, pet the dog to show that you mean no harm to its owner.
  - **A.** True
  - **B.** False

29. A quadriplegic patient has been paralyzed from the waist down.
  - **A.** True
  - **B.** False

30. It is not uncommon for children with juvenile rheumatoid arthritis (JRA) to suffer complications involving the spleen or liver.
  - **A.** True
  - **B.** False

31. If a cancer patient has an implanted infusion port, you can generally hook up your IV fluids to this port.
  - **A.** True
  - **B.** False

32. It is not uncommon for people with more obvious disabilities and who have accepted their impairments to neglect to include this in their pertinent medical history.
  - **A.** True
  - **B.** False

33. One of the most effective means of communication with a deaf patient is the use of writing.
  - **A.** True
  - **B.** False

34. If not treated, glaucoma leads to peripheral vision loss and blindness.
  - **A.** True
  - **B.** False

35. One should always pretend to understand speech impairment patients, even when you do not.
  - **A.** True
  - **B.** False

Matching

Write the letter of the term in the space provided next to the appropriate description.

A.	labyrinthitis	**F.**	sensorineural deafness
B.	conductive deafness	**G.**	sensory aphasia
C.	motor aphasia	**H.**	otitis media
D.	deafness	**I.**	neutropenic
E.	diabetic retinopathy	**J.**	colostomy

_____ **36.** an inability to hear

_____ **37.** middle ear infection

_____ **38.** occurs when the patient cannot speak but can understand what is said

_____ **39.** a surgical diversion of the large intestine through an opening in the skin where the fecal matter is collected in a pouch

_____ **40.** a condition that results in an abnormally low white blood cell count

_____ **41.** occurs when a patient cannot understand the spoken word

_____ **42.** inner ear infection that causes vertigo, nausea, and an unsteady gait

_____ **43.** caused when there is a blocking of the transmission of the sound waves through the external ear canal to the middle or inner ear

_____ **44.** caused by the inability of nerve impulses to reach the auditory center of the brain because of nerve damage either to the inner ear or to the brain

_____ **45.** slow loss of vision as a result of damage done by diabetes

Chapter 46

Acute Interventions for the Chronic-Care Patient

Review of Chapter Objectives

After reading this chapter, you should be able to:

1. **Compare and contrast the primary objectives of the paramedic and the home care provider. pp. 1108, 1112-1113**

The paramedic's primary role is to identify and treat any life-threatening problems and transport as necessary. Home care providers, on the other hand, assume responsibility, in varying degrees, for managing a chronic condition in the home setting and for helping the patient to live as normally as possible. A paramedic provides acute interventions; a home care provider provides ongoing care per medical directives, usually from a physician.

2. **Identify the importance of home health care medicine as it relates to emergency medical services. pp. 1107-1108**

The shift to home health care has important implications for emergency medical services. As patients assume greater responsibility for their own treatment and recovery, the likelihood of ALS intervention for the chronic-care patient increases. Calls may come from the patient, the patient's family, or a home health care provider.

In home care settings, you can expect to encounter a sometimes dizzying array of devices, machines, and equipment designed to provide anything from supportive to life-sustaining care. The failure or malfunction of this type of equipment has the potential to become a life-threatening or life-altering event.

In a call involving a home care patient, you are responding to a patient who is already sick or injured in some way. A previously manageable condition may have suddenly become unmanageable or more complicated. Unlike in a hospital, the patient or home care provider cannot push a button and summon immediate help. Instead, they often summon you, the ALS provider.

3. **Differentiate between the role of the paramedic and the role of the home care provider. pp. 1108, 1112-1113**

As noted in objective 1, the paramedic provides acute interventions for the chronically ill patient who relies in some way on a home care provider who helps to manage his or her condition. Remember that the home care provider—whether it be a nurse, nurse's aide, family member, or friend—usually knows the patient better than anyone else. The provider will often spot subtle changes in the patient's condition that may seem insignificant to the outsider. In assessing the patient, it is crucial that you listen carefully to what this person says.

4. Compare and contrast the primary objectives of acute care, home care, and hospice care. pp. 1108, 1112-1113, 1138

• **Acute care**—focuses on short-term intervention aimed at identifying and managing any immediate life-threatening emergencies, using transport as needed.

• **Home care**—involves the ongoing care and supportive assistance required to help a patient manage an injury or a chronic condition, usually according to a physician's instructions or written orders; home care may be either short-term or long-term.

• **Hospice care**—provides a program of palliative care and support services that address the physical, social, economic, and spiritual needs of terminally ill patients and their families.

5. Discuss aspects of home care that enhance the quality of patient care and aspects that have the potential to become detrimental. pp. 1107-1123

Supporters of home health care offer several arguments in its favor. First, they point out that patients often recover faster in the familiar environments of their homes than in the hospital. They also emphasize the differences in the cost of home care versus hospital care. However, the technological devices required by many home care patients can—and do—fail. Family members may either willingly accept the responsibilities of home care or succumb to the pressure. Finally, as noted in objective 6, home care patients are susceptible to a wide variety of complications related to their particular treatments and/or conditions.

6. List pathologies and complications in home care patients that commonly result in ALS intervention. pp. 1108-1113

A number of situations can involve you in the treatment of a home care patient—equipment failure, unexpected complications, absence of a caregiver, need for transport, the inability to operate a device, and more. Many of the medical problems that you will encounter in a home care setting are the same ones that you would encounter elsewhere in the field. Some of the typical responses involve airway complications, respiratory failure, cardiac decompensation, alterations in peripheral circulation, altered mental status, GI/GU crises, infections and/or septic complications.

In providing ALS intervention, you must always keep in mind that the home care patient is in a more fragile state to begin with. A member of the medical community has already decided that the person needs extra help. A home care patient is more likely to decompensate and go into crisis more quickly than a member of the general population. As a result you need to monitor the home care patient carefully and be ready to intervene at all times.

7. Compare the cost, mortality, and quality of care for a given patient in the hospital versus the home care setting. pp. 1107-1108

The steady rise in hospital charges and the cost of skilled nursing facilities prompted the growth of home health care, along with other factors such as the enactment of Medicare, advent of HMOs, increased medical acceptance, and improved medical technology. With total health expenditures expected to rise by an estimated 7.5 percent in the first decade of the 2000s, the savings promised by home health care continues to speed the dismissal of patients from hospitals and nursing homes. As indicated in objective 5, there are tradeoffs to be made in treating a patient in the hospital versus a home care setting.

8. Discuss the significance of palliative care programs as related to a patient in a home health care or hospice setting. pp. 1112-1113, 1138

A patient in the home care setting is usually receiving curative care aimed at healing the patient's illness or injury. If a patient's condition is terminal, treatment switches to palliative or comfort care. The goal is relieve symptoms, manage pain, and give patients control over the end of their lives. Palliative care may be provided by hospice workers in the patient's home or in homes or apartments managed by hospices.

9. **Define hospice care, comfort care, and DNR/DNAR as they relate to local practice, law, and policy. pp. 1112-1113, 1118, 1138-1140**

Hospice care provides a program of palliative or comfort care as well as support services that address the physical, social, economic, and spiritual needs of terminally ill patients and their families. The goal of hospice care is very different than the goal of most other branches of the health care professions, including EMS. For an ALS team, care is usually geared toward aggressive and life-saving treatment. A hospice team, on the other hand, seeks to make the patient as comfortable as possible.

For the most part, patients in hospice situations have already exhausted or declined curative resources. As a rule, family members, caregivers, and health care workers have been instructed to call a hospice rather than EMS. However, you may be summoned for intervention, particularly in situations involving transport. In such cases, you should keep in mind that the hospice patient is in an end-stage disease and has already expressed wishes to withhold resuscitation. In all likelihood the patient will probably have a Do Not Resuscitate (DNR) or Do Not Attempt Resuscitation (DNAR) order in place. However, such orders should not prevent you from performing palliative or comfort care.

Local protocols may vary in respect to DNRs, DNARs, living wills, and durable power of attorney documents. Be sure that you are familiar with these legal statements and their implications for care of the terminally ill.

10. **List and describe the characteristics of typical home care devices related to airway maintenance, artificial and alveolar ventilation, vascular access, drug administration, and the GI/GU tract.   pp. 1112-1112, 1119, 1123-1135**

You can expect to encounter a vast number of machines and devices in the home care situation—anything from a home dialysis unit to personal care items such as a long-handled shoehorn to wheelchairs, canes, and walkers. Examples of typical equipment aimed at airway maintenance and/or ventilation include portable suctioning devices, nebulized and aerosolized medication administrators, incentive spirometers, home ventilators, apnea monitors, tracheostomy tubes or collars, and oxygen delivery systems (oxygen concentrators, oxygen masks, liquid oxygen reservoirs, regulator-flow meters, nasal cannulas, tubing, and sterile water).

Patients may also have any variety of vascular access devices (VADs). Patients may have a peripherally inserted central catheter (PICC line) or a surgically implanted medication delivery system such as a Port-A-Cath or Medi-Port. Some VADs have been permanently implanted, such as a dialysis shunt or a Hickman, Broviac, or Groshong catheter.

Yet other patients may have various long-term devices to support gastrointestinal or genitourinary functions. These include urinary catheters (Texas/condom catheters or internal/Foley catheters), urostomies, nasogastric feeding tubes, or gastrostomy tubes (with a colostomy).

As these examples show, home care devices range from the simplicity of a nasal cannula to the complexity of a home ventilator. If you encounter an unfamiliar device—which may happen at some time in your career—don't panic. Find out what it's used for, and you will then have an idea how to proceed. Don't be afraid to look foolish by asking questions. You won't. You will be foolish, and endanger the patient, if you pretend to understand a device but don't. (For more detailed descriptions of the devices named, see information on pages listed in the objective.)

11. **Discuss the complications of assessing each of the devices described above. pp. 1123-1135**

Discussion of the complications for the various devices can be found on the pages indicated with this objective. However, in general, keep in mind these points.

Oxygen delivery systems
Very few problems arise from oxygen delivery systems themselves. When they do occur, patients or home care providers can usually correct the situation on their own. Some technical problems include impeded oxygen flow (faulty tubing/dirty or plugged humidifier), activation of the warning buzzer on the oxygen concentrator (unplugged unit or power failure), and hissing or rapidly depleted oxygen tank (leak).

In terms of the oxygen therapy itself, follow these guidelines:
• Ensure the ability of the patient/home care provider to administer oxygen.
• Make sure the patient knows what to do in case of a power failure.
• Evaluate sterile conditions, especially disinfections of reusable equipment.
• Remain alert to signs and symptoms of hypoxemia.

Artificial airways/tracheostomies

The most common problems faced by tracheostomy patients include blockage of the airway by mucus and a dislodged cannula. Children can also have their stoma blocked by foreign objects that enter by accident or are put there by a sibling or playmate. Other complications include infection of the stoma, drying of the mucus leading to crusting or bleeding, and tracheal erosion from an overinflated cuff (causing necrosis).

If EMS is called, it means that neither the patient nor the caregiver has been able to solve the problem. If the tracheostomy patient is on a ventilator, you must rapidly determine if the problem is with the ventilator or with the airway itself. If the problem is simply a loose fitting or disconnected tube, fix it. If the problem is not immediately apparent, do not waste time trying to troubleshoot the machine—unless you are qualified to do so. Your bag-valve device will connect directly to where the ventilator tubing connects. Remove the tubing, connect the bag-valve device to the trach connector, and ventilate.

If the problem is with the patient's airway, you will need to clear it. If the patient is hypoxic, always hyperventilate before suctioning. Remember to ensure that ventilations are directed downward toward the lungs. If you are unable to ventilate, clearing the airway is your first priority. If it appears that the inner cannula is blocked or dislodged, you may remove it. If necessary, you may intubate the stoma. Once the airway is secure, you may proceed with the rest of your assessment. It is inappropriate to proceed until you have protected the airway.

Ventilators

Ventilatory problems are traditionally easy to remedy, such as in the case of unplugged power cords or a temporary loss of electricity. If you are familiar with the ventilator, you can remedy other problems by adjusting the settings to restore or improve ventilations. However, if you are unfamiliar with the ventilator, play it safe and support ventilations with your own equipment. Remember—if a home ventilator fails, begin manual positive-pressure ventilation immediately. Whatever interventions you choose, you will have to make arrangements for home devices to be transported with you to the hospital.

Vascular access devices

In the case of patients with VADs, the most common complications result from various types of obstructions. A thrombus may form at the catheter site, or an embolus may lodge there after formation elsewhere in the body. Other obstructive problems include catheter kinking or catheter tip embolus. With central venous access devices, always be aware of the potential for an air embolus. Of course, any device implanted in the body has a risk for infection. Because these catheters provide a channel into the central circulation, patients may quickly become septic, especially if they are weakened or immunosuppressed.

Urinary devices

Most complications related to urinary tract support devices result from infection or device malfunctions. Infection is a very common problem with urinary tract devices because the area is rich with pathogens and because the catheter provides a pathway directly into the body. Remain alert to foul-smelling urine or altered urine color, such as tea-colored, cloudy, or blood-tinged urine. Also look for signs and symptoms of systemic infection, or urosepsis, as urinary infections can quickly spread in the immunocompromised patient.

Device malfunctions typically include accidental displacement of the device, obstruction, balloon ruptures in devices that use a balloon as an anchor, or leaking collection devices. Changes in the patient's anatomy, such as a shortened urinary tract or tissue necrosis, can also cause malfunctions. Ensure that the collection device is empty and record the amount of urine output. Look for kinks or other obstructions in the device and make sure the collection bag is placed below the patient.

Gastrointestinal tract devices

Complications from GI tract devices include tube misplacement, obstruction, or infection. Because misplaced tubes can obstruct the airway or GI system, you should always ensure device patency if you have any doubts about placement of the tube. First, have the patient speak to you. If he or she cannot speak, the tube may be in the airway and need to be removed. Second, to ensure patency of an NG tube, use a 60 mL syringe to insert air into the stomach. Use your stethoscope to listen over the epigastrium for air movement within the stomach. A low-pitched rumbling should be heard. You may also note stomach contents spontaneously moving up the tube or they may be aspirated with a 60 cc syringe. In such cases, patients may be repositioned to return patency, or the device reinserted.

Tubes are also prone to obstruction. Colostomies may become clogged or otherwise obstructed. Feeding tubes can become clogged due to the thick consistency of supplemental feedings or pill fragments. As a result, the tubes may require irrigation with water. In addition, the thick consistency of food may cause bowel obstructions or constipation.

As might be expected, ostomies can become infected or lose skin integrity from pressure. Look for signs and symptoms of skin or systemic infection. In addition, remember that digestive enzymes may leak from various ostomies and begin to digest the skin and abdominal contents.

12. Describe indications, contraindications, and techniques for urinary catheter insertion in the male and female patient in an out-of-hospital setting.   pp. 1132

There are various medical devices designed to support patients with urinary tract dysfunction. External devices, such as Texas catheters or condom catheters, attach to the male external genitalia to collect urine. Because these devices are not inserted into the urethra, they reduce the risk of infection. However, they do not collect urine in a sterile manner, nor are they adequate for long-term use.

Internal catheters, such as Foley or indwelling catheters, are the most commonly used devices for urinary tract dysfunction. They are long catheters with a balloon tip that is inserted through the urethra into the urinary bladder. The balloon is then inflated with saline to keep the device in place. Internal catheters are well tolerated for long-term use and are frequently found in hospitals, skilled nursing facilities, or home care situations.

Suprapubic catheters are similar in purpose to internal catheters. However, they are inserted directly through the abdominal wall into the urinary bladder. Suprapubic catheters may be used instead of indwelling catheters in the event of surgery or other problems with the genitalia or bladder. In nearly all cases, insertion of urinary catheters is performed in a medical setting.

13. Identify failure of GI/GU, ventilatory, vascular access, and drain devices found in the home care setting.   pp. 1123-1135

See appropriate portions of points listed in objective 11.

14. Discuss the relationship between local home care treatment protocols/SOPs and local EMS protocols/SOPs.   p. 1113

In responding to a call involving a home care patient, remember that you may not be the first person to provide intervention. If home care patients have a good relationship with their home health care practitioner or physician, they may contact this person first. If fact, they may be required to do so in order to receive reimbursement for medical services. As a result, be sure to ask whether a patient has called another health care professional. If so, find out what instructions or medications have been issued. Also inquire about written orders from the physician or the physician-approved health care plan. Health care agencies resubmit these plans to physicians at least every 62 days. So check the date to see when the plan was last revised.

If the call involved a hospice patient, the situation will almost always require intervention by specially trained health care professionals. Find out the names of these people as quickly as possible and determine the advisability of consultations versus rapid transport.

15. Discuss differences in the ability of individuals to accept and cope with their own impending death. p. 1140

Each patient deals with his or her impending death in a different manner. Some can come to grips with it, while others refuse to believe they are going to die. Remember that while hospice prepares patients for their death, patients without hospice may be ill-prepared for the end stages of life. Don't assume that all terminally ill patients are under hospice care. A simple question to determine the presence of hospice may alter your course of treatment and approach to the patient.

16. List the stages of the grief process and relate them to an individual in hospice care. p. 1140

Regardless of whether a patient is in hospice or not, keep in mind the stages of the grief process—denial, anger, depression, bargaining, and acceptance. Remember that both the patient and the family will go through these stages, and, in the case of the terminally ill, the patient may have reached acceptance well ahead of those who will remain behind.

17. Discuss the rights of the terminally ill patient. pp. 1138-1140

In treating a terminally ill patient, you need to establish communication with the home care worker as quickly as possible. Your inclination may be to intubate, start a line, or administer medications. However, palliative care supersedes curative care. A hospice worker, when faced with the end stage of a disease, may do nothing in accordance with the patient's wishes, whether those wishes are expressed through a family member or a written document. If you are called to the house, it is your responsibility to respect the wishes of the patient and the ideas of hospice care.

18. Summarize the types of home health care available in your area and the services provided. pp. 1107-1112

There is a wide variety of home health care services provided in every community, ranging from professional home care agencies to unpaid volunteers. Find out what services operate in your area, using sources such as local hospitals (which arrange referrals) or county health departments (which certify and/or regulate many agencies).

19. Given a series of home care scenarios, determine which patients should receive follow-up home care and which should be transported to an emergency care facility. pp. 1113-1118

During your classroom, clinical, and field training, you will assess real and simulated patients and decide which patients should be transported to the hospital and which should receive additional care in the out-of-hospital setting. Use the information in this text chapter, the information on chronic home care patients in the field presented by your instructors, and the guidance given by your clinical and field preceptors to develop good assessment and decision making skills in regard to patient transport. Continue to refine these skills once your training ends and you begin your career as a paramedic.

20. Given a series of scenarios, demonstrate interaction and support with the family members/support persons for a patient who has died. pp. 1138-1140

Approaching the family members/support persons left behind after a patient has died is never easy, even if they have had the help of hospice. As noted in the text, many times the terminally ill patients are more prepared for their impending death than their family or caregivers. However, they, too, must go through the stages of grieving—denial, anger, depression, bargaining, and acceptance. Use practice scenarios to draw upon the information in this text chapter and suggestions presented by your instructors and clinical and field preceptors to develop the communication skills needed to manage this difficult situation. Continue to refine these skills once your training ends and you begin your career as a paramedic. Also find out about stress management programs provided by your agency so that you can get support after such a call has ended.

CONTENT SELF-EVALUATION

Multiple Choice

1. All of the following factors have promoted the growth of home care in recent years EXCEPT:
   A. enactment of Medicare.
   B. the advent of HMOs.
   C. an increase in malpractice lawsuits.
   D. changes in the attitudes of doctors and patients toward hospital care.
   E. improved medical technology.

2. Common reasons for ALS intervention in the treatment of a home care patient include all of the following EXCEPT:
   A. inability to operate a device.
   B. absence of a caregiver.
   C. equipment failure.
   D. need for transport.
   E. pain management.

3. Home care providers can be of great assistance to EMS crews because they:
   A. have more experience in the field of prehospital medicine.
   B. will often spot subtle changes in the patient's condition.
   C. will easily grasp technical medical language.
   D. have legal authority to speak for the patient.
   E. both C and D

4. Common causes of cardiac decompensation—a true medical emergency leading to shock—include all of the following EXCEPT:
   A. acute myocardial infarction.
   B. stroke.
   C. cardiac hypertrophy.
   D. sepsis.
   E. heart transplant.

5. Signs and symptoms of sepsis in a patient with an indwelling device can include:
   A. cyanosis at the infection site.
   B. fever.
   C. increased urination.
   D. cool skin at the insertion site.
   E. all of the above

6. The ability of the skin to return to normal appearance after being subjected to pressure is called:
   A. capillary refill.
   B. tenting.
   C. turgor.
   D. diaphoresis.
   E. hypertrophy.

7. Conditions that may be treated in a home care setting include:
   A. brain or spinal trauma.
   B. arthritis.
   C. AIDS.
   D. both B and C
   E. all of the above

8. Examples of commonly used medical devices in the home care setting includes all of the following EXCEPT:
   A. glucometers.
   B. tracheostomies.
   C. apnea monitors.
   D. heart/lung machines.
   E. dialysis units.

9. The matrix for injury prevention developed by William Haddon includes all of the following steps EXCEPT:

A. prevent the creation of the hazard in the first place.

B. counter the damage done by the hazard.

C. increase the release of an already existing hazard.

D. modify the basic qualities of the hazard.

E. separate the hazard and that which is to be protected by a barrier.

10. In responding to any home care situation, you should remember that:

A. any bed-bound patient may have pressure sores.

B. hospital beds, wheelchairs, or walkers may be contaminated by body fluid.

C. medical wastes may not be properly contained.

D. sharps may be present.

E. all of the above

11. Of the following acute home care situations, the one LEAST commonly encountered by paramedics is:

A. respiratory disorders.

B. end stages of a hospice patient.

C. cardiac problems.

D. GI/GU disorders.

E. use of vascular access devices.

12. In treating home care patients with cystic fibrosis (CF), the patient will probably be:

A. over age 65.

B. between 40 and 60 years old.

C. of almost any age.

D. under age 40.

E. an infant.

13. Which of the following is an advantage of oxygen therapy for the home care patient?

A. It is relatively easy to manage.

B. Most patients tolerate it easily.

C. Oxygen therapy adds to the quality of life.

D. Oxygen prevents hypoxic states.

E. all of the above

14. If a buzzer goes off on an oxygen concentrator, you would mostly likely suspect:

A. faulty tubing.

B. a leak in the tank.

C. a dirty or plugged humidifier.

D. power failure.

E. either A or C

15. Routine care of a tracheostomy includes all of the following EXCEPT:

A. keeping the stoma clean and dry.

B. removing the device daily.

C. frequent suctioning.

D. changing the ventilator hose routinely.

E. periodically changing/cleaning of the inner cannula.

16. Which of the following ventilatory options are you LEAST likely to find in a home care setting?

A. PEEP

B. CPAP

C. BIPAP

D. poncho-wrap

E. both A and C

17. The most common complication found in patients with VADs results from:

A. an embolus.

B. dehydration.

C. a thrombus.

D. hypertension.

E. both A and C

18. The most commonly used device for urinary tract dysfunction is a(n):

A. Texas catheter.

B. urostomy.

C. Foley catheter.

D. suprapubic catheter.

E. condom catheter.

19. The most common complications related to urinary tract support devices result from:
- **A.** obstructions.
- **B.** device malfunctions.
- **C.** infections.
- **D.** misplacement of devices.
- **E.** both B and C

20. If you have any doubts about the placement of a nasogastric feeding tube, your first step should be to:
- **A.** listen for air movement within the stomach.
- **B.** use a 60 mL syringe to insert air into the stomach.
- **C.** have the patient speak to you.
- **D.** irrigate the tube with water.
- **E.** immediately remove the tube.

21. The stages in the grief process for both the patient and those left behind are:
- **A.** depression, bargaining, guilt, anger, acceptance.
- **B.** anger, denial, bargaining, guilt, acceptance.
- **C.** denial, bargaining, anger, acceptance, guilt.
- **D.** bargaining, denial, anger, guilt, acceptance.
- **E.** denial, anger, depression, bargaining, acceptance.

22. In utilizing drains for the treatment of acute infections of open wounds, which type of drain includes a suction bulb?
- **A.** Penman .
- **B.** Wrenford .
- **C.** Jackson-Pratt
- **D.** Pickford
- **E.** Thibault

23. Which of the following is NOT a sign of respiratory or cardiac insufficiency in a infant?
- **A.** tachycardia
- **B.** cyanosis
- **C.** respiratory distress
- **D.** bradycardia
- **E.** crackles

24. In cases of respiratory and/or cardiovascular insufficiency in an infant with a heart rate of 50, the most appropriate resuscitative measures include.
- **A.** ventilation with a bag valve mask
- **B.** CPR
- **C.** chest thrusts
- **D.** oxygen delivery by blow-by device
- **E.** none

25. Common diseases that you can expect to see in a hospice include which of the following:
- **A.** AIDS
- **B.** cystic fibrosis
- **C.** congestive heart failure
- **D.** cancer
- **E.** all of the above

True/False

26. As patients assume greater responsibility for their own treatment and recovery, the likelihood of ALS intervention for the chronic-care patient increases.
- **A.** True
- **B.** False

27. A home care patient is less likely to decompensate and will go into crisis less quickly than the general population.
- **A.** True
- **B.** False

28. One reason that diabetics get gangrene is due to slowed circulation to the extremities.
A. True
B. False

29. Home interventions such as peritoneal dialysis can alter electrolytes.
A. True
B. False

30. It is a serious mistake to arrive on the scene with a "take-over" mentality that all but eliminates the home care provider.
A. True
B. False

31. In assessing home care patients, the focus of your physical exam should be on the patient's chronic condition.
A. True
B. False

32. When providing intervention to home care patients with chronic respiratory diseases, remember that they usually have a low dosing regimen, which may make them more responsive to their medications.
A. True
B. False

33. Patients with VADs will be much more prone to bleeding disorders than the general population.

A. True
B. False

34. In terms of providing care, the goal of hospices closely resembles the goal of EMS services.
A. True
B. False

35. When assessing a chronic-care patient, tailor your questions to the home care setting.

A. True
B. False

Matching

Write the letter of the term in the space provided next to the appropriate description.

A.	hypertrophy	**F.**	cellulitis
B.	hemoptysis	**G.**	gangrene
C.	exocrine	**H.**	turgor
D.	demylenation	**I.**	cor pulmonale
E.	emesis	**J.**	sensorium

36. destruction or removal of the myelin sheath of nerve tissue; found in Guillain-Barré syndrome

37. death of tissue or bone, usually from an insufficient blood supply

38. disorder involving external secretions

39. an increase in the size of an organ or structure caused by growth rather than by tumor

40. ability of the skin to return to normal appearance after being subjected to pressure

41. sensory apparatus of the body as a whole; also that portion of the brain that functions as a center of sensations

_____ **42.** inflammation of cellular or connective tissue

_____ **43.** expectoration of blood arising from the oral cavity, larynx, trachea, bronchi, or lungs

_____ **44.** vomitus

_____ **45.** congestive heart failure secondary to pulmonary hypertension

Answer Key

59.	J	*p.* 40
60.	C	*p.* 36

Chapter 18: Penetrating Trauma

Multiple Choice

1.	C	*p.* 44
2.	C	*p.* 45
3.	C	*p.* 46
4.	B	*p.* 46
5.	E	*p.* 46
6.	E	*p.* 50
7.	A	*p.* 53
8.	C	*p.* 53
9.	E	*p.* 54
10.	A	*p.* 53
11.	C	*p.* 55
12.	B	*p.* 56
13.	A	*p.* 57
14.	D	*p.* 58
15.	C	*p.* 59
16.	E	*p.* 60
17.	D	*p.* 61
18.	C	*p.* 62
19.	B	*p.* 57
20.	A	*p.* 52
21.	B	*p.* 53
22.	E	*p.* 57
23.	B	*p.* 57
24.	D	*p.* 62
25.	E	*p.* 56

True/False

26.	A	*p.* 46
27.	A	*p.* 48
28.	A	*p.* 48
29.	A	*p.* 51
30.	A	*p.* 57
31.	A	*p.* 58
32.	B	*p.* 59
33.	A	*p.* 51
34.	A	*p.* 60
35.	A	*p.* 63

Matching

36.	J	*p.* 46
37.	G	*p.* 62
38.	D	*p.* 46
39.	A	*p.* 46
40.	E	*p.* 46
41.	H	*p.* 47
42.	F	*p.* 47
43.	I	*p.* 47
44.	C	*p.* 62
45.	B	*p.* 55

Chapter 19: Hemorrhage and Shock

Multiple Choice

1.	D	*p.* 66
2.	B	*p.* 66
3.	A	*p.* 66
4.	D	*p.* 66
5.	D	*p.* 66
6.	E	*p.* 68
7.	B	*p.* 71
8.	B	*p.* 73
9.	A	*p.* 72
10.	B	*p.* 73
11.	C	*p.* 73
12.	E	*p.* 74
13.	D	*p.* 74
14.	A	*p.* 74
15.	C	*p.* 77
16.	B	*p.* 78
17.	E	*p.* 79
18.	E	*p.* 79
19.	E	*p.* 80
20.	D	*p.* 80
21.	B	*p.* 81
22.	B	*p.* 84
23.	B	*p.* 84
24.	A	*p.* 84
25.	C	*p.* 86
26.	E	*p.* 86
27.	D	*p.* 87
28.	B	*p.* 88
29.	E	*p.* 89
30.	C	*p.* 89
31.	E	*p.* 90
32.	B	*p.* 90
33.	E	*p.* 91
34.	A	*p.* 92
35.	E	*p.* 68

True/False

36.	B	*p.* 66
37.	A	*p.* 68
38.	A	*p.* 74
39.	A	*p.* 76
40.	B	*p.* 86
41.	A	*p.* 86
42.	B	*p.* 66
43.	B	*p.* 69
44.	B	*p.* 73
45.	B	*p.* 78

Matching

46.	I	*p.* 65
47.	D	*p.* 78

48.	E	*p.* 73
49.	C	*p.* 69
50.	B	*p.* 84
51.	G	*p.* 83
52.	A	*p.* 65
53.	H	*p.* 72
54.	J	*p.* 84
55.	F	*p.* 71

Chapter 20: Soft-Tissue Trauma

Multiple Choice

1.	B	*p.* 95
2.	E	*p.* 99
3.	B	*p.* 96
4.	C	*p.* 96
5.	D	*p.* 100
6.	E	*p.* 97
7.	B	*p.* 98
8.	A	*p.* 100
9.	D	*p.* 100
10.	B	*p.* 102
11.	B	*p.* 103
12.	B	*p.* 104
13.	A	*p.* 104
14.	E	*p.* 105
15.	C	*p.* 105
16.	E	*p.* 106
17.	E	*p.* 107
18.	E	*p.* 107
19.	A	*p.* 108
20.	A	*p.* 108
21.	C	*p.* 109
22.	E	*p.* 110
23.	D	*p.* 112
24.	A	*p.* 113
25.	E	*p.* 115
26.	B	*p.* 120
27.	E	*p.* 121
28.	C	*p.* 122
29.	B	*p.* 122
30.	C	*p.* 124
31.	D	*p.* 124
32.	A	*p.* 125
33.	C	*p.* 125
34.	E	*p.* 127
35.	E	*p.* 128
36.	D	*p.* 129
37.	E	*p.* 129
38.	B	*p.* 130
39.	A	*p.* 130
40.	E	*p.* 130
41.	C	*p.* 130
42.	E	*p.* 132

43.	E	*p.* 108
44.	A	*p.* 104
45.	B	*p.* 104

True/False

46.	B	*p.* 101
47.	B	*p.* 103
48.	A	*p.* 106
49.	B	*p.* 109
50.	A	*p.* 106
51.	A	*p.* 114
52.	A	*p.* 118
53.	B	*p.* 125
54.	A	*p.* 121
55.	A	*p.* 122

Matching

56.	C	*p.* 97
57.	J	*p.* 104
58.	A	*p.* 96
59.	I	*p.* 102
60.	H	*p.* 108
61.	E	*p.* 96
62.	B	*p.* 107
63.	D	*p.* 98
64.	F	*p.* 105
65.	G	*p.* 96

Chapter 21: Burns

Multiple Choice

1.	D	*p.* 136
2.	D	*p.* 137
3.	B	*p.* 137
4.	A	*p.* 137
5.	C	*p.* 139
6.	E	*p.* 140
7.	B	*p.* 141
8.	C	*p.* 143
9.	A	*p.* 143
10.	E	*p.* 143
11.	D	*p.* 144
12.	C	*p.* 144
13.	E	*p.* 144
14.	C	*p.* 145
15.	D	*p.* 146
16.	B	*p.* 147
17.	C	*p.* 147
18.	B	*p.* 147
19.	C	*p.* 148
20.	D	*p.* 148
21.	E	*p.* 148
22.	E	*p.* 148
23.	E	*p.* 150
24.	B	*p.* 152

25.	B	*p. 155*
26.	E	*p. 155*
27.	A	*p. 155*
28.	D	*p. 155*
29.	D	*p. 155*
30.	D	*p. 155*
31.	A	*p. 157*
32.	B	*p. 157*
33.	B	*p. 158*
34.	A	*p. 158*
35.	B	*p. 158*
36.	B	*p. 158*
37.	B	*p. 159*
38.	A	*p. 159*
39.	E	*p. 160*
40.	C	*p. 160*
41.	D	*p. 162*
42.	E	*p. 162*
43.	C	*p. 162*
44.	D	*p. 163*
45.	A	*p. 164*

True/False

46.	A	*p. 136*
47.	A	*p. 136*
48.	A	*p. 140*
49.	B	*p. 140*
50.	B	*p. 140*
51.	A	*p. 153*
52.	A	*p. 153*
53.	B	*p. 153*
54.	A	*p. 157*
55.	B	*p. 158*

Matching

56.	F	*p. 149*
57.	J	*p. 137*
58.	H	*p. 163*
59.	I	*p. 145*
60.	C	*p. 140*
61.	B	*p. 138*
62.	G	*p. 145*
63.	A	*p. 137*
64.	D	*p. 147*
65.	E	*p. 141*

Chapter 22: Musculoskeletal Trauma

Multiple Choice

1.	E	*p. 168*
2.	C	*p. 170*
3.	B	*p. 170*
4.	B	*p. 171*
5.	A	*p. 171*
6.	E	*p. 173*

7.	B	*p. 173*
8.	A	*p. 175*
9.	E	*p. 175*
10.	C	*p. 176*
11.	A	*p. 177*
12.	D	*p. 177*
13.	A	*p. 179*
14.	E	*p. 179*
15.	E	*p. 179*
16.	C	*p. 182*
17.	C	*p. 182*
18.	A	*p. 184*
19.	E	*p. 185*
20.	A	*p. 187*
21.	D	*p. 187*
22.	C	*p. 189*
23.	D	*p. 189*
24.	B	*p. 190*
25.	E	*p. 190*
26.	E	*p. 190*
27.	D	*p. 190*
28.	E	*p. 191*
29.	D	*p. 192*
30.	E	*p. 193*
31.	B	*p. 194*
32.	A	*p. 195*
33.	C	*p. 195*
34.	C	*p. 196*
35.	A	*p. 196*
36.	A	*p. 197*
37.	E	*p. 198*
38.	E	*p. 200*
39.	D	*p. 201*
40.	B	*p. 202*

True/False

41.	A	*p. 168*
42.	A	*p. 174*
43.	B	*p. 176*
44.	A	*p. 176*
45.	B	*p. 183*
46.	A	*p. 184*
47.	A	*p. 184*
48.	B	*p. 189*
49.	B	*p. 196*
50.	B	*p. 198*

Matching

51.	F	*p. 173*
52.	G	*p. 177*
53.	J	*p. 171*
54.	D	*p. 176*
55.	C	*p. 172*
56.	I	*p. 175*
57.	A	*p. 171*
58.	B	*p. 175*

| 59. | H | *p.* 174 |
| 60. | E | *p.* 171 |

Chapter 23: Head, Facial, and Neck Trauma

Multiple Choice

1.	A	*p.* 206
2.	D	*p.* 206
3.	E	*p.* 209
4.	C	*p.* 209
5.	D	*p.* 210
6.	B	*p.* 210
7.	B	*p.* 210
8.	D	*p.* 212
9.	E	*p.* 212
10.	B	*p.* 213
11.	C	*p.* 213
12.	E	*p.* 214
13.	C	*p.* 214
14.	B	*p.* 215
15.	C	*p.* 215
16.	C	*p.* 215
17.	A	*p.* 216
18.	E	*p.* 217
19.	A	*p.* 217
20.	C	*p.* 218
21.	A	*p.* 219
22.	B	*p.* 219
23.	E	*p.* 221
24.	E	*p.* 221
25.	A	*p.* 222
26.	C	*p.* 223
27.	C	*p.* 224
28.	B	*p.* 227
29.	E	*p.* 227
30.	A	*p.* 227
31.	C	*p.* 228
32.	B	*p.* 229
33.	E	*p.* 229
34.	B	*p.* 230
35.	D	*p.* 230
36.	E	*p.* 231
37.	C	*p.* 233
38.	A	*p.* 233
39.	A	*p.* 234
40.	E	*p.* 236
41.	D	*p.* 238
42.	C	*p.* 239
43.	B	*p.* 240
44.	D	*p.* 241
45.	B	*p.* 242
46.	E	*p.* 243
47.	C	*p.* 243
48.	B	*p.* 246
49.	D	*p.* 216

| 50. | A | *p.* 224 |

True/False

51.	A	*p.* 208
52.	B	*p.* 208
53.	B	*p.* 210
54.	A	*p.* 211
55.	A	*p.* 214
56.	A	*p.* 219
57.	A	*p.* 219
58.	A	*p.* 233
59.	B	*p.* 236
60.	A	*p.* 236

Matching

61.	C	*p.* 220
62.	H	*p.* 213
63.	I	*p.* 217
64.	J	*p.* 219
65.	B	*p.* 241
66.	A	*p.* 214
67.	D	*p.* 211
68.	E	*p.* 222
69.	F	*p.* 215
70.	G	*p.* 217

Chapter 24: Spinal Trauma

Multiple Choice

1.	E	*p.* 251
2.	A	*p.* 253
3.	A	*p.* 253
4.	E	*p.* 255
5.	A	*p.* 255
6.	D	*p.* 256
7.	C	*p.* 258
8.	C	*p.* 258
9.	A	*p.* 260
10.	E	*p.* 260
11.	A	*p.* 263
12.	E	*p.* 262
13.	B	*p.* 263
14.	B	*p.* 265
15.	E	*p.* 266
16.	B	*p.* 270
17.	E	*p.* 273
18.	D	*p.* 273
19.	B	*p.* 274
20.	B	*p.* 254
21.	B	*p.* 273
22.	B	*p.* 264
23.	D	*p.* 268
24.	C	*p.* 273
25.	E	*p.* 253

True/False

26.	A	*p.* 252
27.	A	*p.* 254
28.	B	*p.* 253
29.	B	*p.* 257
30.	A	*p.* 258
31.	A	*p.* 262
32.	B	*p.* 263
33.	A	*p.* 267
34.	A	*p.* 269
35.	A	*p.* 269

Matching

36.	H	*p.* 252
37.	G	*p.* 254
38.	J	*p.* 254
39.	I	*p.* 255
40.	B	*p.* 260
41.	F	*p.* 254
42.	E	*p.* 259
43.	A	*p.* 254
44.	C	*p.* 260
45.	D	*p.* 269

Chapter 25: Thoracic Trauma

Multiple Choice

1.	A	*p.* 278
2.	C	*p.* 279
3.	D	*p.* 281
4.	B	*p.* 281
5.	A	*p.* 281
6.	A	*p.* 282
7.	E	*p.* 282
8.	B	*p.* 283
9.	D	*p.* 284
10.	B	*p.* 285
11.	E	*p.* 283
12.	D	*p.* 287
13.	B	*p.* 287
14.	D	*p.* 287
15.	D	*p.* 288
16.	D	*p.* 288
17.	E	*p.* 289
18.	C	*p.* 289
19.	A	*p.* 290
20.	A	*p.* 290
21.	D	*p.* 292
22.	A	*p.* 292
23.	E	*p.* 293
24.	B	*p.* 293
25.	D	*p.* 293
26.	C	*p.* 294
27.	B	*p.* 294

28.	E	*p.* 294
29.	C	*p.* 294
30.	A	*p.* 295
31.	B	*p.* 296
32.	E	*p.* 296
33.	E	*p.* 297
34.	A	*p.* 298
35.	D	*p.* 299
36.	E	*p.* 299
37.	B	*p.* 300
38.	B	*p.* 301
39.	D	*p.* 302
40.	B	*p.* 303
41.	C	*p.* 303
42.	A	*p.* 304
43.	A	*p.* 305
44.	E	*p.* 307
45.	D	*p.* 307

True/False

46.	B	*p.* 284
47.	A	*p.* 289
48.	A	*p.* 293
49.	B	*p.* 295
50.	A	*p.* 302
51.	A	*p.* 303
52.	B	*p.* 283
53.	A	*p.* 287
54.	A	*p.* 281
55.	A	*p.* 285

Matching

56.	G	*p.* 290
57.	H	*p.* 277
58.	C	*p.* 291
59.	E	*p.* 293
60.	A	*p.* 277
61.	D	*p.* 285
62.	B	*p.* 285
63.	I	*p.* 293
64.	J	*p.* 288
65.	F	*p.* 283

Chapter 26: Abdominal Trauma

Multiple Choice

1.	B	*p.* 311
2.	D	*p.* 312
3.	C	*p.* 312
4.	E	*p.* 313
5.	C	*p.* 313
6.	A	*p.* 313
7.	C	*p.* 314
8.	B	*p.* 315
9.	D	*p.* 315

10.	E	*p. 315*
11.	E	*p. 315*
12.	D	*p. 316*
13.	C	*p. 316*
14.	A	*p. 317*
15.	E	*p. 317*
16.	D	*p. 318*
17.	D	*p. 318*
18.	C	*p. 319*
19.	A	*p. 319*
20.	D	*p. 321*
21.	E	*p. 322*
22.	C	*p. 325*
23.	C	*p. 325*
24.	D	*p. 325*
25.	B	*p. 326*
26.	D	*p. 326*
27.	E	*p. 313*
28.	D	*p. 314*
29.	C	*p. 323*
30.	E	*p. 313*

True/False

31.	A	*p. 311*
32.	B	*p. 311*
33.	B	*p. 313*
34.	A	*p. 315*
35.	A	*p. 317*
36.	A	*p. 319*
37.	A	*p. 319*
38.	A	*p. 326*
39.	A	*p. 326*
40.	A	*p. 321*

Matching

41.	E	*p. 316*
42.	D	*p. 313*
43.	J	*p. 316*
44.	H	*p. 314*
45.	F	*p. 313*
46.	G	*p. 318*
47.	A	*p. 313*
48.	I	*p. 313*
49.	B	*p. 313*
50.	C	*p. 315*

Chapter 27: Pulmonology

Multiple Choice

1.	C	*p. 331*
2.	A	*p. 332*
3.	A	*p. 332*
4.	D	*p. 332*
5.	E	*p. 333*
6.	C	*p. 335*

7.	D	*p. 336*
8.	B	*p. 337*
9.	B	*p. 337*
10.	E	*p. 339*
11.	B	*p. 339*
12.	A	*p. 339*
13.	C	*p. 340*
14.	B	*p. 340*
15.	A	*p. 340*
16.	B	*p. 340*
17.	A	*p. 341*
18.	C	*p. 341*
19.	E	*p. 341*
20.	D	*p. 342*
21.	D	*p. 342*
22.	D	*p. 342*
23.	B	*p. 343*
24.	E	*p. 343*
25.	B	*p. 343*
26.	E	*p. 344*
27.	D	*p. 344*
28.	C	*p. 344*
29.	C	*p. 346*
30.	E	*p. 355*
31.	C	*p. 349*
32.	A	*p. 351*
33.	A	*p. 353*
34.	B	*p. 355*
35.	B	*p. 356*
36.	B	*p. 357*
37.	D	*p. 358*
38.	D	*p. 358*
39.	B	*p. 358*
40.	B	*p. 360*
41.	B	*p. 362*
42.	A	*p. 364*
43.	D	*p. 365*
44.	C	*p. 366*
45.	A	*p. 367*
46.	C	*p. 365*
47.	D	*p. 362*
48.	A	*p. 371*
49.	C	*p. 372*
50.	B	*p. 373*
51.	B	*p. 374*
52.	E	*p. 375*
53.	D	*p. 375*
54.	C	*p. 377*
55.	C	*p. 379*
56.	C	*p. 382*
57.	D	*p. 384*
58.	B	*p. 385*
59.	A	*p. 386*
60.	C	*p. 387*
61.	C	*p. 389*
62.	C	*p. 389*

63.	A	p. 391
64.	E	p. 392
65.	B	p. 393
66.	B	p. 394
67.	D	p. 394
68.	E	p. 394
69.	A	p. 395
70.	C	p. 390
71.	B	p. 411
72.	C	p. 414
73.	A	p. 416
74.	A	p. 418
75.	E	p. 420
76.	E	p. 431
77.	B	p. 433
78.	C	p. 434
79.	C	p. 436
80.	D	p. 436
81.	D	p. 438
82.	D	p. 439
83.	A	p. 440
84.	D	p. 440

True/False

85.	A	p. 341
86.	A	p. 360
87.	A	p. 364
88.	B	p. 364
89.	A	p. 365
90.	A	p. 368
91.	A	p. 368
92.	B	p. 374
93.	B	p. 380
94.	A	p. 385
95.	B	p. 389
96.	B	p. 391
97.	B	p. 393
98.	B	p. 363
99.	A	p. 405
100.	B	p. 412

Matching

101.	C	p. 351
102.	F	p. 353
103.	A	p. 355
104.	E	p. 358
105.	G	p. 362
106.	B	p. 363
107.	D	p. 366
108.	I	p. 361
109.	H	p. 364
110.	J	p. 368

Chapter 28: Cardiology (Part I)

Multiple Choice

1.	C	p. 448
2.	A	p. 448
3.	D	p. 450
4.	E	p. 451
5.	B	p. 452
6.	E	p. 465
7.	C	p. 469
8.	D	p. 474
9.	B	p. 484
10.	E	p. 487
11.	C	p. 489
12.	D	p. 489
13.	B	p. 495
14.	E	p. 499
15.	C	p. 497
16.	D	p. 502
17.	A	p. 503
18.	C	p. 453
19.	A	p. 455
20.	B	p. 456
21.	E	p. 471
22.	C	p. 479
23.	C	p. 488
24.	D	p. 504
25.	D	p. 507

True/False

26.	B	p. 461
27.	A	p. 484
28.	A	p. 489
29.	A	p. 468
30.	B	p. 461
31.	A	p. 497
32.	B	p. 499
33.	A	p. 484
34.	B	p. 477
35.	A	p. 497

Matching

36.	B	p. 450
37.	G	p. 450
38.	D	p. 450
39.	A	p. 450
40.	H	p. 450
41.	C	p. 450
42.	F	p. 450
43.	E	p. 450
44.	B	p. 451
45.	C	p. 451

Chapter 28: Cardiology (Part II)

Multiple Choice

1. D   *p.* 526
2. E   *p.* 526
3. B   *p.* 526
4. B   *p.* 531
5. A   *p.* 537
6. E   *p.* 549
7. B   *p.* 552
8. D   *p.* 558
9. D   *p.* 515
10. C   *p.* 524
11. B   *p.* 525
12. D   *p.* 526
13. D   *p.* 528
14. E   *p.* 528
15. B   *p.* 528
16. A   *p.* 531
17. B   *p.* 532
18. D   *p.* 537
19. C   *p.* 545
20. D   *p.* 556
21. A   *p.* 551
22. C   *p.* 560
23. B   *p.* 553
24. D   *p.* 562
25. C   *p.* 550

True/False

26. A   *p.* 512
27. A   *p.* 555
28. B   *p.* 513
29. A   *p.* 517
30. B   *p.* 519
31. A   *p.* 533
32. A   *p.* 540
33. A   *p.* 536
34. B   *p.* 546
35. A   *p.* 520

Matching

36. E   *p.* 527
37. D   *p.* 533
38. A   *p.* 525
39. B   *p.* 531
40. C   *p.* 536
41. A   *p.* 542
42. C   *p.* 540
43. B   *p.* 540
44. B   *p.* 540
45. C   *p.* 541
46. D   *p.* 545
47. B   *p.* 546
48. F   *p.* 555
49. E   *p.* 545

50. A   *p.* 547
51. G   *p.* 549
52. H   *p.* 550
53. B   *p.* 513
54. C   *p.* 549
55. A   *p.* 560

Chapter 29: Neurology

Multiple Choice

1. C   *p.* 570
2. C   *p.* 575
3. E   *p.* 580
4. C   *p.* 583
5. B   *p.* 584
6. D   *p.* 586
7. C   *p.* 588
8. B   *p.* 590
9. B   *p.* 590
10. C   *p.* 591
11. C   *p.* 595
12. C   *p.* 600
13. E   *p.* 603
14. E   *p.* 570
15. E   *p.* 571
16. D   *p.* 572
17. B   *p.* 575
18. D   *p.* 576
19. D   *p.* 578
20. A   *p.* 579
21. B   *p.* 580
22. E   *p.* 590
23. B   *p.* 594
24. E   *p.* 593
25. A   *p.* 600

True/False

26. B   *p.* 571
27. A   *p.* 594
28. A   *p.* 587
29. B   *p.* 590
30. B   *p.* 600
31. A   *p.* 594
32. A   *p.* 601
33. B   *p.* 592
34. B   *p.* 603
35. A   *p.* 593

Matching

36. H   *p.* 597
37. C   *p.* 601
38. I   *p.* 590
39. D   *p.* 578
40. A   *p.* 599
41. E   *p.* 598

42.	G	*p. 587*
43.	F	*p. 601*
44.	J	*p. 590*
45.	B	*p. 579*

| 44. | A | *p. 609* |
| 45. | H | *p. 610* |

Chapter 30: Endocrinology

Multiple Choice

1.	C	*p. 607*
2.	C	*p. 608*
3.	C	*p. 609*
4.	E	*p. 608*
5.	B	*p. 611*
6.	D	*p. 612*
7.	E	*p. 612*
8.	A	*p. 613*
9.	A	*p. 613*
10.	C	*p. 615*
11.	E	*p. 615*
12.	B	*p. 617*
13.	A	*p. 617*
14.	E	*p. 618*
15.	B	*p. 619*
16.	A	*p. 620*
17.	A	*p. 617*
18.	D	*p. 609*
19.	B	*p. 609*
20.	A	*p. 610*
21.	D	*p. 610*
22.	B	*p. 613*
23.	A	*p. 616*
24.	B	*p. 621*
25.	A	*p. 607*

True/False

26.	A	*p. 613*
27.	A	*p. 616*
28.	A	*p. 619*
29.	B	*p. 620*
30.	A	*p. 616*
31.	A	*p. 608*
32.	A	*p. 609*
33.	A	*p. 610*
34.	B	*p. 611*
35.	B	*p. 607*

Matching

36.	F	*p. 608*
37.	B	*p. 610*
38.	J	*p. 609*
39.	E	*p. 611*
40.	C	*p. 616*
41.	D	*p. 607*
42.	G	*p. 615*
43.	I	*p. 611*

Chapter 31: Allergies and Anaphylaxis

Multiple Choice

1.	B	*p. 624*
2.	D	*p. 624*
3.	B	*p. 624*
4.	C	*p. 625*
5.	D	*p. 625*
6.	C	*p. 626*
7.	C	*p. 626*
8.	C	*p. 626*
9.	B	*p. 627*
10.	A	*p. 628*
11.	B	*p. 628*
12.	C	*p. 630*
13.	D	*p. 629*
14.	D	*p. 629*
15.	B	*p. 627*

True/False

16.	A	*p. 623*
17.	B	*p. 623*
18.	A	*p. 623*
19.	B	*p. 625*
20.	A	*p. 625*
21.	B	*p. 627*
22.	A	*p. 627*
23.	A	*p. 629*
24.	A	*p. 629*
25.	A	*p. 632*

Matching

26.	F	*p. 627*
27.	J	*p. 623*
28.	E	*p. 624*
29.	B	*p. 625*
30.	G	*p. 626*
31.	A	*p. 624*
32.	I	*p. 626*
33.	C	*p. 624*
34.	D	*p. 626*
35.	H	*p. 628*

Chapter 32: Gastronenterology

Multiple Choice

1.	D	*p. 634*
2.	A	*p. 635*
3.	E	*p. 639*
4.	C	*p. 639*

5.	D	*p. 640*
6.	E	*p. 642*
7.	C	*p. 647*
8.	D	*p. 650*
9.	B	*p. 654*
10.	D	*p. 635*
11.	B	*p. 643*
12.	C	*p. 656*
13.	C	*p. 643*
14.	B	*p. 637*
15.	B	*p. 644*
16.	A	*p. 638*
17.	D	*p. 653*
18.	E	*p. 646*
19.	C	*p. 642*
20.	C	*p. 654*
21.	D	*p. 644*
22.	D	*p. 642*
23.	E	*p. 647*
24.	B	*p. 646*
25.	A	*p. 644*

True/False

26.	A	*p. 635*
27.	A	*p. 639*
28.	B	*p. 640*
29.	A	*p. 642*
30.	A	*p. 647*
31.	B	*p. 644*
32.	B	*p. 635*
33.	B	*p. 636*
34.	B	*p. 645*
35.	A	*p. 655*

Matching

36.	C	*p. 641*
37.	H	*p. 650*
38.	E	*p. 640*
39.	B	*p. 647*
40.	G	*p. 643*
41.	D	*p. 649*
42.	I	*p. 641*
43.	J	*p. 647*
44.	F	*p. 639*
45.	A	*p. 640*

Chapter 33: Urology and Nephrology

Multiple Choice

1.	B	*p. 659*
2.	C	*p. 659*
3.	D	*p. 661*
4.	B	*p. 661*
5.	E	*p. 662*
6.	B	*p. 664*

7.	A	*p. 664*
8.	C	*p. 669*
9.	D	*p. 671*
10.	C	*p. 674*
11.	E	*p. 675*
12.	C	*p. 676*
13.	C	*p. 677*
14.	A	*p. 677*
15.	B	*p. 666*
16.	A	*p. 671*
17.	A	*p. 674*
18.	B	*p. 670*
19.	D	*p. 673*
20.	E	*p. 679*
21.	B	*p. 664*
22.	A	*p. 678*
23.	E	*p. 666*
24.	D	*p. 666*
25.	C	*p. 664*

True/False

26.	A	*p. 664*
27.	A	*p. 665*
28.	A	*p. 667*
29.	A	*p. 670*
30.	B	*p. 677*
31.	A	*p. 677*
32.	A	*p. 664*
33.	A	*p. 671*
34.	B	*p. 666*
35.	A	*p. 668*

Matching

36.	I	*p. 677*
37.	J	*p. 659*
38.	D	*p. 665*
39.	B	*p. 670*
40.	G	*p. 659*
41.	H	*p. 678*
42.	C	*p. 677*
43.	E	*p. 678*
44.	F	*p. 677*
45.	A	*p. 665*

Chapter 34: Toxicology and Substance Abuse

Multiple Choice

1.	C	*p. 682*
2.	D	*p. 684*
3.	B	*p. 684*
4.	E	*p. 685*
5.	E	*p. 686*
6.	B	*p. 687*
7.	B	*p. 687*
8.	C	*p. 688*

9.	D	*p. 690*
10.	A	*p. 691*
11.	E	*p. 694*
12.	B	*p. 696*
13.	A	*p. 696*
14.	A	*p. 696*
15.	E	*p. 696*
16.	C	*p. 698*
17.	E	*p. 701*
18.	B	*p. 700*
19.	D	*p. 704*
20.	E	*p. 699*
21.	C	*p. 716*
22.	A	*p. 719*
23.	A	*p. 718*
24.	B	*p. 721*
25.	C	*p. 704*

True/False

26.	A	*p. 683*
27.	A	*p. 685*
28.	B	*p. 688*
29.	A	*p. 688*
30.	B	*p. 691*
31.	A	*p. 694*
32.	A	*p. 699*
33.	A	*p. 704*
34.	A	*p. 707*
35.	A	*p. 718*

Matching

36.	B	*p. 684*
37.	H	*p. 715*
38.	F	*p. 681*
39.	D	*p. 684*
40.	A	*p. 681*
41.	G	*p. 698*
42.	E	*p. 683*
43.	I	*p. 721*
44.	C	*p. 705*
45.	J	*p. 685*

Chapter 35: Hematology

Multiple Choice

1.	B	*p. 725*
2.	B	*p. 725*
3.	D	*p. 725*
4.	C	*p. 726*
5.	D	*p. 729*
6.	E	*p. 730*
7.	A	*p. 731*
8.	C	*p. 731*
9.	D	*p. 732*
10.	C	*p. 733*

11.	C	*p. 735*
12.	E	*p. 737*
13.	D	*p. 737*
14.	B	*p. 738*
15.	B	*p. 740*

True/False

16.	B	*p. 725*
17.	B	*p. 729*
18.	A	*p. 731*
19.	A	*p. 731*
20.	A	*p. 734*
21.	A	*p. 735*
22.	A	*p. 735*
23.	B	*p. 737*
24.	B	*p. 738*
25.	A	*p. 739*

Matching

26.	G	*p. 734*
27.	A	*p. 733*
28.	H	*p. 737*
29.	F	*p. 735*
30.	I	*p. 739*
31.	B	*p. 725*
32.	J	*p. 739*
33.	D	*p. 735*
34.	E	*p. 733*
35.	C	*p. 736*

Chapter 36: Environmental Emergencies

Multiple Choice

1.	C	*p. 743*
2.	E	*p. 744*
3.	B	*p. 748*
4.	D	*p. 753*
5.	C	*p. 758*
6.	E	*p. 760*
7.	D	*p. 763*
8.	C	*p. 765*
9.	C	*p. 764*
10.	B	*p. 764*
11.	E	*p. 770*
12.	D	*p. 771*
13.	C	*p. 775*
14.	B	*p. 777*
15.	B	*p. 745*
16.	C	*p. 746*
17.	A	*p. 746*
18.	D	*p. 746*
19.	C	*p. 749*
20.	B	*p. 768*

21.	A	*p.* 743
22.	B	*p.* 749
23.	A	*p.* 752
24.	B	*p.* 752
25.	A	*p.* 755
26.	B	*p.* 762
27.	B	*p.* 761
28.	A	*p.* 764
29.	B	*p.* 774
30.	A	*p.* 779

Matching

31.	I	*p.* 749
32.	D	*p.* 760
33.	E	*p.* 774
34.	J	*p.* 755
35.	G	*p.* 773
36.	F	*p.* 749
37.	H	*p.* 770
38.	A	*p.* 754
39.	C	*p.* 767
40.	B	*p.* 774

Chapter 37: Infectious Disease

Multiple Choice

1.	B	*p.* 784
2.	E	*p.* 787
3.	C	*p.* 787
4.	D	*p.* 788
5.	D	*p.* 788
6.	E	*p.* 789
7.	C	*p.* 790
8.	B	*p.* 790
9.	C	*p.* 793
10.	E	*p.* 796
11.	D	*p.* 801
12.	A	*p.* 798
13.	A	*p.* 801
14.	B	*p.* 804
15.	D	*p.* 807
16.	C	*p.* 810
17.	D	*p.* 811
18.	E	*p.* 831
19.	A	*p.* 813
20.	E	*p.* 813
21.	B	*p.* 820
22.	C	*p.* 825
23.	A	*p.* 820
24.	C	*p.* 808
25.	C	*p.* 808

True/False

26.	B	*p.* 783
27.	B	*p.* 795
28.	A	*p.* 821
29.	A	*p.* 830
30.	B	*p.* 828
31.	A	*p.* 825
32.	A	*p.* 823
33.	A	*p.* 818
34.	B	*p.* 814
35.	B	*p.* 808

Matching

36.	I	*p.* 810
37.	D	*p.* 784
38.	E	*p.* 830
39.	A	*p.* 829
40.	B	*p.* 818
41.	F	*p.* 824
42.	G	*p.* 815
43.	H	*p.* 812
44.	C	*p.* 816
45.	J	*p.* 828

Chapter 38: Psychiatric and Behavioural Disorders

Multiple Choice

1.	B	*p.* 835
2.	C	*p.* 836
3.	C	*p.* 837
4.	B	*p.* 839
5.	D	*p.* 838
6.	E	*p.* 842
7.	C	*p.* 843
8.	C	*p.* 843
9.	A	*p.* 839
10.	C	*p.* 841
11.	A	*p.* 841
12.	A	*p.* 838
13.	B	*p.* 853
14.	A	*p.* 835
15.	D	*p.* 837
16.	B	*p.* 841
17.	B	*p.* 840
18.	A	*p.* 841
19.	B	*p.* 842
20.	E	*p.* 847
21.	C	*p.* 846
22.	D	*p.* 845
23.	A	*p.* 847
24.	D	*p.* 849
25.	A	*p.* 843

True/False

26.	B	*p. 835*
27.	B	*p. 856*
28.	B	*p. 834*
29.	B	*p. 841*
30.	A	*p. 841*
31.	A	*p. 849*
32.	B	*p. 850*
33.	A	*p. 838*
34.	B	*p. 840*
35.	A	*p. 841*

Matching

36.	J	*p. 847*
37.	A	*p. 841*
38.	D	*p. 841*
39.	I	*p. 848*
40.	E	*p. 841*
41.	H	*p. 845*
42.	F	*p. 841*
43.	C	*p. 841*
44.	G	*p. 842*
45.	B	*p. 841*

Chapter 39: Gynecology

Multiple Choice

1.	D	*p. 858*
2.	C	*p. 859*
3.	C	*p. 859*
4.	C	*p. 860*
5.	A	*p. 861*
6.	E	*p. 862*
7.	D	*p. 862*
8.	C	*p. 862*
9.	B	*p. 863*
10.	A	*p. 864*
11.	A	*p. 865*
12.	D	*p. 865*
13.	B	*p. 863*
14.	D	*p. 863*
15.	E	*p. 860*

True/False

16.	B	*p. 858*
17.	B	*p. 862*
18.	B	*p. 863*
19.	A	*p. 861*
20.	B	*p. 866*
21.	A	*p. 866*
22.	B	*p. 864*
23.	A	*p. 864*

24.	A	*p. 859*
25.	A	*p. 860*

Matching

26.	D	*p. 858*
27.	H	*p. 862*
28.	B	*p. 862*
29.	J	*p. 863*
30.	A	*p. 858*
31.	F	*p. 861*
32.	G	*p. 862*
33.	E	*p. 858*
34.	I	*p. 862*
35.	C	*p. 859*

Chapter 40: Obstetrics

Multiple Choice

1.	A	*p. 868*
2.	D	*p. 869*
3.	E	*p. 872*
4.	D	*p. 871*
5.	A	*p. 874*
6.	C	*p. 874*
7.	E	*p. 876*
8.	C	*p. 885*
9.	B	*p. 879*
10.	A	*p. 880*
11.	A	*p. 880*
12.	C	*p. 883*
13.	B	*p. 884*
14.	E	*p. 885*
15.	C	*p. 889*
16.	B	*p. 902*
17.	C	*p. 901*
18.	C	*p. 897*
19.	A	*p. 889*
20.	B	*p. 896*
21.	C	*p. 901*
22.	D	*p. 902*
23.	D	*p. 891*
24.	A	*p. 896*
25.	D	*p. 885*

True/False

26.	B	*p. 889*
27.	A	*p. 895*
28.	B	*p. 894*
29.	A	*p. 870*
30.	A	*p. 870*
31.	B	*p. 872*
32.	A	*p. 876*

33.	A	p. 879
34.	B	p. 880
35.	B	p. 882

Matching

36.	D	p. 870
37.	E	p. 868
38.	A	p. 873
39.	C	p. 870
40.	B	p. 871
41.	G	p. 887
42.	J	p. 887
43.	H	p. 876
44.	I	p. 888
45.	F	p. 889

Chapter 41: Neonatology

Multiple Choice

1.	B	p. 908
2.	A	p. 908
3.	C	p. 909
4.	E	p. 909
5.	B	p. 909
6.	A	p. 910
7.	E	p. 911
8.	D	p. 911
9.	C	p. 911
10.	B	p. 912
11.	E	p. 912
12.	E	p. 914
13.	A	p. 914
14.	B	p. 915
15.	D	p. 916
16.	A	p. 916
17.	C	p. 919
18.	B	p. 910
19.	C	p. 911
20.	E	p. 911
21.	C	p. 911
22.	D	p. 922
23.	A	p. 922
24.	A	p. 921
25.	C	p. 921

True/False

26.	A	p. 909
27.	B	p. 911
28.	B	p. 911
29.	B	p. 912
30.	B	p. 915
31.	B	p. 915

32.	A	p. 916
33.	A	p. 922
34.	A	p. 910
35.	A	p. 915

Matching

36.	J	p. 909
37.	A	p. 907
38.	F	p. 911
39.	C	p. 909
40.	E	p. 914
41.	H	p. 908
42.	G	p. 933
43.	I	p. 935
44.	D	p. 911
45.	B	p. 912

Chapter 42: Pediatrics

Multiple Choice

1.	C	p. 939
2.	D	p. 939
3.	C	p. 939
4.	B	p. 940
5.	E	p. 940
6.	C	p. 941
7.	C	p. 942
8.	B	p. 943
9.	C	p. 947
10.	E	p. 947
11.	A	p. 947
12.	B	p. 948
13.	B	p. 948
14.	B	p. 948
15.	E	p. 952
16.	E	p. 953
17.	E	p. 956
18.	D	p. 958
19.	C	p. 958
20.	D	p. 961
21.	E	p. 962
22.	C	p. 965
23.	E	p. 966
24.	C	p. 967
25.	D	p. 969
26.	C	p. 972
27.	C	p. 980
28.	E	p. 981
29.	C	p. 983
30.	A	p. 984
31.	D	p. 987
32.	A	p. 991
33.	B	p. 997
34.	C	p. 999
35.	C	p. 1003

36.	C	*p.* 1006
37.	C	*p.* 1011
38.	E	*p.* 1013
39.	D	*p.* 1015
40.	C	*p.* 1018

True/False

41.	B	*p.* 951
42.	A	*p.* 957
43.	A	*p.* 970
44.	B	*p.* 974
45.	B	*p.* 988
46.	A	*p.* 943
47.	A	*p.* 955
48.	B	*p.* 960
49.	A	*p.* 988
50.	B	*p.* 996

Matching

51.	B	*p.* 998
52.	F	*p.* 948
53.	A	*p.* 983
54.	E	*p.* 985
55.	H	*p.* 980
56.	D	*p.* 1010
57.	J	*p.* 972
58.	I	*p.* 988
59.	G	*p.* 982
60.	C	*p.* 980

Chapter 43: Geriatric Considerations

Multiple Choice

1.	B	*p.* 1023
2.	C	*p.* 1024
3.	C	*p.* 1026
4.	A	*p.* 1026
5.	C	*p.* 1026
6.	D	*p.* 1027
7.	E	*p.* 1027
8.	B	*p.* 1027
9.	B	*p.* 1027
10.	C	*p.* 1027
11.	D	*p.* 1028
12.	E	*p.* 1029
13.	C	*p.* 1028
14.	A	*p.* 1030
15.	E	*p.* 1030
16.	E	*p.* 1030
17.	D	*p.* 1031
18.	A	*p.* 1031
19.	A	*p.* 1032
20.	E	*p.* 1033
21.	E	*p.* 1034
22.	D	*p.* 1035

23.	E	*p.* 1040
24.	A	*p.* 1035
25.	C	*p.* 1036
26.	B	*p.* 1036
27.	C	*p.* 1037
28.	C	*p.* 1037
29.	B	*p.* 1038
30.	E	*p.* 1039
31.	A	*p.* 1039
32.	B	*p.* 1043
33.	E	*p.* 1043
34.	A	*p.* 1044
35.	B	*p.* 1044
36.	C	*p.* 1044
37.	C	*p.* 1045
38.	B	*p.* 1046
39.	B	*p.* 1047
40.	A	*p.* 1048
41.	B	*p.* 1049
42.	D	*p.* 1050
43.	C	*p.* 1051
44.	D	*p.* 1053
45.	A	*p.* 1054
46.	B	*p.* 1056
47.	B	*p.* 1056
48.	B	*p.* 1056
49.	E	*p.* 1057
50.	A	*p.* 1059

True/False

51.	B	*p.* 1026
52.	A	*p.* 1027
53.	A	*p.* 1029
54.	A	*p.* 1031
55.	B	*p.* 1033
56.	A	*p.* 1038
57.	A	*p.* 1038
58.	A	*p.* 1037
59.	B	*p.* 1038
60.	A	*p.* 1043

Matching

61.	J	*p.* 1052
62.	G	*p.* 1060
63.	A	*p.* 1048
64.	H	*p.* 1047
65.	E	*p.* 1056
66.	F	*p.* 1067
67.	I	*p.* 1051
68.	B	*p.* 1049
69.	C	*p.* 1066
70.	D	*p.* 1051

Chapter 44: Abuse and Assault

Multiple Choice

1.	A	*p.* 1076
2.	E	*p.* 1076
3.	C	*p.* 1075
4.	B	*p.* 1077
5.	B	*p.* 1078
6.	C	*p.* 1078
7.	C	*p.* 1079
8.	D	*p.* 1080
9.	E	*p.* 1081
10.	E	*p.* 1082
11.	B	*p.* 1082
12.	B	*p.* 1082
13.	A	*p.* 1086
14.	C	*p.* 1087
15.	A	*p.* 1087

True/False

16.	B	*p.* 1075
17.	A	*p.* 1077
18.	A	*p.* 1084
19.	B	*p.* 1084
20.	B	*p.* 1086
21.	B	*p.* 1075
22.	A	*p.* 1076
23.	A	*p.* 1077
24.	B	*p.* 1079
25.	A	*p.* 1081

Matching

26.	F	*p.* 1078
27.	D	*p.* 1076
28.	B	*p.* 1084
29.	E	*p.* 1079
30.	G	*p.* 1080
31.	A	*p.* 1075
32.	J	*p.* 1078
33.	H	*p.* 1081
34.	C	*p.* 1084
35.	I	*p.* 1077

Chapter 45: The Challenged Patient

Multiple Choice

1.	B	*p.* 1090
2.	A	*p.* 1091
3.	A	*p.* 1091
4.	B	*p.* 1091
5.	B	*p.* 1092
6.	B	*p.* 1092
7.	A	*p.* 1093
8.	D	*p.* 1093

9.	B	*p.* 1094
10.	E	*p.* 1095
11.	A	*p.* 1096
12.	E	*p.* 1097
13.	A	*p.* 1098
14.	B	*p.* 1099
15.	C	*p.* 1101
16.	E	*p.* 1102
17.	D	*p.* 1101
18.	C	*p.* 1103
19.	B	*p.* 1098
20.	D	*p.* 1104
21.	E	*p.* 1103
22.	A	*p.* 1104
23.	E	*p.* 1105
24.	B	*p.* 1105
25.	C	*p.* 1093

True/False

26.	B	*p.* 1105
27.	A	*p.* 1105
28.	B	*p.* 1093
29.	B	*p.* 1097
30.	A	*p.* 1099
31.	B	*p.* 1100
32.	A	*p.* 1089
33.	A	*p.* 1091
34.	A	*p.* 1092
35.	B	*p.* 1094

Matching

36.	D	*p.* 1090
37.	H	*p.* 1090
38.	C	*p.* 1094
39.	J	*p.* 1096
40.	I	*p.* 1100
41.	G	*p.* 1093
42.	A	*p.* 1091
43.	B	*p.* 1090
44.	F	*p.* 1090
45.	E	*p.* 1092

Chapter 46: Acute Interventions for the Chronic-Care Patient

Multiple Choice

1.	C	*p.* 1107
2.	E	*p.* 1108
3.	B	*p.* 1108
4.	B	*p.* 1109
5.	B	*p.* 1110
6.	C	*p.* 1110
7.	E	*p.* 1112
8.	D	*p.* 1112
9.	C	*p.* 1113

10.	E	*p.* 1115
11.	B	*p.* 1119
12.	D	*p.* 1121
13.	E	*p.* 1123
14.	D	*p.* 1124
15.	B	*p.* 1126
16.	D	*p.* 1127
17.	E	*p.* 1131
18.	C	*p.* 1132
19.	E	*p.* 1133
20.	C	*p.* 1134
21.	E	*p.* 1140
22.	C	*p.* 1135
23.	A	*p.* 1137
24.	B	*p.* 1137
25.	E	*p.* 1139

True/False

26.	A	*p.* 1107
27.	A	*p.* 1108
28.	A	*p.* 1109
29.	A	*p.* 1110
30.	A	*p.* 1114
31.	B	*p.* 1116
32.	B	*p.* 1120
33.	A	*p.* 1131
34.	B	*p.* 1139
35.	A	*p.* 1117

Matching

36.	D	*p.* 1122
37.	G	*p.* 1109
38.	C	*p.* 1121
39.	A	*p.* 1109
40.	H	*p.* 1110
41.	J	*p.* 1110
42.	F	*p.* 1110
43.	B	*p.* 1121
44.	E	*p.* 1114
45.	I	*p.* 1121